AROUND THE WORLD WITH
NEPHROLOGY
AN AUTOBIOGRAPHY

To Dear Madge and Betsy

[signature]

December 2012

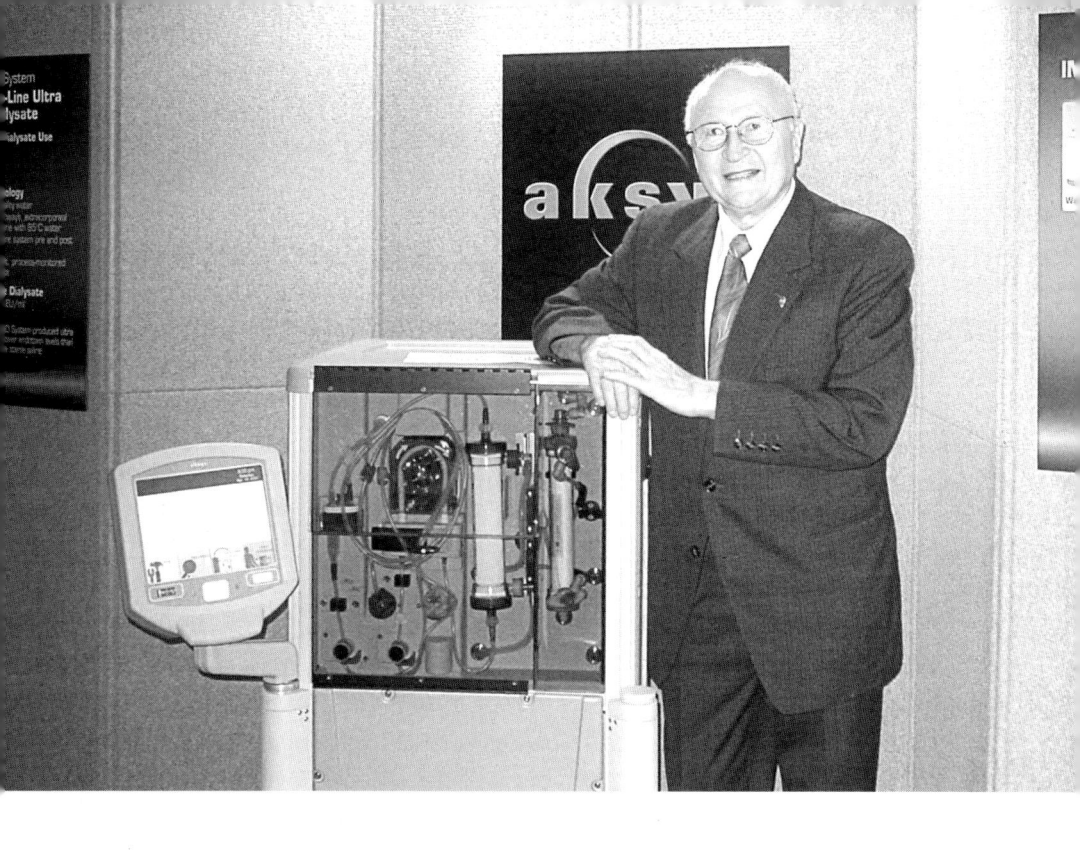

AROUND THE WORLD WITH
NEPHROLOGY
AN AUTOBIOGRAPHY

Zbylut J. Twardowski

University of Missouri-Columbia, USA

World Scientific

NEW JERSEY · LONDON · SINGAPORE · BEIJING · SHANGHAI · HONG KONG · TAIPEI · CHENNAI

Published by

World Scientific Publishing Co. Pte. Ltd.
5 Toh Tuck Link, Singapore 596224
USA office: 27 Warren Street, Suite 401-402, Hackensack, NJ 07601
UK office: 57 Shelton Street, Covent Garden, London WC2H 9HE

Library of Congress Cataloging-in-Publication Data
Twardowski, Zbylut J.
   Around the world with nephrology : an autobiography / Zbylut J. Twardowski.
   p. ; cm.
   Includes bibliographical references and index.
   ISBN 978-9814390026 (hardcover : alk. paper)
   I. Title.
   [DNLM: 1. Twardowski, Zbylut J. 2. Nephrology--Missouri--Autobiography. 3. Nephrology--Poland--Autobiography. 4. Nephrology--United States--Autobiography. 5. Physicians--Missouri--Autobiography. 6. Physicians--Poland--Autobiography. 7. Physicians--United States--Autobiography. 8. History, 20th Century--Missouri. 9. History, 20th Century--Poland. 10. History, 20th Century--United States. 11. History, 21st Century--Missouri. 12. History, 21st Century--Poland. 13. History, 21st Century--United States. WZ 100]

   616.6'10092--dc23
   [B]
                                                               2012028813

British Library Cataloguing-in-Publication Data
A catalogue record for this book is available from the British Library.

Copyright © 2013 by World Scientific Publishing Co. Pte. Ltd.

All rights reserved. This book, or parts thereof, may not be reproduced in any form or by any means, electronic or mechanical, including photocopying, recording or any information storage and retrieval system now known or to be invented, without written permission from the Publisher.

For photocopying of material in this volume, please pay a copying fee through the Copyright Clearance Center, Inc., 222 Rosewood Drive, Danvers, MA 01923, USA. In this case permission to photocopy is not required from the publisher.

Typeset by Stallion Press
Email: enquiries@stallionpress.com

Printed by Fulsland Offset Printing (S) Pte Ltd Singapore

I will prepare and some day my chance will come

Abraham Lincoln

To my wife Halina and my family

Foreword

I have had the honor, privilege and pleasure of being a friend and colleague of Zbylut Twardowski for over 36 years. He is one of the most brilliant, creative, industrious and personable persons that I have ever known. When he arrived at the University of Missouri to work as a Nephrology Fellow in 1976, it was not long until I realized that my life as Division Director would be more exciting than I had ever imagined — because we had a highly motivated and productive genius in our midst. I am very pleased that he has written his auto-biography. It is a personal history of life under German occupation and then communist rule in Poland; it is a heartwarming story of separation from family and ultimate reunification; it is an opportunity to examine how the creative mind can endure under challenging circumstances; it is the amazing story of how one single individual can contribute enormously to the betterment of life for those suffering from chronic illness; it is an example of a human life well-lived; it is a history of the progress of dialysis therapy over the past 60 years and how the contributions to that progress have often been made by Zbylut Twardowski or can be attributed to his ideas.

Zbylut grew up in a German-occupied Poland while his father was in a Nazi concentration camp. Times were very hard for him and his family. The years of his education, training and early career in nephrology were during the long rule of Russian-controlled communism in Poland. Nevertheless, Zbylut was able to pioneer the early development of chronic hemodialysis and peritoneal dialysis in Poland. It seems to be a recurring theme in history whereby creative energy and great accomplishments emerge from adversity. As you read about his early years, you will be impressed with what he was able to do under the conditions in which he lived and worked.

His early experiences with hemodialysis and peritoneal dialysis prompted him to do what he has done all of his career when he is exposed to existing clinical techniques and practices –that is to question how they can be improved or replaced with something better. In the early 1960s, he conceived of the hollow fiber dialyzer and successfully patented this idea in Poland in 1964. He was unable to produce a hollow fiber dialyzer under the conditions in which he worked and the resources that he had available, and abandoned his efforts to do so in the late 1960s when he learned of the successful production of the hollow fiber dialyzer by the Cordis Dow Company in the USA. Nevertheless, Zbylut should be given credit for being an early inventor, perhaps the first inventor, of the hollow fiber dialyzer.

Very early in his career in Poland, Zbylut became intrigued with the concept of more frequent (more than three times weekly), or even daily, dialysis. In the Polish literature, he published some of the earliest, if not the first, experiences with more frequent hemodialysis.

Zbylut was well on the way to becoming a highly regarded full professor In Poland when he made his first visit to Missouri as a "nephrology fellow" in 1976. It was an interesting twist for our Division to have such a highly-experienced nephrologist in the role of a fellow — but this was the visa door that was open to give him the opportunity to participate in an academic program in the USA. All of us were more students than teachers of this distinguished "fellow." He had extensive knowledge of dialysis kinetics, blood access techniques, membrane transport, and dialysis adequacy as well as extensive nephrological expertise.

He happened to arrive at Missouri, when we were just getting starting in our NIH sponsored studies of continuous ambulatory peritoneal dialysis (CAPD) in collaboration with Drs. Jack Moncrief and Robert Popovich in Austin, Texas. It was at this time that Zbylut first became intrigued with peritoneal equilibration curves and how the differences between patients might distinguish patient membrane transport characteristics and help in planning peritoneal dialysis prescriptions with different techniques and patients. After returning to Missouri in 1981, he eventually completed equilibration curves in 100 patients and published one of his most quoted papers; this paper describes the peritoneal equilibrium test ("The PET"). The PET or modifications thereof are the worldwide standard ways of characterizing peritoneal transport characteristics in peritoneal dialysis patients and tailoring prescriptions to provide better outcomes in terms of clearances and ultrafiltration.

In 1977, after one year at the University of Missouri, he returned to Poland to a very prestigious position. However, under communism, opportunities for clinical or laboratory research were very limited. Nevertheless, he was able to publish the first report on CAPD with high volume exchanges — another paper that impacted on how CAPD would be practiced. His frustrations worsened with the declaration of martial law in Poland in 1981. He returned to the University of Missouri as a Visiting Associate, but his family was not allowed to accompany him. Little did he, his wife and two sons realize that many years would pass until they would see one another again. Eventually, the family was allowed to leave Poland. His sons were already in medical school in Poland and matriculated into the University of Missouri School of Medicine. Both of them graduated at or near the top of their class. One is now a cardiologist and the other an oncologist living in the USA. The genes carrying intelligence and the desire to study medicine must have been passed from Zbylut and his wife, Halina (a psychiatrist), to their sons.

We were pleased when Zbylut accepted an offer to join our faculty in 1983. We learned that there would be delays in obtaining a green card so that he could receive a salary as a faculty member (he had been coming to Missouri on educational visas). A contact at NIH mentioned to me that green cards could be obtained quickly if someone were designated by the NIH as an internationally renowned scientist. We put together a package of Zbylut's many publications from his work in Poland and some from his time in the USA along with letters explaining his talents, situation and potential. A committee met at NIH and shortly thereafter, in 1983, an official letter came to Missouri declaring that Zbylut was "an internationally renowned scientist." The green card was issued very promptly when the application was accompanied by this letter. I often tease Zbylut about the fact that many people consider themselves as internationally renowned, but he is the only one that I know that has an official letter to prove it.

After joining the faculty at the University of Missouri School of Medicine, Zbylut quickly rose to the rank of full professor. His productivity continued at a fast pace and now, even in retirement, he continues to share his ideas in multiple publications. This autobiography is an example of his desire to continue sharing his thoughts and experiences through writing. He has 23 patents, has published 390 scientific papers and has delivered 532 scientific presentations at national and international meetings.

His contributions to the dialysis field cover a large number of areas. I will highlight a few in addition to those mentioned above. Publications on the kinetics of nightly intermittent peritoneal dialysis and tidal peritoneal dialysis helped to increase understanding of how best to apply these therapies.

He pioneered many of the early studies on alternative osmotic agents for peritoneal dialysis; these studies explored the use of various polymers and collagen derivatives. These worked well in *in vitro* models of peritoneal dialysis, but were toxic to the rat peritoneum. Nevertheless, an understanding of ultrafiltration kinetics using these larger molecular weight agents was helpful in advancing the interest in polymer osmotic agents.

Dr. Twardowski and the late Barbara Prowant, RN (she was another major reason for successes of all of us in the Division of Nephrology at the University of Missouri) studied and photographed large numbers of peritoneal catheter exit sites in various stages of healthy healing or inflammation. Together, they published an extensive paper on the classification of exit site health and pathology. This work contributed enormously to the better diagnosis and treatment of exit site problems around the world and has become the standard guide for exit site care.

He has markedly impacted on how peritoneal access and blood access are practiced. In peritoneal dialysis, the Missouri Swan Neck Catheter and the Missouri Pre-Sternal Swan Neck Catheter are now used extensively in many countries. In hemodialysis, the Swan Neck Internal Jugular Catheter and the palindrome modification of internal jugular catheters are in extensive use around the world.

One of his patents later in his career was for a hemodialysis machine for daily or nocturnal hemodialysis. The ideas incorporated in his machine are being used in artificial kidney machines now being developed. This may become one of his major contributions.

I have only touched briefly on some of his contributions to the dialysis field. He discusses many of these in great detail and generously shares credit with colleagues. In reading the book, one becomes fascinated with how his ideas take seed and then come into their own as practical applications. The publication references related to these efforts can be found in his curriculum vitae that is part of the book.

For the past 32 years, Zbylut has been extensively involved as a speaker, program planner, abstract reviewer and manuscript editor for the Annual Dialysis Conference (ADC). He has served as chair of the hemodialysis program of the ADC for many years; in recent years, he has co-chaired the hemodialysis program of the ADC with Dr. Madhukar Misra. Madhukar is a Professor in the Division of Nephrology at the University of Missouri and, over the past several years, has been President of the International Society for Hemodialysis. Zbylut began editing the hemodialysis proceedings of the ADC as a parallel publication with the *Advances in Peritoneal Dialysis* edited by Dr. Ramesh Khanna (Director of the Division of Nephrology at the University of Missouri since I retired). Eventually, the hemodialysis journal became *Hemodialysis International* and was acquired by the International Society for Hemodialysis as their official journal — of which Dr. Twardowski is listed as the Founding Editor.

I have focused mainly on the contributions of Zbylut to the field of dialysis. Although his interests in dialysis have been broad (he even has delved into comparisons of the metabolisms and dialysis adequacy requirements in elephants and hummingbirds), I would like to close with examples of how his creative mind has explored diverse interests beyond the realm of dialysis.

Zbylut has some familiarity with four languages and he enjoys studying word origins and language comparisons. He has become an authority on the evolution of the English language. He loves to quote philosophers, theologians, historians, and ancient scientists — often translating their original works into English.

Once his curiosity is stimulated, his analysis of the question at hand is always extensive and precise. Our fellows and residents used to often say, "If you ask Dr. Twardowski the time, he will teach you how to make a watch." I recall that one time a common housefly landed on an indoor motion detector that is part of my home security system and set off the alarm. I asked Zbylut how that was possible since the motion detector detects differences in the temperature of objects compared to room temperature and I have always presumed the fly to be cold-blooded and at room temperature. The next day, Zbylut reported back to me that his study of the literature revealed that the body temperature of a fly is at room temperature when the fly has been sitting for several minutes; however, after a period of flight, the body temperature of the fly will rise above environmental temperature briefly. Thus, if the fly landed on the heat-motion detector after being in flight, it could trigger the alarm. This is an example of the Zbylut Twardowski curiosity and his relentless pursuit of knowledge.

In retirement, he has been invited to Turkey several times to lecture and to consult on a research project. Being a devout Catholic and a religious scholar, Zbylut decided to follow the journeys of St. Paul and St. John throughout Turkey. He put together a series of Power Point presentations titled "In the Footsteps of St. Paul and St. John." It is a presentation of beautiful photographs (taken by Zbylut) along with detailed descriptions of the history, architecture, and art of each site visited. For me, his presentations had enough information to qualify as a college course.

Zbylut Twardowski is an extraordinary human being. I hope that this Foreword gives you an appreciation of the great influence he has had on me and on all others privileged to know him. Reading this book will teach you many things about history, perseverance, and a life devoted to the search for knowledge. Most of all, it will provide a sterling example of the triumph of the human spirit.

Karl D. Nolph, M.D.
Curators' Emeritus Professor of Internal Medicine
University of Missouri School of Medicine
Columbia, Missouri

Contents

Foreword vii

Chapter 1	Childhood	1
Chapter 2	Medical School and the Beginning of My Career in Kraków	21
Chapter 3	Professional Progress in Bytom	45
Chapter 4	Fellowship in America	97
Chapter 5	Return to Poland: The Lublin Years	111
Chapter 6	Return to Columbia: Migrating to the U.S.	127
Chapter 7	Cooperation with Fellows, Laboratory Visitors, Nurses and Technicians	141
Chapter 8	Major Research in the 1980s	151
Chapter 9	Patients Who Inspired or Contributed to Progress	169
Chapter 10	Patents in Columbia	185
Chapter 11	Major Research in the 1990s	241
Chapter 12	Teaching and Consulting	269
Chapter 13	Vacations and Travel Unrelated to Business	391
Epilogue		587
Letters to the Editor		593
Patents		595

Publications	603
Selected Abstracts	633
Selected Presentations	651
Videos	697
Index	699

CHAPTER 1

Childhood

My parents were children of farmers and devout Catholics. My father, Józef Twardowski,[1] was born in Damienice, Bochnia County, Cikowice Parish, on February 1, 1900. His primary education started in Damienice. At that time, grade 1 lasted one year; grade 2, one year; and grade 3, two years. Because he was an exceptional student, his teacher urged his parents to send him for further education to a better school in Bochnia. His mother and father agreed and he continued his primary education in a school there (Szkoła im. Kazimierza Brodzińskiego). He then attended high school in Bochnia, graduating in 1920. Shortly after his graduation, a war broke out between Poland and the newly established Soviet Union, and he volunteered in the Polish Army's cavalry division. He fought from July 15 to September 17, when he was shot in his right foot at the battle of Klewań in Wołyń.[2] A bullet pierced his heel bone and hit his horse in the right femoral artery, killing it within minutes. The injury was not life threatening and he was released after a two-week stay at a hospital in Skierniewice. He was discharged from the army and started his education in the Medical Faculty of the Jagiellonian University in Kraków. He earned money to pay for his education by administering vaccinations and other injections on the order of doctors. Graduating in 1927, he assumed residency at a hospital in Chorzów.

---

1. Regarding my surname, one of my ancestors was most likely from Twardowo in Greater Poland (near Poznań). Until the end of 15th century, the names of Polish nobles were related to their place of residence. They would write their name, say, *Jan z Twardowa*, meaning "Jan from Twardowo," similar to *van* in Dutch and *von* in German. At the end of the 15th century, the surnames of Polish nobility assumed an adjectival form (Twardowski for men and Twardowska for women). The estates of many nobles were gradually divided among descendents into small farms. This was probably the case regarding my ancestors. I do not know any stories, famous or infamous, pertaining to my immediate family; however, there are many famous people with the name "Twardowski" — a poet, a philosopher, and a mathematician. There is also a legend about Piotr or Jan Twardowski, a magician, who sold his soul to the devil, but there is debate about whether he was really a Pole. Some report that he was a German with the name Durus (from the Latin for "hard"; in Polish: *twardy*) and he assumed the name Twardowski. He lived in Kraków, and according to a legend, his most notable achievement was evoking the soul of late Queen Barbara, the beloved wife of Zygmunt August (Sigismundus Augustus), the last king of the Jagiellonian Dynasty.

2. Klewań is in Volhynian Voivodeship, which belonged to Poland before 1939 but is now in Ukraine.

My mother was born in Stanisławice, Bochnia County, Cikowice Parish, on September 12, 1903. She was educated to be a teacher. My parents married on August 3, 1930. My mother worked as a teacher until my elder brother, Lesław Andrzej, was born, on September 18, 1931. In 1932 my parents moved to Szack in Eastern Poland. As Poland regained its political independence after World War I, professionals were encouraged to work in Eastern Poland to provide services for the population. My father was the only physician there within a 60-mile radius. In this region, communication was usually made possible by buggies, as public transportation was not available at that time. He practiced all medical specialties, including internal medicine, pediatrics, obstetrics-gynecology, and surgery in acute cases. There was not enough supporting staff, so my mother frequently assisted my father by administering ether anesthesia in emergencies, and my father often performed appendectomies and other surgeries.

I was born in Szack on June 2, 1934. My parents had already decided to leave that town and had me baptized in Cikowice. There were two reasons: firstly, there were no Catholic parishes, only Eastern Orthodox ones, nearby; secondly, my parents wanted my place of birth to be recorded in Central Poland, where they were born. Ultimately, I was baptized in Cikowice on September 1, 1935, and my godfather was Antoni Siemdaj and my godmother, Matylda Zborowska (Fig. 1). My birthplace was recorded in Stanisławice, the same as my mother's. Szack was separated from Poland in 1939 and has since become part of Ukraine.[3] In

---

3. Eastern Poland was annexed by the Soviet Union in September 1939, following the clandestine Molotov–Ribbentrop Pact of August 23, 1939, which resulted in an attack on Poland by Germany on September 1, 1939, and by the Soviet Union on September 17, 1939. The attack by the Soviet Union on Poland was a complete surprise for the Polish Army, given the existence at the time of the Soviet–Polish Non-Aggression Pact, signed in 1932. It was a stab in the back, culminating later in the murder of thousands of Polish officers by the Soviets at Katyń — a typical example of treaty observation by dictatorial regimes.

It is reported that Stalin was surprised and devastated when Hitler broke the Molotov–Ribbentrop Pact and invaded the Soviet Union (during Operation Barbarossa) on June 22, 1941. He should not have been. After World War II and following the Yalta Conference (February 5–February 14, 1945), the eastern part of Poland was handed to the Soviet Union by the United States and Great Britain. After the collapse of the Soviet Union, Ukrainian independence was proclaimed on July 16, 1990. Thus, Szack (Ukrainian: *Šac'k*; English spelling: Shatsk), at Lake Świtiaź (Ukrainian: *Svitjaz*; English spelling: Svityaz), located about 20 kilometres from the Byelorussian border and about 20 kilometres from the Polish border, near the source of the Prypeć river (Ukrainian: *Pryp'jat*; English spelling: Pripyat), became a Ukrainian town.

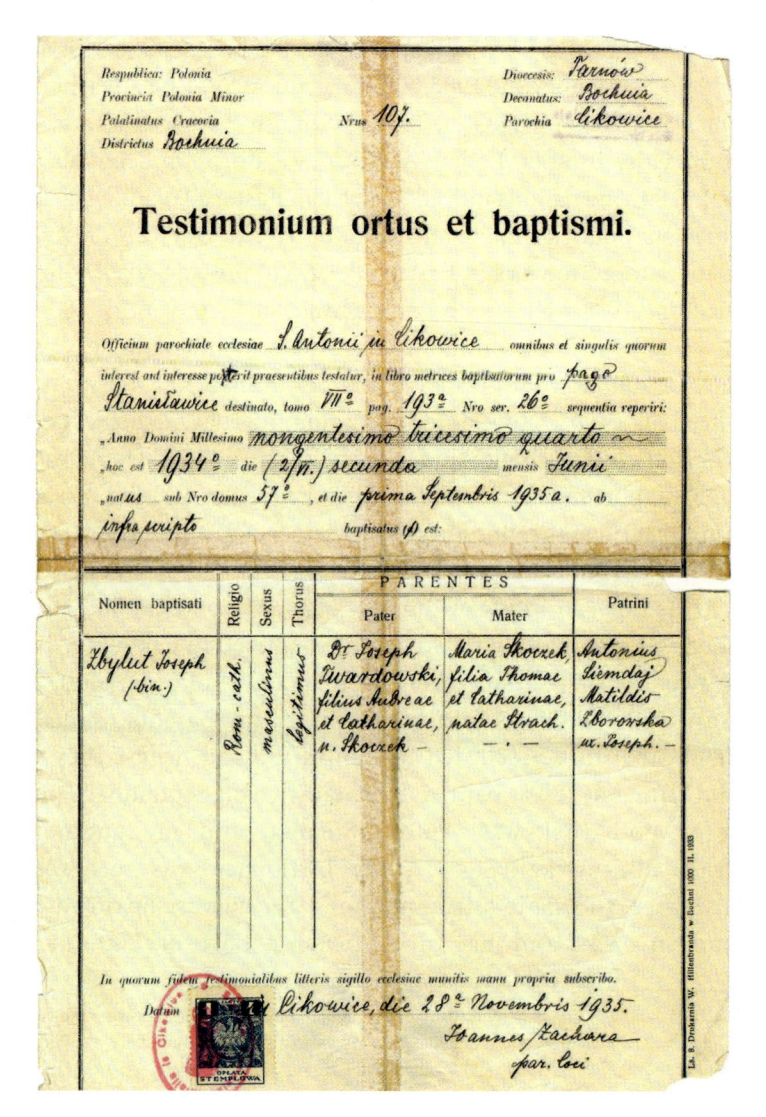

Figure 1. *Testimonium ortus et baptismi* (Certificate of birth and baptism).

retrospect, one could say that moving was a good idea, since if I had ever required official documents such as my birth certificate, I would have had to have communicated with officials of the Soviet Union. I was given the names Zbylut and Józef, the latter obviously coming from my father. My father chose old Polish names for his sons.[4] Later, he told me that the priest, Jan Zachara, was reluctant to give me the name Zbylut, as there was no saint with this name. But when my father argued that I could be the first saint with the name Zbylut, the priest relented.

My parents moved to Szopienice, near Katowice, in Upper Silesia, where my father started a private practice as a general practitioner. Doctors and other professionals were eagerly sought after in Upper Silesia. I have few recollections from Szopienice. My earliest childhood memory — I think that I was about three at the time — concerned a scooter (one propelled by foot) that I had learned to ride. We had a nice four-bedroom apartment with a balcony, a bathroom, indoor plumbing, and a telephone. I remember how I loved playing on that balcony with my brother (Fig. 2).

We were living quite a comfortable life before World War II. Our vacations were spent in a little thatched roof cottage that belonged to my mother's sister, Joanna Siemdaj, in Stanisławice. We also spent the summer of 1939 in Stanisławice. My elder brother had started primary school the year before and the family was supposed to return to Szopienice in September, but the situation changed completely when German troops attacked Poland on September 1, 1939, igniting World War II. Together with other civilians, we escaped into Niepołomice Forest (Puszcza Niepołomicka), north of Stanisławice. We were lucky because we were not shot at, whereas those who used the roads to flee were shot and bombed by Stukas, dive-bombers equipped with machine guns, bombs, and special cardboard sirens. As they dove at high speed to attack, the sirens made a terrifying screaming noise. Apparently, they were installed on the orders of Germany's highest level of command to enhance the psychological effect of the bombings, particularly on civilians. We were fortunate to have only heard the Stukas' sirens from a distance, as they did not fly over the forest.

When the initial fighting stopped at the end of September, we returned to Szopienice, only to find that this was part of Poland annexed into the Third Reich of Nazi Germany. My father was

---

4. The meaning of Zbylut is derived from *zby* (short for *zbądź się*), which means "to get rid of," and *lut* (short for *lutość*), which means "anger, cruelty, and bad temper." The word is now used only in the name of the month *luty* (February), meaning "cruel." My brother's first name, Lesław, is also an old Polish name, whose meaning is almost identical to Bolesław: *bolej* or *lej*, which means "more," and *sław*, which means "fame." So Lesław means "to be famous."

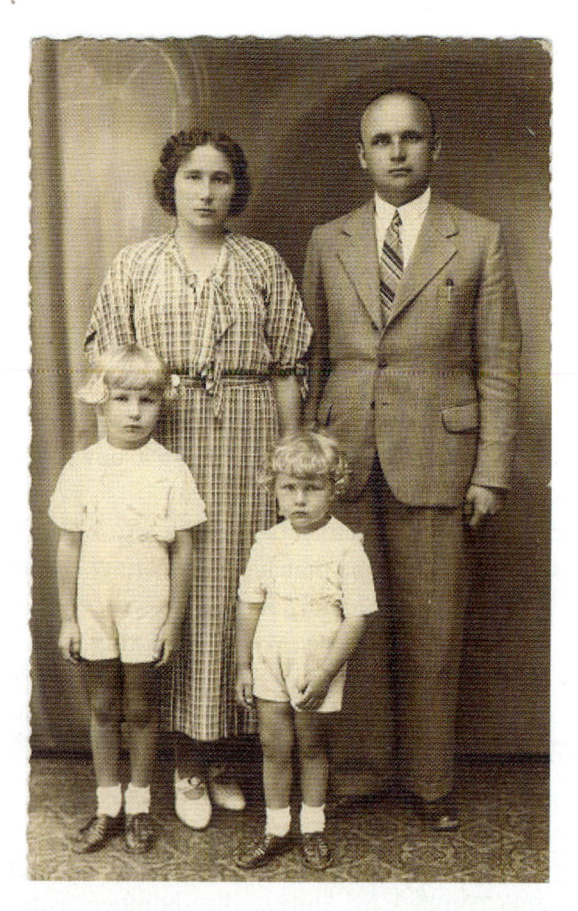

Figure 2. The author with his parents and brother in Szopienice before WWII.

arrested and later interned at various concentration camps, first Dachau, and then Mauthausen. Many educated Poles, like my father, were arrested for no other reason than that they were educated. Our apartment was confiscated, and we moved to Stanisławice and lived in the same cottage we had stayed in during our prewar vacations. My father was released in 1941, but he was arrested again in 1943 when he was found to be a member of the underground resistance AK, or Armia Krajowa ("Home Army"). He was then taken to Montelupi Prison in Kraków and was scheduled for execution, his part in collective punishment for attacks on Germans or those who collaborated with the Germans. He was listed as number 32 out of 72 in an announcement published on January 29, 1944, and signed by "Der

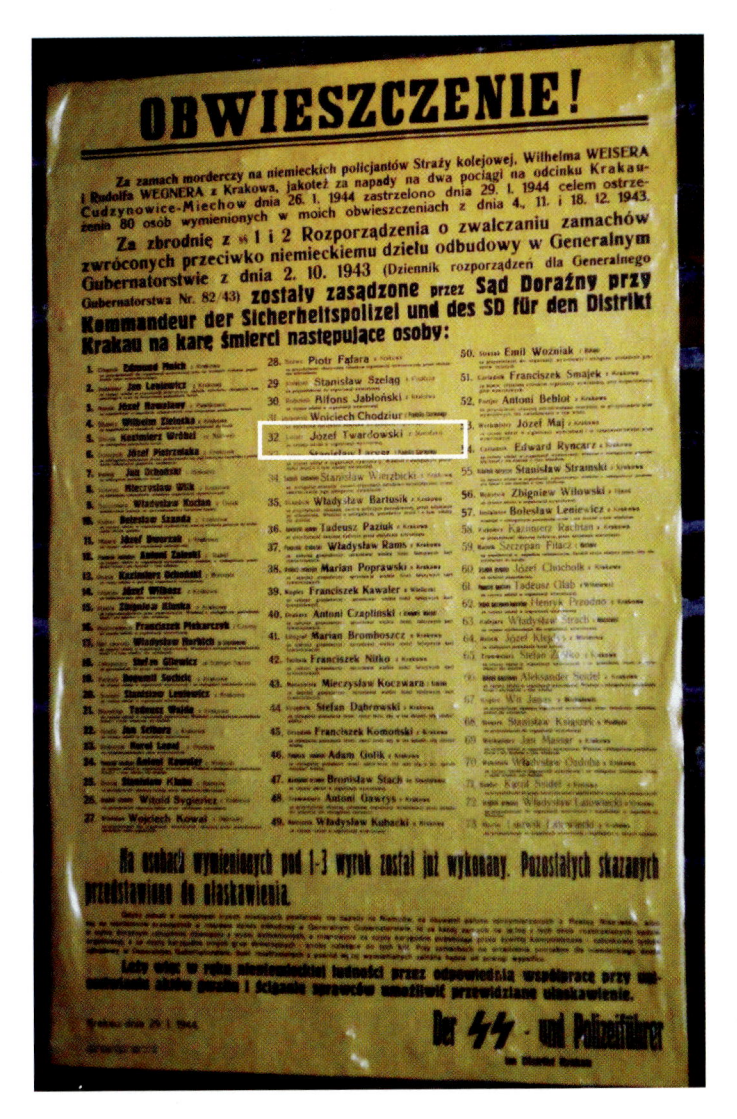

Figure 3. Józef Twardowski, sentenced for execution.

SS-und Polizeiführer" (Fig. 3). On the same list there were several Poles taken hostage because they hid Jews by providing them shelter. The announcement stated that for each German casualty at least 10 persons from the list would be executed within three months.

As it was for so many, it was a terrible time for our family. When the day came for my father to be taken away for execution, my mother succeeded in arranging for his transfer to a concentration camp in Gross Rosen (near Breslau, now Wrocław) by bribing a high-ranking official through a Volksdeutsch lady. It was considered a triumph, because there was at least a chance of survival in a concentration camp, whereas the people held in the prison were ultimately destined to be killed. My father was transferred to Gross Rosen in 1944. As the war front moved westwards, he was transferred to concentration camps in Litoměřice on Labe (German: Elbe), presently located in the Czech Republic, and finally to Flossenbürg (Bavaria, Germany), where he was freed by the advancing American soldiers. Found unconscious and suffering from typhus, he spent several months in an American military hospital, but finally recovered and returned to Poland in 1946.

Life was pretty tough for my brother and me. Winters were very cold and there was never enough coal or wood to heat the cottage. We had no electricity or running water, but we had sufficient clothes to keep warm. Local farmers were obliged to deliver quotas of grain, potatoes, cows, and pigs for the Germans, but there was enough left, so we were not starving. Breakfast was usually a slice of bread with jam, cheese or butter, and ersatz coffee (made of burned grain) with milk; dinner was typically potato soup, sometimes chicken with potato; supper was often boiled or fried potatoes with cultured milk. Meat was rather rare, as farmers were not supposed to butcher animals, under penalty of death, but we did this clandestinely during Easter or Christmas. There were no mills operating during the war, so we used a quern to grind grains. The ground grain — rye or wheat — was sifted through a sieve; people used the flour and the remainder was used in animal feed. Some bran "contaminated" the flour, but that was not a bad thing. The bread made with this flour was very tasty; it was a real farmer's bread. Our staple foods were potatoes with cultured milk.[5]

---

5. The combination of potatoes and milk is excellent, as potatoes contain all exogenous amino acids, with the exception of methionine. On the other hand, milk also has all exogenous amino acids, with a surplus of methionine. Thus, Polish farmers, even in very tough times (as during the wars), had enough exogenous amino acids despite the lack of meat in their diets. I would only appreciate this many years later when I was a nephrologist and became aware of the "potato diet" used in Poland for the treatment of advanced renal failure. [Połeć R, Liwski R, Kociszewski J. (1968) Dieta ziemniaczana w leczeniu przewłekłej niewydolnoiści nerek (Potato diet in the treatment of chronic renal failure). *Pol Arch Med Wewn* **40**(4): 449–458. Reprinted in *Pol Med J.* **8**(2): 284–293 (1969).]

The room I slept in was unheated, so during winter I had to breathe under the covers for about twenty to thirty minutes to warm up the bed enough to be able to sleep. My uncle (Antoni Siemdaj) and aunt did not have kids, so my brother and I had to perform various chores that were typical for village children, such as tending the animals, shepherding cattle, and flailing and winnowing. For most of the year, "shepherding cattle" entailed keeping the cows to a small pasture and preventing them from going into the grain field. We were also warned not to let the cows graze on the dew-covered clover, as it could lead to very dangerous bloat.[6] Only late in September, after the crops were harvested, was it possible to allow the cows to graze anywhere. That was the time I liked to be a shepherd. Several of us gathered together, built a fire, baked potatoes, and played games while the cows roamed and grazed. As we grew up and became stronger, we were allowed to plow and even scythe.[7] During the summer months I did not wear shoes, so the skin on my soles became very thick and I was even able to walk barefoot on stubble. After the end of the war, machines were available for cutting cereal grasses, and for threshing. However, to obtain good straw for repairing a thatched roof, flailing by hand was necessary.

In spite of these chores, there was enough time for swimming in the nearby Raba River and playing soccer. In the winter, the Raba was usually completely frozen and ice skating became our beloved sport. Indeed, there was much more time for sport in the winter. There were no skates available to buy, so we made them ourselves using an iron wire, filed to create something resembling a proper edge, fixed to the

---

6. Bloat is a digestive disorder characterized by an accumulation of gas in the first two compartments of a ruminant's stomach (the rumen and reticulum). Dew-covered clover induces excessive fermentation with the production of gas (primarily carbon dioxide and methane). In more severe bloat, the animal's rumen is distended and pressure on the diaphragm may lead to restricted breathing and death. In advanced cases, experienced farmers treated it by puncturing the rumen through the left flank with a sharp knife.

7. Scything, at that time a basic method of reaping fields of grain, was a very demanding job. Usually, scything was done by two or three men, or even more, working together at the same speed on the same field, keeping a distance of 10 to 15 yards. There were two methods of scything: on a swath or on a wall (uncut cereal grass). In the first method, the cut grain could be collected later; in the second, the cut grain had to be taken immediately by helpers (young boys or women) to enable the next mower to scythe. Young boys were not able to keep up with adults and could only handle the scythe for short periods, but helping with the work was a good way to learn.

bottom of a piece of wood. We had to file the edges frequently to keep them as sharp as possible, as they were made of iron, not steel. Even skiing was a possibility if you were prepared to improvise. Stanisławice is a completely flat place, but just across the Raba River were small hills in the village of Chełm suitable for skiing. We would make primitive skis from old barrel staves with straps to fix them to our boots. It was not the easiest equipment to use, but the joy it brought outweighed any shortcomings in terms of practicality.

As my father was away, my mother and my aunt played the major roles in bringing me up during those formative years (ages five to twelve). Both were disciplinarians and it was very good for my character. My mother always encouraged me to work hard and be as good a student as possible. Before the war, when my father was at home, he would be rather easy-going, devoting his time to his work while my mother focused her efforts on raising my brother and me. I remember my mother spanking me, but never my father, though I do not recall being spanked after the age of four. As a hard-working farmer, my uncle's only role in my upbringing was by example: working hard from sunrise to sunset, attending church services every Sunday, praying, and being pleasant to just about everyone — animals included. My uncle had a very skittish mare named Sawka. It took him several years to calm that horse, but eventually she was obedient enough that even my brother and I were able to guide her to plow the soil.

In 1940, when I was six, my mother decided to send me to primary school in Stanisławice. It was a small school with only four grades, and classes for the 1st and 2nd grades were held together, as were the classes for the 3rd and 4th grades. We were mainly taught reading, writing, and arithmetic. I had to go to the neighboring village of Kłaj for the 5th and 6th grades. In addition to "the three Rs," classes included biology, geography, history, painting, singing, and religion. I do not think that the Germans interfered with the program, at least in any way that I was aware of, and I remember being well stimulated by the teachers. The only real downside was the three miles that separated our cottage from the school; with no available transport, I had to walk or ride my bicycle to school every day.

On the other hand, the exercise — cycling, walking, sometimes running — helped me develop some useful athletic skills. For the 7th grade I had to cover a distance of about five miles to a school in the neighboring town, Bochnia, as the school in Kłaj only had six grades. I was extremely impressed with the level of teaching at the primary school in Bochnia (Szkoła im. Stanisława Jachowicza),[8] but I attended the school for less than two months.

My mother wanted to have her sons educated in music. So she arranged piano lessons for my brother and me. Our teacher soon suggested that teaching my brother music was futile because, as she put it, "an elephant stepped on his ear."[9] By contrast, the teacher praised my abilities. It is possible that I could have displayed a little more aptitude than my brother, but I think I was also rather lamentable. However, my teacher could have had an interest in keeping me as a student, as I not only took lessons but also practiced at her house. There was no piano in my aunt's cottage, so my parents had to pay for lessons. I was an altar boy at the Cikowice parish and I loved attending the Tridentine Mass, which was in Latin. To this day I like to attend Latin Mass, even in the post-Vatican II rite, wherever they are available. I had my First Communion at the Cikowice parish when I was seven. My Confirmation was later, in Chorzów Batory, and I received the name Andrzej (after my paternal grandfather).

Thus, my real childhood was during World War II. My father was interned in concentration camps throughout the war and my mother worked underground to have him released. In retrospect, life was difficult, but at that time it seemed completely natural to me; I did not know any different.

In October 1946 my parents moved to Chorzów Batory, in Silesia. My father resumed his practice as a physician and our standard of living improved markedly, the most important development being that my father was no longer victimized. Although the communists who came to power in Poland after the war persecuted members of the AK, my father was left alone as he had worked only briefly in the resistance and had spent most of his time in concentration camps. In spite of his awful treatment at the hands of the Germans, my father

---

8. The level of teaching in this school was always very high. It was originally founded as a parochial institution in the 12th century, and in the 16th century it was connected with the Jagiellonian University in Kraków, which was established in 1364.

9. This Polish expression means that somebody is completely musically deaf.

was more critical of the Soviet Union than of Nazi Germany. From the very beginning, he predicted the economic ruin of the whole Soviet Bloc, as he considered the communist system to be *praeter naturam* — "against human nature" in Latin. As he saw it, the major problem with communism was the disconnection between remuneration and the quality of work. People have no real incentive to work diligently or efficiently. Most expect to be paid appropriately for what they do. Only a small minority work for the real love of their job, and the economy cannot rely on only a fraction of the population. My father expected the communist system to collapse in short order, before his death, and I would frequently argue with him, pointing out that the communists had enough power to subdue the population. It turned out that he was right concerning the ultimate result, but it took much longer than he had predicted. He passed away on June 29, 1975, and it was not until June 4, 1989, that communism in Poland finally collapsed with the completion of the first "semi-free" elections in the entire Soviet Bloc.

My father did not talk much about his years in prison and in the concentration camps. He once mentioned that in prison he developed a generalized reaction after an injection of some experimental drug. He spoke of his constant hunger, as the food rations he received were extremely small. My father was rather "well nourished" before his arrest, and he believed that his survival was partly related to his low metabolism and high fat storage. He used to say that in the concentration camps "before fat people lost weight, skinny people had died". My father lost about 50 percent of his body weight in Dachau and Mauthausen-Gusen, and he was lucky to have been out of the concentration camps for almost two years, regaining his natural weight before being arrested again.

One of worst experiences he talked about was the Sisyphean work[10] he had to endure. He was forced to fill a wheelbarrow with dirt, push it up a ramp, empty the dirt out, and repeat the task over and over again. It was particularly difficult for him to bear, knowing that with the small food rations they were given, any expenditure of extra

---

10. The term comes from the legend of Sisyphus, an ancient king of Corinth, who was sent to Hades for crimes against his subjects and condemned forever to roll a huge stone up a steep hill, only to have it roll downhill again.

energy was highly detrimental. Besides, he was the son of a Polish farmer. Farmers were very deliberate with energy expenditure, as food production was difficult. Any physical activity was supposed to be done for a useful task. With such a mindset, this Sisyphean work was, for my father, a form of torture far worse than any beating. He also taught me that the most important thing one can do is doing something of value for other people — or at least for oneself (physical exercise for one's health being of obvious value).

I attended the 7th grade in Chorzów-Batory, and the level of teaching was markedly inferior to Bochnia — even worse than in Kłaj during my 6th grade. One of the reasons was that during the war classes were held in German, and there was a tremendous lack of Polish teachers in Silesia at that time. After finishing primary school I was enrolled in the Liceum Muzyczne (Musical Lyceum) in Katowice. As I have already mentioned, my mother believed that I had a talent for music because some of my teachers had enthused over my abilities. So it was only natural for my mother to enroll me in the Musical Lyceum, which taught both music and general classes. There was another reason: there was no high school in Chorzów-Batory at that time. The high school in Chorzów Miasto (Chorzów City) did not teach religion, so my mother was not eager to send me there. I was enrolled in bassoon and piano classes, and proved to be a rather poor music student. (But I was the best student in general classes — Polish, history, geography, biology, mathematics, and so on — and by my own reckoning, I had learned enough in Kłaj and Bochnia that I did not need to study too much for those classes.) I did not have a musical ear, but some of my classmates had perfect pitch. One of those with perfect pitch was Ireneusz Wikarek, who later became Director of the Great Orchestra of the Polish Radio in Katowice. I was stunned when in a solfeggio classroom test — without blinking an eye — he was able to write down the notes that were played. I simply could not do it. Ultimately, I came to the conclusion that I would never become an accomplished musician, so I quit trying. Instead, I spent a lot of time playing bridge, chess, and various other sports, and ultimately excelled at all of them.

I practiced the bassoon at home, but my playing left a lot to be desired. The bassoon requires a good musical ear, and mine was just average. My mother was unconvinced when I tried to explain this to her, apparently preferring instead to believe the people who insisted that I had some musical talent. Then one fine day, as I was playing my bassoon, one of the neighbors came and asked my mother whether we were keeping a goat in our apartment. That was the moment she finally accepted that I had, after all, not been endowed with a gift for music. After two years attending the Liceum Muzyczne, my general education was so poor that I could not enter the 10th grade in the newly opened high school in Chorzów-Batory, Szkoła Ogólnokształcąca Męska im. Stefana Batorego,[11] which was a very good school. Even as I entered 9th grade instead, I struggled to keep up with the rest of the class. But I was determined to study hard, and after a full year, I was getting straight A's. It was a very intensive program, including languages (Polish, English, and Latin), mathematics, logic, chemistry, physics, biology, history, geography, geology, astronomy, religion, and others. Interestingly, religious classes were not forbidden at that time (1949–1952).

In the early 1950s there was still a dearth of teachers, and when a teacher was sick or could not come to class for any reason, the director of the school asked me to substitute. I taught in all classes from grade 1 to 10. The students in 9th and 10th grades were my peers, so maintaining discipline was quite a challenge. For grades 1 to 3, keeping the attention of the class also proved very difficult, and I enjoyed these classes the least. My best teaching experience was in grades 5 to 7, but the chore of teaching often kept me from attending my own classes and I had to compensate by doing more homework. There was also a program designed to pair struggling students with more advanced ones. I had to help six students in mathematics, and I consumed much more time than I would have liked. Overall, I felt like I was not cut out to be a teacher.

As I entered my final year before graduation, I was uncertain about where to go for further study. My favorite subjects were in science, particularly mathematics, but I was not quite sure whether my

---

11. Stefan Batory (English: Stephen Báthory), Prince of Transylvania, and King of Poland (1576–1586), is considered by many historians to be one of the greatest elected rulers of Poland. Together with his chancellor Zamoyski, he led the army of the Commonwealth in a brilliant decisive campaign during the Livonian War against the Muscovite army of Tsar Ivan the Terrible.

mathematical abilities were good enough for a career in academia. Computer science as a subject was decades away, and I was afraid that after study mathematics I would become a schoolteacher, a career path which had little appeal for me. It was then I decided I would try to become a doctor like my father. I was sure that medicine was such a broad field that I would end up making use of my love of science to some satisfying end. That would turn out to be true.

Our high school class was made up mostly of male students: there were 33 of us, but only seven female students. Gradually, in such a big class, smaller groups of students with similar interests formed. Five of us formed a group that we called Geruzja (after Gerousia, council of elders[12]). We were not the oldest, but we had some authority among the class. In addition to me, the members were Wiesław Ciemiński, Mieczysław Kalisz, Tadeusz Lazar, and Kazimierz Pędziński. All of us continued on to university: Ciemiński, medicine; Lazar, sports education; Kalisz and Pędziński, engineering. (Unfortunately, three members are already deceased at the time of writing: Ciemiński in 1971, Lazar in 1980, and Kalisz in 2008.) I represented my class in basketball and volleyball. My basketball teammates were Joachim Giec and Jan Więcek — there were just three members of the team, due to the small size of the basketball court. I also trained in track and field. My favorite distance was 800 meters. Many of my school records in track and field — long jump, triple jump, 400 meters, and 800 meters — were not surpassed by other students for many years. I also joined the track and field section of Ruch Chorzów.[13]

I was the only student graduating with "A" grades in all subjects (Fig. 4). Two of the best graduates received special certificates that came with free admission to a university. When the awards went to two other graduates, my mother was very upset. At that time, children

---

12. The Gerousia was the Spartan Senate, its council of elders. It consisted of 30 members in total, two of which were the ruling kings. Sparta had two kings in order to manage its large military based government, an arrangement that allowed one to wage a military campaign while the other ruled Sparta. If one died, the people would immediately elect a replacement. Of the other 28 elders, several would usually belong to one of the two royal Spartan houses. Members had to be over the age of 60 and were elected for life.

13. Ruch Chorzów, 14-time national champion, is one of the most successful football teams in Poland. Its track and field section, however, was not particularly good.

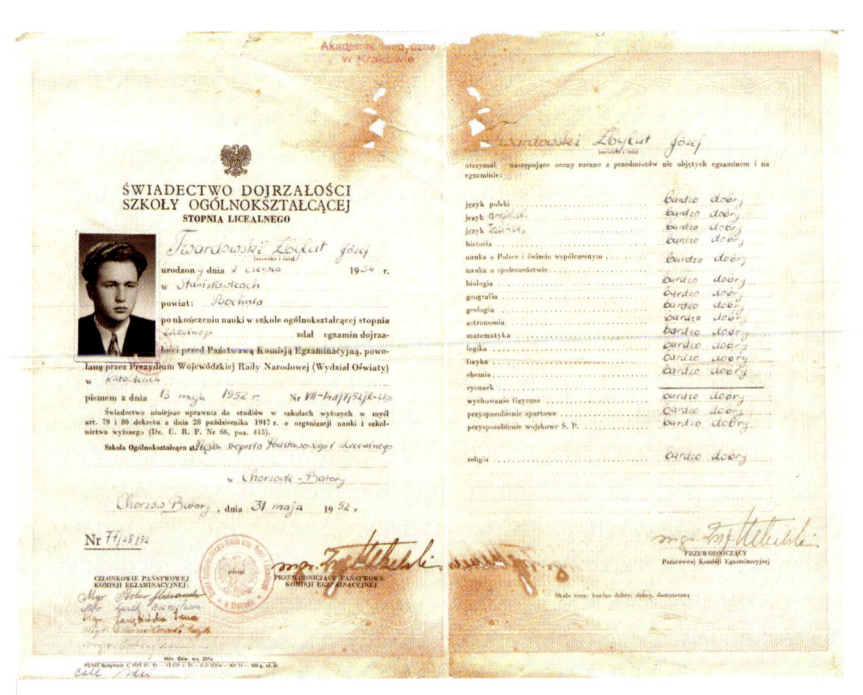

Figure 4.   High School Certificate of Graduation.

of the intelligentsia were rather discriminated against, and preference for university admissions was given to workers' and farmers' children. When my mother asked the director of the school why I did not get this "free admission" certificate, the answer she was given was that other students needed it more, as I could get into a university by getting good results in the entrance examination. It was perverse reasoning, but it turned out to be prophetic. After passing its entrance exam, I would be accepted to the Medical Academy in Kraków.[14]

I did not get this special diploma. Instead, as a token of appreciation for helping other students, I received a book on Leonardo da Vinci (Fig. 5). Published in October 1951, this was the Polish edition of Antonina Vallentin's *Leonardo da Vinci: The Tragic Pursuit of*

---

14. Communism took hold in Poland following World War II, and one of the communists' administrative decisions — for reasons I do not understand — was to separate the Medical Faculty from the Jagiellonian University and establish a medical academy under the Ministry of Health, instead of the Ministry of Education. Following the collapse of Polish communism, the Medical Academy was transformed into the Collegium Medicum, as part of the Jagiellonian University once more.

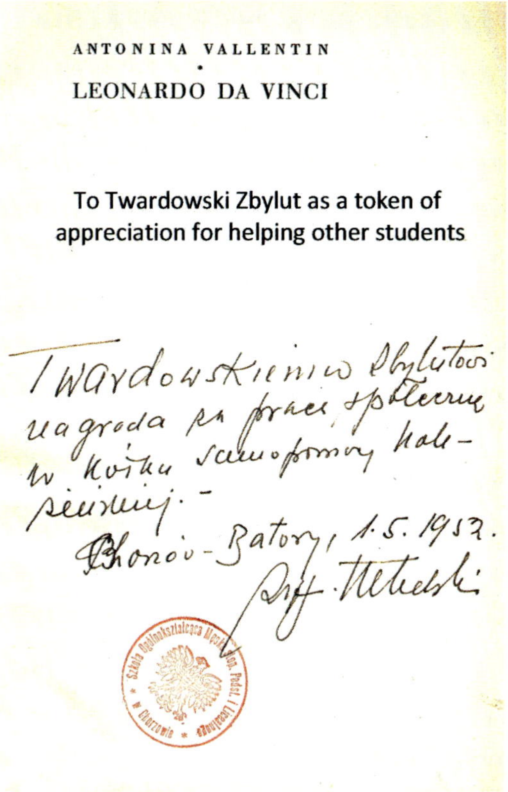

Figure 5. Book on Leonardo da Vinci, a token of appreciation for helping other students.

Perfection, translated by Stanisław Sielski. As it happened, it was a well-received gift, as I was fascinated with the life and accomplishments of da Vinci, not only in painting but also his multiple inventions. I learned that the only painting of da Vinci's that could be found in Poland, *Lady with an Ermine*, was housed in the Czartoryski Museum, incorporated into the National Museum in Kraków in 1950.

The history of *Lady with an Ermine* was fascinating, highlighting not only da Vinci's broad knowledge but also the hidden cryptograms in his paintings. The painting, a portrait of Cecilia Gallerani, was commissioned by Lodovico "il Moro" Sforza, Duke of Milan, at a time when she was his mistress. Some time ago the painting was called *Lady with a Weasel*, referring to the species *Mustela nivalis*, or least weasel. Thus, the term "weasel" is used to denote the species rather than the genus. All species of the *Mustela* genus are similar in appearance. *Mustela erminea* (ermine) is mainly differentiated from the very similar *Mustela nivalis* by its characteristic black tailed tip. Also, weasels have a serrated border between the brownish upper part of the body and their white belly, while in ermines this border is straight. Looking at da Vinci's painting, it is difficult to say whether it is an ermine or a weasel in the arms of the lady, as we do not see the tail. Also, the animal has winter fur, which is white, and the border is not visible anyway. It is now generally accepted that it is an ermine, and there are several interpretations of the significance of the ermine in the painting. The ermine, a stoat in its winter coat, was a traditional symbol of purity, because it was believed that an ermine would face death rather than soil its white coat. Ermines were kept as pets by the aristocracy, and their white pelts were used to line or trim aristocratic garments. For Ludovico Sforza, the ermine had a further personal significance in that he had been in the Order of the Ermine in 1488 and used it as a personal emblem "L'Ermellino." The association of the ermine with Cecilia could have multiple meanings, alluding to her purity and to the status of her lover. The depiction of the ermine could also have been a pun on her name, because the Greek for ermine is γαλεμ (*galée*).

The provenance of the painting is equally fascinating. It was bought by Prince Adam Kazimierz Czartoryski, probably from Marquis Boursane at Milan in 1798, and brought to Poland in 1800. The painting traveled extensively in the 19th century. After a failed November uprising, Princess Czartoryska rescued it in advance of the invading Russian army in 1830, sent it to Dresden, Germany, and on to the Czartoryski place of exile in Paris, the Hôtel Lambert. It subsequently returned to Poland in 1882. In 1939, it was seized by the Nazis and placed in Berlin's Kaiser Freidrich Museum. In 1940, Hans Frank, the Governor General of Poland, managed to have it returned to Kraków, where it hung in one of his offices. At the end of the war it was discovered by Allied troops in Frank's country home in Bavaria and was returned to the Czartoryski Museum in Kraków, which is where I saw it when I arrived in Kraków in the summer of 1952. After seeing the painting, I dreamed of being able to visit, at some point in my life, the places where Leonardo da Vinci had lived and worked. In

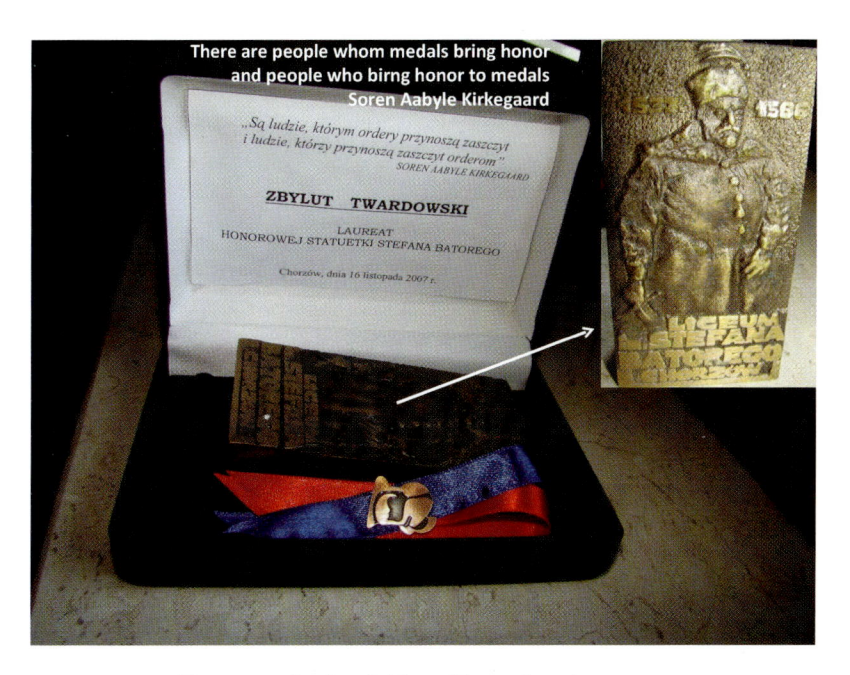

Figure 6. Stephen Báthory Honor Award statuette.

communist Poland, that prospect did not seem likely, as travel abroad was very difficult for ordinary citizens. Many years later, on November 16, 2007, I would receive another token of appreciation from my school: a Stephen Báthory Honor Award statuette for my professional achievements after graduation, presented to me on June 20, 2008 (Fig. 6).

CHAPTER 2

Medical School and the Beginning of My Career in Kraków

Medical school in Poland started immediately after high school graduation and lasted six years. Five years were devoted to lectures and study and the sixth to final exams and internships in internal medicine, surgery, pediatrics, and gynecology/obstetrics. At the time of my entrance into medical school, I was told that students with mostly "A" grades — and no "C" grades — would receive the so-called "Red Diploma,"[1] or Diploma with Distinction, corresponding to *summa cum laude* (with highest praise) or *cum eximia laude* (with special praise). This kind of diploma was supposed to guarantee employment as a teaching assistant in any department of the Medical Academy. I thought that I would be able to achieve that if I studied hard enough.

In Poland, medical students did not work to support their studies, and I did not plan to work either. My parents were able to provide for my room and board. I shared the room with my brother, who studied engineering in the Kraków Academy for Mining and Metallurgy.[2] So my time was divided between study and sport. When my brother graduated, I shared the room with Jacek Hawiger, who, after finishing two years in the Silesian Medical Academy, decided to continue in the Medical Academy in Kraków, which was supposed to be a better school.

I was convinced that I would be able to achieve some measure of success in track and field, especially in the 800 meters. As a matter of fact, my personal record was 1:55.8 sec, which was 13th best time in Poland in 1956. In the Medical School in Kraków I did not have any real competition in sport. In local meetings I was the best in 800 meters, 400 meters (51.4 sec), 400 meters hurdles (55.5 sec), 200 meters (23.0 sec), 100 meters (11.5 sec), long jump (6.66 m), triple jump (13.21 m), and 50 meters freestyle swimming (39.6 sec). During our recent reunion (June 6, 2009), one of our colleagues, Barbara Harasiewicz,[3] reminded me that I competed against the women, including her, in the 100 meters dash, where I was running backwards and they were running forwards, and I beat all of them.

---

1. The Red Diploma had a red cover; all other diplomas had a black cover.

2. Akademia Górniczo-Hutnicza im. Stanisława Staszica in Kraków.

3. Her brother was Adam Harasiewicz, a well-regarded pianist who won the first prize in the fifth International Chopin Competition in 1955.

Still, combining sport and medical study was rather tough. In 1956–1957, my fifth year of medical school, I decided to spend less time training, but rather maintaining my level from the summer season of 1956. My training was shorter, but more intense. It turned out that it was not such a good idea, as I devoted less time to warming up, cooling down, and stretching. As a consequence I pulled some muscles and ultimately could not train at all. So my engagement in competitive sports ended in 1957. I did not exercise for some time, but my appetite was pretty much the same as during intense training. Within two years I had gained almost 40 lbs. In retrospect I do not think that my interest in sports was futile, as I learned to be competitive and win, and accept defeat as well. After a few years I returned to recreational exercise, which I continue to this day. With sports like volleyball and swimming, and by maintaining an appropriate diet, I started to lose the excess weight I had put on, but it took almost 10 years.

I had little time for other extracurricular activities. In the first two years I had three *celujące* (excellent or "A+"), nine "As" and only one "B". By the third year I had been accepted by Prof. Jerzy Kaulbersz, Chair of the Department of Physiology, as a volunteer to do some research in the department. I prepared a presentation on the life and work of Napoleon Cybulski, the most prominent Polish physiologist at the turn of 20th century, and presented it during a student meeting,[4] a presentation that was never published. I also worked under the direction of Stanisław Jan Konturek,[5] a teaching assistant in the Department of Physiology. He asked me to conduct a study on the influence of hypophysectomy on the development of gastric ulcers. First, I was supposed to learn how to perform transnasal hypophysectomy in rats, but I was unable to master the technique, and unfortunately,

---

4. Napoleon Nikodem Cybulski (1854–1919). One of Cybulski's greatest achievements was the development of the photohemotachometer, a device used for the precise measurement of blood flow in the vessels, which provided a better insight into the physiology and pathophysiology of the circulatory system. To pursue this work, he was granted a PhD placement in the St. Petersburg Military Academy in 1885. A decade later, Cybulski, together with Władysław Szymonowicz, discovered that adrenal extracts contain biologically active substances that elevate blood pressure. The St. Petersburg Military Academy had an excellent track record in the study of blood flow and blood pressure. In 1905 Nikolai Korotkoff presented his famous Korotkoff's sounds for measuring systolic and diastolic blood pressures.

5. Stanisław Jan Konturek (born 1931), who chaired the Department of Physiology after Prof. Jerzy Kaulbersz retired, made significant contributions to gastroenterology.

almost all my rats died during surgery. Ultimately, we discontinued the study, and I do not know whether anybody mastered the technique later.

Due to time constraints, I also gave up my volunteer work. My goal was to get as many "A" grades as possible and obtain the Red Diploma, giving me a teaching assistant position in one of the departments. At the time I was not sure what specialty I would pursue, but I gradually began to think about clinical work in one of the big specialties — surgery, pediatrics or internal medicine. I passed all of them with an "A" grade, completing my final exams in December 1957. Taking my medical courses as a whole, I had four "A+" (*celujące*) grades, 30 "A" grades, and 7 "B" grades.

I wanted my sixth-year internships to be in the Kliniki Akademii Medycznej (departments of the Medical Academy) in Kraków, but I encountered my first surprise. I found out that I could not take an internship in Kraków, because it was a "closed city," which meant that it did not accept interns who were not permanent residents of Kraków. I brought up the matter with the Dean of the Medical School, Prof. Mieczysław Kubiczek, who decided that an exception should be made for me because of my grades. I could select departments of my choice, so I chose the Second Department of Internal Medicine, the Department of Pediatrics, and the Department of Obstetrics/Gynecology at the Medical Academy Hospital (St. Lazarus Hospital), and the First Department of Surgery.

In 1952 there were about 500 students in the first year of medical school in Kraków. They were divided into 20 groups: ten in "Year A" and the remainder in "Year B." I was in Group 10 of Year A. Year B had four groups in the School of Medicine and six in the School of Stomatology. In the first two years of study, lectures were separate for Years A and B, though medical and stomatology students had the same lectures. Exercises were undertaken within groups, so group members knew one another much better than they did the remaining students. During our third year of study, the six groups from "Year B" continued with stomatology studies alone, while the remaining four groups were combined with the 10 "Year A" groups, forming a single entity. There was some attrition during these first two years, so the total number of students was about 320 in year three. All the lectures were available for every student. Attendance was not mandatory, but many students attended anyway, particularly as medical books were not readily available and lectures were basic sources of knowledge.

Some professors were excellent teachers. I remember being impressed by lectures in anatomy (Prof. Tadeusz Rogalski), biology (Prof. Stanisław Skowron[6]), histology (Prof. Jadwiga Ackerman), biochemistry (Prof. Bolesław Skarżyński, 1901–1963), and physiology (Prof. Jerzy Kaulbersz). To this day I remember a brilliant lecture by Prof. Bolesław Skarżyński about the discovery of insulin by Banting and Best in the laboratory of Prof. MacLeod. It was fascinating to hear him describe how Banting was inspired to acidify a pancreas specimen to prevent the digestion of Langerhans islands before isolating them and he recounted all his discussions with the skeptical MacLeod. It was also extremely interesting to listen to Prof. Skowron as he faked his criticism of the theories of Mendel and Morgan, as it was obvious that he did not believe in the Stalin-approved theories of Michurin and Lysenko.

In the third year, my favorite lectures were in pharmacology (Prof. Janusz Supniewski), pathological anatomy (Prof. Janina Kowalczykowa[7]), pathology (Prof. Bronisław Giędosz), and microbiology (Prof. Zdzisław Przybyłkiewicz). Over the next two years, I was most impressed with the lectures in surgery (Prof. Józef Bogusz, Chairman of the First Department of Surgery, and Prof. Kornel Michejda, Chairman of the Second Department of Surgery), dermatology/venereolgy (Prof.

---

6. Stanisław Skowron (1900–1976) had been granted the title of professor in 1938, but his career was interrupted by the outbreak of World War II and his arrest, together with other professors of the Jagiellonian University during the so-called Sonderaktion on November 11, 1939. After being released from the concentration camp, and upon his return to Kraków, he started teaching in the underground Jagiellonian University. After the war, he became the head of the Department of Biology and Embryology, which after the reorganization of medical universities in 1950 and its subsequent separation from the Jagiellonian University, was included under the Medical Academy. He studied biology and embryology under the direction of the eminent Thomas Hunt Morgan (1866–1945) but was forced by the authorities to teach the theories of Soviet gurus in biology such as Ivan Vladimirovich Michurin, Trofim Lysenko, Olga Lepieszynska, and Aleksander Iwanowicz Oparin, who were approved by Stalin and were considered sacrosanct in the Soviet Bloc.

7. Prof. Janina Kowalczykowa was a survivor of concentration camp at Auschwitz (Nr. 32212).

Kazimierz Lejman[8]), forensic medicine (Prof. Jan Stanisław Olbrycht, 1886–1968), infectious diseases (Prof. Józef Karol Kostrzewski, 1883–1959[9]), otorhinolaryngology (Prof. Jan Miodoński, 1902–1963) and internal medicine (Prof. Leon Tochowicz, 1897–1965, Chairman of the First Department of Internal Medicine; Prof. Tadeusz Tempka,[10] Chairman of the Second Department of Internal Medicine; Prof. Julian Aleksandrowicz, Chairman of the Third Department of Internal Medicine).

In the fourth year, I met my future wife, Halina Anna Nowosielska, who was in the 14th group, so we had lectures together starting in the third year. We were engaged in July 1957 and married in the Church of Saint Nicholas in Kraków on October 11, 1958 (Fig. 7). When we were married, we lived in one room of my wife's parents' apartment on 26 Wielopole Street in Kraków. My wife gave birth to our first son, Radomysł (Radek) Marian, on December 8, 1959, and our second, Przemysław (Przemek) Wiktor, was born on July 28, 1963. Both were baptized in the Church of Saint Nicholas. Radomysł's godparents were my brother Lesław and Halina's younger sister Joanna. Przemysław's godparents were Jacek Hawiger (my former roommate) and Halina's youngest sister Barbara. My wife's parents, Karol Nowosielski and

---

8. The famous lecturer Prof. Kazimierz Lejman (1907–1987) was very popular among medical students. To this day I remember his lecture on venereology and the problems with sexual stimulants. He started his lecture with these words: "Count Orlov, elevated to this honor by the grace of Czarina Catherine, died of renal failure because of overuse of Spanish fly, which contained cantharidine, a popular aphrodisiac." For those who were aware of the Czarina's sexual appetite, it was very revealing how it was possible to make a career in Russia at that time.

9. Prof. Kostrzewski was famous for using only Polish names or Latin names for infectious diseases, but never polonized Latin or Greek names. For example, for scarlatina, he never used "szkarlatyna," only "płonica" (from Polish *płonąć*, meaning "to burn"); for diphtheria, not "dyfteria" but "błonica" (from *błona*, meaning "membrane"); for typhus or typhoid, not "tyfus" but "dur" (from *odurzyć*, meaning "daze, stupefy"). Even for other polonized Latin words, he insisted using words of Polish origin, like "ciepłostka" (calorie) instead of "kaloria" (from *ciepło*, meaning "heat"); "ciepłota" instead of "temperature"; "deszczochron" instead of "parasol," because in Poland nobody uses an umbrella to protect against the sunshine like in Italy (Italian: *parasole*), but to protect (*chronić*) against the rain (*deszcz*).

10. Kraków-born Tadeusz Tempka (1885–1974) was Professor of Internal Medicine at the Jagielonian University and Medical Academy in Kraków from 1928 to 1974. He created a very strong hematological center there, introducing bone marrow biopsy, immunohematology, cytochemistry, and coagulology. He determined that pernicious anemia is actually a panmyelopathy and for the first time described giant band cells in this disease. He mentored many specialists in internal medicine, including future professors Julian Aleksandrowicz, Julian Blicharski, Aleksander Skotnicki, Jan Fenczyn, Zygmunt Hanicki, Stanisław Kirchmayer, and Mieczysław Kubiczek.

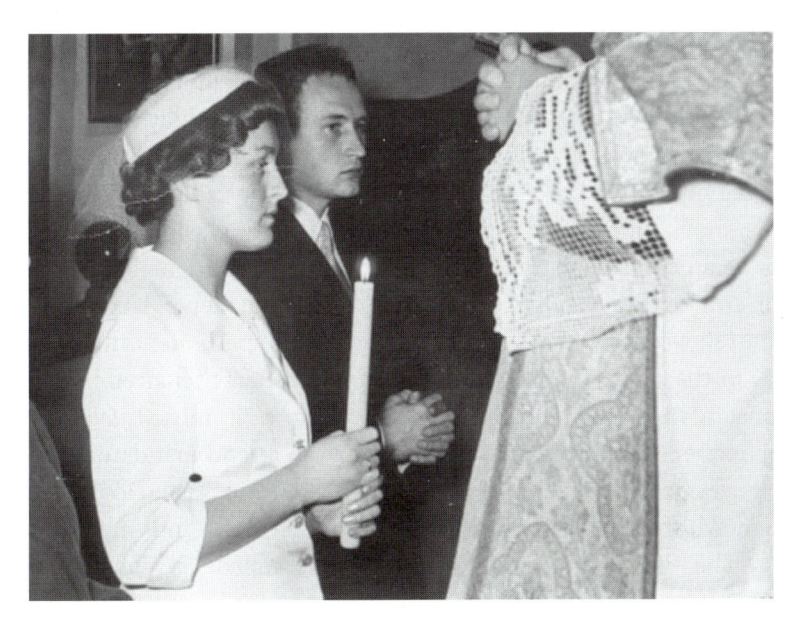

Figure 7. The author married Halina on October 11, 1958.

Eugenia (Gena), were extremely nice people, and they helped us a great deal in the early years of our marriage. Karol did not want to be called *dziadek* (grandpa) by his grandsons, but preferred to be called "Lolek" (the diminutive form of Karol in Polish).

I started my internship on February 6, 1958, in the Second Department of Internal Medicine, with Prof. Tadeusz Tempka as the chairman. I was extremely impressed with the quality of service and knowledge, not only of the professors, but also of the assistants and adjuncts. The department's main interest was in hematology, but there were also gastroenterology and pulmonology wards. After completion of this internship I was convinced that internal medicine would be my future specialty. Initially, I thought about a subspecialty in hematology, particularly coagulology.

The next internship, which began on April 18, 1958, was in the Department of Pediatrics on Strzelecka Street. The chairman of the department at that time was Prof. Stanisław Giza. I liked pediatrics and was very much impressed with the quality of the service. I even thought about continuing pediatrics after graduation. But something happened that changed my mind completely. During my internship, there were two girls about seven years of age, Ania Amborska, and another whose name I do not remember. Both had acute leukemia. Initially, they were in reasonable health and liked to play with me. At that time there was only symptomatic treatment for leukemia, and during my internship both died of fulminant sepsis. It was a tremendous shock for me, and I quickly came to the conclusion that I could not be a pediatrician and be so close to the suffering of children; by the end of the 1950s there was no hint that acute leukemia in children would be treatable during my lifetime. My next internship was in the Department of Gynecology/Obstetrics (chaired by Doc. Konstantynowicz), and was in two parts, June 27–July 31, 1958, and September 1–October 4, 1958 (as we had to attend mandatory military service in between). Mostly, interns stayed in obstetrics, accepting newborns, and I soon realized that this was also not my calling.

The First Department of Surgery, so-called "White Surgery" because the building was white, was the venue for my next internship, from October 22, 1958, to January 7, 1959. It was located on 40 Mikołaja Kopernika Street, opposite the Second Department of Surgery, otherwise known as "Red Surgery," as it was housed in a red brick building. I eagerly assisted in operations, enjoying the immediate and visible results, and seriously considered surgery as my final specialty. There was, however, one serious problem. In July 1955, I had a summer practice in Red Surgery, and the summer was very hot that year. With no air conditioning in the operating rooms at the time, I was inclined to sweat profusely under the shadow-free operating lamp, and the nurses had to constantly wipe my forehead. It was problematic enough that I decided against this specialty, too, although my love of procedures persisted and would turn out to be useful later.

After finishing my last internship, I received my Red Diploma, or Diploma with Distinction (Fig. 8), corresponding to *summa cum laude* (with highest praise) or *cum eximia laude* (with special praise), on January 7, 1959. This kind of diploma was supposed to guarantee employment as a teaching assistant in any department in the Medical Academy. As I was already a resident of Kraków, I thought that there would be no problem obtaining a position in my preferred department, the Second Department of Internal Medicine. But contrary to what I had been told at the start of my medical education, I learned

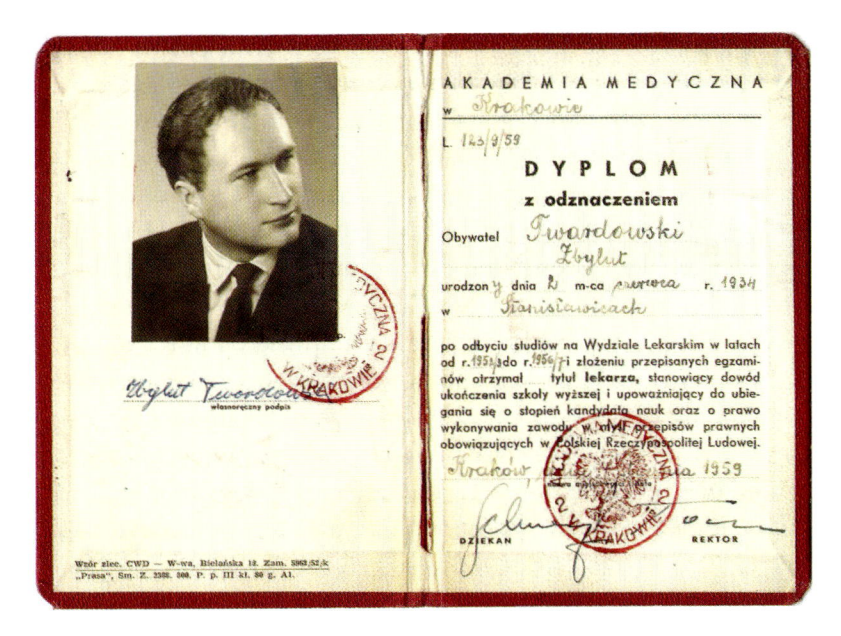

Figure 8. The author's Diploma with Distinction, or "Red Diploma."

that my special diploma did not, in fact, guarantee any such position, and there was indeed no position available for me.

My wife received her diploma on January 31, 1959. For some time we were uncertain about what to do. She knew that I wanted to pursue an academic career, and she was ready to help in any way she could, taking on extra jobs, in addition to looking after our sons. There was a possibility of my getting a position outside Kraków, even one with a better salary and an apartment supported by an employer. So one option was to take a better-paid position in the provinces, save some money, and return to Kraków later. The risk associated with this option was that after earning more money, it would have been difficult to adjust to a lower salary and more modest living conditions, so this route might have put my academic career in jeopardy. Another option was to stay in Kraków by taking any job and then get a volunteer academic position. After lengthy deliberation and discussions with my wife and her parents, we decided that this was what we would do — with our parents' help. My wife's parents allowed us to continue living with them. Getting an apartment in Kraków was very difficult, and although my parents gave us money to cover most of the cost, we had to wait until an apartment was available. As it turned out, this never happened, as our situation had changed by 1963.

In 1957, my father bought a new Warszawa, a car built by Fabryka Samochodów Osobowych, or FSO (literally, "Factory for Passenger Automobiles") in Żerań (a district in *Warszawa*, Polish for Warsaw). The car was based on the Soviet "Pobeda," whose design lines were clones of American cars of the 1940s. My father did not drive, but he allowed my brother and me to use the car. I used it for vacation trips to the seaside and the Mazury Lakes. It was a primitive car by today's standards — no power steering, no servo brakes, no air conditioning, and so on — but it did have some advantages. It was sturdy and mechanically unsophisticated, so in the case of a breakdown, it was possible to fix certain problems if the driver had some knowledge about the car's construction. At the time, when one undertook to learn how to drive, it was also necessary to learn some fundamentals about the workings of the car. The knowledge turned out to be very useful, as road service was not easily available. On one occasion when we were out driving, a good distance away from the nearest village, I discovered that a fuel injection pump had a broken pin and I was able to fix it using a wire, allowing us to return to Kraków, where the fuel pump could be professionally fixed. Another time, an ignition distributor rotor arm broke and I was able to fix it using a container for a greasepaint stick. Some of my experience with fixing cars would come in handy later for fixing kidney machines.

In July 1960, we drove to Mazury with my wife's friends Maria Starzycka[11] and her husband Zbyszek Starzycki, while our eldest, Radomysł (Radek), stayed in Kraków with my wife's mother, Eugenia. Our Warszawa was big enough to accommodate the four of us and all the necessary equipment, including tents. In Giżycko, at Lake Niegocin, we left the car, rented two canoes, and kayaked through Lake Kisajno, and from Lake Łabap to Lake Dobskie and back. On this last leg of our trip, a tremendously powerful squall suddenly developed. There was little we could do, but luckily we were pushed northward and were able to enter a narrow canal connecting Łabap

---

11. Maria Starzycka was later Professor of Medicine as well as Chairman of the Ophthalmology Department.

Lake with the small Sztynort Lake, where the waves were more manageable.

Years later, we used the Warszawa to take the whole family on vacation to Chałupy, a little village on the Hel Peninsula that had a wonderful beach. We went for walks on the sand and in the forest and swam in the Baltic Sea. The temperature of the water was not bad — usually around 17–21°C (62–70°F) and sometimes as high as 23°C (73°F), but sometimes as low as 14°C (57°F), which made it impossible to swim. Occasionally, there were very nice waves that broke about 50 to 80 yards from the shore. Radek, Przemek, and I learned how to bodysurf and always looked forward to the northwest winds, when the waves were at their best. My sons and I continued bodysurfing for many years in the Baltic, as well as other seas and oceans. We established a rule that we had to *earn* the right to have sweet treats during these vacations; for a cake providing 300 calories, we had to burn an extra 300 calories. And the rule was observed very strictly.

My wife got a position at the psychiatry hospital in Kobierzyn and started her specialization in psychiatry. At that time, a specialization was granted after a minimum three-year residency in a chosen specialty and after successfully passing an examination. Exams were usually oral and questions were posed by a commission of three specialists in the field, the chairman of the commission usually being a chairman of some academic department who was also appointed as a voivodeship[12] consultant in the field.

In 1959, I started to look for a job and found a locum position as a physician in the Mateczny Spa in Kraków, a position that I held for two months. The remaining time I spent on intensive self-education in English, as my English language education in school had been somewhat lacking. It was a good way of improving my reading and writing skills, but less useful for learning pronunciation. In the meantime, I applied to the emergency services for the position of emergency physician and I was accepted on July 1, 1959. I also applied for

---

12. Voivodeship (Polish: *województwo*), also spelled voivodship, is a type of administrative division dating to medieval Poland, Romania, Hungary, Lithuania, Latvia, Russia, and Serbia, ruled by a voivode (Polish: *wojewoda*). The voivode (literally, "the one who leads the warriors," equivalent to the Latin *Dux Exercituum* or the German *Herzog*) was originally the military commander next to the ruler. The voivodeships of modern Poland are sometimes called simply "provinces" or "regions."

the position of volunteer physician in the Second Department of Internal Medicine and I was accepted at the same time. I worked 48 hour weeks (usually Tuesday 7 am to Thursday 7 am) and one Sunday (24 hours) per month as an emergency physician as part of an ambulance crew.[13] My volunteer work was Mondays, Thursdays, Fridays, and Saturdays from 8 am to 2 pm. All in all, I worked about 216 hours per month in the emergency services and about 100 hours per month as a volunteer. There was not too much time left, as a month is about 730 hours on average. I also enrolled in an English language course with Mr. Chlamtacz (a British citizen living in Poland with a Polish last name; his father was Polish and his mother, British), who was an excellent teacher and grammarian and spoke with a beautiful British accent. They were only once-a-week classes, but my English pronunciation still improved a little within a year.

I was only 25 years old, so I could manage this kind of schedule. Most of the night I slept in the ambulance and was woken only when we arrived at the patient's home. Sometimes we went to villages outside Kraków, so I could sleep an extra hour, sometimes more. However, after a year, I started to experience some difficulties in keeping alert after about 44 hours of continuous duty, so I decided to reduce my schedule to 24-hour blocks. After two years of working in an ambulance, I knew Kraków's geography and the surrounding villages pretty well. Some calls were not for emergencies, and sometimes drivers would be upset and complain about it to me. I did not like to listen to their constant complaining, so I decided to drive by myself when I did not expect the need to transport the patient to the hospital. I was sometimes wrong and after examining a patient, I had to take him or her to the emergency room. On those occasions, I would have to manage to carry the patient on a stretcher with a nurse or get help from the family. Visits to patients with psychiatric disorders could be scary, as they resisted being moved and even threatened to kill us with an ax! But despite the occasional unnerving moment, I never had any serious incidents.

---

13. At that time in Poland doctors without specialization went to accidents and other emergencies in ambulances. Sometimes an emergency was not reallu urgent, but rather was more like home call. Usually a team was composed of a physician, a nurse (usually male), and a driver. When needed the nurse and driver would transport a patient on a stretcher.

My volunteer work also counted as a residency in internal medicine. I was impressed by the clinical acumen of almost all the assistants and adjuncts in the department — and, of course, the docents and professors. Dr. med. Tadeusz Struzik, Doc. Zygmunt Hanicki, Doc. Stanisław Kirchmayer, Prof. Mieczysław Kubiczek, and Prof. Tadeusz Tempka were excellent diagnosticians and overall clinicians. Dr. Struzik had an excellent memory. During rounds with residents, when an attending physician asked about some laboratory test, and the resident could not find it quickly in the notes, Dr. Struzik provided the figure without hesitation. He was also mathematically inclined. One of his papers was on the physical model explaining the Ellis–Damoiseau line in pleural effusion.[14] Prof. Tempka was an expert in differentiating various cells in bone marrow and peripheral blood. As I was thinking about being a hematologist, I learned a great deal from Prof. Tempka, who was kind enough to teach me how to recognize bone marrow cells.

There were two more young physicians, Jacek Hawiger (my former roommate) and Przemysław (Przemek) Hirszel, who were interns in the department at the time. Jacek Hawiger worked in the Department of Medical Microbiology, while Przemysław Hirszel was employed in the Department of Anatomy. Doc. Zygmunt Hanicki had a patient with almost a complete lack of γ-globulin. He asked us to help him with the patient as well as the publication of a related article. The first scientific paper that I coauthored, it was submitted in 1962 and published in 1963 [Pu 1].

In 1961, Przemek and I received good news: there would be positions for physicians in a newly built artificial kidney unit. The opening was scheduled for the fall of 1962, but we were to study hard in the new field and be ready before the deadline. We agreed immediately, as it appeared to be something fascinating and completely new to us. Besides, I would be paid for my work in the department. I had never heard about artificial kidneys during my five years in medical school. Nephrology did not exist as a branch of medicine in Poland at that time. There were other subspecialties of internal medicine, but in

---

14. Struzik T. (1962) A simple physical model interpreting the course of the upper limit of free fluids in the pleural cavity in the form of the Ellis–Damoiseau line. *Pol Arch Med Wewn* **32**: 391–400 (in Polish).

Kraków, lectures in diseases of the kidney were only rarely given. Doc. Hanicki gave us reprints of numerous papers by Nils Alwall,[15] as the department was supposed to get Alwall's Kidney. We were also required to help with the final stages of room remodeling and machine assemblage. To become acquainted with the procedure, we were sent to the First Department of Internal Medicine of the Warsaw Academy of Medicine, Poland,[16] where they already had Alwall's Kidney and had been using it for the treatment of acute renal failure since January 1959. The most helpful of our instructors was Dr. Zbigniew Fałda.[17]

Our unit was scheduled to open in September 1962. However, on Monday, June 11, Jasiu Różycki, a young patient with acute renal failure, was admitted to the department and Doc. Hanicki decided to perform dialysis, if possible, as no artificial kidney center was able to admit him and he was afraid that the patient would die without dialysis. The diagnosis was acute glomerulonephritis, but no biopsy was done, as renal biopsies were not done at that time. The patient was oliguric, but metabolic derangement was progressing slowly. Przemek and I were required to inspect the adaptation of the rooms and all the equipment. Alwall's spiral dialyzer consisted of two metal cylinders (inner and outer), a 140 L tank (Fig. 9), where the assembled metal cylinders were contained, and a huge 700 L tank located in the adjacent room, high above the floor. Dialysis solution was prepared in the huge tank and transferred via a hose to the 140 L tank. There were additional parts, like cellophane and latex tubing, glass cylinders, blood pump (sigma or finger pump), glass bubble catcher, and manometer. Water softener[18] was needed for the preparation of the dialysis solution, as well as a gas bottle

---

15. Nils Alwall (1906–1986), from Lund, Sweden, designed a spiral artificial kidney suitable for hydrostatic ultrafiltration.

16. The Chairman of the Department was Prof. Andrzej Biernacki; the Director of the Artificial Kidney Center was Prof. Tadeusz Orłowski.

17. Although Prof. Tadeusz Orłowski was Director of the Dialysis Center, Dr. med. Zbigniew Fałda was involved in the nitty-gritty work at the center. He knew all about Alwall's Kidney and gave us excellent instructions. Nurses were also trained in the unit.

18. In Kraków we had neither deionizer nor reverse osmosis units at that time. However, the water was high in calcium, so water softener was necessary.

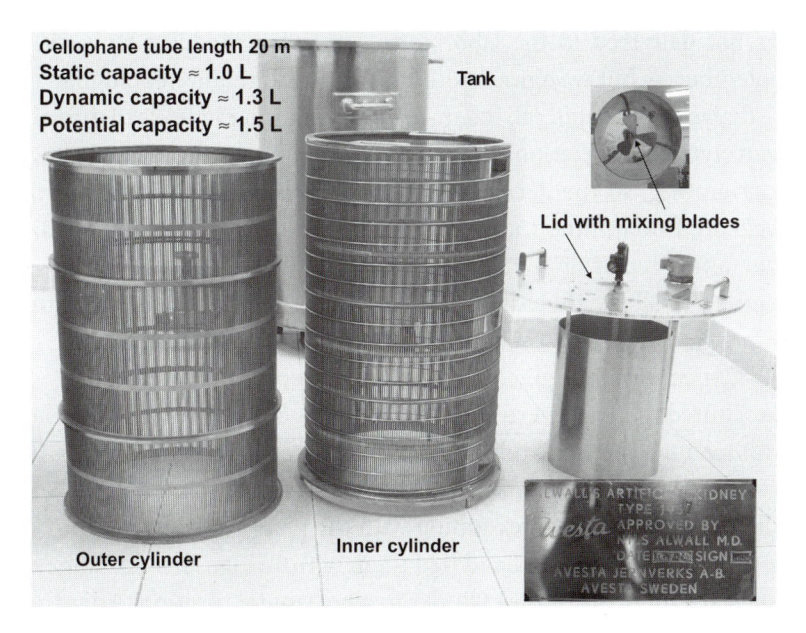

Figure 9. Alwall's dialyzer. (Modified from Fig. 3 in Pu 375.)

with carbogen.[19] Cellophane tubing was wrapped spirally around the metal cylinder and connected with latex tubing (bloodlines). Glass cylinders were inserted into the ends of the latex tubes so that a connection with the cellophane could be made, and the ends of the cellophane tube were then tied with string over the latex tubing stiffened with the glass cylinders. (More details on design of artificial kidneys, including Alwall's, can be found in my recently published paper [Pu 375].)

We determined that we had all the necessary parts, except the glass bubble catcher, which was not delivered. My father-in-law, the director of a glass manufacturing plant, agreed to make one for us and coat it with silicone. I also asked him to coat the glass cylinders with silicone. In two days, everything was ready. The flame photometer

---

19. Carbogen, also called "Meduna's mixture," after its inventor, Ladislas Meduna, is a mixture of carbon dioxide and oxygen gas. Various proportions of CO_2 and O_2 were used for various purposes. In dialysis, commonly a mixture 5% of CO_2 and 95% of O_2 was used. In the early years of dialysis, sodium bicarbonate was added to the dialysis solution, causing its pH level to exceed 7.8. With such alkaline pH, calcium and magnesium carbonate precipitated from the solution. Carbon dioxide kept the pH of the dialysis solution below 7.4 and the precipitation of calcium was markedly decreased or eliminated.

was not delivered to the laboratory — it was scheduled to work in September — but we agreed with Doc. Hanicki that we could manage the dialysis without it, relying instead on titration methods to measure electrolyte concentrations. The patient's uremic syndrome was slowly deteriorating, so the decision was made to begin dialysis before the weekend: Friday, June 15, 1962. I was tasked with assembling the dialyzer and preparing the dialysis solution. It was Przemek's job to ensure that all the ingredients in the dialysis solutions were prepared by our pharmacy and that the water softener was ready to use.

Expecting some glitches, I started to prepare the dialyzer early on the Thursday. And there were indeed glitches. I inserted the glass cylinder into the latex tubing and tied the cellophane tubing to the latex with string. Then I wrapped the cellophane tubing on the inner cylinder, inserted the latex tubing with the glass cylinder into the cellophane on the other end and tied them with string. This was done on a special support with the cylinder in a horizontal position. After that, I put the cylinder in an upright position and took the outer cylinder and placed it over the inner cylinder. This had to be done very carefully, as any deviation from the ideal direction would have damaged the cellophane tubing. Some centers had a hoist to help with the procedure; we did not, so the maneuver relied on my strength and skill. I subsequently placed the assembled dialyzer into the tank filled with water. The next step was to attach a manometer to the upper latex tubing and pump air into the lower latex tubing; the cellophane tubing had to tolerate over 150 mm Hg of pressure.

I was very disappointed when I saw air bubbles coming from several places. I tried to localize them as carefully as I could, because their location would indicate where the "spikes" were. I disassembled the dialyzer and started to look. They were tiny and therefore difficult to feel with the fingers, but I found a few of them and removed them with my wife's nail file, repeating the process four times until the reassembled dialyzer could withstand a pressure of 150 mm Hg. Then I tried to boil water in the tank. The water was supposed to boil for at least 30 minutes to sterilize the dialyzer and remove glycerol from the cellophane to make it more permeable. I put a hose from a steam outlet to the tank and opened a stop valve. Very little steam was coming out, and the water was not boiling after about an hour. I went downstairs to the boiler room and asked a stoker to increase the steam pressure, but it did not help. I again asked the stoker to increase the pressure, but he refused, explaining that he could not go over the prescribed safety level. Our dialysis room was on the second floor and the boiler room was in the basement. As I was heading from the basement, I noticed steam coming from a locked room located on the first floor. It turned out that during the building's remodeling, one steam pipe was not plugged but covered with mortar. I eventually found a helper who plugged the pipe. The steam went to the dialysis room and finally the dialyzer was sterilized. From what I remember, I filled the huge tank with 700 liters of softened water and heated it to 39°C (102.2°F). I also attached a hose with carbogen and bubbled through the water. It was about 7 o'clock in the morning on Friday, June 15, 1962. As a final preparation, Przemek put all the ingredients already prepared by the pharmacy into the water. I also checked whether all the ingredients were added in proper amounts (double-checking of this step was absolutely necessary), and we mixed them with a huge, wooden spade. Then we drained the water from the 140 L tank, filled it with dialysis solution, and attached a hose with carbogen to keep the solution's pH level below 7.4. The tank was covered with a plastic lid provided with a heater, thermometer, and mixing blades (Fig. 9).

Once everything was prepared, the patient was brought to the dialysis room by nurses Krystyna (Krysia) Piotrowska and Michalina (Misia) Pacut, who were also tasked with helping with the dialysis procedure in addition to their usual nursing tasks. One nurse frequently checked blood pressure, while the other monitored blood clotting time by the Lee–White method. Doc. Hanicki supervised the whole procedure. We filled the dialyzer with one liter of donor blood. I remember that we did not add heparin to the donor blood, which was a mistake, because the citrate was dialyzed out and the blood was prone to clotting. Przemek inserted polyethylene cannulas for the Fałda–Deczkowski shunt.[20] We connected them with latex tubing, injected heparin into the venous line and started the dialysis. Unfortunately, we observed that blood clots appeared in the bubble catcher,

---

20. This shunt was designed in 1959 by Zbigniew Fałda, from the First Department of Medicine of the Warsaw Academy of Medicine, Poland (I Klinika Chorób Wewnętrznych Akademii Medycznej w Warszawie) and Juliusz Bogdan Deczkowski, from the Institute of the Organic Technology I of the Warsaw University (Zakład Technologii Organicznej I, Politechniki Warszawskiej). The shunt was patented and manufactured in 1961.

and we had to disconnect the venous line from the venous cannula to remove the clots. We restarted the blood pump and noted a drop in blood pressure due to blood loss outside and into the dialyzer.[21] We did not have more donor blood (we ordered two more bottles immediately), so the patient's blood pressure dropped. It was impossible to do a venipuncture because of venoconstriction, so we hooked up an infusion line with saline to the latex line before the sigma pump, where the pressure was negative. As the patient's blood pressure was so low, a decision was made to administer norepinephrine until more blood became available. We could not connect the infusion line to the latex venous (outflow) line because of high outflow pressure.[22] These arrangements created more problems, as we had a delay of about five minutes (transfer of blood through the dialyzer) after we provided a particular dose of norepinephrine. We observed a seesaw of blood pressure for about an hour. We had difficulties with blood clotting monitoring as the Lee–White method gives results with a delay.

Eventually, we stabilized the patient's blood pressure, received more blood and were able to finish the 6-hour dialysis. It was an exhausting procedure. I went home to get some sleep while Przemek stayed on duty. The patient's condition was stable and his blood urea nitrogen (BUN) dropped by about 60 percent. In the evening Przemek called to inform me that he received the result of the post-dialysis potassium level, which was 8.3. I was stunned, as we had used dialysate potassium of 3.0. I made my way back to the hospital, and in the meantime Przemek was able to organize an electrocardiogram (the EKG laboratory was closed that afternoon). The EKG turned out to be normal; there were absolutely no signs of hyperkalemia. More blood was drawn to allow us to check the patient's potassium level, which was found to be 4.0. Apparently, there had been hemolysis in the first blood sample. The patient was dialyzed two more times, regained renal function and was discharged from the hospital within four weeks. From what I remember, the patient had erythrocyturia for

---

21. The static capacity of the Alwall dialyzer was about one liter (depending on how tight the cellophane tubing was wrapped), dynamic capacity (during regular blood flow of 200 mL/min and outflow pressure of <50 mmHg) was about 1200 mL, and potential capacity (with high outflow pressure for maximal ultrafiltration) was 1500 mL.

22. We did not have infusion pumps at that time.

almost a year, which was consistent with the diagnosis of acute glomerulonephritis, but his kidneys regained normal function. In retrospect, we were convinced that the patient would have died without dialysis, so all our efforts had been absolutely necessary. It was also very rewarding. I was told that the patient lived many more years.

There were no more dialyses until after the official opening of the Artificial Kidney Unit on August 1, 1962. Przemek and I filled the positions and I stopped working in emergency medicine in September 1962. There were other physicians employed in the Second Department of Medicine with the responsibility of working in the dialysis unit. These were Zuzanna Pączek, Krystyna Dużyk, Józef Bogdał, and Adam Wiernikowski. I coauthored two papers describing the experience gathered during treatment of patients with acute renal failure in the unit [Pu 3, Pu 4].

In the early 1960s, my wife's Scottish relatives came to visit us in Poland. Włodzimierz Nowosielski, a brother of my wife's father, Karol, escaped to the West during World War II and served in the Polish Army in Scotland. He married a Scottish lady, Grace, and decided to stay in Edinburgh. They had three daughters, Alexandra, Barbara, and Anna, and a son, Charlie. We had never been to the West before, so we were stunned when we saw their car, a Vauxhall Victor, which was so different from my father's Warszawa. We planned to visit them sometime, but it was not easy for Polish citizens to travel abroad at the time. We needed special permission, and usually the whole family was not allowed to go. Citizens in communist countries were considered property of the state, something similar to feudal times when peasants were *glebae adscripti* (assigned to the land) and could not easily leave the place where they lived and worked. Regardless, we hoped that it would be possible to go at some point in the future.

The problems I encountered during that first dialysis, especially regarding blood pressure, influenced me profoundly. It was obvious to me that with this kind of dialyzer, the future of dialysis was not very bright. The only hope was that the usually bulky machines would be reduced in size and their services simplified. The most important issue for me was the reduction of dialyzer capacity without reducing dialysis efficiency. I theorized that it would be ideal to have a capacity of less than 250 mL, so there would be no need for donor blood and the drop in blood pressure. I thought about this issue almost constantly. I read about other dialyzers manufactured at that time, and they did not seem optimal to me. The solution came to me suddenly as I was falling asleep at 11 o'clock on Sunday, November 11, 1962. I awoke with the thought that a capillary artificial kidney should maintain high efficiency with low internal capacity. Later, in a paper I wrote (Pu 2), I mentioned that "the 'capillary' artificial kidney resembles the body capillaries, which, in fact, are also hemodialyzers." However, on that night I did not think about tissue capillaries; it was some recollection from geometry that the ratio of a circle's surface area ($A = \pi r^2$) to its circumference ($C = 2\pi r$) gets smaller with smaller circles ($A/C = r^2/2r$). The implications of this realization were profound: if I could make a dialyzer from capillaries instead of larger tubes, then its capacity would be lower while maintaining a high surface area.

I could not sleep that night. I tried to emulate the efficiency of Alwall's kidney by keeping the capacity at about 250 mL. After several trials I calculated that a dialyzer composed of 400 cellophane capillaries 50 cm long with internal diameter of 1 mm would have surface area of 6,280 cm^2 and a capacity of 157 mL. I figured out that about 100 mL would be sufficient for the capacity of arterial and venous lines. The surface area of Alwall's dialyzer was 13,000 cm^2, and the wall thickness of the cellophane tube was 23 μm, so to match its efficiency I assumed that the wall thickness of the capillaries should be decreased to 10 μm. I then calculated the differences in pressure between the inflow to the capillaries and outflow from the capillaries at a blood flow of 200 mL/min. I calculated that this would be about 5 mm Hg, a minuscule pressure easily tolerated by cellophane tubes. It was already early morning, so I went to the department and shared the news with Przemek and Doc. Hanicki. They told me to have my figures checked, so I asked our mathematical guru, Dr. Tadeusz Struzik, to verify my calculations. Everything was OK, except for the fact that he calculated the drop in pressure along the capillaries to be 515 mm Hg, which was very disappointing as this would lead to the rupture of the tubes. Such a dialyzer could not work. I decided to recalculate everything again in the evening, and I also sent a request to my brother, an engineer, to recalculate the data. Both my calculations and my brother's indicated that the drop in pressure would be slightly above 5.15 mm Hg. Dr. Struzik rechecked his calculations, admitting that he had made a mistake of two orders of magnitude.

I decided that this project would be good for a PhD thesis.[23] For the next four months, I digested literature related to available dialyzers, reviewed general principles of rheology and studied bursting strengths of various materials. I also made detailed calculations and wrote a manuscript entitled "O zaletach i możliwości zbudowania sztucznej nerki kapilarnej" (On the advantages and possibility of constructing a capillary artificial kidney). I went with this manuscript to Doc. Stanisław Kirchmeyer, Interim Chairman of the Department following Prof. Tempka's retirement, and asked him to be my adviser in the dissertation defense. He said that I was eligible, as it was not my first manuscript, but that he needed a physicist as one of the reviewers. I did not know any physicists in Kraków, so I asked a friend of mine and my wife, Maria Starzycka, whose family friend was a famous physicist, Prof. Mięsowicz. He promised to have somebody review my thesis. He asked his assistant, Doc. dr. Jerzy Massalski,[24] to agree to be a reviewer if the Council of the Faculty would ask him to do so. Thus, I wrote an application to the Dean of the Faculty with the approval of Doc. Kirchmeyer on April 5, 1963. On May 17, 1963, the Council of the Faculty appointed Doc. Massalski and Prof. dr. hab. Tadeusz Orłowski as referees of my thesis. As Doc. Massalski was not a medical doctor, the Council of the Faculty additionally appointed Prof. dr. hab. Ździsław Wiktor (1911–1970) from the Department of Nephrology, Medical Academy in Wrocław, as the third referee, on June 21, 1963.

Prof. Wiktor's review was positive, but Prof. Orłowski declined, explaining that he did not know enough about the topic. This

---

23. Unlike in the United States, graduates of Medical School in Poland did not receive the title of MD (Doctor of Medicine), but the title of physician. Customarily, physicians are addressed as "Doctor." If one wants to go into academic medicine, one needs to write a thesis and pass a special exam. If one passes the exam and the thesis is accepted, then one is conferred the degree of *"Doktor Medycyny"* (Doctor of Medicine). The title "Dr. med." is written before the name. This corresponds to the PhD degree in the United States. At the time, the rules stipulated that a dissertation could not be the first manuscript published by the candidate.

24. Prof. dr. hab. Jerzy Michał Massalski (1919–2008) was the author of several books, including *Physics for Engineers* and *Legal Measure Units and Physical Constants*.

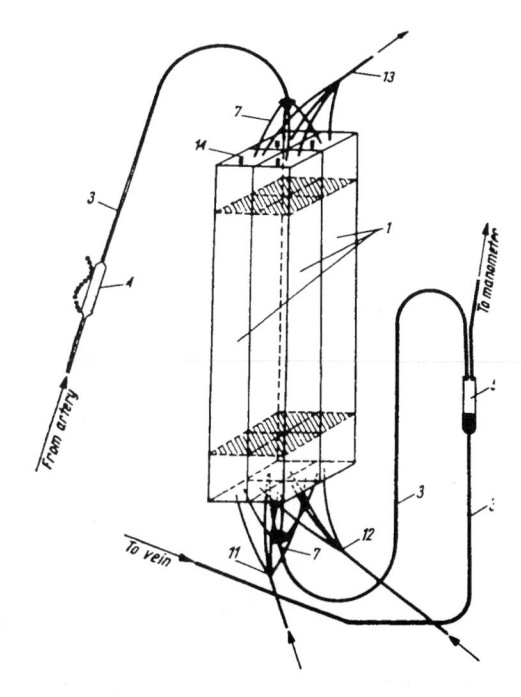

Figure 10. Schematic of the dialyzer consisting of four units. (Reprinted from Pu 2.)

surprised me because I knew that he was working on the so-called Warsaw Artificial Kidney, a replica of the Skeggs–Leonards dialyzer, built more than a decade earlier but considered obsolete by the early 1960s.[25] On November 11, 1963, the Council appointed Prof. dr. hab. Jan Roguski from Poznań[26] as the third reviewer, and he accepted the thesis for review, but he wanted me to come to Poznań and present my concept to him and his collaborators. I also submitted my thesis for publication in *Acta Medica Polona*, and it was published in 1964 [Pu 2] with all the calculations and figures.

---

25. This dialyzer consisted of multiple units connected in parallel, each consisting of a single sheet of cellophane placed between grooved rubber pads. [Skeggs LT Jr, Leonards JR. (1948) Studies on an artificial kidney. Preliminary results with a new type of continuous dialyser. *Science* **108**: 212–213.]

26. The first Artificial Kidney Center in Poland was at the Second Department of Internal Diseases of the Medical Academy in Poznań; Chairman: Prof. dr. hab. Jan Roguski (1900–1971).

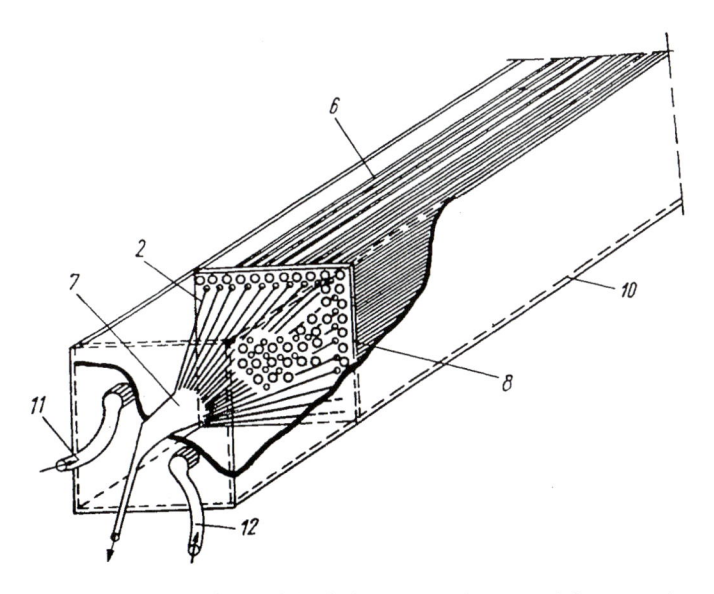

Figure 11. Schematic of the dialyzing unit. (Reprinted from Pu 2.)

The dialyzer was supposed to consist of four units (Fig. 10). I assumed that blood should flow down and dialysis solution counter currently up. Each unit was supposed to have 100 capillaries, each 50 cm long and 1 mm in diameter, with a wall thickness of 10 µm (Fig. 11).

CHAPTER 3

Professional Progress in Bytom

My professional life began to be impacted by forces beyond my control. Firstly, I was told that I would be drafted for two years to serve in military medicine, the prospect of which did not thrill me, as it was to be very basic service for mostly healthy soldiers. As my medical studies would be interrupted for two years, I considered it to be a waste of my time. Przemek was dealing with the same problem. Around the same time, Doc. Hanicki told Przemek and me that the Ministry of Mining had decided to buy an artificial kidney, as they were disappointed with the treatment of miners with crush syndrome.[1] They requested the opening of an artificial kidney center in the Hospital for Miners in Bytom. He asked us to coordinate the process, make sure that all the equipment was delivered and the dialysis room was properly constructed. When it was ready, he was to come and direct the center. As a token of gratitude for our coming to Bytom, the Ministry of Mining promised us a release from military duty and offered apartments provided by the employer. It was a very appealing offer, of course, from all points of view. In addition to the exemption from military duty, the free accommodation was very attractive, as our second son, Przemysław Wiktor, was born on July 28, 1963, and my wife's parents' apartment was getting crowded. Besides, we could not find another apartment in Kraków. Przemek and I already had some experience with opening a kidney center, so Doc. Hanicki promised to come and we expected to have an excellent learning experience. The Ministry of Mining had the financial resources to buy better dialysis equipment. We suggested that they avoid buying Alwall's kidney, as there were newer machines available. Instead, we proposed buying a tank system with coil dialyzers from Fischer-Freiburg in West Germany. This system did not require a huge 700 L tank in a separate room, so the construction of the center would be easier. Rather than water softener, we requested deionizer, for a better quality of water, which was purchased from the Berkefeld Company.

---

1. Roof collapse in mine galleries frequently causes so-called crush syndrome, with internal bleeding, muscle damage, rapid release of toxic substances into the blood stream and acute renal failure. Such patients may require very early use of an artificial kidney.

Przemek and I were supposed to move to Bytom on September 1, 1963. However, Przemek's call for military duty was already in effect, as the recommendation to relieve him of this obligation was delayed by the preoccupation of officials with the visit to Poland of Walentina Tiereszkowa, the first female cosmonaut. He eventually came to Bytom in November 1963. My exemption had come through, so I had started coordinating construction of the artificial kidney center and the Fourth Department of Internal Medicine in the Hospital for Miners. Przemek and I were the only ones who had experience with dialysis, and we had to teach our assistants and nurses the fundamentals relating to dialysis.

In December 1963, I went to Poznań to present my concept of the capillary artificial kidney for my PhD thesis. On the panel, in addition to Prof. Roguski, was Dr. med. Kazimierz Bączyk, later Prof. dr. hab., Chairman of the Nephrology Department after Prof. Roguski's retirement, and Dr. med. Andrzej Wojtczak, later Prof. dr. hab., and Director of the Personnel Department in the Ministry of Health. This was, in fact, very important to the defense of my thesis, as they were very knowledgeable in the subject matter. My defense at the Faculty Council Meeting of the Medical Academy in Kraków was less demanding and I received the degree on March 6, 1964 (Fig. 12). A formal ceremony to confer the title of Doktor Medycyny (PhD) was held on June 14, 1964 (Fig. 13).

During this time, I tried to build a capillary artificial kidney. The main problem was that there were no semipermeable capillaries available in Poland at the time. I asked the Ministry of Mining for help and they wanted to be helpful. I first received advice from Mr. Gaweł, an engineer at the Ministry of Mining, to patent my idea.[2] I submitted a patent application on January 11, 1964, before my article was published in *Acta Medica Polona*. I paid the application fee myself, which was about 3,300 zł, twice my monthly salary, but my wife agreed to the expense. In the meantime, I visited the Cellophane Factory in Tomaszów Mazowieckiand tried to convince them that it would be a good idea to make an extruder (die) for cellophane capillaries. It was

---

2. Mr. Gaweł had a very witty adage: "It takes a smart person to invent something, but a smarter one to sell it. However, a true genius is somebody who can profit from the invention — and that may be a different person."

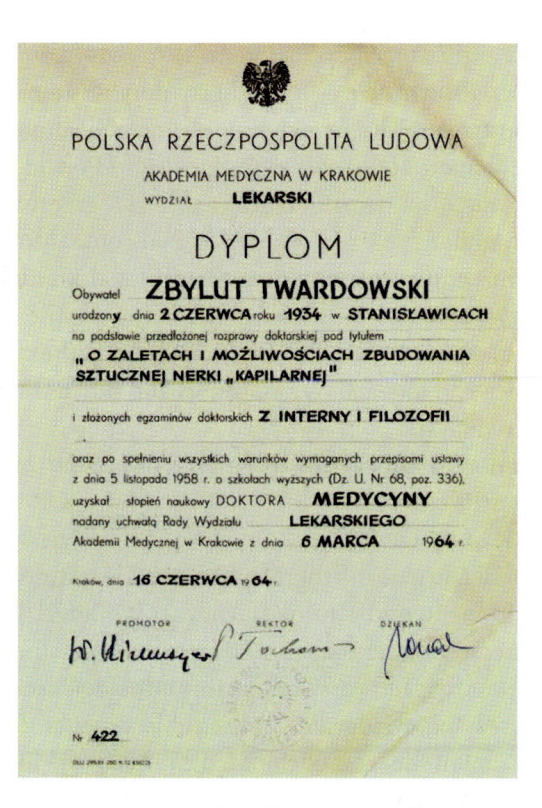

Figure 12. Doktor Medycyny certificate.

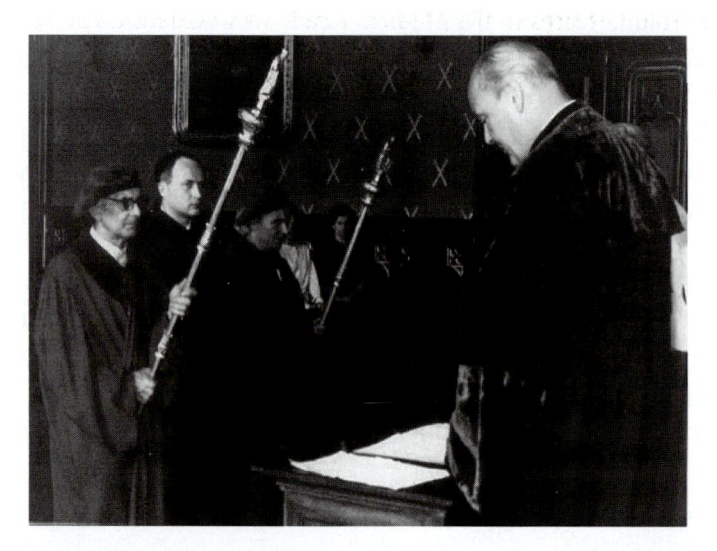

Figure 13. Formal ceremony conferring the title of Doktor Medycyny (PhD).

markedly more difficult than extruding cellophane sheets, but they agreed to take up the project.[3]

In the meantime, Doc. Hanicki told me that there was an engineer, Dr. Lindeman, at Wrocław University, who was working on extrusion of acetylcellulose hollow fibers, which were much easier to extrude compared to cellophane. After saponification,[4] such fibers could be made semipermeable, like cellophane. I started to correspond with Dr. Lindeman, but shortly thereafter he passed away and nobody took over his work. It became quite obvious to me that this project could not be brought to fruition in Poland. Mr. Gaweł again advised me to submit a patent abroad — and I had to hurry up, as a foreign patent had to be submitted within one year of submission to the Polish Patent Office. This was a very expensive undertaking (more than US$1,000), and I simply did not have the funds for it; in fact, it would have cost me more than what I earned in six years! Instead, I decided to give the rights to my patent to the Ministry of Health, asking them to submit the patent application abroad.

Before spending the money on the application, the bureaucrats involved needed some support from outside experts. The first was Prof. Tadeusz Orłowski, who offered a negative opinion regarding the possibility of constructing such a dialyzer. The second expert was Prof. Jakub Penson (1899–1971), Chairman of the Second Department of Internal Diseases in the Medical Academy in Gdańsk. His opinion was that hemodialysis would not be used much in the future, as peritoneal dialysis was becoming an established method. Subsequently notifying me about these negative opinions, the Ministry of Health refused to submit the patent abroad.

I was not prepared to give up. I presented my predictions regarding the future of hemodialysis. (These predictions were very optimistic, of course, but they were pretty much confirmed in future years.) I urged them to send requests for opinions to Prof. Wiktor and Prof. Roguski, who had given positive judgments about my PhD. I also urged them to expedite the process, as the foreign submission had to be received before January 11, 1965. Unfortunately, the review

---

3. It turned out to be an extremely difficult project. They were ready some four years later, but the quality of the cellophane capillaries was not good enough for the capillary kidney.

4. Saponification of acetylcellulose relies on using alkaline solution to remove acetyl esters.

process was extremely slow and the commission whose task it was to apply for foreign patents was only assembled a day later, on January 12. The chairman of the commission declared that the meeting had been called too late and that there would be no further action on the matter. I was very disappointed. I started thinking of a solution, and during a train ride from Warsaw I came up with the idea of a divisional patent with some new claims. I figured out that the optimal distribution of capillaries should be similar to a honeycomb with capillaries in the vertices of the hexagons. I received a patent, but I learned that the priority of the divisional patent was till January 11, 1964, and foreign patents could not be acquired. So I had two Polish patents [Pa I-1, Pa I-2] of no real value, as they could not be used in practice. Many years later, when interviewed by Sue Salzer for an article in the *Missouri Medical Review*, I confessed that, "It angered me at that time, but looking back, it's probably a good thing I didn't get the foreign patent for my hollow-fiber dialyzer back in 1964; if I had made a big hit then, when I was very young, I might never have done anything else."[5]

I still tried to come up with another idea. I discovered that there are structures in certain plants that might be useful for the capillary kidney. One such plant was the ramie (*Boehmeria nivea*), a tropical Asian perennial herb, and another was hemp (*Cannabis sativa*). The flax-like fibers from the stem of these plants were used in making fabrics and cordage. These fibers are, in fact, hollow fibers of various lengths. Unlike flax, which is used in the production of linen and has very short fibers (2–4 cm), ramie and hemp fibers are longer and may even be as much as 20 cm long or more. I began looking for someone who could collaborate with me on this new project, but after an entire year I could not find anybody. In any event, I found that the lengths and diameters of fibers were highly variable, so it would be extremely difficult to use them to make a capillary dialyzer.

I finally stopped working on the capillary artificial kidney in 1968 when I came across a paper indicating that the Dow Chemical Company in Midland, Mich., U.S., had been working on a capillary dialyzer for a few years and had succeeded in constructing one.

---

5. Sue Salzer. (1998) Home hemo redux. Experts say: There's no place like home. *Missouri Med Rev* Summer: 3–7.

The company had originally started manufacturing hollow fibers made from saponified cellulose triacetate. Henry I. Mahon, who had created this technology, initially used the fibers in reverse osmosis systems.[6] Later, he had suspected that they could be used for hemodialysis and had asked doctors for help. Richard D. Stewart and Joseph C. Cerny from the Section of Urology, Department of Surgery, University of Michigan in Ann Arbor, joined Henry I. Mahon to pursue the idea of a hollow-fiber dialyzer. The first dialysis apparatus consisted of a bundle of 800 capillaries, each of which was 10 cm long, with an inside diameter of 55 mm and a wall thickness of 14 mm. The capillary ends were sealed in phenolic tubing with Silastic RTV 601 (Dow Corning Corporation, Midland, Mich.). With an internal surface area of 138 cm^2 and a volume of 0.19 mL, the dialyzer had a urea extraction ratio[7] of 51 percent at a blood flow of 9.0 mL/min. These figures come from an *in vitro* study reported in 1964,[8] but it was published in a journal not available in Poland at the time.

Over the next four years, the project progressed thanks to the cooperation of the Department of Environmental and Internal Medicine, Marquette School of Medicine in Milwaukee, Wisconsin; Western Division Research Laboratories, The Dow Chemical Company in Walnut Creek, California; and the Wood Veterans Administration Hospital in Milwaukee, Wisconsin. In 1968, they reported the initial results with the first capillary artificial kidney or the "hollow-fiber artificial kidney" (HFAK), used for treatment of a patient with chronic renal failure.[9] The capillary artificial kidney was made of about 10,000 deacetylated cellulose acetate hollow fibers

---

6. Reverse osmosis is a filtration process that is often used for the purification of water. It works by using pressure to force a solution through a membrane, retaining the solute on one side and allowing the pure solvent to pass to the other side. This is the reverse of the normal osmosis process, which is the natural movement of solvent from an area of low solute concentration, through a membrane, to an area of high solute concentration when no external pressure is applied. Nowadays, reverse osmosis is one of the components of the water purification system for hemodialysis.

7. The extraction fraction is calculated by subtracting outflow tubing concentration (O) from the inflow tubing concentration (I) and dividing by the inflow tubing concentration $[(I - O)/I]$. The clearance is calculated by multiplying the extraction fraction by the blood flow.

8. Stewart RD, Cerny JC, Mahon HI. (1964) The capillary "kidney": Preliminary report. *Univ Michigan Med Center J (Med Bull-Ann Arbor)* **XXX**: 116–118.

9. Stewart RD, Lipps BJ, Baretta ED, *et al.* (1968) Short-term hemodialysis with the capillary kidney. *Trans Am Soc Artif Intern Organs* **XIV**: 121–125.

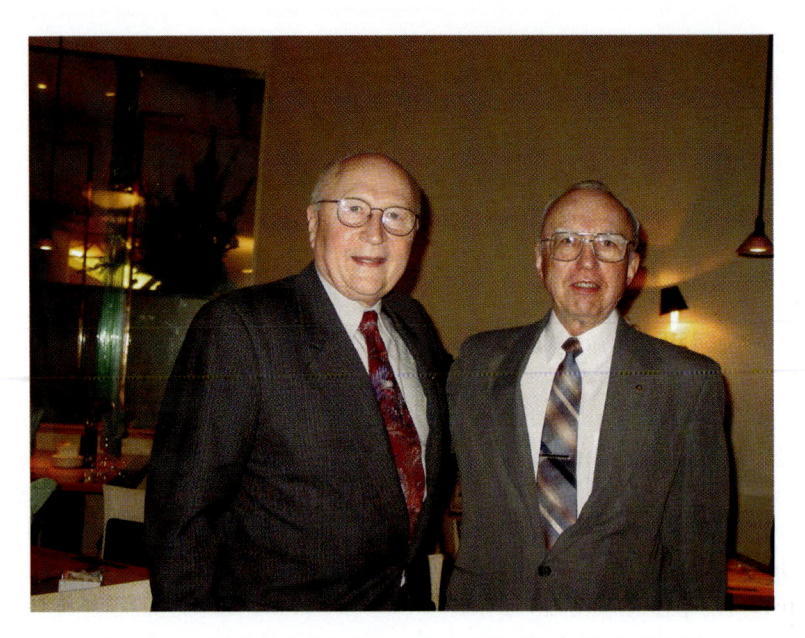

Figure 14. The author (left), and Richard D. Stewart, MD, during the Annual Dialysis Conference in Seattle, Washington, on March 2, 2003.

sealed at each end into a tube sheet with silicone rubber and jacketed in a plastic cylinder. This report was available in Poland and I discovered that they had started to work on the project shortly after I did, but they were successful and I was not. Given the extensive cooperation required to make the project succeed, it seems that I was naïve to think that I would manufacture a capillary dialyzer in Poland at the time. When I met Dr. Richard Stewart during the Annual Dialysis Conference in Seattle on March 2, 2003 (Fig. 14), he told me that he had not been aware of my publication for several years, admitting that had they used my calculations, it would have taken them markedly less time to come up with the dialyzer described in 1968. Indeed, papers published in *Acta Medica Polona* were not widely read, but my paper was cited in a book written by Yukihiko Nose,[10] who was working in the Cleveland Clinic, Ohio, at that time. The book was

---

10. Yukihiko Nose, educated at the University of Hokkaido (1951–1958), performed the first home hemodialysis in 1961, came to the U.S. in 1962, and initially worked in Brooklyn, NY, then in Cleveland Clinic, OH, under the direction of Willem J. Kolff, who had performed the first successful hemodialysis in a patient in 1946.

published in 1969,[11] after most of the work on the capillary artificial kidney had been completed with funds from the Dow Chemical Company. How slowly the information was disseminated at that time is illustrated by Clark Colton,[12] who asked me how to get cellophane capillaries for his work toward his PhD thesis in 1968. I advised him to contact the Dow Chemical Company. I do not know how he learned about my interest in cellophane capillaries; either he read the title from Index Medicus, which cited the work in the 1965 issue, or *Acta Medica Polona* was available in the U.S. at the time. Stewart's paper was cited in Index Medicus in 1964.

Before leaving Kraków I passed an examination for the first degree specialization in internal medicine. Immediately after my arrival in Bytom, I was given the keys to the apartment in the building owned by, and located very close to, the hospital. The apartment was located on the third floor.[13] It was unfurnished, so we withdrew the money we received from my parents for the apartment in Kraków and dedicated it to the purchase of furniture. I bought some essential items, but the apartment's real furnishing started after Halina's arrival in November 1963. She got a position in the Psychiatry Department of the Hospital for Miners and took an additional job in an outpatient clinic. One major disadvantage of our arrangement at the time was the location of our apartment on a very high floor. The water pressure was very low and as we only had running water at night, we had to collect water in a tub and other containers during the night in order to have it for the daytime. The lack of a lift was another major headache; the baby carriage with our younger son had to be carried up the stairs, which Halina mostly had to do by herself. We kept a lookout for a more convenient apartment and after a few years we managed to find one on the first floor,[14] which alleviated the water pressure and baby carriage issues. By then, our younger son was able to walk. With both of us working long hours, we hired a babysitter. Both of our boys attended preschool after they reached the age of three.

---

11. Nose Y. (1969) *Manual on Artificial Organs: Volume I — The Artificial Kidney*. C.V. Mosby Co., St. Louis, pp. 343.

12. In 1969, Clark Colton developed the equations governing mass transport in hemodialysis in his PhD Thesis at Massachusetts Institute of Technology. At that time, hollow-fiber dialyzers were not yet commercially available.

13. In American terminology it was the fourth floor.

14. In American terminology it was the second floor.

During the first half of 1964, Przemek (Dr. Hirszel) and I were busy teaching nurses and physicians, organizing the dialysis center and the Fourth Department of Internal Medicine. We were ready by the middle of 1964, expecting Doc. Hanicki to join us soon, so it was a surprise when we learned that he had changed his mind. I was older than Przemek and I had the title of Doctor of Medicine, having already passed an exam for the first degree specialization in internal medicine, so I was supposed to become Interim Chairman of the Department and Dialysis Unit. Being only 30 at the time, I was scared. I asked Dr. Zbigniew Fałda from Warsaw to take the position of Chairman, but he declined. I confessed to him about my fear that all dialyzed patients under my care would die. He told me, "Don't be scared; your results will be similar to others," which was somewhat encouraging. It was certainly very fortunate that the calm and knowledgeable Przemek was by my side.

The first patient with acute renal failure was treated in Bytom at the end of that year. Very early on, we adopted a policy of prophylactic dialysis, particularly for those with crush syndrome, as waiting for a so-called "classical indication for dialysis" seemed to be obsolete for us. We followed the recommendations and excellent results of Paul Teschan.[15] Over seven years (June 1964 to May 1971), we treated 11 cases of crush syndrome using prophylactic dialysis. Two died, one of myocardial infarction and one of sepsis, so mortality in our series was 18.2 percent, similar to others' using prophylactic dialyses [Pu 15]. For blood access we were using Fałda–Deczkowski polyethylene arteriovenous shunts, 1963 version, or Teflon catheter inserted into the femoral artery and vein by the Seldinger method. In 1966 we acquired Quinton–Scribner arteriovenous shunts manufactured by the Sweden Freezer Company in Seattle, Washington, and used them for acute and chronic dialysis.

In 1964, a new artificial kidney center opened in nearby Katowice, in the Third Department of Internal Medicine at the Silesian Medical Academy. The Chairman of the Department was

---

15. Teschan PE, Baxter CR, O'Brien TF, et al. (1960) Prophylactic hemodialysis in the treatment of acute renal failure. *Ann Intern Med* **53**: 992–1016. Recognizing his pioneering work in frequent prophylactic hemodialysis in acute renal failure, Paul Teschan was a recipient of the Special Award for Lifetime Achievements at the 5th International Symposium on Home Hemodialysis at the Annual Dialysis Conference in Charlotte, NC, on February 28, 1999. [Twardowski ZJ. (1999) Laudatio: Professor Paul E. Teschan. *Home Hemodial Int* **3**: 1–4.]

Prof. dr. hab. Kornel Gibiński.[16] Doc. Franciszek Kokot[17] became the center's Director and I asked him to become a scientific consultant for our Department and Dialysis Center. He agreed and we started working together on various projects, as well as established weekly teaching conferences alternately in Bytom and Katowice.

The founding of two artificial kidney centers in one region in a single year created some problems with regard to the number of patients requiring dialysis for acute renal failure. Prof. Gibiński, who was the voivodeship (regional) consultant in internal medicine, sent a letter to hospitals announcing the opening of two dialysis centers, but requested that the cases should be transferred preferentially to Katowice; only in the case that the Katowice center was unable to accept the patient should such a patient be referred to Bytom. As a result, in 1964 we had only one case of acute renal failure, and by early 1965 only a few cases had been referred to us.

In 1965, we treated a young nurse from our hospital with acute hepatic failure (*Atrophia hepatis acuta flava*). At that time there was nothing to offer except an exchange transfusion. I created a Fałda–Deczkowski arteriovenous shunt. Employees from the whole hospital offered blood and we treated her for 19 days with daily exchange transfusions. Ultimately, she died, and in the autopsy she had typical acute hepatic atrophy with minimal rim (a few millimeters) of liver tissue; the rest was necrotic. The hepatitis B virus had not yet been discovered. I also developed hepatitis in 1965 and spent a few months hospitalized before being sent to a sanatorium. (I think that I stuck myself while creating an arteriovenous fistula.) The diagnosis was hepatitis B, without serologic confirmation.[18] I was quite sick for some time, with bilirubin exceeding 24 mg/dL and transaminases over 1,500, but within a few days I felt a good deal better despite my poor

---

16. Prof. dr. hab. Kornel Gibiński (1915–) was a gastroenterologist arrested by the Gestapo in 1943 for working in the AK (Armia Krajowa, or Home Army). My father told me that he saw him in Montelupich Prison in Kraków; after being severely beaten, he was thrown into the cell where my father was kept. Both Gibiński and my father were transferred to the Gross-Rosen concentration camp. Gibiński was liberated from Gross-Rosen by the advancing Soviet Army in 1945; my father had been transferred earlier to Litoměřice on Labe.

17. Prof. dr. hab. Franciszek Kokot, (1929–), Doc. dr. hab. 1962, Associate professor 1969, Professor 1982. His main interests were in nephrology and endocrinology.

18. It was, in fact, hepatitis B, as to this day I have the isolated antibody to hepatitis B core antigen (anti-HBc).

laboratory results. I had a lot of time to read, and I consumed most of the available literature related to dialysis, particularly chronic dialysis, and also a book on transplantation by Thomas E. Starzl from the University of Colorado School of Medicine and Surgical Service, Veterans Administration Hospital in Denver, CO.[19] After reading that book, I came to the conclusion that we had the capability in our hospital to start a transplant program. We had a dialysis center, and departments of general surgery and neurosurgery, but we did not have a urology service or a vascular surgery service.

During my absence, Przemek acted as Interim Chairman of the Department. After returning from medical leave, Przemek informed me that he would be returning to Kraków. That was unhappy news, but I understood that he preferred to work in academic medicine under the guidance of Doc. Hanicki. By then, we had quite a large team of physicians who could help with everyday work, among them: Lech Orawski, Roman Lebek, Alfred Hakuba, and Bolesław Kłosowski. Shortly thereafter, the Department of Internal Medicine expanded by 25 beds and new physicians, Henryk Nowak and Cecylia Gajdzik, were hired. Gradually, four physicians acquired first degree and two of them second degree specializations in internal medicine. Henryk Nowak left to work in a leprosy center in Buluba, Uganda. In later years, two more physicians were hired: Ludmiła Pohorecka-Zagroba and Jerzy Sobczyk. All of them participated in research and were coauthors of published papers. The head nurse of the Dialysis Center was Helena Kubara.

In 1965, we acquired Vim–Silverman biopsy needles[20] and introduced kidney and liver biopsy. The Vim–Silverman needle, originally invented for renal biopsy, was also used for liver biopsy. Tissue samples were sent to Prof. dr. hab. Janina Kowalczykowa, Chairwoman of the Department of Pathological Anatomy, Medical Academy in Kraków, as the Pathology Department of the Silesian Medical Academy was not providing this service in 1965. Since the Radiology Department of our hospital had vascular diagnostic capabilities, we

---

19. Starzl TE. (1964) *Experience in Renal Transplantation*. Philadelphia, W. B. Saunders Co.
20. Silverman I. (1954) Improved Vim–Silverman biopsy needle. *J Am Med Assoc* **155**(12): 1060–1061.

were able to make a diagnosis of kidney diseases very precisely. I did not have to go anywhere to learn kidney or liver biopsies. There was no ultrasound available at the time, but the kidneys could be located very precisely in the Radiology Department by taking an X-ray of a supine patient lying on a rolled towel under the abdomen. The Vim–Silverman needle consisted of an outer cannula and inner needle with a side groove in which the tissue is retained when the needle and cannula are withdrawn. After the needle tip is introduced to the kidney, the position of the needle tip is confirmed by asking the patient to breathe — the needle's head moving up with inspiration and down with expiration — and then hold the breath. Then a very fast maneuver must be performed: the needle is advanced, and then held, and the outer cannula is advanced and then both are withdrawn; the whole maneuver should last no more than two seconds. The tissue is retained in the groove. As this was the most important maneuver to avoid tearing the tissue and causing bleeding, I trained repeatedly on an apple. The method seemed to work effectively, as we did not have any serious bleeding even in patients with advanced chronic renal failure. We also did liver biopsies and bone biopsies when needed.

In 1964 and 1965, we were using Fałda–Deczkowski shunts as blood accesses. The shunts were created on the forearm by cutting down the radial artery and basilic vein, and on the lower extremity by cutting down the posterior tibial artery and saphenous vein, or by insertion into the femoral vein and artery using the Seldinger method. Shunts could function for one to three dialyses. All blood accesses were created by Przemek or me, as we did not have a vascular surgery service in the hospital. After Przemek's departure, I did all the catheter insertions myself.

There were not a great many cases referred to us, as most were going to Katowice. This prompted me to think about starting a chronic dialysis program, but I hesitated to establish such a program, as we used Fischer–Freiburg or Travenol twin-coil 1.8 m^2 dialyzers with a static capacity of 800–900 mL. This would have required a rather large amount of donor blood being given to chronic dialysis patients. Moreover, we had only one kidney machine (Fischer–Freiburg), and cases of acute renal failure would be priorities with the possible interruption of the chronic patient treatment. On the other hand, because most acute cases went to Katowice, our machine was frequently idle, sometimes for long periods, and there was the risk that the personnel would lose out on experience. Training without a patient was consuming supplies without providing real service. Ultimately, the program started incidentally. In December 1965, a 25-year-old woman, a bricklayer's helper, fell from a scaffold and suffered severe trauma to the right lumbar region with subsequent rupture of the right kidney. A right nephrectomy was performed in a trauma hospital, and because of anuria, the patient was referred to us for treatment of acute renal failure. The case looked unusual, as the patient did not have prolonged hypotension, which would be responsible for damage to the other kidney, so I decided to request further diagnostic tests. Renal arteriography and retrograde pyelography revealed a polycystic and atrophic left kidney. The patient had eight dialyses via polyethylene catheters inserted into femoral vessels. As her brother offered to donate a kidney, we also looked into the possibility of a kidney transplant. We were not prepared for a kidney transplant program, so I contacted Prof. Ździsław Wiktor from the Department of Nephrology in Wrocław, who had opened a kidney center in 1964. The patient was transferred to Wrocław, where she received more dialysis treatment, and was subsequently transferred to the Second Department of Surgery of the Medical Academy in Wrocław. Prof. dr. hab. Wiktor Bross, Chairman of the Department, transplanted the kidney from the patient's brother on March 31, 1966, with immediate diuresis and survival at least until October 6, 1966, when the case report was sent for publication [Pu 5].

In 1966, we acquired Silastic-Teflon Quinton–Scribner cannulas[21] manufactured by Sweden Freezer Company in Seattle, Washington Initially, we used a Teflon connector between arterial and venous cannulas as originally described by Quinton and coauthors. The tubing was heated with a torch to over 300°C and bent into an appropriate shape using a Teflon tube bender until cooled by running cold water through the bender.[22] Bending the Teflon tube was real trial, as

---

21. Quinton WE, Dillard DH, Cole JJ, Scribner BH. (1962) Eight months' experience with the Silastic-Teflon bypass cannulas. *Trans Am Soc Artif Intern Organs* **VIII**: 236–243.

22. Quinton W, Dillard D, Scribner BH. (1960) Cannulation of blood vessels for prolonged hemodialysis. *Trans Am Soc Artif Intern Organs* **VI**: 104–113.

I frequently burned my fingers during the procedure. At the end of 1966 we acquired 30 ft (9 m) of Silastic tubing, which was used as a connector between arterial and venous cannulas. Our method of shunt creation and care was described in detail in a paper published in 1969 [Pu 8]. We were very happy with the results, as some of the shunts functioned without interruption for over a year. We even expressed the opinion that, "[A]t this time we see no need for the use of other means of access to the blood vessels, e.g., the arteriovenous fistula of Brescia *et al.*" [Pu 8]. At the same time, we did have some exit-site infections and needed to reinsert some shunts after a few months due to clotting.

The decision to continue the chronic dialysis program was prompted by the March 1966 admission of a patient with suspected acute renal failure. The patient was Alicja Balicka, and I will describe her story in detail later. We obtained very impressive results with this patient. I was so impressed with the results that I had no doubts about the value of chronic hemodialysis and went ahead with the development a chronic dialysis and renal transplantation program in the hospital. Though I had the approval of the Director of the Hospital for Miners, Dr. med. Jerzy Dutkiewicz, his ability to support the program through the purchase of equipment and by expanding the dialysis center was very limited.

Shortly after, we accepted another patient with chronic renal failure, but there were difficult organizational issues, as we still had patients with acute renal failure and we had only one kidney machine. "At times, we had three patients with chronic renal insufficiency, under treatment simultaneously, but one of the patients usually died" [Pu 8]. Initially, we had only two trained nurses, but with a large number of successfully performed hemodialyses, the training was rapid. Hemodialyses became nursing procedures. One nurse was fully trained, while the other was in training. I was giving weekly theoretical lectures, and Helena Kubara, the head nurse, did most of the practical training. Unfortunately, the kidney machine was not very reliable and needed to be constantly observed for ruptures in the latex tubing in the blood pump and clot formation in the bubble trap. Between December 1965 and May 1968 we performed 515 hemodialyses and had 105 latex tubing ruptures. Clot formations in the glass bubble traps, also called clot catchers, were so frequent (197 times in 393 procedures) that we called them clot formers and replaced them with a simple polyvinyl branch connected with a manometer to control outflow pressure. After this modification, clots formed only twice in 122 procedures. The change allowed us also to reduce heparin use by 50 percent. Cellophane tubing ruptures, on the other hand, were rather rare. Initially, dialyses were performed only during the day, but gradually we were able to start an overnight program, once we had more trained nurses and physicians able to deal with complications. Indeed, they could handle most situations, but I was essentially on call all the time. For more than two years I was constantly exhausted, and at one point I experienced asystole for several seconds at home. Thankfully, my wife was able to resuscitate me, but the scare, a direct result of exhaustion, forced me to take more breaks. Fortunately, my deputy and assistants had become experienced enough that I did not need to be on call constantly by the beginning of 1969.

I remember being very upset about the discrepancy between the number of patients needing dialysis and our capabilities, and I sometimes became depressed. I figured out that the best treatment for my depression was to recharge by going to a western, among them *High Noon*, with Gary Cooper, *3:10 to Yuma*, with Glenn Ford, *The Magnificent Seven*, with Yul Brynner, Steve McQueen, Charles Bronson and the others, and *Rio Bravo*, with John Wayne. After a good western, I always felt uplifted and reassured that the good guys always win — if enough energy is devoted to the problem. After a good movie, I could return to my struggle.

There was indeed a constant battle to optimize dialysis with only one machine and the twin-coil 1.8 m^2 dialyzers. Initially, dialysis was performed twice weekly for 6 hours using two coils. There were two problems with use of two coils: we had a limited number of dialyzers, and the usage of donor blood was very high. We decided to use only one coil, store the dialyzer in a sterinol solution, and use the other coil for the following dialysis in the same patient. With this scheme we could increase dialysis time to 8 hours. It was obvious within a few weeks that the patients were developing uremic symptoms, so the dialysis time was increased to 10 hours, and ultimately to 12 hours, twice weekly for most patients and three times weekly for some. The capacity of one coil was about 400–450 mL, so the use of donor blood was markedly reduced. During the initial two-and-a-half years of our chronic program, we accumulated a tremendous number of observations. Ultimately, we were able to dialyze day and night and published our experience in 1969 [Pu 8]. The most salient observations were that longer and more frequent dialyses provided better clinical and laboratory status of patients. We also found that in the treatment of hypertension, salt balance was of the utmost importance. Some patients had multiple complications; some were rehabilitated to a degree that they could resume employment.

Two of our patients underwent kidney transplants [Pu 6]. Alicja Balicka received a kidney from her father, and the surgery was performed in our hospital on September 5, 1966. The transplant surgeon was Prof. dr. hab. Józef Gasiński, the Chairman of the Second Department of Surgery at the Silesian Medical Academy. The patient died 26 days after transplant because of rejection and sepsis. Another patient in this series was Zbigniew Kaczmarek, a 27-year-old male nurse who was admitted with chronic glomerulonephritis and malignant hypertension associated with complete blindness on June 8, 1966. After treatment with peritoneal dialysis and hemodialysis, as well as careful regulation of sodium balance, the patient's condition markedly improved. As a preparation for the transplant, a double nephrectomy was performed by Dr. Łotkowski on September 8, 1966. The patient recovered his vision (0.9 on the left eye, 0.7 on the right). Prof. Gasiński performed the kidney transplant from the patient's father on November 7, 1966, and the patient had five acute rejections, the last one severe, which ultimately destroyed the kidney 132 days after transplant [Pu 7, Pu 7a]. When the patient was feeling better after recovering from one transplant rejection, he told me that the medical profession was very lucky. "All of its successes bathe in the sunshine; all of its failures are hidden in the ground."

Having only one kidney machine created another severe problem. When a patient was transplanted, the space was immediately filled by another patient, and if there was transplant rejection, the patient had no opportunity to return to hemodialysis. As a consequence, patients on dialysis who were well did not want to undergo kidney transplant and felt safer on dialysis. With the increased frequency and duration of dialysis, no patients died in 1969 or 1970. It was extremely difficult, as there was constant pressure to accept new patients into the program, but we just did not have the capacity. At a certain point I was desperate and I fretted over how we could best find a solution to the problem. Should I admit everybody and dialyze with short and infrequent dialyses, accepting a high mortality rate, or should I dialyze the best way I could determine and restrict the number of admissions? The first approach was entirely unacceptable, as it would contradict the aim of treatment, i.e., prolongation of useful patient life. I came to the conclusion that it was better to dialyze in the best possible way to show the authorities that the method was good and deserved support and development. Although it was terribly difficult for me to turn away new candidates, I was convinced that this had to be our approach. The medical criteria for admission were rather straightforward: the patient had to be between the ages of 20 and 40 and have no primary renal disease (no systemic disease). I tried to establish a committee to enforce these criteria (similar to the "Life or Death Committee" in Seattle[23]), but I had no candidates willing to serve, and when I learned that the Seattle Committee had been disbanded, I stopped trying. I decided that the best criterion for accepting patients for chronic dialysis, in addition to the medical specifications mentioned, was the order of appearance. This last criterion was also very difficult to determine. Should priority be given to a patient under my care in an outpatient clinic who may require dialysis in a few weeks, or to somebody sent to our ward requiring dialysis immediately? The selection of patients for chronic dialysis was the most difficult problem for me during all the time I worked in Poland.

A better solution to the problem of selection would have been expanding the chronic dialysis program, but that would not have been an easy task. The results we achieved in our program were met with

---

23. The "Life or Death Committee" established in Seattle in 1961 was comprised of community representatives including a banker, a surgeon, a lawyer, a minister, a labor leader, a housewife and a government official. The committee decided who was deserving of treatment. Criteria were medical and social; however, social criteria were rather vague. An article written by journalist Shana Alexander and published in *Life* magazine in 1962 explained the committee's decision-making process. The public was outraged at the committee's unfair selection process and random qualifications based on its own judgments. It was alarming to the public that citizens were responsible for "playing God." The Committee was disbanded in 1967. Many scholars consider the role played by the "Life or Death Committee" to be the beginning of bioethics (medical ethics).

accolades from the hospital administration and the Department of Health in the Silesian Voivodeship, as our program achieved the best results in the country. At the same time, with the declining economic situation during the last years of General Secretary Gomułka's regime, it was impossible to acquire new machines and expand or remodel the hemodialysis center.

One of the possible solutions was to use peritoneal dialysis for the treatment of acute and chronic renal insufficiency. In 1966 we introduced peritoneal dialysis for treatment of acute renal failure and in chronic renal failure patients with very high urea levels as a preparation for hemodialysis to avoid disequilibrium syndrome.[24] We acquired a stylet catheter manufactured in Poland[25] very similar to the Weston–Roberts catheter.[26] Since 1968 we also used peritoneal dialysis for a prolonged period as a preparation for eventual transplant or "as a means of keeping patients alive until a hemodialyzer becomes available" [Pu 10]. Peritoneal dialysis solutions were originally bought from the Pharmaceutical Cooperative "Inlek" (Farmaceutyczna Spółdzielnia Pracy "Inlek") in Lublin, Poland. Unfortunately, the cost of dialysis was so high that we were forced to obtain solutions from the hospital pharmacy. There were many downsides to the solutions at that time, but the disadvantages were greater in our center. Firstly, the solutions were prepared in 0.5 L bottles, so for each 2 L exchange, four stopper punctures were needed. Each puncture was associated with a risk of bacterial contamination. Secondly, the solutions were autoclaved for sterilization, but our pharmacy did not have a rapid cooling system, so the solutions stayed warm for a prolonged period of time. Consequently, even with acidification of the solution before sterilization, caramelization of the solution (brownish color) was visible with the naked eye. Such solution caused abdominal pain, which

---

24. With very high urea levels (over 250 mg/dL), high efficiency hemodialysis quickly lowering blood urea level causes rapid decrease in blood osmolality. Urea is removed slowly from the brain and consequently water enters the brain due to the osmotic pressure gradient. The prevention of disequilibrium syndrome relies on lower efficiency hemodialysis or peritoneal dialysis. [Kennedy AC, Linton AL, Eaton JC. (1962) Urea levels in cerebrospinal fluid after haemodialysis. *Lancet* **1**(7226): 410–411.]

25. Luniak J. (1966) Cewniki z tworzyw sztucznych do dializy otrzewnowej. (Peritoneal catheters made of plastic materials.) *Tworzywa Sztuczne w Medycynie* **III**(4): 161–163.

26. Weston RE, Roberts M. (1965) Clinical use of stylet-catheter for peritoneal dialysis. *Arch Intern Med* **115**: 659–662.

was severe in some patients. This forced us to use neuroleptanalgesia in 25 percent of patients [Pu 13], but the situation was unacceptable. We insisted on receiving solutions from Pharmaceutical Cooperative "Inlek" in Lublin. This alleviated one problem: severe pain after infusion of the solution into the abdominal cavity. However, multiple punctures of 0.5 L bottles contributed to high peritonitis rates in our program. "[W]e believe that the peritoneal infections were caused mainly during piercing the stoppers of the bottles many times, each puncture being connected with the hazard of infecting the dialysis fluid. In the patient L. Ch. the stoppers of the bottles were punctured more than 7,000 times in the whole treatment course" [Pu 10]. In the late 1960s, Inlek manufactured dialysis solutions in a limited number of 2 L bags made from Sicron CR/S3 (polyvinyl chloride),[27] but we did not receive them.

In 1968, a chronic peritoneal dialysis program was established. The results, from five patients treated between April 1968 and June 1969, were published in 1970 [Pu 10]. One advantage of peritoneal dialysis was that we were not restricted by the need to use a machine. Another was the minimal blood loss, so blood transfusion requirements were markedly lower than in hemodialysis. Initially, I did all the peritoneal catheter insertions, but gradually other physicians performed the procedure. The nurses carried out other functions. With our system, a single nurse was able to attend to two peritoneal dialyses in the general ward. If peritoneal dialysis was performed in the artificial kidney room, it was carried out by the nurses who performed hemodialysis.

We mostly used peritoneal dialysis for acute renal failure. The exception was in patients with high catabolic rate, such as those with crush syndrome, or in patients who had undergone abdominal surgery. With this approach we were able to cover for other dialysis centers from time to time. In 1968 the Dialysis Center in Warsaw stopped admitting patients, so we accepted a patient from the First Department of Internal Medicine of the Voivodeship Hospital in Warsaw. The patient was a 29-year-old white male, a professional driver with paroxysmal nocturnal hemoglobinuria, who developed acute renal

---

27. Falda Z. (1968) *Dializa otrzewnej* (*Peritoneal Dialysis*), printed by Farmaceutycznea Spółdzielnia Pracy (Pharmaceutical Cooperative) "Inlek", Lublin, ul. Króla Leszczyńkiego 11, 1–46 (p. 12).

failure after hemolytic crisis. During the period of acute renal failure, the Ham test (acidified serum lysis) was negative, indicating the presence of such severe hemolysis that all abnormal red blood cells were destroyed and the remainder did not lyse in acidified serum. Only after 33 days did the Ham test became positive. After 36 days of therapy, including transfusions of red blood cells washed in physiologic saline and peritoneal dialyses, the patient was transferred back to Warsaw in the polyuric stage of acute renal failure [Pu 9].

Many patients experienced psychiatric disturbances and we asked our Department of Psychiatry for consultations. Evaluations were frequently performed by my wife, Halina Twardowska. The most salient observations were that patients with elevated levels of urea (218 mg/dL) and creatinine (12.4 mg/dL) did not have any discernible mental disturbances. Oneiroid disturbances or paranoid syndrome with delusions were observed in patients with brain edema due to malignant hypertension or massive fluid overload. Quantitative disturbances of consciousness, like sleepiness, semicoma or coma, were associated with acidosis [Pu 11].

In 1966, I passed an examination for the second degree specialist certification in internal medicine, and by 1968 my position had changed from Interim Chairman to Chairman of the Fourth Department of Internal Diseases with the Dialysis Unit. This was associated with a small increase in salary. All my assistants pursued specializations in internal medicine, four achieving first degree and two getting second degree specialization. After Przemek's departure, my deputy was Lech Orawski, and when he left in 1970 to become a chairman of a department of internal medicine in another hospital, Roman Lebek became my deputy.

In 1966, I presented our two cases of kidney transplantation in the Hospital for Miners at the meeting of the Polish Academy of Science, Department of Medical Science, Renal Section [Pr 3]. After the presentation I was appointed as a member of the Transplantation Committee of the Ministry of Health and as a member of the Nephrology Committee of the Polish Academy of Science.

The Chairman of the Transplantation Committee of the Ministry of Health was Prof. Tadeusz Orłowski. I do not recall all of the members, but I remember that a director of the Finance Department of the Ministry of Health participated in our meetings. I insisted on the development of chronic dialysis, whereas Prof. Orłowski maintained that Poland could not afford it, that we should spend more money on the prevention of renal failure and transplantation. My point of view was that there was no way to prevent chronic renal failure, so we should spend money on what works, which meant dialysis and transplantation. During one of the meetings, I pointed out to Prof. Orłowski that the Director of the Finance Department was participating and he was best qualified to indicate whether the Ministry of Health could afford a chronic dialysis program or not, and our role as physicians was to indicate that the results of chronic dialysis were very good and worthy of dissemination in Poland.

At that time we also opened an outpatient clinic, and as our reputation grew, we admitted more patients with various kidney diseases. Some of the prominent Communist Party officials from the Ministry of Mining asked us to monitor their family members in the clinic. Compared to other employees, these officials were given tremendous benefits. In addition to a decent salary, they had a pool of tickets to buy various goods that were difficult to get, such as a car,[28] TV set, washer, and so on. As a token of appreciation for the care of a VIP's mother, I received a ticket for a Škoda 1000 MB and bought one in 1968. Manufactured in Mladá Boleslav (hence MB) in Czechoslovakia, the car was markedly better than the Warszawa, but still quite basic and easy to repair. In 1968, I could finally stop using my father's car.

Protein losses during peritoneal dialysis were considered to be a major obstacle for the widespread use of chronic peritoneal dialysis. We observed that some patients did not show any decrease in serum protein after months of peritoneal dialysis. I started to wonder whether protein losses may vary in individual patients [Pu 12, Pu 12a]. One female patient had nephrotic syndrome before she developed end-stage renal disease. I did not mention that in our paper related to protein losses in peritoneal dialysis, but I was curious whether patients with nephrotic syndrome could have higher protein losses than others. I observed that protein losses did not depend on the

---

28. The prices of new cars were relatively low, but they could not be purchased without a ticket. A car bought in this way and immediately put on the used car market was worth at least twice the price paid with a ticket — a rather different situation to the 20 percent depreciation new cars typically undergo in the free market economy.

number of exchanges, only on the duration of dialysis, and that peritonitis increases protein losses, but leaving the catheter in the peritoneal cavity between dialyses did not increase protein losses. The most important observation was that there was individual proneness to protein losses due to unknown factors. Our patient with nephrotic syndrome had the lowest peritoneal protein losses, which was surprising to me, as I did not know at that time that in nephritic syndrome only glomerular capillaries were leaky to proteins and that other capillaries were not. The determination that there were individual differences in protein losses was very important in my later studies on the peritoneal equilibration test. Another very interesting observation was that the protein losses in consecutive exchanges were decreasing, so from the protein loss point of view, prolonged single dialysis is more favorable than more often repeated dialyses of short duration.

This observation led us to perform a study on the kinetics of protein loss during consecutive exchanges [Pu 14, Pu 14a]. In the first two exchanges there was some protein in the peritoneal cavity at time zero, and during these two exchanges protein present in the peritoneal cavity was completely washed out. We determined that there was a linear increase in protein concentration in peritoneal dialysate taken every 10 min. In each consecutive exchange this increase showed a downward tendency. It suggested to us that protein transfer from serum to the peritoneal cavity was almost constant regardless of the presence or absence of fluid in the peritoneal cavity.

As I mentioned previously, we usually spent our vacations in the seaside resort of Chałupy. In 1969 we were in Chałupy when the first landing of a man on the moon occurred on July 20. We were originally uncertain as to whether there would be TV coverage in Poland. In many other countries under Soviet rule, transmissions of the event were forbidden, but Władysław Gomułka, the First Secretary of the Polish United Worker's Party, decided to allow the spectacle to be broadcast. It's anybody's guess why he decided to do so on this occasion; a year later he decided against broadcasting the World Soccer Championship in Mexico, an action for which he was very much criticized, as neighboring Czechoslovakia had decided to air the event. Some Poles traveled to the south of the country to catch reports from Czechoslovakian transmitters. I remember going to Szczyrk, a city close to the border, to watch — paying particular attention to the Brazilian team and their exceptional star Pele. There was also resentment in Poland about the decision to participate in the Soviet Union's invasion of Czechoslovakia in 1968. The Polish population was aware of the moon landing and many people wanted very much to see the triumph of American technology over that of the Soviet Union. I remember the landing being at night, Polish time, and all of us, including our children, were enthralled to witness the event. It certainly served to put in the shade all the Soviet propaganda following Yuri Gagarin's first orbit of the Earth in 1961.

In 1969, an opportunity to visit some dialysis centers in Great Britain suddenly arose. Adolf Nowosielski, a brother of Halina's father, Karol Nowosielski, emigrated with his wife, Wira,[29] to Israel and later to the U.S. in the late 1950s and became American citizens. He visited Poland in the mid-1960s and decided to give my father-in-law some money (US$100) to visit Scotland to meet their brother Włodzimierz and his family. Adolf wanted to be in Edinburgh at the same time as Karol. My father-in-law wanted Halina and me to go with him. We were rather unsure because of the cost of the trip, but Adolf promised to provide more money later. Tragically, both Karol's brothers, Adolf and Włodzimierz, died in the meantime.

Left with the US$100, we decided that going in our new Škoda 1000 MB would be much more reliable than taking the Warszawa, and its much better mileage would make the trip possible. Before issuing passports,[30] the authorities wanted to know whether potential travelers had enough funds, so we went to the Orbis (travel agency) and got an estimate that the funds we had were sufficient. We were skeptical, but happy to be eligible to get passports, and we also got permission to buy foreign currency, the equivalent of US$5 per person. Our sons had to stay in Poland — to guarantee that we would come back — and our mothers took care of them whilst we were away.

One of my goals during the trip was to visit some dialysis and transplant centers in London (Royal Free Hospital and Hammersmith

---

29. Polish citizens, with the exception of Jews, were not permitted to emigrate. Wira was of Jewish origin, so she and her whole family (her non-Jewish husband and her two children, Barbara and Zbigniew) could emigrate to Israel.

30. Polish citizens, like citizens of other communist countries, were not permitted to keep their passports with them at home. A passport was handed over for a particular trip and had to be returned to the Passport Office upon one's return to Poland.

Hospital) and Edinburgh (Royal Infirmary and Western General Hospital). Just after World War II, Eric George Lapthorne Bywaters (1910–2003), discoverer of crush syndrome (or Bywaters' syndrome caused by traumatic rhabdomyolysis with consequent renal failure), worked in Hammersmith Hospital and received one of the first rotating drum dialyzers from Willem Johann Kolff in 1946. It occurred to me that there should be a tradition of knowledge related to crush syndrome, a syndrome so common in victims of roof collapse in mine galleries. Royal Free Hospital was famous for its dialysis center and I was aware of many papers related to dialysis from this institution. I wrote a letter to the Department of Health in London to receive recommendations for visiting these places. In particular, I asked to meet Stanley Shaldon, John F. Moorhead and Rosemary Baillod in the Royal Free Hospital in London, while in Edinburgh I wanted to meet James S. Robson, from the Artificial Kidney Unit in the Royal Infirmary. I was informed that the department did not have contact with Dr. Shaldon, and that their advice was not to meet him, as he was about to leave the country. Only later I learned that Dr. Shaldon did not have a good relationship with the Department of Health and he was relocating to Germany to work, anyway.

As a preparation for the trip, I bought some spare parts for the car that the mechanic had told me were likely to break. These were a wedge belt, a line connecting the accelerator pedal with the throttle valve, spare bulbs, and the whole ignition distributor. Having so little foreign money, it was important to be able to fix the car by myself. As it turned out, a wedge belt did indeed break during our trip, destroying the ignition distributor, and I was able to replace them without having to payout any foreign currency. A line also broke in the region close to the throttle valve where it was subjected to bending with each application of pressure to the accelerator pedal, and I replaced it without difficulty. I was very happy that we took all the spare parts with us. We also took a tent, food, fluids, and some items that could be sold abroad, such as vodka, amber and a fur collar. I also had some contact with Mr. Elphic, a representative of Burroughs Wellcome & Company, who had visited me in Bytom. After learning that I was going to Britain, he asked me to visit him in London and record an advertisement in Polish related to the treatment of urinary tract infection with nalidixic acid (Negram)[31]; as this would bring in some extra money, I agreed. We had also hoped to borrow some money from Grace. However, after the death of her husband, she did not have any money to spare.

We started from Kraków, and on the first day we found some camping areas in East Germany and slept in the tent, which did not cost too much. By the next day we were already driving through West Germany. The Škoda's top speed was about 105 km/hr (65 mi/hr), so nearly every car overtook us on the autobahns; most were driving at least twice as fast as us. We stopped in Leuven, Belgium, where Wira and Adolf's daughter Barbara studied medicine at the university. She accommodated us for the night. The next day we drove to Ostend, Belgium, to take a ferry to Dover, England. The ferry ticket cost US$65, which was a surprise as the travel agent in Kraków told us that the price was about US$30. I asked at the ticket office whether the price included the return trip and the clerk laughed, informing me that there were no round-trip tickets. We were suddenly rather scared as it dawned on us that we would not have enough money for the return ferry. We had to be as thrifty as possible, and Halina and I got into an argument when she wanted to buy some matchbox cars for our sons, as I considered our return ticket to be the most important expense. On the ferry many people had soft drinks, and we looked on with a degree of envy. But we abstained, as we had to conserve every penny. From Dover we went to Canterbury, visiting the cathedral and meeting with Mr. Elphic in the Burroughs Wellcome office. Then we drove to the campsite close to Heathrow Airport and slept in the tent. I was quite surprised that I did not have any difficulty driving on the left. While our car had a steering wheel on the left-hand side, I did not overtake anybody, as I was the slowest driver, so the position of the steering wheel was not a problem.

The following day we donned our best attire and drove to London. The Department of Health had kindly arranged my visit to Hammersmith Hospital, but I spent a rather short time there; they

---

31. Nalidixic acid was manufactured by Burroughs Wellcome & Company under the brand name Negram. Burroughs Wellcome and Glaxo merged in 1995 to form Glaxo Wellcome. In 2000, Glaxo Wellcome and SmithKline Beecham merged to form GlaxoSmithKline. The company now markets nalidixic acid under the name NegGram.

were not too excited about Bywaters' legacy.[32] We visited Madame Tussauds museum on Baker Street, Hyde Park, Buckingham Palace and the home of Sherlock Holmes. We put on our best clothes again next morning; I went to the Royal Free Hospital and spent about four hours talking with Dr. John Moorhead and Dr. Rosemary Baillod, and I also visited a dialysis room and saw some patients. I have to say that I learned a lot. First of all, they confirmed my impression about the importance of sodium balance to achieve blood pressure control without blood pressure medications or recourse to bilateral nephrectomy. Their method, described to me in our discussions, was elucidated in detail in a 1972 publication.[33] Most patients were dialyzed two or three times weekly on Kiil dialyzers.[34] Secondly, I noticed that most patients were dialyzed with the use of Cimino–Brescia fistulas. There were patients over 60 years old on chronic dialysis. The results with fistulas were excellent, and I became convinced about their superiority over Quinton–Scribner shunts.

In the afternoon we went north on the M1 highway to Edinburgh. The last part of the drive, in the evening, was very impressive with beautiful cat's eyes on twisty roads. In Edinburgh we were looking for Grace's house on Sciennes Road and asked passersby, pronouncing the name similar to the way one pronounces "science," but people did not understand what we were saying. We had to write the name down before we discovered that the proper pronunciation was "shins." Eventually, we arrived at our destination.

During our stay in Edinburgh I visited the Royal Infirmary's Artificial Kidney Unit, and the Nuffield Transplant Unit at the Western General Hospital, where all kidney transplant patients were treated. The most impressive aspect for me was the tremendous effort

---

32. Bywaters introduced the Kolff artificial kidney in the UK, but was not convinced of its value [Bywaters EG, Joekes AM. (1948) The artificial kidney; its clinical application in the treatment of traumatic anuria. *Proc R Soc Med* **41**(7): 420–426.] He left Hammersmith Hospital in 1947 to become a rheumatologist.

33. Craswell PW, Hird VM, Judd PA, *et al.* (1972). Plasma renin activity and blood pressure in 89 patients receiving maintenance haemodialysis therapy. *Br Med J* **4**: 749–753.

34. In 1960, Frederik Kiil from Ullevål Hospital, Oslo, Norway, modified the Skeggs–Leonards sheet dialyzer by replacing rubber pads with plastic boards made of an epoxy resin compound with talcum as a filler. Cellophane sheets were replaced with more permeable cuprophane (Bemberg Cuprophan PT-150). The dialyzer had low internal resistance so could be used without a blood pump if an arteriovenous shunt was used, and it had a low static capacity of about 150 mL. More than 90 percent of the blood could be returned to the patient after dialysis.

to maintain the sterility of the air in areas housing post-transplant patients. If a patient needed dialysis, the kidney machine was outside the room, the bloodlines from a patient were threaded through an opening in the window. All meals were delivered with special elevators going very slowly to avoid air movement. Entry to a patient's room was via a clean room and those entering had to wear sterile gowns, masks and gloves.

In addition to my visits to hospitals, my father-in-law, Lolek, and I tried to sell some of the goods we brought with us for sale, successfully accumulating about US$150. I figured that we had enough money to visit a few places of interest and return to Kraków. We paid a visit to the Royal Palace and Princes Street Gardens, and we visited Selkirk, where the famous Selkirk Bannock[35] is made. One of the highlights of the trip was the Edinburgh Military Tattoo, which takes place on the esplanade at Edinburgh Castle. Pipers and drummers supplied a rousing soundtrack, and there was a performance by the Royal Canadian Mounted Police. The most moving part was the climactic close as the Lone Piper, high on the castle ramparts, played a haunting lament, the Highland Cradle Song. It was one of the most spectacular shows we had ever seen.

After two weeks in Edinburgh we began our trip home, stopping at the same camping area near Heathrow Airport on the first day. We met with Mr. Elphic in London the following day and I recorded my Polish advertisement for Negram. He paid an honorarium of £20, which was almost US$60 with the exchange rate at the time, and we had enough money to buy our sons matchbox, and some other items. We kept US$65 for the ferry ticket and US$130 just in case something went wrong on the drive back. The ferry took us from Dover to Ostend and then we drove to Nuremberg, West Germany. We found a very nice camping area there and stayed the night. Nuremberg was very close to the Czechoslovakian border, so we could safely spend almost all of our money there. Lolek bought Karl May's collection of books in German, which pleased him greatly as he had bought them before World War II and was forced to sell them after the war when he needed to raise some money. The next day we drove to Poland

---

[35]. A rich fruit bun made the traditional way with oatmeal, with butter and plenty of sultanas. It looks rather like a large oatcake.

through Czechoslovakia. The car needed an oil change and a lubrication service, so we stopped at a service station. It was then we discovered the distaste some Czech people had for Poles in 1969 — the Polish Government having supported the Soviet invasion of Czechoslovakia the previous year. I also found out that the Polish and Czech languages are close but not identical. I asked that they lubricate (*smarować*) the car, but they could not understand the Polish word (and they did not speak English). Resorting to sign language, I finally explained what I wanted, and I was told that the word I should have used was *mazanie*. In Polish, *mazanie* means "to smear"— something similar but not the same. In any event, we returned in high spirits from our first visit abroad. I was 35 at the time.

After the trip, I had lots of ideas to implement in our work. I was very skeptical about the possibility of creating a transplant ward similar to the one in Nuffield Western General Hospital, but I thought about expanding our dialysis capabilities and maybe even create a transplant center. It would not be as sophisticated as the one in Edinburgh, but it would be sufficient to prevent hospital-acquired infections. Doc. Paliwoda, a vascular surgeon, and Doc. Adamkiewicz, a urologist, both from the Silesian Medical Academy, wanted to work with me to create a transplant service in Bytom. For some time, we went every week to Koźle near Opole, where an animal laboratory was in operation. We did some renal transplants on dogs. After about six months, we realized that there was no way we could create a transplant service in the Hospital for Miners in Bytom, as there was simply no money for such an endeavor and the hospital was not affiliated with the Medical Academy. Prof. dr. hab. Tadeusz Paliwoda (1922–1981) would later become a pioneer in cardiac surgery in Silesia. Prof. dr. hab. Kazimierz Adamkiewicz (1928–2004) moved to Gdańsk in 1971 and became Chairman of the Department of Urology in the medical academy there.

I was criticized by the hospital administration for having a high budget, higher than those of other departments. For this and other reasons I became very cost conscious, believing that this would be the best way of expanding our program. As mentioned previously, I tried to use only one of the coils of the Fischer and Travenol 1.8 m² twin coil dialyzers. This was not the ideal strategy because although we prolonged the dialysis, patients had clinical symptoms of uremia. In 1969 we tried reusing a dialyzer using the method of Shaldon *et al.*,[36] but we had to abandon this because of frequent pyrogenic reactions. The method relied on using both coils but keeping the dialyzer with lines in the refrigerator between dialyses.

The situation was soon to change markedly. In 1969 we were able to obtain Ultra-flo 145 dialyzers with the Hoeltzenbein net,[37] which allowed an almost complete recovery of blood after dialysis. There were some other developments that forced us to work on dialyzer reuse. In our outpatient clinic we were monitoring Maria Zieleniec, a young lady with chronic glomerulonephritis who was a daughter of a prominent official in the Ministry of Mining. It was obvious that she would need chronic dialysis in 1971 at the latest. Informing her father that all the available spaces in the dialysis ward were occupied, he offered to provide resources for new kidney machines and remodel our dialysis center if we would consider taking his daughter into the program. The work on remodeling started, and we received five Travenol RSP kidney machines, but there were two obstacles to utilizing the unit to its full capacity. Firstly, our hospital did not have facilities to repair the equipment. I decided to buy spare parts for those likely to break frequently, like dialysate pumps or heaters, and my training in fixing cars paid off, as I could fix a machine during dialysis by exchanging a broken part. From what I remember, it took us a few years to establish equipment maintenance facilities in the hospital. Secondly, the Department of Health, which was supposed to provide dialyzers, told us that we would get only 1,200 dialyzers per year. It was obvious that if we wanted to use all our machines at full capacity, we would perform at least 3,000 dialyses per year.

As a consequence, we started to focus our efforts on dialyzer reuse, adopting the method of Pollard *et al.* for Kiil dialyzers.[38] It soon became clear that the method needed modification. We noted

---

36. Shaldon S, Silva H, Rosen SM. (1964) Technique of refrigerated coil preservation haemodialysis with femoral venous catheterization. *Br Med J* **ii**(5406): 411–413.

37. Hoeltzenbein J. (1966) A new disposable coil system. *Proc Eur Dial Transplant Assoc* **III**: 390–391.

38. Pollard TL, Barnett BMS, Eschbach JW, Scribner BH. (1967) A technique for storage and multiple re-use of the Kiil dialyzer and blood tubing. *Trans Am Soc Artif Intern Organs* **XIII**: 24–28.

a higher rupture rate of the membrane when sodium hypochlorite was used, so we decided to use only tap water and 2 percent formaldehyde for rinsing dialyzers. The dialyzers with arterial and venous lines were kept in canisters with 2 percent formaldehyde between dialyses. We also noted that reused coil dialyzers tended to telescope when removed from the container in the RSP machine; this damaged the cellophane tubing with reuse. The reason for this phenomenon was related to the welding of the mesh at the bottom of the coils: the manufacturer welded only about half of the mesh at the bottom. We decided to weld the whole mesh (Fig. 15), which prevented telescoping and increased the number of reuses. After the reuse method was finally established, urea dialysance was measured for consecutive uses. Dialyses were carried out twice weekly for 11 hours with blood flow of 200 mL/min and recirculating dialysate; the measurements were done at the second, sixth, and eleventh hours of dialysis. The differences in dialysance values were minuscule and mostly insignificant. Only dialysance values at 2 hours with first use (133 ± 26 mL/min) and fifth use (113 ± 29 mL/min) were significantly different [Pu 16].

Our method was presented at the meeting of the Nephrology Section of the Polish Society of Internal Medicine in Gdańsk in the fall of 1971 [Pr 12]. It was met with skepticism, the main criticism being

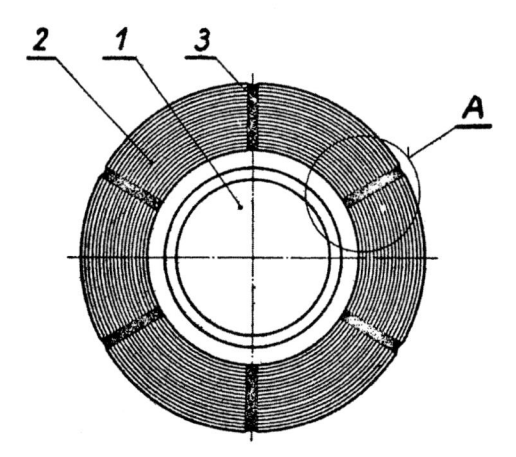

Figure 15. Mesh welded at the bottom to prevent telescoping. (Reprinted from Pa I-3.)

the risk of transmission of viral infections. Even my assertion that the reused dialyzer was for the same patient did not change the minds of the majority of physicians in the audience. I had hoped to receive some reward for saving the hospital administration money, but they did not have funds for such a purpose. Administrative Director Mr. Henryk Kosecki advised me to patent the idea, which I did, with Roman Lebek as a coauthor [Pa I-3]. The method was only used in our hospital and we received five percent royalties from the savings over five years. The reuse of dialyzers was not practiced in other hospitals in Poland for many years.

Another way to lower the cost of dialysis was modifying the composition of the dialysis solution. The most expensive constituent was glucose. The initial idea of using a high glucose concentration in dialysis solution stemmed not only from the need for osmotic ultrafiltration in rotating drum dialyzers, but also from Kolff's belief that glucose may prevent hemolysis in extracorporeal circulation.[39] High glucose concentration was continued in dialyzers capable of hydrostatic ultrafiltration, for various reasons, which I described in a letter to the editor of *Hemodialysis International* in 2009 [Le 26].

In the late 1960s, we were using coil dialyzers and tank systems [Fischer–Freiburg, West Germany] and glucose in concentrations from 1.0 to 1.4 percent. Growth of bacteria in the tank system was very high and we were surprised to find extremely low glucose concentrations in the dialysate at the end of a 10-hour dialysis session, as bacteria used glucose as a source of energy. This led us to lower the glucose concentration in dialysis solution to 0.2 percent in 1967 [Pu 8]. Reports[40,41] of no side effects with glucose-free dialysis solution prompted us to compare the effects of low glucose concentration (0.1 percent) and no glucose in dialysis solution during 8- or 12-hour dialysis [Pu 17]. From the 1970s, dialyses were performed on a recirculating single pass (RSP)

---

39. Kolff WJ. (1965) First clinical experience with the artificial kidney. *Ann Intern Med* **62**(3): 608–619.

40. Eschbach JW Jr, Barnett BM, Cole JJ, *et al.* (1967) Hemodialysis in the home. A new approach to the treatment of chronic uremia. *Ann Intern Med* **67**(6): 1149–1162.

41. Hübner W, Sieberth HG, Pottreck KH. (1971) Chronisch-intermittierende Hämodialyse mit zuckerfreien Dialysat. (Chronic intermittent hemodialysis with a sugar-free dialysate.) *Med Welt* **3**: 86–88.

artificial kidney[42] with a tank of 120 L, and Ultra-flo 145 dialyzers (Travenol, Morton Grove, Ill.), reused four to six times with blood flow always 200 mL/min. The aim of the study was to examine glucose losses during dialysis and bacterial growth with the use of 0.1 percent and 0.0 percent glucose in dialysis solution. It was found that glucose concentration in the recirculating dialysate compartment decreased from 100 mg/dL to 54 mg/dL in the sixth hour and to 22 mg/dL in the eleventh hour of dialysis. The dialysis solution flow to the recirculating compartment was 500 mL/min. The bacterial growth in glucose-free dialysate was four times lower than in dialysate containing glucose. The average glucose level in arterial blood dropped at the end of the eleventh hour of dialysis by 22 mg/dL with glucose-free dialysate and by 13.5 mg/dL with 100 mg/dL glucose in dialysis solution. Glucose losses averaged 60 mg/min (3.6 g/hr) with glucose-free dialysate. Thus glucose-free dialysate decreased the cost of dialysis, decreased bacterial growth, and was associated with minimal glucose losses during dialysis. We never observed hypoglycemia in any of our patients.

By 1972 we had four chronic hemodialysis stations, and each station was used during the day and the night. There were two half-days left (Thursday and Sunday) for thorough cleaning of the kidney machines and the room. We had 14 patients on chronic hemodialysis and various numbers of cases of acute renal failure. Among our chronic hemodialysis patients, we had a case of familial nephropathy (Alport's syndrome) with hearing impairment, myopia due to lenticonus, and albipunctate retinitis. We followed the patient's whole family; his mother and two daughters had some features of Alport's syndrome but not advanced renal failure. We noted that our patient on dialysis had hematocrit higher than most of our hemodialysis patients, similar to patients with polycystic renal disease [Pu 19].

We also treated acute poisoning cases, as some of them might require dialysis, though most did not. I remember that many cases of ethanol poisoning were referred to us as methanol poisoning. These

---

42. In this system the dialysis solution is taken from the tank to the dialysis compartment containing a dialyzer. The solution is recirculating to increase the contact of the solution with the dialyzing membrane and prevent streaming through the limited part of the dialyzer. Fresh solution is taken from the tank to the dialysis compartment usually at the rate of 500 mL/min and is not returned to the tank, but removed to the drain — hence the term "recirculating single pass."

were patients who had consumed so-called Denaturat (contaminated spirit), which was much cheaper than vodka and was sold for various domestic uses, like cleaning or for use as fuel. Years ago, to prevent people from drinking it, Denaturat was contaminated with methanol. This method of contamination was abandoned for decades, but contamination with methanol lingered in the memory of many people, including physicians. In the late 1960s and early 1970s Denaturat was contaminated with acetylsalicylic acid to give it a very bitter flavor, and dyes were added to indicate that it was not meant for drinking. We had two patients with blood ethanol levels of 0.72 percent and 0.73 percent, the highest levels I had ever seen. Both recovered without dialysis after a prolonged period of unconsciousness. On the other hand, we had some patients poisoned with methanol and polyethylene glycol who required intensive dialysis.

We also had a case of mixed poisoning with carbon monoxide and metholo-hydroquinone developer. This patient had initially attempted suicide by ingesting 12 g of photographic developer (a mixture of methol and hydroquinone), but because he had not observed any symptoms of poisoning, he had decided to inhale carbon monoxide as well. There was some difficulty in making a full diagnosis because the patient only admitted to breathing in carbon monoxide. The poisoning was found to be mild, with an initial HbCO of only 15 percent, so the patient was just sent for treatment of the broken nose he received when he fell. In the Laryngology Department, the patient developed jaundice, cyanosis, dyspnea and passed dark urine, and he was transferred to our center. We determined that he had liver and kidney damage, methemoglobinemia and hemolysis. The patient was treated with exchange transfusions and supportive therapy. Only after two days did the patient admit to poisoning himself with developer. At the time a urine test for hydroquinone was negative. Ultimately, the patient recovered, but the recovery process was very long [Pu 20].

After returning from my visit to Great Britain, I decided to use arteriovenous fistulas as blood accesses for chronic hemodialysis. As there was no vascular surgery in our hospital, I decided to create them by myself. We did not have an appropriate procedure room in the department, so I made an agreement with Dr. med. Stanisław Stawiński, Chairman of the Department of Laryngology, to allow us to use one of their operating rooms. Fortunately, one of the rooms was

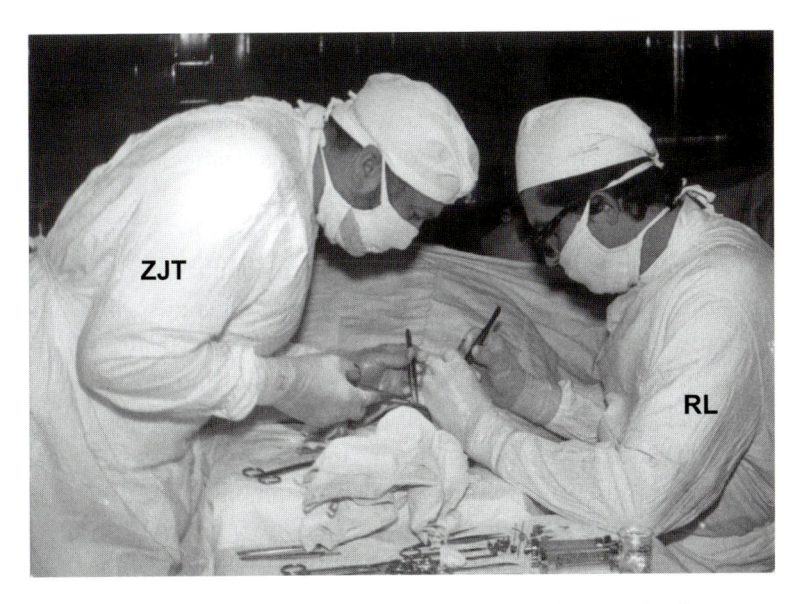

Figure 16. Roman Lebek (RL) assisting the author (ZJT) during fistula creation.

usually unoccupied when we needed to use it for the procedure. After acquiring all the necessary equipment for the procedure, I carefully studied the literature related to the procedure and began creating fistulas in September 1969. Dr. Roman Lebek assisted me during surgery (Fig. 16). The procedure underwent some small modifications, but it was very similar to that reported by Brescia *et al.* in 1964.[43] Only local anesthesia with 0.5 percent lignocaine was used. By semicircular cut with distal pole 1–3 cm from the styloid process, the radial (or ulnar) artery and the cephalic (or basilic) vein were exposed. The vessels were liberated from all tributaries and fascia on a long stretch to avoid tension after anastomosis. Both vessels were clamped and turned 90° to bring up surfaces that would be anastomosed. The next step was to make 8–10-mm cuts on the surfaces facing up. The anastomosis was made with a round-bodied needle attached to a 7–0 absorbable suture. To avoid excessive bleeding, the site of anastomosis was wrapped with fibrin membrane. After the clamps were released,

---

43. Brescia MJ, Cimino JE, Appel K, Hurwich BJ. (1966) Chronic hemodialysis using venipuncture and a surgically created arteriovenous fistula. *N Engl J Med* **275**(20): 1089–1092.

the vessels were turned back 90° so that the anastomosed artery and vein were not twisted. An immediate blood flow through anastomosis was almost always achieved. In a few instances local papaverine or intravenous dextran infusion were used to overcome venous spasm. The wound was closed with subcutaneous absorbable sutures.

I created 37 fistulas in 27 patients from 1969 to 1976. During this time seven patients had Quinton–Scribner shunts, five on upper extremities and two on the tibial arteries and saphenous veins. Since 1972 only arteriovenous fistulae were created for chronic dialysis. Twenty-three fistulas were created on the left radial artery, 10 on the right radial artery, three on the left ulnar artery, and one on the right ulnar artery. Creating side-to-side anastomosis fistulas was supposed to have two limbs, proximal and distal; however, ulnar fistulas did not usually develop distal limbs. Failure of one limb was not considered fistula failure. Figure 17 shows survival probabilities of distal limb, proximal limb and overall (either one), which was 86.7 percent at 6.5 years. Almost all fistulas allowed achieving 200 mL/min blood flow through the dialyzer. In any event, we did not use higher blood flow. We started using fistulas 14 days after implantation with blood flow of 100–150 mL/min; then within a week or two the blood

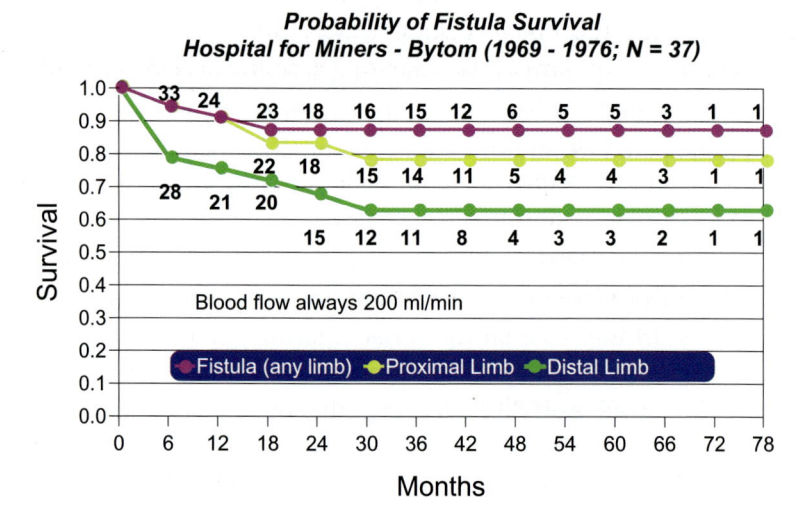

Figure 17. Survival probabilities of distal limb, proximal limb and overall (either one). (Modified from Pu 27.)

flow was increased to 200 mL/min. I did the first cannulations in 1969, but shortly thereafter nurses were doing needle insertions. The most skillful was the head nurse, Helena Kubara, and she did all needle insertions for at least a month after fistula creation. Only later were other nurses sufficiently skilled to insert needles.

In 1972, I visited my wife's family in Edinburgh again and, of course, spent some time as a Visiting Doctor in the Medical Renal Unit of the Royal Infirmary. One observation that did not impress me was that water was not treated, as it was thought that Edinburgh's water had low enough levels of calcium and magnesium. However, most patients had calcium and phosphorus disturbances, and I observed many patients with obvious metastatic calcifications. Another problem was an epidemic of hepatitis B in the personnel. I remember that they had some unique method of keeping open arterial and venous cannulas in patients with acute renal failure. Instead of connecting them and creating a shunt, they infused heparin to both cannulas very slowly. During my short visit, none of the cannulas clotted. In spite of the fact that I did not have a British license to practice medicine, they allowed me to insert arterial and venous cannulas. I spent some time in the Pathology Department, where they were working on glomerulonephritis. I recall that they were one of the first to blame fibrin leak into the Bowman space as a stimulant for Bowman capsule proliferation and formation of crescents.

From 1969 onwards, I was keen to determine the best method of dialysis to achieve "adequate" results.[44] At the time I did not even think about optimal[45] results. To this day, according to guidelines, the goal is to achieve *adequate* dialysis; people will sometimes talk about *optimal* treatment, but this is not the realistic goal of those who pay for dialysis. As a matter of fact, it would be difficult to say that some method is "optimal," as something may be developed in the future that is slightly better.

My goal was to find out the best duration and frequency of dialysis that would eradicate all symptoms and signs of uremia and lead to full rehabilitation. I would consider this an adequate dialysis. However, we were, of course, limited by the equipment and facilities at our

---

44. According to dictionaries, *adequate* means "barely satisfactory" or "sufficient."
45. According to dictionaries, *optimal* means "most favorable" or "desirable."

disposal. The following signs and symptoms were considered as caused by uremia if no other etiology could be determined:

- Gastrointestinal and nutritional:
    - nausea, vomiting
    - anorexia
    - dysgeusia
    - hypoalbuminemia
- Neurological:
    - peripheral neuropathy
    - restless leg syndrome
    - burning feet syndrome
    - insomnia
    - depression
    - pruritus
    - decreased nerve conduction velocities
- Skeletal:
    - bone pain
    - bone fractures
    - osteomalacia
    - cystic fibrosis
    - pseudogout
    - metastatic calcifications
    - elevated P, low Ca, high Ca × P
- Cardiovascular:
    - hypertension
    - arrhythmia related to electrolyte disturbances
    - pericarditis
    - dyspnea
    - sleep apnea
- Hematological:
    - hemorrhagic diathesis
    - anemia[46]

---

46. Erythropoietin was unavailable, and anabolic steroids were available but were not used in our patients.

The following symptoms were considered as related to inappropriate dialysis technique (essentially too short dialysis with too high ultrafiltration rate):

- Intradialytic and postdialytic hypovolemia:
  - during dialysis — cramps, hypotension, backache, "crash"
  - after dialysis — dizziness, hangover (thirst, headache, fatigue)

In all patients treated from March 1969 to May 1973, the amount (duration and frequency) of dialysis was adjusted to eradicate all symptoms and signs of uremia and achieve full rehabilitation. All of these patients had isolated renal diseases [glomerulonephritis: 10; pyelonephritis: 2; polycystic renal disease: 1; hereditary nephritis (Alport's syndrome): 1]. The average composition of dialysis solution in mEq/L was Na^+ : 140.1; K^+ : 2.75; Ca^{++} : 3.5; Mg^{++} : 1.2; Cl^- : 110.0; HCO_3^- : 37.5; no glucose. However, the composition for some patients needed adjustment depending on the average predialysis serum electrolyte levels. Sodium ranged from 135 to 145 mEq/L, bicarbonate from 35 to 40 mEq/L, potassium from 1.5 to 3 mEq/L, and calcium from 3.25 to 3.75 mEq/L.

The conclusions of the study were as follows:

1. Most patients with renal failure caused by isolated renal diseases can be relieved of the clinical symptoms of uremia (except anemia) by the proper selection of the amount of dialysis (duration and frequency), which equates to achieving adequate dialysis.
2. In patients with diuresis exceeding 500 mL/24 hours, adequate dialysis may be expected by performing two dialyses weekly of 12 hours each using the Ultra-flo 145 dialyzer repeatedly. Endogenous creatinine clearance is a worse indicator than diuresis.[47]
3. Using the same dialysis technique, adequate dialysis is achieved in patients with lower diuresis by means of three dialyses weekly of 8–9 hours each.

---

47. Simple diuresis may be a better indicator due to the fact that in the residual urine there are many more toxic substances (e.g., sodium, phosphorus) than urea or creatinine, and they do not correlate well with creatinine clearance. I am amazed that many nephrologists still use creatinine or mean creatinine and urea clearance as a measure of renal function in patients on dialysis. Simple urine output is a better measure.

4. Four patients with uremic symptoms refractory to treatment required four dialyses weekly of 6–7 hours each.
5. The body weight after dialysis in the studied range of 47–75 kg does not permit the duration and frequency of dialyses to be predicted.
6. In clinically adequate hemodialysis the hematocrit after dialysis is above 20 percent (without blood transfusion), albumin before dialysis above 3.00 g/dL,[48] and nerve conduction velocity usually above the lower normal range.
7. Weight gain between dialyses of up to 3.5 kg does not rule out achieving adequate hemodialysis.
8. There is no correlation between the clinical condition of the patient and serum urea before dialysis in the range 86–172 mg/dL, and after dialysis in the range 18–64 mg/dL, and serum creatinine before dialysis in the range 6.7–14.3 mg/dL, and after dialysis in the range 2.3–6.8 mg/dL.
9. Frequent and short duration dialyses are much more effective in the treatment of uremic manifestations than longer but less frequent dialyses.
10. Increased frequency of dialyses has a very favorable effect on hematocrit value, albumin concentration, conduction velocity in motor nerves (Fig. 18), and dry body weight.
11. Prolongation of dialysis duration without changing frequency of dialysis improves the value of hematocrit and albumin concentration, although this improvement is less pronounced than after increasing frequency of dialyses.
12. Increase in the frequency as well as duration of dialyses causes a drop in arterial blood pressure, particularly in hypertensive patients.
13. Increased frequency and duration of dialyses in the ranges used does not have a significant influence on urea and creatinine concentrations before and after dialysis, as better removal is counter

---

48. Serum albumin concentration was calculated from determinations of total protein by the burette method [Richterich R. (1971) *Klinische Chemie. Theorie und Praxis*. S. Karger, Basel] and proteinograms were obtained by paper electrophoresis and read from a Zeiss densitometer [Scheiffarth F, Berg G, Götl H. (1962) *Papierelektrophorese in Klinik und Praxis*. Urban and Schwartzenberg, Munich]. This method gives much lower albumin concentrations than by a dye-binding technique using bromocresol green or purple as it is commonly done nowadays.

balanced by higher protein intake increasing urea generation and increased muscle mass increasing creatinine generation.

There were a lot of calculations for this study. Needless to say, I had neither computer nor calculator, only an abacus, slide ruler, and arithmometer. The latter we called *kręciołek*, meaning "spinner," as it used a crank to perform calculations; to multiply by 57, one had to spin the crank 57 times. To make sure that calculations were accurate, I compared different methods of calculation and then asked my mother-in-law, who was very skilled and fast at addition and subtraction, to confirm the figures. I wrote the manuscript in Polish and asked my secretary to type it out on an Olivetti typewriter using perforated ribbons. This was an advanced typewriter that allowed retyping if needed after checking spelling and grammar. I asked Barbara, my sister-in-law — who was a chemist and not familiar with medicine, hemodialysis in particular — to check whether she could understand what I had written and correct any spelling or grammatical errors. She let me know that she could indeed understand the manuscript.

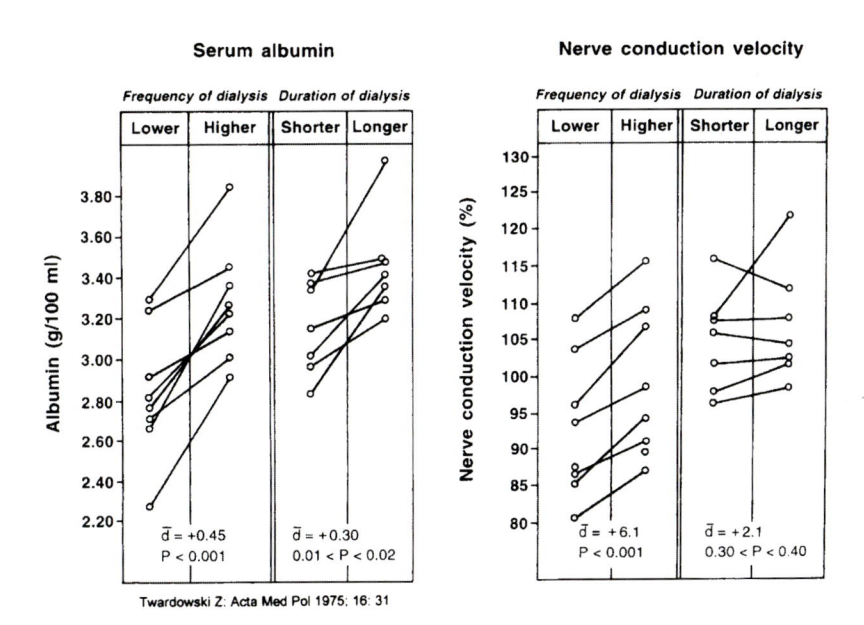

Figure 18. Effect of frequency and duration of dialysis on serum albumin and nerve conduction velocity. (Modified from Pu 352.)

After retyping all of the corrections, I presented the manuscript to Prof. dr. hab. Franciszek Kokot, to see if it would be good for a habilitation thesis.

In Poland, at the time, if you wanted to become a docent,[49] or later a professor, you needed to write and defend a habilitation thesis. The word comes from Latin *habile* (able) and means "to qualify oneself for a post or office." Prof. Kokot told me that it would be suitable and agreed to be my "patron" for the habilitation procedure. The first step was to publish an abstract of the thesis, which I sent to the Przegląd Lekarski, and the abstract was published in 1974 [Pu 18]. As I already had a PhD and had published 19 papers (as well as two reprinted in the *Polish Medical Journal*), I had a good deal more qualifications than the necessary minimum for eligibility. I also had teaching experience, as I had trained three assistants for the second degree specialization in internal medicine and two for the first degree specialization, and I lectured students, nurses and physicians, and had given many presentations at meetings. On the basis of my submitted C.V., the published abstract, and the manuscript, the Faculty Council of the Medical Academy in Katowice decided to open a habilitation procedure and appointed reviewers on June 20, 1974. I also submitted an English version of the work to *Acta Medica Polona* and it appeared in three parts [Pu 21, Pu 22, Pu 23]. The appointed reviewers of my thesis were Doc. dr. hab. Leszek Giec, Prof. dr. hab. Zygmunt Hanicki and Prof. dr. hab. Tadeusz Orłowski. Professor Orłowski excused himself, as he was scheduled for a trip abroad, and Prof. dr. hab. Andrzej Wojtczak was appointed as the third reviewer.

The reviews were extremely positive, so the committee formed by the council and composed of Prof. Kornel Gibiński, Doc. dr. hab. J. Sroczyński, and Doc. dr. hab. Adam Szkodny decided to admit me to the habilitation colloquium on February 26, 1975. All reviewers, especially Prof. Wojtczak, stressed my scientific achievements before the habilitation procedure, my three patents, my ongoing search for the least expensive dialysis methods (which had saved the Hospital for Miners over 4,000,000 zł), and my appointments to the Nephrology

---

49. In Poland, "docent" has been an established faculty position and title. The name comes from Latin *docens*, the present participle from *docere*, which means "to teach."

Committee of the Polish Academy of Science and the Transplantation Committee of the Ministry of Health. I successfully defended my thesis before the Faculty Council on May 22, 1975. The examiners were the reviewers, with the exception of Prof. Wojtczak, who was abroad at that time, and Prof. dr. hab. Józef Japa substituted for him. The questions they submitted were related mostly to chronic renal failure and its treatment, particularly anemia, hypertension, and acute renal failure related to pregnancy. I stressed the need for long and frequent dialysis. I was very much against indiscriminate use of blood transfusions. On the question of the difference between chronic dialysis and transplantation, I stressed that my results on chronic dialysis were better than transplantation at that time. The major problem with transplantation was the selection of donors and immunosuppression. The major problem with chronic dialysis was cost.[50]

Only with respect to one question would I answer differently today than I did then. On the question on the removal of middle molecules, my answer was that high surface and high permeability dialyzers would be very efficient in their removal even within a short time. I was impressed, at the time, with the "square-meter hour hypothesis" of Les Babb and others from Seattle.[51] Today, knowing about intercompartmental transport, I would stand by the value of long and frequent dialysis for the removal of middle molecules as well. Following the colloquium, the vote was 64 out of 64 in favor of granting the degree. The decision was sent to the Central Qualifying Committee at the Ministry of Health for final approval on June 16, 1975. Owing to the vacation period, the "super reviewer" appointed in September 1975 declined the assignment, and the Committee appointed another super-reviewer, whose opinion was positive. The Committee subsequently offered their positive opinion on March 29, 1976. Prof. Kokot recently told me that the first reviewer, who declined to undertake the task, was Prof. Tadeusz Orłowski, and

---

50. Since that time, transplantation has made tremendous progress, but chronic dialysis has not. I will return later to the notion that the approach to chronic dialysis has even regressed somewhat when compared to the method presented in my thesis.

51. Babb AL, Popovich RP, Christopher TG, Scribner BH. (1971) The genesis of the square meter-hour hypothesis. *Trans Am Soc Artif Intern Organs* **17**: 81–91.

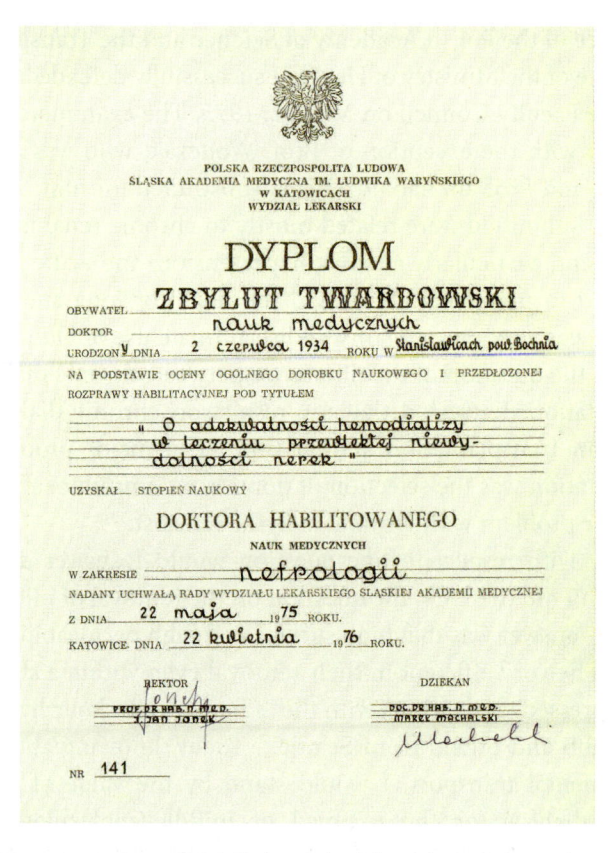

Figure 19. Doctor Habilitowany (Habilitated Doctor) certificate.

the other was Prof. dr. hab. Andrzej Manitius,[52] who gave a very positive opinion. Ultimately, the certificate was issued on April 22, 1976 (Fig. 19). On the basis of the thesis, I was also certified as a Specialist in Nephrology by the Center for Postgraduate Medical Education in Warsaw.

In the meantime, in April 1974, I was invited by Italian firm Bellco to visit their company in Mirandola as well as their dialysis centers in Bologna, Parma and Milan in northern Italy. I had a very fruitful conversation with Prof. Vittorio Bonomini in Bologna, who

---

52. Prof. dr. hab. Andrzej Manitius (1927–2001) was Chairman of the Department of Nephrology of the Medical Academy in Gdańsk, and the Country Consultant in Nephrology from 1984–1992.

just two years earlier had published his results on five-times weekly dialysis (work that I cited in my thesis.[53]) One of the early proponents of frequent dialysis,[54] he already had experience with the Cordis Dow Artificial Kidney capillary dialyzer (CDAK 4), which he considered superior to other types of dialyzers. I had a long discussion with Prof. Vicenzo Cambi in Parma, who was an advocate of clinical assessment of dialysis adequacy and introduced intensive utilization of dialysis unit by short (3-hour) but every-other-day dialysis. (I also cited his work in my thesis.[55]) I remember he had hung a funny sign on his office door: *CAUTION: GENIUS AT WORK*. In Mirandola I met with Mr. Bellini, President of the Bellco Company, and his advisers. I suggested making 2 L plastic bags for peritoneal dialysis fluid and a special connector with a bacteriological filter for inflow and bypassing for outflow. I put forward the idea of doing a few (6) hourly exchanges every day, supposing that this technique would be associated with markedly lower peritonitis rates than with 500-mL bottles. Bellco was not so taken with this idea at the time, as their interest lay not in peritoneal dialysis but in single-needle hemodialysis and manufacturing coil dialyzers. I learned a few years later that a bacteriological filter for fluid inflow, very similar to my idea, was attempted with very poor results due to high peritonitis rates. Bellco provided me with a little money to cover expenses, which I used to buy a *judogi* (traditional judo uniform) for our elder son Radek, who had just started judo training.

In 1973, Dr. William Newnam, Director of the Psychiatry Hospital in Leicester, England, invited my wife, Halina, to work as a house officer there for a year. During World War II, Dr. Newnam had served as a pilot with Polish fighters during the Battle of Britain[56] and befriended many of them. Such was the warmth he felt towards the

---

53. Bonomini V, Mioli V, Albertazzi A, Scolari P. (1972) Daily-dialysis programme: Indications and results. *Proc Eur Dial Transplant Assoc* **9**: 44–52.

54. Recognising his early support for frequent dialysis, I presented him with a Special Award for Lifetime Achievement at the 4th International Symposium on Home Hemodialysis, a part of the Annual Dialysis Conference, in Nashville, Tenn., on February 23, 1998. I also wrote a *Laudatio* [Pu 272].

55. Cambi V, Arisi L, Buzio C, *et al.* (1973) Intensive utilisation of a dialysis unit. *Proc Eur Dial Transplant Assoc* **10**: 342–348.

56. The story of the Polish fighters in the Battle of Britain is brilliantly presented in the book *A Question of Honor. The Kosciuszko Squadron: Forgotten Heroes of World War II* by Lynne Olson and Stanley Cloud, published by Alfred A. Knopf, New York, 2003.

Poles that he typically invited one Polish psychiatrist to work in his department for a year. After his own stint in Leicester, Dr. Robert Hese, Halina's colleague, was asked whom he would recommend for the following year, and Dr. Hese recommended Halina. The Ministry of Health wanted to send somebody else, so they initially did not give permission for Halina to go. That upset Dr. Newnam greatly and he contacted the Ministry of Health to warn them that if Halina did not get their permission, nobody from Poland would be invited to work in his department again. Halina eventually got the permission she needed and went to Leicester in September 1974 — though the rest of the family had to remain in Poland to ensure that she would indeed return.

Our boys were old enough and doing well at school, so I had no problems with them. Our younger son, Przemek, had a passion for swimming and became rather good at breaststroke. On March 1 and 2, 1975, he competed among boys younger than 12 years of age in the Polish Winter Championships in Zielona Góra, winning silver medals in 200 meters and 100 meters breaststroke. In June that same year, in the Summer Championships in Bydgoszcz, he won bronze in the 100 meters breaststroke. He definitely had a talent for swimming, but he had a dilemma. By his assessment, there were two arguments against continuing swimming. Firstly, to compete in later years he would need to at least double or triple the time he devoted to training, and this would decrease the time available for study, which he was not inclined to do. Secondly, he had started to get some shoulder pain and he was afraid that the extra training would lead nowhere. Both of us agreed that it would not be a good idea to pursue competitive swimming any further.

Meanwhile, there were several developments that would completely change the direction of my career. My roommate, Przemek's godfather and later coauthor of my first paper, Jacek Hawiger,[57] immigrated to the U.S. and got a position in the Microbiology Department of Vanderbilt University in Nashville, Tenn. At the same time my colleague Przemek (Przemysław Hirszel, MD) was looking for a fellowship in the U.S., and Jacek recommended him to Dr. Charles Mengel, Chairman of the Department of Medicine at the University of Missouri in Columbia,

---

[57]. Prof. Jacek Hawiger is famous for his work related to staphylococcal infections, immunology and intracellular signaling. He discovered the staphylococcal clumping factor.

Mo. Dr. Mengel in turn recommended Przemek to John F. Maher,[58] Director of the Division of Nephrology at the University of Missouri from 1969. Przemek was accepted and worked there from August 1971 to August 1972. Dr. Maher moved from Missouri to the University of Connecticut at Hartford, Conn., and Dr. Karl D. Nolph[59] became Director of the Division in 1974. Przemek was greatly appreciated for his contributions to the division, so when he was about to leave Columbia, Dr. Nolph asked him to suggest a candidate for the fellowship who was "as good as he was." He recommended me. When he returned to Kraków, he called to inform me that Dr. Nolph was going to send me an invitation for a fellowship at the Division of Nephrology. I immediately applied for an Educational Commission for Foreign Medical Graduates (ECFMG) examination. The cost was not very high, only US$20, with an additional US$100 or so due after arriving in the U.S. I passed the examination in 1975 and applied to the Ministry of Health for permission to go. I remember being in Bydgoszcz to cheer on Przemek, who was competing in a swimming championship, and driving directly to Warsaw for the ECFMG exam in the morning. I recall being extremely tired afterwards, but fortunately I was able to get back to Bytom without incident. My wife was to return from Leicester in August 1975.

One of my habilitation thesis reviewers was Prof. Andrzej Wojtczak, Director of the Personnel Department in the Ministry of Health. His opinion was extremely important when it came to getting permission for temporary work abroad. He was also a patron of the Department of Nephrology of the Medical Academy in Lublin. The problem was that the department did not have an "independent research worker" or a person with the title of "doktor habilitowany medycyny" (habilitated doctor of medicine), and there was no hope of having one in the near future.

---

58. John F. Maher, MD, FACP, FRCP(I) 1929–1992, was Director of the Division of Nephrology, Department of Medicine, University of Missouri, Columbia, Mo. (1969–1973); Director of the Division of Nephrology, University of Connecticut (1974–1979); and Director of Nephrology Division in the Uniformed Services University of the Health Sciences (1979–1992). He also served as President of the American Society of Artificial Internal Organs (1975–1976) and of the International Society for Peritoneal Dialysis (1983–1987).

59. Karl Nolph, MD, FACP, FRCP (Glasgow) was born on February 6, 1937, and completed his nephrology fellowship at the University of Pennsylvania before working with Dr. Paul Teschan at Walter Reed Army Medical Center using his experience with acute peritoneal dialysis. Dr. Nolph and his wife, Georgia, also a physician, came to the University of Missouri in 1969. He became Director of the Division of Nephrology in 1974.

Up to 1975, Dr. med. Lidia Perlińska-Sznajder was Interim Chairwoman of the Department, but her habilitation thesis on pyelonephritis was rejected by reviewers, largely because her conclusions were against popular belief at the time. For instance, her analysis indicated that pyelonephritis was markedly less prevalent than reported, because other diseases were mislabeled. When I read her thesis a few years later, I thought that she was right in many respects. In any event, she left the department and Dr. med. Anna Gutka became Interim Chairwoman, but she did not want to write a habilitation thesis. Prof. Wojtczak had other plans and did not want to move to Lublin. The agreement between Prof. Wojtczak and me was that I would get a permission to go to Columbia, Mo., for a year, but after my return I would move to Lublin to become Chairman of the Department of Nephrology.

In 1975, I published a paper entitled "Criteria for the choice of optimal hemodialysis equipment for patients with chronic renal failure" [Pu 24]. In this work I presented my vision of the perfect equipment for hemodialysis, based mostly on my personal experience. I stated that the most important features of effective hemodialysis equipment were low cost, reliability, noncomplicated design of the kidney machine, small static, dynamic and potential capacity of the dialyzer, almost complete recovery of blood, good efficiency for small and larger molecules, and good ultrafiltration. I was very impressed with the Travenol RSP tank system, which was easy to repair even for a physician, and Ultra-flo 145 dialyzers, which were easy to reuse and with excellent recovery of blood. I was obviously in favor of capillary dialyzers, which I considered to be perfect, if their cost would decline and reuse would become possible.

As mentioned previously, my efforts to create a transplant center in Bytom in 1970 turned out to be futile, as there was no money for such an endeavor and the hospital was not really interested. As we essentially did not have any mortality, our hemodialysis center was unable to admit any new patients. Our peritoneal dialysis program was growing, but we could not admit more patients for dialysis in the hospital, so we tried to send some patients for home peritoneal dialysis. We also tried to send patients to centers providing transplant services. The most advanced transplant service was in Warsaw, but they did not have the capacity to admit patients from us at the time. I remember that they started to take patients from other places in 1976. We started to cooperate with Prof. dr. hab. Zygmunt Hanicki, Chairman of the Nephrology Department of the Institute of Internal Medicine, Medical Academy in Kraków and Prof. dr. hab. Mieczysław Politowski, Chairman of the Third Department of Surgery of the Medical Academy in Kraków.

The first of our patients to have a renal transplant in Kraków was a 23-year-old white male with slowly developing chronic renal failure without hypertension who was admitted to our department in Bytom for diagnosis and treatment in February 1973. Arteriography of the abdomen did not indicate kidneys, and it was assumed that the patient had an ectopic kidney located in the pelvis. For two reasons, we decided not to do another arteriogram (ultrasound was not available then) in order to locate the kidney and attempt a kidney biopsy. Firstly, any diagnosis of slowly developing chronic renal failure would not be amenable to anything other than supportive therapy like treatment of acidosis and electrolyte disturbances. Secondly, another arteriography could precipitate deterioration of renal function, very important for conservative therapy and in patients on dialysis. Because of deteriorating acidosis and subjective symptoms of uremia, the patient started peritoneal dialysis in February 1974. The patient initially came to the hospital for twice-weekly 24-hour peritoneal dialysis sessions, then three times weekly treatments lasting 16 hours each, and later performed peritoneal dialysis at home. He maintained a good urine output of slightly below 1000 mL/24 hours. In retrospect I suspected some kind of interstitial renal disease in his ectopic kidney. A cadaveric kidney transplant was performed in the Surgery Department on March 15, 1975. The patient had two acute rejection episodes treated with high doses of corticosteroids and local irradiation. The patient was discharged from Kraków and returned for follow-up in Bytom on maintenance doses of Imuran (azathioprine) and Encorton (prednisone). It was the first renal transplant in Kraków [Pu 25].

My last study in Bytom was geared toward saving blood in patients on peritoneal dialysis. In nine patients on chronic peritoneal dialysis, 50 determinations were carried out comparing the concentrations of urea, creatinine, uric acid, sodium, potassium and chloride in plasma, and the fluid accumulating in the peritoneal cavity between dialyses at least 30 hours after previous dialysis. It was found that under these conditions a complete equilibration of the concentrations of all these substances in plasma occurred according to the Gibbs–Donnan effect. We postulated that determination of all these biochemical indices in the peritoneal fluid instead of plasma would save about 500 mL of blood per year, which would ameliorate anemia to some degree in these patients [Pu 26].

In May 1975, I was invited to present our experience with chronic hemodialysis at the 15th Congress of the Polish Society of Urology in Wisła-Jawornik, Silesian District. My presentation, "Treatment of chronic renal failure with hemodialysis," was delivered on May 28 and published in the proceeding of the congress [Pu 28]. I presented all my experiences with chronic hemodialysis. I insisted on using reusable dialyzers, permitting almost complete recovery of blood after dialysis. In my experience, the symptoms and signs of uremia, not amenable to conservative treatment, occurred with diuresis below 1000 mL/24 hours. My experience also indicated that those patients taken for dialysis while having some uremic symptoms appreciated therapy and were more likely to follow dietary and other instructions. I insisted on long and frequent hemodialysis sessions using Ultra-flo 145 dialyzers:

1. twice-weekly for 10–12 hours in patients with diuresis over 500 mL/24 hours;
2. three times weekly for 8–9 hours in patients with diuresis below 500 mL/24 hours;
3. four times weekly for 6–8 hours in patients with resistant uremic symptoms;
4. five to six times weekly for 3–4 hours in the post-surgical period or in patients with additional diseases like acute infections.

My experience indicated that such a schedule enabled the eradication of all symptoms and signs of uremia, the achievement of real dry body weight to control blood pressure in at least 80 percent of patients without antihypertensive drugs, and the avoidance of blood transfusion, except in cases of acute blood loss. This schedule permitted one to achieve normal predialysis phosphorus with the addition of aluminum hydroxide of 0–12 g/day, and calcium carbonate 0–6 g/day. I mentioned that daily dialysis would be most physiological, but because of organizational and financial restrictions, such as wide use of such a schedule was not possible at the time. We used only arteriovenous fistulas as blood accesses with constant sites of needle insertions and achieved over 86 percent fistula survival at six years (Fig. 17) [Pu 27, Pu 41]. Our selection criteria were very strict, as we accepted only patients with isolated renal diseases in an age range between 20 and 50. These admission criteria and our hemodialysis technique provided a very good survival rate of 77 percent at seven years, better than European data for home hemodialysis (64 percent), living related donor transplant (52 percent), hospital hemodialysis (49 percent), and cadaveric transplant (27 percent) [Pu 28].

I remember that during the presentation the fan in the projector broke and my slides got burned after having shown only about half of them. Fortunately, the most illustrative ones had been shown at the beginning, but I had to speak without slides for the remainder of the session. In spite of this mishap, my presentation was well received. In a report on the conference published in *Urologia Polska* in 1978, Prof. Kazimierz Adamkiewicz stated: "*Bardzo interesujący I wartościowy referat wygłosił Z. Twardowski ze szpitala Górniczego w Bytomiu 'Leczenie powtarzanymi hemodializami przewlekej niewydolności nerek'. Ośrodek nefrologiczny w Bytomiu ... stosuje hemodializy w przewlekej niewydolnoci nerek i należy do tych ośrodków w Polsce, które mają najdłuższe obserwacje i największe doświadczenie w tym zakresie* (A very interesting and valuable lecture was presented by Doc. Z. Twardowski from the Hospital for Miners in Bytom: 'Treatment of chronic renal failure with hemodialysis.' The nephrology center in Bytom ... applies hemodialysis for chronic renal failure and belongs to centers with the longest observations and the highest experience in this area)."[60]

---

60. Adamkiewicz K. (1978) http://www.urologiapolska.pl/artykul.php?247. Sprawozdanie z XV Zjazdu Naukowego Polskiego Towarzystwa Urologicznego (Report from the XVth Scientific Congress of the Polish Society of Urology). *Urologia Polska* 31(3).

CHAPTER 4

Fellowship in America

On September 1, 1976, I headed to Columbia, Mo., through New York and St. Louis. It was my first flight to another continent and I was a little apprehensive. I spoke and understood English, but with a mostly British accent, and I had difficulties understanding American speakers, especially over the phone. I stayed one night in St. Louis and took a Greyhound bus to Columbia in the morning. Dr. Nolph's secretary, Ms. Midge Kellerhaus, gave me a ride to Dr. Nolph's office. After introducing me to other faculty members and fellows, Dr. Nolph showed me the Nephrology Laboratory in the Veterans Administration Hospital and the Chronic Dialysis Unit in a barrack addition to the Hospital called TD4. At the time the faculty members were John C. Van Stone, MD; Michael Sorkin, MD; John F. Bauer, MD; and Steve Brooks, MD. The fellows were Ahad J. Ghods, MD, from Iran, and Wallace C. Gauntner, MD. Carole A. Hopkins worked in the laboratory. In the afternoon Dr. Nolph's secretary tried to help me find locum accommodation. I had decided not to have a car — indeed, I did not have the money to rent or buy one — so I wanted a place to stay close to the hospital and as inexpensive as possible. There was nothing immediately available. I was told about another Polish fellow in the Gastroenterology Division who worked in the GI Laboratory in Virginia: Andrzej S. Tarnawski, MD,[1] who was from the Gastroenterology Department of the Medical Academy in Kraków. I contacted him and he invited me to stay with him until I could find a place. Unfortunately, his apartment had no air-conditioning, and with my poor tolerance for the extremely hot weather, especially the uncomfortably warm nights, I soon had to redouble my efforts to find more suitable accommodation. I settled upon the Tiger Motor Hotel on 8th Street. The room came with rather too many cockroaches, but it had air-conditioning, it was inexpensive, and it was within walking distance of the hospital.

I thought that I knew English before coming to Columbia, but I quickly realized that my accent was difficult to understand and I had my own difficulties understanding people. I resolved to improve my English, making an effort to study the American Heritage Dictionary,

---

1. Prof. Andrzej S. Tarnawski later moved to California, where he became Division Chief and Fellowship Program Director, University of California, Irvine, and Chief, Gastroenterology Section, VA Medical Center in Long Beach, University of California.

watch TV and listen to the radio, and converse with as many people as possible. For a period of time, I stopped speaking Polish. My approach left me feeling uncomfortable initially, but it eventually began to produce results. Progress was gradual, with small improvements every month, and after six months I felt much more at ease. I still did not fully grasp what some patients were saying — "hillbillies" in particular[2] — but there was always a nurse or somebody else to repeat what a patient said in an accent I could understand. One negative aspect of this method of learning (i.e., not translating into Polish) was that I had, and still have, difficulty translating from Polish to English and *vice versa*. I really admire interpreters, who can translate almost instantaneously; I have to think for several seconds before I can translate something. I'm not sure what the mechanism is for me; sometimes I wonder whether my Polish and English language processing takes place in different parts of my cortex and it takes some time to connect them.

Dr. Nolph had me on clinical duty. I served as a fellow in the Internal Medicine ward and as a resident in Nephrology Service. Patients on chronic dialysis were under my direct care with the supervision of a faculty member. Coming to the U.S. from Poland, I was quite unfamiliar with the system and had to learn a lot. For one thing, in the U.S. nurses could not administer any medication or undertake any kind of procedure, even something like an enema, without a physician's order. In Poland minor complaints were routinely taken care of by nurses without a physician's order. Interns and residents in the U.S. were familiar with this (since they were educated in the U.S.), so they would deliver conditional orders like "In case of constipation, give an enema" or "Tylenol 600 mg if temperature is over 37.5°C; call me if temperature is over 38°C." This was not something that I did initially, so I would be paged in the middle of the night with questions. It took me some time before I learned how to avoid being awakened to take care of such minor complaints.

---

2. "Hillbilly" is an American term for a person from the backwoods or a remote mountain area, like of the Ozarks in southern Missouri. Some consider the term derogatory, but for me it is not. I spent my childhood in rural Poland and I admire the people who live there — and I can still speak their dialect. Nevertheless, hillbilly English was a real challenge.

I was extremely busy with my clinical duties and on call around the clock. I did all the renal biopsies in the hospital, as well as peritoneal catheter insertions for acute dialysis and intravenous catheter insertions for acute hemodialysis. Dr. John Bauer taught me one very valuable trick with regard to peritoneal dialysis catheter insertion. Usually, before the insertion of the stylet catheter, I filled the abdominal cavity with dialysis solution through a trocar to avoid the possibility of wounding the intestines. Dr. Bauer advised me to use, instead of the trocar, a ventricular needle,[3] which was much blunter and better suited to this purpose. Having done all the procedures in Bytom, I wanted to create fistulas, insert Tenckhoff catheters and do all the procedures for chronic dialysis access. However, we did not have a procedure room and the surgery department was rather reluctant to rent us one, as they preferred doing chronic dialysis insertions themselves. Besides, the nephrology faculty and fellows were not interested in undertaking these procedures, and in any event, doing all the procedures by myself would have definitely been too much, as I was already extremely busy. In the end I gave up trying to create interventional nephrology in Columbia.

The chronic hemodialysis program was located in the TD4 freestanding building. The dialysis technique was markedly different than that in Bytom. The patients were dialyzed three times weekly for between 2.5 and 4 hours and not kept on scales during dialysis. I was a little surprised by this, but Dr. John C. Van Stone, Director of the Chronic Hemodialysis Program, explained that short dialysis was becoming popular in the U.S. and there were ongoing studies which seemed to support that. He told me that scales were very expensive and they could not afford them. They also did not reuse dialyzers, and I tried to explain that the savings from reuse would be more than enough to pay for scales. However, there was no change in policy during my stay between 1976 and 1977.

The Christmas period brought the only respite from work, and I decided to visit Jacek Hawiger, who lived in Nashville, Tenn. He took me to Huntsville, Alabama, to show me the U.S. Space & Rocket

---

3. A ventricular needle is used in neurosurgery for drainage of fluid from the cerebral ventricle. It is relatively blunt and it is provided with a side entrance hole.

Center and I was really impressed with Huntsville's role in the space race, the creation of a Moon rocket, and the Apollo missions. My Greyhound bus had some difficulty because of a blizzard, but I eventually made it back to Columbia.

I continued my clinical duties until the middle of February 1977, but by then I was so exhausted that I had to inform Dr. Nolph that it would be extremely difficult for me to continue such a busy schedule. He asked me why I did not come to him earlier, and I told him that I had presumed that every fellow had such a heavy workload and did not want to appear incapable. He informed me that I was the first with such extensive clinical duties and he decided to move me into research. For a long time he never tried such a schedule on other fellows.

While in the Research Service, I recalled some unusual cases, which I had observed in Bytom in 1969 and 1975, of psoriasis clearing during peritoneal dialysis for chronic renal failure and never reappearing after patients continued on hemodialysis. The first case, in 1969, was a 40-year-old white female with a 20-year history of psoriasis. After two weeks of peritoneal dialysis her psoriasis disappeared, and she asked me whether dialysis could have been responsible. I told her that I had not heard of anything that could support this, but I kept her intriguing case in my mind. In 1975 a 35-year-old white male was admitted into the chronic peritoneal dialysis program. His psoriasis, present for a decade, almost cleared after two months of peritoneal dialysis and never reappeared during 12 months of peritoneal dialysis and subsequent hemodialysis. I found a case report from the *Ulster Medical Journal*[4] of psoriasis clearance after only three hemodialysis sessions in a patient with chronic renal failure. I thought that it would be justified to perform peritoneal dialysis in cases of psoriasis without renal failure. Dr. Nolph agreed that this would be justified, but he asked me whether I had been reading *Ulster Medical Journal* regularly to be able to find this particular article. Obviously I had not, but I had been looking in the Index Medicus for dialysis and psoriasis and had found this one article. He advised me to send a letter to the *Annals of Internal Medicine*, which I did [Le 1], and then

---

4. McEvoy J, Kelly AMT. (1976) Psoriatic clearance during hemodialysis. *Ulster Med J* **45**: 76–78.

talk to Dr. Philip C. Anderson,[5] the Director of the Division of Dermatology, University of Missouri. He agreed to cooperate with me on the project. It was only after many years that I learned there was another early paper on hemodialysis and psoriasis, published in 1970 in the Russian literature.[6]

Dr. Anderson selected three patients with severe, refractory, long-standing psoriasis, but with normal renal functions, to undergo weekly peritoneal dialysis treatments of 32 to 48 hours. Two patients began to improve after the first dialysis with nearly complete resolution after four and nine treatments. The third patient, with erythrodermic psoriasis, showed no objective changes after four dialyses. The report added to the anecdotal reports of psoriasis improving with dialysis, and they were cases without renal failure [Pu 30]. Dr. Anderson, a dermatologist with tremendous experience in the treatment of psoriasis, was very impressed with the results obtained by dialysis and later published a few short reports on this topic.[7]

At that time Dr. Nolph was cooperating with Robert P. Popovich, PhD, and Jack W. Moncrief, MD, from Austin, Texas, on a new method of peritoneal dialysis. Their preliminary findings were submitted as an abstract to the American Society of Artificial Internal Organs,[8] but as sometimes happens, their idea was so new that it was not deemed suitable for presentation during the meeting. The concept was indeed highly innovative. Instead of doing frequent exchanges for 24 or 48 hours once or twice weekly, they postulated the continuous presence of the fluid in the peritoneal cavity with infrequent exchanges (24 hours a day, 7 days a week). Dr. Nolph immediately recognized the potential of this method and decided to get involved with the project. I had ideas along similar lines and discussed them with the Bellco Company in 1974. At the time I was not considering the continuous presence of

---

5. Philip C. Anderson, MD (1930–2000), Director, Division of Dermatology, University of Missouri.

6. Shimkus EM, Malygina TA, Kalenkovich NI. (1970) Treatment of a psoriasis patient with hemodialysis (in Russian). *Vestn Dermatol Venerol* **44**(2): 69.

7. Anderson PC. (1978) Dialysis for psoriasis. *Artif Organs* **2**(2): 202; Anderson PC. (1978) Treatment of psoriasis with dialysis. *Arch Dermatol* **114**(6): 966.

8. Popovich RP, Moncrief JW, Decherd JB, et al. (1976). The definition of a novel portable/wearable equilibrium peritoneal dialysis technique. *Am Soc Artif Intern Organs Abstracts* **5**: 64.

fluid, as I was afraid there would be ultrafiltration issues related to the excessively lengthy presence of fluid in the peritoneal cavity.

When Moncrief and Popovich demonstrated that there were no problems with ultrafiltration, I became very enthusiastic. In 1977 a continuous dialysis program with four exchanges per day was started in three Missouri patients. In each patient, Tenckhoff peritoneal dialysis catheters had been inserted by W. Kirt Nichols, MD, a vascular surgeon who cooperated with the Division of Nephrology and was doing almost all the procedures for patients on dialysis. The first patient selected for the technique was a 35-year-old white male with a history of recent myocardial infarction and cardiac arrest who had one prior 48-hour intermittent peritoneal dialysis. The second was a 50-year-old white female who, after four years of hemodialysis and a failed kidney transplant, was on intermittent peritoneal dialysis following a loss of blood access. The third was a 76-year-old black male who was on intermittent peritoneal dialysis for two months after blood access failure. The experience with these three cases, as well as six from Austin, Texas, which started the program in 1976, was reported in 1978 [Pu 31]. The regimen was renamed continuous ambulatory peritoneal dialysis (CAPD), and it immediately caught the attention of numerous centers. I did an equilibration study during an 8-hour exchange overnight in the Clinical Research Center on a 37-year-old patient (Fig. 20). Urea was equilibrated after 6 hours, and dialysate-to-plasma concentration ratios at 8 hours were 0.7 for creatinine, 0.3 for inulin, and 0.02 for protein. The laboratory tests were run by Paul Brown and Harold F. Moore, MS, a recent addition to the laboratory. I was impressed with the data points nicely located on the equilibration curves with minimal deviations, indicating excellent laboratory technique and proper timing of sample taking. Protein losses were rather small and in line with my previous studies in Bytom, where we showed in intermittent peritoneal dialysis that protein transfer from the serum to the dialysate is almost constant and that most protein in the initial exchange is a washout from the period off dialysis [Pu 12, Pu 12a, Pu 14, Pu 14a].

According to the Division of Nephrology's rules, every fellow was eligible to receive free travel expenses to attend one meeting per year. I chose the American Society for Artificial Internal Organs (ASAIO) Meeting in Montreal, Quebec, Canada, in April 1977. Bob Popovich

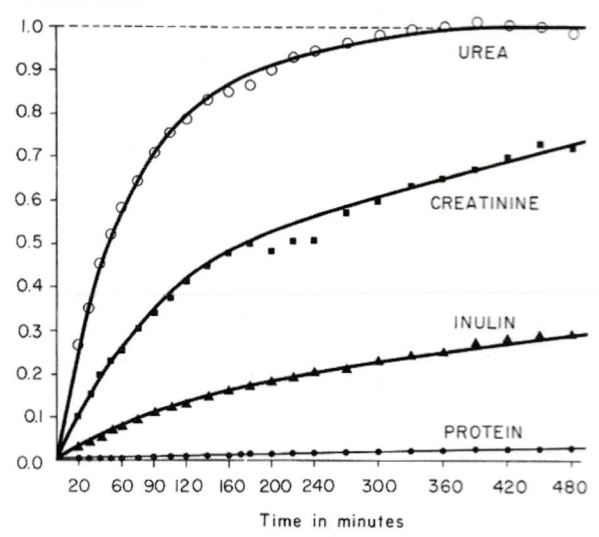

Figure 20. Equilibration curves during an 8-hour dwell in a single exchange. (Reprinted from Pu 31.)

was very concerned about protein losses in CAPD, and during the Montreal meeting, I had a long discussion with him about this problem, presented my previous studies and tried to console him that protein losses in CAPD should not be higher than in intermittent peritoneal dialysis (IPD). It turned out later that protein losses were not the major problem in CAPD.

In the Research Service, I spent most of my time in the VA Laboratory doing *in vitro* studies on dialyzers, in the Clinical Research Center of the University of Missouri Medical Center conducting studies in peritoneal dialysis patients, and reviewing the literature related to peritoneal dialysis. I was one of the coauthors of a very comprehensive review on the determinants of low clearances in peritoneal dialysis [Pu 29], a part of which was a presentation of transport of CO_2 and bicarbonate into the peritoneal cavity. Transport of CO_2 was much faster than that of urea. The conclusion of the review was that the limitation of the urea mass transfer coefficient (MTC),[9] which

---

9. The mass transfer coefficient is the maximum clearance that may be achieved in a dialysis system. It can never be higher than blood flow or dialysate flow or membrane resistance to a particular solute.

corresponds to maximal achievable clearance (about 30 mL/min), was related to total membrane resistance rather than to effective capillary blood flow, which is probably in excess of 60 mL/min. I was amazed at the speed of CO_2 transport but also with the slow transport of bicarbonate and the pH rise to 7.0 (more than 30 min) after infusion of regular dialysis solution, the pH of which was about 5.0.

A comparison of two hollow-fiber dialyzers with either regenerated cellulose or thinner walled cuprophan fibers was performed *in vitro* and in clinical studies. The results showed that per square meter of surface area, the cuprophan dialyzer has higher rates of ultrafiltration (UF) per transmembrane pressure (TMP) and greater clearances, particularly of larger solutes; also, with cuprophan the sieving coefficient[10] for vitamin B_{12} was higher. Thus all the findings suggested greater permeability of cuprophan fibers. In both dialyzers, total clearances increased with UF by amounts compatible with predicted increases in convective transport; diffusive transport remained stable as TMP was increased [Pu 34].

A very comprehensive and time-consuming project was to determine whether the sodium salt of a large-molecular-weight anionic polymer could generate a large amount of ultrafiltration in a dialysis system without crossing the membrane and to establish the mechanism of less efficient convective transport with glucose as compared to hydrostatic pressure-induced ultrafiltration. Previous studies showed that glucose-induced ultrafiltration was associated with lower sieving coefficient compared to that achieved with hydrostatic ultrafiltration. For this study, ultrafiltration was induced by (i) poly (sodium acrylate), (ii) glucose, and (iii) hydrostatic pressure. A high concentration of poly(sodium acrylate) was obtained by dialysis of the solution against deionized water in a hollow-fiber dialyzer with high hydrostatic pressure on the polymer side. Vitamin B_{12} was added to the solution subjected to ultrafiltration. It was found that the mean sieving coefficients with polymer-induced ultrafiltration and hydrostatic ultrafiltration were almost identical (0.72 vs. 0.69), whereas the

---

10. Sieving coefficient S is a measure of the equilibration between two solutions separated by a membrane and subjected to ultrafiltration. If C_d is the concentration of a solute on the side of a membrane subjected to hydrostatic ultrafiltration and C_r is the concentration of the same solute on the other side of the membrane, then $S = C_r/C_d$. A sieving coefficient of 1.0 indicates that the membrane does not restrict the passage of the solute; a coefficient of 0.0 indicates no transfer of the solute.

mean sieving coefficient with glucose-induced ultrafiltration was 0.37. Our interpretation of the data was that the lower sieving coefficient with glucose was dependent on the movement of glucose molecules in the opposite direction to the studied solute (vitamin B$_{12}$). This phenomenon is not observed with polymer, which cannot cross the membrane and holds sodium on the same side (Fig. 21). We speculated that it would be worthwhile to evaluate polymers as osmotic agents for peritoneal dialysis, as glucose was not without clinical problems. The study was presented in part at the Meeting of the American Society of Nephrology, Washington, DC., November 1977 [Pr 16] and at the 24th Meeting of the American Society for Artificial Internal Organs [Pr 20]; the complete study was published later [Pu 32, Pu 33].

I participated in two more studies related to the influence of various modifications of dialysis solution composition on microvasculature and clearances in rats and in patients. The most striking observation was that peritoneal dialysis solution caused a transient constriction of small arteries on the mesothelial surface followed by prolonged dilation. An addition of nitroprusside to the dialysis solution decreased the time to maximal dilation. Since nitroprusside

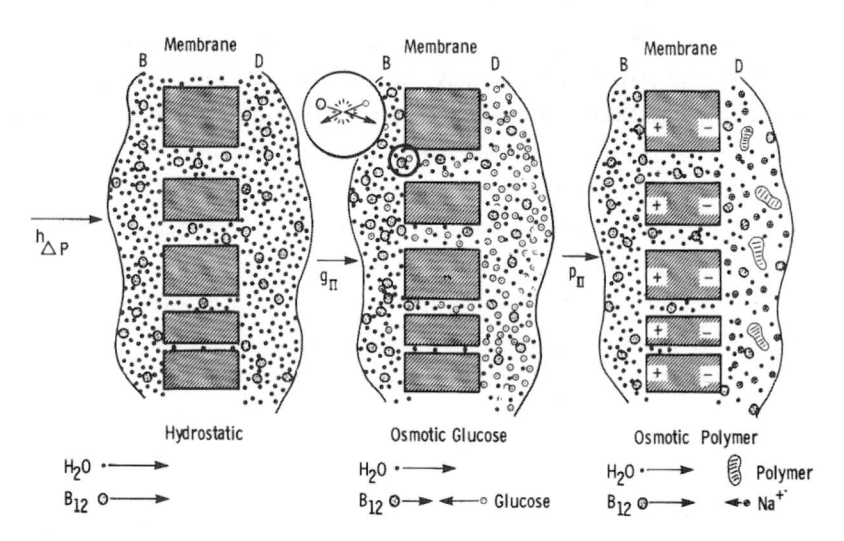

Figure 21. Simplified diagram of sieving with ultrafiltration in a membrane with heterogeneous pores. (Reprinted from Pu 32.)

increased clearances of larger molecules proportionally more than of the smaller molecules, we speculated that nitroprusside increases solute clearances by both the vasodilatory effect and by an effect on vascular membrane permeability and area of solute exchange [Pu 39]. Another study during 400 exchanges in 10 patients showed increases in clearances and protein losses were seen with 1 mg of nitroprusside per liter of dialysis solution; the maximum effect was seen at 4.5 mg/L. There were no increases in serum thiocyanate, a major metabolite of nitroprusside. One disturbing observation regarding the possibility of clinical use of nitroprusside was that protein losses were disproportionately higher than increases in clearances of small molecular weight solutes [Pu 40].

My last study in Columbia was on equilibration of peritoneal dialysis solutions during long-dwell exchanges. I started performing equilibration studies in the Clinical Research Center of the University of Missouri Medical Center in March 1977. From March to May I performed equilibrations in five 8-hour exchanges with 1.5% glucose solution and four 4-hour exchanges with 4.25% glucose solution in three patients. Barbara ("Barb") Friscoe Prowant, RN,[11] helped me with the collections of dialysate and blood samples, while Paul Brown and Harold F. Moore analyzed the samples. Following my departure, Jack Rubin (a new fellow who came to Columbia from Toronto in July 1977) and Barb, in April 1978, performed four more equilibration curves in two patients. This study showed that transport from plasma to the dialysis solution was dependent on molecular weight of solutes: the fastest for urea, then creatinine and uric acid, and markedly slower for phosphorus and inulin. For small solutes, dialysate-to-plasma (D/P) ratios fell most dramatically with dwell times beyond 3 hours. The study confirmed our previous observation in one patient that for very large solutes like inulin and protein the equilibration curves took on an almost linear appearance [Pu 31]. Sodium and chloride sieving was seen after many hours and was more pronounced with 4.25% glucose solution [Pu 35].

---

11. Barbara Friscoe Prowant (1953–2009), or "Barb" to her many friends, started to work in the Division of Nephrology in 1977. She contributed immensely to the field of nephrology, especially to dialysis, and became one of the most well known and most highly respected nephrology nurses in the world.

Up to this point, I have been concentrating primarily on my professional work, but I was also involved in a number of other activities in Columbia. I volunteered for a study by John Bauer, MD, a principal investigator, and Steve Brooks, MD, who wanted to see the response of renin and aldosterone in human subjects on a daily diet with zero sodium and 300 mEq of potassium — the so-called 7000-J diet. Apart from the changes in sodium and potassium, this was a normal adult diet with enough calories and protein. Every morning blood samples were taken for electrolytes and other measurements. On the first day I noted a very small diuresis while I was working and mostly in the upright position. A huge diuresis was noted during the night when in a supine position. After one day on the diet, electrolytes were normal; after the next day my potassium in the morning was high-normal. I lost about 4 kg. On the third day of the diet, in the evening I felt some tingling around the mouth and some muscle numbness, so I suspected elevated potassium. Barb was in the Clinical Research Center and she took my blood for electrolytes. The potassium was 7.2, but all other electrolytes were within the normal range; there was no acidosis and no hypocalcemia. Barb became very concerned and notified Dr. Bauer and Dr. Nolph. An EKG was ordered and showed minimal changes consistent with slight hyperkalemia: low P, slightly prolonged PQ and peaked T wave, but QRS was not widened. I felt that stopping the diet would suffice to lower potassium within a few hours. However, they decided to keep me in the Clinical Research Center overnight. In fact, I had a good night's sleep and a huge diuresis, and by the next morning my potassium had dropped to 5.4. The next day, when everything was fine, they joked that the worst thing, should something have happened to me, would have been notifying my wife that her husband had died for science. There were no problems in the other volunteers, but their electrolytes were only checked in the morning. In any event, John decided to stop the study. I regretted hearing later that the results of the study had never been published, as, in my opinion, they were very interesting.

During that time, I was very busy and spent only a little time on personal activities. All my laundry was done at Sudden Service Cleaners on the corner of 8th Street and Locust, close to the Tiger

Motor Hotel. I devoted little time to meals, drinking only a cup of coffee for breakfast, skipping lunch, and essentially having only one meal a day. In the evening I would frequent various fast food restaurants, like the House of Pancakes, Dairy Queen, and Pizzeria. They would each have special deals once or twice a week, and I would patronize them on those specific days. On Wednesdays Dairy Queen offered three braziers for the price of two and additionally a banana split ice cream for US$0.49. On Fridays the House of Pancakes offered an unlimited number of pancakes for the price of one order.[12] At the end of my stay, the Tiger Motor Hotel was offering smorgasbord in the evening for US$2. Ultimately, I spent very little on food and I lost about 6 lb in weight, which was good for me, as I managed to reach 83 kg (183 lbs) — only 8 kg more than during my track and field days. At that time I was still a smoker, but I could buy a pack of cigarettes for US$0.37 in the VA canteen. All in all, my expenses were very small, about US$300 per month, and my salary was tax free, about US$1,125 per month, so I could save some money. I made only one major and very important purchase in Columbia: A Hewlett Packard HP-65 programmable calculator, which cost about US$650. From that point onwards, I could permanently retire my slide rule, abacus and *kręciołek* (arithmometer).

Almost all faculty members and fellows were relatively young, so the Division of Nephrology organized physical activities, like basketball and football. Opposing teams were usually composed of mixed fellows and faculty members. Some of the games were very tough, especially water football. In July 1977, after one of the last football games, I suffered some back pain, which became much worse following my return to Poland in September that year.

Overall, my stay in Columbia was very pleasant. I learned new things and my English improved tremendously. I was impressed by how eager Americans were to help foreigners, which may surprise some people. I was particularly impressed that Americans appeared to share their knowledge without reservation. Dr. Nolph suggested that

---

12. When I returned to Columbia four years later, none of the specials were available. Dairy Queen, in the vicinity of the Tiger Motor Hotel, was closed. Pizzeria was closed. And the House of Pancakes no longer had such deals. When I told my wife, she concluded that I must have put them out of business. I also learned that shortly after my departure the deal on cigarettes came to an end, and later cigarettes were not available in the VA canteen.

I stay in the Division of Nephrology as a faculty member, but I had to decline the offer. Firstly, my wife was resolutely against permanent relocating to the U.S. Secondly, I had promised Prof. Wojtczak that I would return to Poland after a year and move to Lublin to become Chairman of the Nephrology Department at the Medical Academy.

CHAPTER 5

Return to Poland: The Lublin Years

After returning to Bytom, I contacted Prof. Wojtczak and the Rector of the Medical Academy in Lublin. My wife and I visited Lublin to see the apartment that was provided for us by the Medical Academy, and within a few days we moved in. There were a few setbacks related to our relocation to Lublin. During the move, I tried to lift a large table, suffered a prolapsed disc (L3/L4) and started experiencing pain with increased abdominal pressure, especially when coughing and with any movement associated with leaning forward. Another problem was that we had no friends in shops and kiosks in Lublin, and we had to wait in line for food, particularly meat, because of the supply problems in the communist system. I remember standing in line for about four hours to buy some ground meat. Toilet paper was not available in shops at all. I later heard that a chronic shortage of toilet paper is characteristic of any communist system, and nobody knows why. Our sons had to change schools, but they adjusted pretty quickly. Halina found employment as a senior assistant in the Department of Psychiatry. Gradually, we were able to function in Lublin, but it took us several months.

I also remember a joke related to toilet paper in Poland. In the early 1950s Israel tried to build a fighter jet, but during every test flight, the wings would break from the fuselage. After various attempts the engineers became frustrated. As it happened, one of the engineers was Polish and he suggested they make holes in the wings close to the fuselage. The other engineers laughed at him, but ultimately, out of desperation, they followed his advice. Amazingly, the first test flight was a success! So they asked him how he came up with his brilliant idea. He answered that it was simple. "When I was in Poland and was able to get toilet paper, I noticed that it never tears at the perforations."

A few days after I settled into my new office, I had to be admitted to the Neurology Department. X-rays confirmed a prolapsed disc, but the treatment was only partly successful. Surgery was deemed unnecessary, but rather rehabilitation in a sanatorium. After treatment I felt a little better, but I had to sleep on a very hard surface — the floor — for about a year. The improvement was very slow. In July 1978 I went with our younger son, Przemek, to Ostrowo at the Baltic Sea, and while bodysurfing, I suddenly realized that the pain had gone. The experience prompted me to believe that such dolphin-like movements during swimming sessions are good when I have back pain.

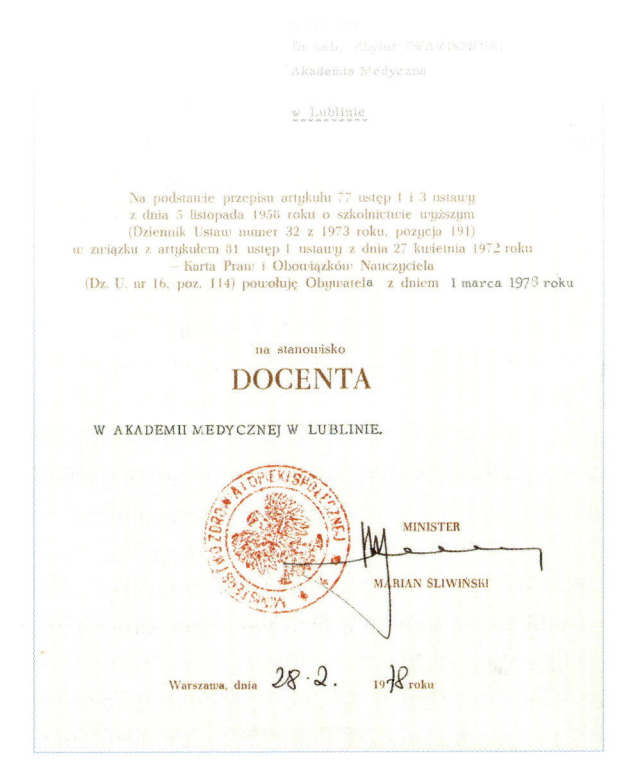

Figure 22. Appointment for a Docent position in Lublin.

I started work in October. I was appointed to the position of Docent of the Medical Academy in Lublin (Fig. 22) and I became Interim Chairman of the Department of Nephrology. The department had three adjuncts: Dr. med. Anna Gutka, Dr. med. Andrzej Książek and Dr. med. Lucyna Janicka. There were also five assistants: Elżbieta Bocheńska-Nowacka, Gabriela Sokołowska, Anna Żbikowska, Maria Majdan and Hanna Marczyńska. There were 40 beds and a dialysis center with six kidney machines — three Unimat (Bellco, Mirandola, Italy), one Travenol RSP and two Rhodial 75 (Rhône-Poulenc, France) — and rooms for peritoneal dialysis. Patients were dialyzed three times weekly for 4 hours on Rhodial 75 machines with

RP-6 dialyzers and 6 hours on RSP and Unimat machines with Vita 2 HF dialyzers (Bellco). I was surprised by the high mortality rate and the poor clinical status of the patients.

There were three major differences in dialysis technique in this institution compared to the one in Bytom. First, the time of dialysis was shorter than in Bytom; second, blood pressure control was not based on strict fluid balance; third, the patients had high bicarbonate levels and easily became hypotensive during dialysis. It surprised me even more when I increased the duration of dialysis and patients were not faring any better. They actually became more alkalotic and had more problems with blood pressure control and more hypotensive episodes. It was completely different than my experience in Bytom. Unlike in Bytom, where the dialysis solution contained bicarbonate, the dialysis solution in Lublin contained acetate. Suspecting that something was wrong with the composition of the dialysis solution, I discovered that it contained acetate in the amount calculated for sodium acetate trihydrate, but anhydrous sodium acetate was used. This explained part of the problems. The Unimat kidney machines were using a proportional system to prepare dialysis solution from concentrate and treated water. I eventually established a standard composition of dialysis solution that contained 35.7 mEq/L of acetate. After changing the composition, the patients tolerated dialysis much better. Blood pressure control was markedly improved and cardiovascular complications decreased. I was able to adjust the duration of dialysis more easily.

There were two shifts on each dialysis station: morning and afternoon. For administrative reasons there was no possibility of doing dialysis overnight. I could not prolong dialysis more than to 7 hours on the Unimat. On Rhodial 75 machines, dialyses were 4 hours; however, the frequency of dialysis was adjusted according to clinical evaluation, a principle established in my habilitation thesis. Out of 20 patients, four were on four times weekly, and patients with infections, surgeries or any other reason for increased catabolism could be dialyzed daily. Dialysis time was longer on the Unimat machine with Vita 2 HF dialyzers, and some patients were dialyzed more than three times weekly. Those starting dialysis with good residual renal function were dialyzed twice weekly. All dialyzers were reused, Vita 2 HF with the method similar to that used for Ultra-flo 145 dialyzers in Bytom. Initially, dialyzers were sterilized with 5 percent formalin. After reports of sufficient sterilization with 3 percent formalin, this latter concentration was used until one patient developed septic shock following dialysis [Pu 42]. After this experience, we returned to sterilization with 5 percent formalin and did not have any more cases of dialysis-related septic shock. RP-6 dialyzers with polyacrylonitrile membrane were cleansed and sterilized with 0.48 percent sodium hypochlorite. I presented my experience with RP-6 dialyzers in Atlantic City, New Jersey, in October 1982, while working in Columbia, Mo. [Pr 42], and my presentation was later published in the proceedings of the meeting [Pu 64]. In any event, there was soon no mortality and all dialysis stations were full. No new patients could be admitted, except to replace those who had received transplants. The patients were transplanted in Warsaw, as there was no transplant program in Lublin.

As we could not enlarge our hemodialysis center, it was important to create satellite dialysis centers. One such center had already been established before my arrival in Lublin, which was in Kraśnik, about 15 miles southwest of Lublin, directed by Dr. med. Stanisław Gottner. As I was the regional (voivodeship) specialist in nephrology, I visited the center from time to time. Dr. Gottner had an excellent reputation and had many friends in various places. (During one visit I asked him whether it would be possible to procure some toilet paper and he promptly arranged it, allowing me to secure enough for the family for about six months.) I attempted to develop another satellite unit, in Puławy, about 16 miles northwest of Lublin, but all my efforts to create new satellite units during my stay in Lublin proved unsuccessful.

With the dearth of hemodialysis stations, there was an urgent need to start a chronic peritoneal dialysis program. Chronic peritoneal dialyses were practiced before my arrival, but the dialyses were performed infrequently and mortality was extremely high. In 1978 I introduced continuous ambulatory peritoneal dialysis (CAPD),[1] presenting the concept and our initial results during the meeting of the Polish Academy of Sciences in Warsaw [Pr 21], and the first paper on this method in Polish literature appeared in 1979 [Pu 38]. There

---

1. In Polish, *ciągła ambulatoryjna dializa otrzewnowa* (CADO).

were tremendous technical problems compared to those in Columbia. The most important was that we had solutions in 0.5 L bottles, whereas in Columbia we used 2 L bottles. This required more punctures for each exchange and, of course, was associated with higher peritonitis rates.

I began working with both the Department of Surgery and the Department of Urology. I had come to the conclusion that it would be better if surgeons created fistulas and inserted chronic peritoneal catheters, as most of my assistants were not surgically inclined. I preferred fistulas with side-to-side anastomosis. For the first fistula I assisted Doc. dr. hab. Jerzy Karski to demonstrate exactly how I wanted the fistulas created. Other surgeons would later do the procedures, but my preferred method was observed as long as I was in Lublin. Most of the fistulas were on the forearm, usually between radial artery and cephalic vein. There was one saphenous vein graft straight-forearm fistula, but no other grafts at that time. Needle insertions used the constant site method, which nurses learned after some short visits to Bytom [Pu 41]. Only needles manufactured in Milanówek were used and blood flow was always 200 mL/min. I was also of the opinion that it would be possible to start a transplant program. However, this did not come to fruition before my departure from Lublin.

In 1977, I was reappointed to the Ministry of Health's Committee for the Development of Dialysis and Transplantation and to the Nephrology Committee of the Polish Academy of Science. The distance between Lublin and Warsaw was only about 100 miles, so I began going there at least once a month. In addition to being kept up to date regarding the state of nephrology in Poland, I could spend some time in the Main Medical Library in Warsaw, which had a rather large variety of useful journals and books. Prof. Orłowski, who continued to serve as Chairman of the Dialysis and Transplantation Committee and the Nephrology Committee of the Polish Academy of Science, offered me a grant to work on a capillary artificial kidney. I was surprised by the offer, as I remembered his negative thoughts on capillary artificial kidneys some 14 years earlier, but I declined, as I already knew that there was no appropriate technology in Poland. Besides, hollow-fiber dialyzers were already commercially available and working on this would be something of a waste of my time.

Shortly after beginning my work in Lublin, I was invited by Prof. dr. hab. Stefania Jabłońska, a famous Polish dermatologist, to present my observations regarding the effects of dialysis on psoriasis [Pr 18]. In discussion Prof. Jabłońska asked me how many white blood cells were lost during dialysis. Informing her that it was about 50 per mm^3, it seemed to me that she suspected that the loss of white blood cells contributed to the alleviation of psoriasis during dialysis. I published two papers on this topic. The first, which appeared in the Polish literature, described data from previous studies as well as my experience with dialysis and psoriasis [Pu 36]. In the second paper I put forward a hypothesis that dialysis removes some factor, which I called epidermopoietin, produced in the epidermis and stimulating the epidermis to increase turnout. I suggested that this substance was not removed efficiently by the kidneys but was removed by dialysis [Pu 37]. Prof. Jabłońska, meanwhile, continued to work on her initial suspicion that removal of white blood cells was responsible for improvement during dialysis and leukopheresis.[2]

I encouraged assistants to publish case reports with interesting observations, and several papers were subsequently published [Pu 45, Pu 46, Pu 55, Pu 60]. The observation of glomerulosclerosis intracapillaris in a patient without carbohydrate disturbances or retinopathy was the first such case reported in the Polish literature [Pu 44].

In 1978, our department started to cooperate with the Department of Hematology in evaluating platelet functions in 18 patients on chronic hemodialysis during repeated use of hemodialyzer before and after dipyridamole administration. It was found that dialyzer reuse had no effect on the platelet system. A significantly lower platelet count was demonstrated in the blood obtained from an arteriovenous fistula in relation to venous blood, and significant platelet retention on the dialyzer membrane was observed. Dipyridamole had no effect on these processes. The drug reduced the number of circulating platelet aggregates but failed to decrease the formation of clots in the dialyzer and failed to improve the reuse of dialyzers [Pu 48]. The most intriguing observation was the difference in platelet count between arteriovenous fistula and vein [Pu 53]. We extended these studies and

---

2. Glinski W, Jablonska S, Imiela J, Daszynski J. (1985) Peritoneal dialysis and leukopheresis in psoriasis: Indications and contraindications (in German). Hautarzt **36**(1): 16–19.

found that there were differences in platelet counts taken from the cubital vein with and without stasis, and arteriovenous fistula with and without stasis. The platelet counts taken from the femoral artery and vein were almost identical but lower than that in the cubital vein without stasis and higher than that in the arteriovenous fistula. Simple calculations ruled out there being a real difference in the platelet content as a possible explanation for our findings. We thought that our finding might be partly explained by a variable tendency to platelet aggregation in different blood vessels. This aggregation might depend on diminished platelet concentration of adenosine 3′,5′-monophosphate related to lower prostacyclin generation in the walls of some vessels. Although other explanations could be hypothesized, the most important conclusion of our study was that an awareness of these differences was important in studies on platelet behavior in hemodialysis patients. The study was presented in part during the Annual Meeting of the Polish Society of Hematology in June 1980 [Pr 27] and published in 1982 [Pu 61]. At the time, I found this interesting, but I was pursuing other studies and had neither time nor the hematology experts with whom to collaborate and study this problem. To this day there is no explanation as to the reason for these differences.

In Lublin we did not have a laboratory. I was very interested in continuing my previous study on osmotic ultrafiltration [Pu 32], but the possibility of creating a laboratory in Lublin was nonexistent at the time. I was constantly thinking about the problems of diffusive and convective transport in dialysis systems. I gave presentations on this area in Warsaw [Pr 17] and Poznań [Pr 19]. At the Congress of the International Society of Nephrology in Amsterdam, I met with Dr. Nolph and described to him some of my ideas on new osmotic agents that I thought would be worthwhile studying. Dr. Nolph suggested I come to Columbia and do the studies in their laboratory. I knew I would not be able to stay for a long time, but I told him might be able to come for six months. He subsequently sent me a formal invitation and I began the process of obtaining permission to go.

During my time in Lublin, I had teaching responsibilities in addition to clinical and research duties. Under my supervision, one of my assistants, Elżbieta Bocheńska-Nowacka, was writing her thesis on iron metabolism in renal failure for her *Doktor medycyny* (Dr. med., the equivalent of a PhD). She successfully defended her thesis in May 1980. A decade later, after communist rule had ended in Poland, she moved to a private dialysis center called Diaverum and became its Deputy Director. I was also a patron for Dr. med. Andrzej Książek for his habilitation procedure. Successfully defending his thesis in 1980, he was soon granted the position of Docent in the Department and became my deputy. I was also a promotor for another assistant, Maria Majdan, who was writing a PhD thesis entitled "Comparison of the effectiveness of peritoneal dialyses conducted by continuous and intermittent methods." The procedure was opened in 1980 but not finished before my departure to the U.S., so the Dean of the School of Medicine appointed Doc. Książek as her promotor. I was asked to approve the change and I gladly agreed as I considered her thesis very valuable but was not able to return to Poland at the time. She defended her thesis successfully in 1983 and it was published in part in 1986.[3] She later became a professor and was appointed Chairwoman of the Department of Rheumatology and Connective Tissue Diseases in Lublin.

I also lectured students in internal medicine and nephrology. At that time it was customary for students to be given oral examinations. In the Institute of Internal medicine, there were several departments (divisions) with various subspecialties, but students had examinations across the whole spectrum of internal medicine. I was responsible for examining about 20 percent of the fifth (and final) year students at the Medical Academy. Some students were very good and I accepted some as teaching assistants in the Department of Nephrology. One such student was Anna Bednarek-Skublewska, who later successfully defended a PhD thesis and went on to coauthor more than 50 papers related to dialysis and nephrology. Another was Krzysztof Marczewski, whose habilitation thesis was approved in 1997 and who subsequently became a professor in 2003. In addition to nephrology, he became an expert in medical ethics, becoming a member of the European Group for Ethics in Science and New Technologies in 2005.

On April 16, 1981, the Faculty Council and Senate of the Medical Academy put my name forward for the title and position of professor.

---

3. Majdan M, Książek A. (1986) Porównanie wydajności dializ otrzewnowych prowadzonych w sposób ciągły i przerywany (Comparison of the effectiveness of peritoneal dialyses conducted by continuous and intermittent methods). *Pol Arch Med Wewn* **76**(1): 27–34.

The recommendation was subsequently approved by the Central Qualification Committee at the Ministry of Health and the approval was sent to the Minister of Health on November 30, 1981. To be promoted to *profesor nadzwyczajny* (associate professor), the application should have been sent to the Council of State, but the procedure was not completed. I recently learned that on March 13, 1982 — after my emigration to the U.S. — the Rector of the Medical Academy in Lublin, Prof. dr. hab. Andrzej Jakliński, sent a letter to the Ministry of Health saying that I had not returned from the U.S. and had not reported for work. This was probably the reason that the Ministry of Health suspended the procedure.[4] After my departure Doc. Książek became the Chairman of the Department of Nephrology. He later became a professor and was appointed to the position of Rector (equivalent to Chancellor) of the Medical University in Lublin. (The name "Medical Academy" was changed to "Medical University" in 2008.)

In September 1980, I organized the Annual Meeting of the Renal Section of the Polish Society of Internal Medicine in Puławy and in Lublin. I held a lecture on the state-of-the-art treatment of acute renal failure [Pr 28].

Gradually I started to change our hemodialysis practice to resemble the one I had developed in Bytom, as I considered the clinical status of Bytom patients to be better than Lublin's. Many patients continued to have hypotensive episodes and other symptoms during dialysis even after I changed the composition of the dialysis solution. At that time it was not possible to use bicarbonate on the Unimat kidney machine; only acetate could be used. I preferred the method of

---

4. At the time the title of "professor" was bestowed by the Council of State (equivalent to the president). Today there are three titles. The more prestigious title is *profesor belwederski* (Belvederian professor), so called because it is conferred in Belvedere (Belweder) Palace, the seat of the President of Poland. There are two levels of Belvederian professor: *profesor nadzwyczajny* (associate professor), and above that, *profesor zwyczajny* (full professor). The third, and least prestigious, title is *profesor uczelniany* (university professor) bestowed by the university without the full procedure involving the Central Qualifying Committee. To differentiate the two main kinds, the title of Belvederian professor is given only before the name. For example, in my case it would be Prof. dr. hab. Zbylut Twardowski for the associate professor, Prof. zw. dr. hab. Zbylut Twardowski for full professor. For the title of university professor, the institution is stated after the name; in my case it would be Prof. dr. hab. Zbylut Twardowski AML (Akademia Medyczna w Lublinie). In the U.S. there is only a single title, that of university professor; in my case it is written Zbylut J. Twardowski, MD, PhD, Professor of Medicine, University of Missouri.

making dialysis solution from dry chemicals and treated water. It was already known that acetate was poorly tolerated on high efficiency dialyzers. Although we used Vita-2 HF dialyzers of medium efficiency, I suspected that bicarbonate would be better, at least in some patients with frequent symptoms during dialysis. We decided to compare bicarbonate and acetate dialysate in eight patients, four of whom had frequent hypotensive episodes during dialysis. This was a prospective, double-blind study with 72 dialysis sessions on the Travenol RSP machine where the composition of dialysate was randomly selected. The study showed a higher incidence of hypotensive episodes and other symptoms like nausea and weakness after dialysis with acetate dialysate. Only muscle cramps were more frequent with bicarbonate dialysate. The study showed that acetate is tolerated more poorly by some patients even on medium-efficiency dialyzers. The results of the study were presented in part at a meeting in Warsaw in 1979 [Pr 23] and published in 1981 [Pu 56]. I was eventually able to buy an additional Travenol RSP kidney machine and use bicarbonate for more patients.

Our department also started cooperating with the School of Pharmacology of the Medical Academy in Lublin and the pharmacological industry at large, particularly the Polfa pharmaceutical factory in Lublin.[5] I delivered a presentation entitled "Pharmacokinetics of drugs in renal failure" during the scientific session of the meeting "35 Years of Schools of Medicine and Pharmacology in Lublin and 20 Years of Cooperation between Pharmaceutical Industry Polfa and the Medical Academy in Lublin" [Pr 24]. The lecture was published in the proceedings [Pu 43] of the conference and republished later in the *Polish Archives of Internal Medicine* [Pu 54]. We also evaluated Vita-2 HF coil dialyzers manufactured by "Polfa" (based on a Bellco license) and compared them to the original Bellco Vita-2 HF dialyzers. Compared to my previous experience with Baxter Ultra-flo 145 dialyzers, both performed worse, especially with regard to first time failures and also to reuse failures. Dialyzers manufactured by Polfa

---

5. On January 1, 1974, the Pharmaceutical Cooperative "Inlek" was taken over by the Association of Pharmaceutical Industry "Polfa," creating a new state-owned enterprise called Lubelskie Zakłady Farmaceutyczne (LPZ) "Polfa" (Lublin Pharmaceutical Industry "Polfa").

were much more difficult to reuse and "resulted in significant decrease of average number of treatments with a single dialyzer" [Pu 47].

For peritoneal dialysis we used solutions in 0.5 L bottles bought from Lublin Pharmaceutical Industry "Polfa." I asked Mgr. Jan Śnieżyński, Director of "Polfa" Lublin to manufacture solutions in bigger glass containers or plastic bags. Solutions in plastic bags were manufactured by the Pharmaceutical Cooperative "Inlek," but shortly after it was transformed into the state-owned Lublin Pharmaceutical Industry "Polfa" they stopped manufacturing solutions in bags. Mgr. Śnieżyński explained to me that they needed titanium for the dies necessary to extrude bags, but all the available titanium was procured by the military and was not available for civilian use. He advised me to ask the Ministry of Health to intervene, but my talks with them were futile. Shortly thereafter Mgr. Śnieżyński passed away, and I decided that I had no option but to use what was available. The composition of dialysis solution (in mEq/L) was as follows: Na 139, Ca 4.0, Mg 1.5, Cl 99.5, acetate 45, and glucose 1.5 percent or 6.0 percent. The pH of the solutions ranged from 6.0 to 6.2.

We subsequently commenced a study on the kinetics of peritoneal dialysis involving 14 patients already on peritoneal dialysis for at least one month. The results were presented in part at the Meeting of the Polish Academy of Science in December 1979 [Pr 25], and the detailed report of the study was published in *Clinical Nephrology* in 1981 [Pu 49]. In all patients four exchanges of 2 L volumes were performed with several different schedules of total exchange time (e.g., 2, 9, 3 and 10 hours; 4, 7, 5 and 8 hours; or four exchanges of 6 hours each). Exchanges of 1.5 percent glucose dialysis solution were alternated with 2.6 percent. To obtain 2.6 percent glucose dialysis solution, three bottles of 1.5 percent and one 6.0% solution were infused intraperitoneally. There were several interesting observations reported for the first time. The number of white blood cells increased from 2 to 5 hours, and then remained essentially unchanged up to 10 hours total exchange time. For small molecular weight solutes (urea, creatinine, sodium, potassium and phosphate), dialysate-to-plasma concentrations tended to be lower with 2.6 percent glucose solution during shorter exchanges. Equilibrium between plasma and dialysate of all these solutes was achieved within 10 hours total exchange time.

Protein concentrations and losses were higher with the 2.6 percent glucose solution. Total protein concentration and losses were markedly lower than those reported for intermittent peritoneal dialysis. Protein losses correlated positively with serum protein concentrations and body surface area. Maximal ultrafiltration volumes were observed after 3 hours with 1.5 percent glucose solution and after 5 hours with 2.6 percent glucose solution. Clearances of inulin also correlated with body surface area, but ultrafiltration volumes did not. Sodium concentrations in dialysate fell below plasma concentration up to 8 hours, and below the concentration in dialysis solutions up to 6 hours with 1.5 percent glucose solution and up to 8 hours with 2.6 percent glucose solution. The results of this study were also reported in three parts in the Polish literature: ultrafiltration [Pu 50], protein losses [Pu 51], and kinetics of inulin and smaller solutes [Pu 52].

Using 0.5 L bottles was obviously disadvantageous, but it did have one positive aspect. I started thinking about how best to decrease the number of connections/disconnections during CAPD, and I came to the conclusion that it would be better to use 2.5 L exchanges three times daily instead of 2.0 L exchanges four times daily if the patients could tolerate the higher volume. If we had 2 L bottles or bags, this idea probably would not have come to my mind. The study on tolerance of higher instilled volume was carried out in 16 patients already tolerating 2 L volumes. By using different number of bottles with 1.5 percent glucose solution and 6.0 percent glucose solution, the overall glucose concentration varied from 1.5 percent to 3.3 percent. Occasionally, a solution with 4.2 percent glucose concentration was used. Tolerance of the 2.5 L volume was subjectively assessed by patients. Three patients did not tolerate 2.5 L volumes: they reported abdominal distension and other symptoms such as vomiting, dyspnea, insomnia or loss of appetite. The remaining patients did tolerate the 2.5 L volumes; however, some reported a diminished appetite and/or abdominal distension for about a week or two weeks. The body surface area of those patients who did not tolerate the higher volume tended to be lower but not statistically different from those who tolerated the higher volume. The most important feature differentiating those tolerating and not tolerating the higher volume was vital capacity. Vital capacity was reduced slightly after infusion of fluid into the peritoneal cavity depending on the volume of instilled fresh dialysis solution. Not only volume but also some source of irritation might have played a role in this reduction because the mean vital capacity before drainage was almost identical to that observed after instillation of 2 L of dialysis solution in spite of a roughly 800 mL higher volume of dialysate present in the peritoneal cavity. After several weeks of dialysis with 2.5 L of fluid, patients did not feel discomfort even if incomplete drainage occurred and during the next exchange the volume of drained dialysate was as high as 3900 mL. The highest ultrafiltration volumes occurred after 4 hours of total exchange time with 1.5 percent and 2.4 percent glucose solutions and after 6 hours with the 3.3 percent glucose solution [Pu 57].

We evaluated the efficiency of three exchanges of 2.5 L volumes in 12 patients who tolerated this volume and wished to participate in the study. These patients had average residual urine output of 297 ± 269 mL. Their dialysis clearances were roughly 0.5 L lower than with four exchanges of 2 L volumes. Nevertheless, with substantial residual renal function they were sufficient for clinically adequate dialysis. We usually did not prolong outflow time beyond 30 minutes even if incomplete drainage occurred. Usually, the retained fluid was drained during the next exchange. The highest drainage volumes during the study period were 4500, 4200, 3900 and 3300 in four different patients. We assumed that if three exchanges were not sufficient, then four 2.5 L volumes might be used. We anticipated that volumes of 3 L or more might be tolerated in some patients and used if needed. The results were presented in part during the 2nd International Symposium on Peritoneal Dialysis in West Berlin on June 18, 1981 [Pr 30], and published later in the symposium's proceedings [Pu 58]. I was a member of the Scientific Committee of the symposium and with Dr. Nolph-co-chaired Session One on Morphology and Physiology on June 17, 1981. I spoke with Dr. Nolph about my visit to Columbia, and we agreed that I would come in August 1981 and stay until February the following year.

Before my trip to Missouri I wrote a book chapter on acute renal failure and the methods of blood purification: peritoneal dialysis and hemodialysis [Pu 76]. I described pathogenesis, the clinical picture, and the treatment of patients with acute renal failure as well as dialysis techniques available at the time.

We also started some kinetic studies on albumin transport from serum to the peritoneal dialysate using radio labeled albumin. We found that the transfer from serum to the dialysate is a very slow process that takes several hours. The results of these studies were published as abstracts long after I left Lublin [Ab 23, Ab 24].

CHAPTER 6

Return to Columbia: Migrating to the U.S.

I came back to Columbia, Mo., in August 1981 and settled in, once again, at the Tiger Motor Hotel. During my absence, the outpatient hemodialysis center had been moved from TD4 to a new building on Walnut Street, which was part of Dialysis Clinic Inc., headquartered in Nashville, Tennessee, the clinic was cooperating with the University of Missouri Hospital. In addition to the hemodialysis center there was also an outpatient peritoneal dialysis center and a clinical laboratory. I began multiple projects in the laboratory located in the Veterans Administration Hospital and in the outpatient peritoneal dialysis unit of Dialysis Clinic Inc. It was a short walk to the laboratory in the VA Hospital, but the clinic on Walnut Street was about three miles from the Tiger Motor Hotel and even further from the University Hospital. I could not afford to buy a car, so I bought a bicycle instead. Cycling came with its own problems, however. When the weather was very hot, I had a tendency to sweat profusely, which meant that I would be drenched upon arrival at my destination. Noticing my suffering and seeing how long it would take for me to cool down, Susan Cooper, the administrative associate of the Division of Nephrology, offered me her car as long as I agreed to pay for the insurance. It was an old Chevy from the late 1960s and the insurance premium was very small — from what I recall, only about US$30 per month. While it did only about six miles to the gallon, the car was big and robust, and I had free parking at the Tiger Motor Hotel, the dialysis clinic and the hospital. The University Hospital was connected to the VA Hospital via a tunnel. The monthly mileage was very low, so my expenses were within my means.

The outlines of my initial areas of work were published in five short articles. The first article, with Dr. Nolph as the first author and published not long after my arrival, indicated areas of interest related to peritoneal dialysis physiology that we wanted to explore [Pu 59]. The second was an opinion in "Open Forum: Peritoneal Dialysis — What's Ahead?" published in *Dialysis and Transplantation* [Pu 62]. The third was on optimal exchange volume in continuous ambulatory peritoneal dialysis [Pu 63], the fourth was on insulin binding to peritoneal dialysis bags [Pu 72], and the fifth was on my preference regarding vascular access [Pu 70]. In this final article I outlined, for the first time in the U.S. literature, my preferred dialysis method: short daily hemodialysis. I will return to this subject later.

At that time, in addition to Dr. Nolph, the division had five faculty members: John Bauer, MD; Stephen Brooks, MD; John Van Stone, MD; Michael Sorkin, MD; and Fred C. Whittier, MD. There were three clinical fellows: Hans Gloor, MD, from Switzerland; Michael Young; and Garry Reams, MD. Dr. Van Stone was also the Medical Director of Dialysis Clinic Inc., which treated end-stage renal disease patients with hemodialysis and peritoneal dialysis. Drs. Bauer and Brooks were mostly interested in hypertension. Dr. Sorkin decided to leave Columbia after being offered a faculty position at the University of Pittsburgh School of Medicine, and Dr. Nolph suggested — as he had done four years earlier — that I accept the position of Associate Professor of Medicine in the Division of Nephrology. I was not ready for several reasons. First of all, my wife and my younger son were reluctant to move to the U.S.; my elder son was open to it, so there was an even split in the family. Secondly, I had already started some research in Lublin and was supervising the doctoral thesis of one of my assistants, Maria Majdan. Thirdly, I was optimistic about the prospects in Poland, as I believed that the new Solidarity movement, of which I was a member, would be able to liberate the country from communism. To be on the safe side, I decided to sit for the Federal Licensing Examination (FLEX), the accepted medical licensing examination in the U.S. at the time. It was not too demanding, as my work as a resident four years previously provided the eligibility I needed to take the exam. Also, the fee then was only US$500, so I figured that it might be useful without being too much of a burden. I took the three-day exam at the Holiday Inn Express at 1716 Jefferson Street in Jefferson City, Mo., from December 1 to 3, 1981.

We had already begun some studies on polymer-induced ultrafiltration in rats and were to present the results in New Orleans in January 1982 [Pr 35]. To try and convince my wife that moving to Columbia was a good idea, Dr. Nolph suggested inviting Halina and taking her to New Orleans and other places. She agreed and made arrangements to obtain a passport and get ready to come. But the situation suddenly changed dramatically. On Sunday, December 13, 1981 martial law was imposed in Poland. When I heard the news, I tried calling my wife, but private telephones in Poland were not working. I wanted to return immediately, but all travel to and from Poland had been suspended. As the days passed, my thoughts about the situation started to change I became afraid that Poland's communist system would remain in place for decades if not half a century. Staying in the U.S., a country with freedoms that Poles might never enjoy, was looking like an increasingly attractive option. I sent several letters to Halina with hints about staying in the U.S. The Polish postal service was very slow at that time and all letters were supposed to be read by the authorities, so caution was needed. The envelope containing one letter I received from Poland was cut off on one side and was stamped with the word *ocenzurowano* (censored), though the letter had not been read as it was glued to the envelope. Thinking about it, I realized that the warning about censoring letters was simply intimidation; it would be impossible, in practice, to read every letter leaving and entering a country. After that realization, I began communicating my plans more explicitly. In February I received a letter from the family in which my elder son insisted that I stay in the U.S. My wife and younger son did not give an opinion either way, so I assumed that the sentiment expressed by my elder son was the position of the whole family. My father-in-law also thought that I should stay in the U.S. In the meantime I received the positive results of the FLEX exam, so I told Dr. Nolph that I would accept his offer. One of my requests was that my sons, who had started medical school in Lublin, would be able to continue their studies in Columbia. Dr. Nolph introduced me to Charles C. Lobeck, the Dean of the School of Medicine, who promised that they would be accepted for the third year of Medical School if they passed the Medical Sciences Knowledge Profile (MSKP) exam. They were very good students so I did not foresee any problems.

It suddenly turned out that there was a problem with my visa status and that my FLEX exam was not sufficient. I still needed to complete the so-called VISA examination, which was less demanding than FLEX but for bureaucratic reasons absolutely necessary. As it happened, I was not able to take this exam in 1982 as the deadline for applications had already passed. Worse still, the next available date to take the exam was late in 1983 with the presentation of the certificate in 1984. After a very long search for a solution, Dr. Nolph learned that a person who is regarded as internationally renowned does not need to take the VISA exam. He then wrote a letter to the Department of Health and Human Services in Washington, DC., attached my CV., and asked for a certificate declaring that I was indeed internationally renowned. The letter confirming this fact arrived on August 10, 1983. Ever since, Dr. Nolph has joked that I am the only person at the University of Missouri who has an official certificate from the Department of Health and Human Services declaring that I am internationally renowned. On November 21, 1983, I received a "green card," which meant that I was "lawfully admitted for permanent residence in the United States."

In 1982, I was given the position of Visiting Associate Professor in the Division of Nephrology and granted staff physician privileges in nephrology at the division and at Dialysis Clinic Inc. in Columbia. The following year I became an Associate Professor of Medicine and granted the privileges of a staff physician in nephrology at the Harry S. Truman Memorial Veterans Hospital in Columbia. In 1985, I was appointed Director of the Outpatient Peritoneal Dialysis Program in the Division of Nephrology and promoted to a full Professor of Medicine in the Department of Medicine. Two years later, I was promoted to full Professor of Medicine with Tenure, and by 1991 I had been added to the roster of investigators at the University of Missouri's Dalton Research Center. My first salary as a Research Fellow in 1981 was US$14,500, but it increased to US$50,000 after I accepted the position of Visiting Associate Professor in 1982. Part of my salary was covered by Dialysis Clinic Inc., for taking care of hemodialysis patients. While my advancement in terms of academic rank was rather rapid, my salary did not increase accordingly, as the Division of Nephrology did not have sufficient funds. However, I was fortunate to have started to gain extra income from consulting and later from patent royalties, both of which I will talk about later.

In 1982, after becoming a Visiting Associate Professor and receiving a higher salary, I decided to buy a car and a house and move out of the Tiger Motor Hotel. In accordance with my deeply-rooted convictions regarding personal finance, I decided to buy the car with cash outright, with only the house requiring a loan. Indeed, I have never taken out a loan for anything but a house. In my entire life, I have never spent more than what I have, paying for all the necessities with check or cash and using a credit card sparingly while always paying the balance in full. After many years I read Dave Ramsey's book *The Total Money Makeover* and found that his advice regarding financial matters was identical. I thanked Susan for the use of her Chevy truck and I bought a Plymouth Champ. I then started to look for an inexpensive house, employing the services of a realtor from House of Brokers Realty in Columbia. She recommended a US$64,000 house at 4012 Defoe Drive, on a low level in the Rothwell Heights neighborhood of Columbia. The owners of the house were in Alaska. At the time the mortgage interest rate was 12 percent, but it was supposed to go down, making refinancing possible. I made an earnest payment of US$1,000, but first asked to rent the house for a few months.

Not long after settling in, there was a torrential downpour and water came into the house through the doors and windows. I was a little upset with my realtor, but she insisted that such a thing had never happened before — and indeed my neighbors confirmed her claim. But concerned that the situation could repeat itself in the future, I decided not to go ahead with the purchase, losing my earnest money but satisfied that I did made the right decision. As a matter of fact, after some time, a bigger sewer was installed under Defoe Drive to drain away the rainwater more quickly, and similar flooding never happened again. In any event, it turned out that a friend of Sobha Sunderrajan, one of the fellows in the Division of Nephrology, wanted to sell a house at 304 Devine Court, also located in Rothwell Heights. Bigger and nicer, the house was only US$8,000 more expensive, and it was situated at the highest point of Rothwell Heights, which was a big plus point after the experience of having my first house flooded. It was for sale immediately and I could assume a mortgage with an interest rate of 10 percent. My first purchases were a refrigerator and a microwave oven. I had no furniture, no cookware, nothing. Fortunately, the division staff organized a housewarming party for me and brought various small necessities. I would never have thought of inviting them, as I had never heard of such a custom, but I was very grateful for their thoughtfulness.

In the meantime I tried to get permission for my wife and sons to join me in Columbia. I asked Senator John C. Danforth of Missouri to help and he wrote to the Foreign Ministry in Poland requesting they allow my family go. It was declined, of course, as were all my direct requests to the Polish Consulate in Chicago. When I complained that their position meant the members of my family were apart, they told me that I could unite the family by going back to Poland. Later that year my wife was finally able to get permission for one person to leave, so we made the decision to let my elder son, Radek, come. Having already finished his fourth year of medical school in Lublin, he arrived in July 1983, passed the MSKP exam with excellent results and could start the third year of medical school in Columbia. He did very well and graduated in 1985, the Missouri State Medical Association conferring on him an Honors Graduate Award "in recognition of outstanding achievement in the study of medicine." In January 1985 his future wife, Małgorzata Kotlińska, arrived in Columbia and they got married in February. She did not want to stay in the U.S. at the time, so she went back to Poland, where their daughter Anna (Ania) was born on December 15, 1985. By the time they returned to the U.S. in 1987, Radek was already completing his third year residency in Hartford, Conn. After finishing the residency program, he became Chief Resident and then came to the University of Missouri for a fellowship in cardiology. His two sons were born while in Columbia: Adam Karol, on August 14, 1990, and Aleksander Marian (Alek), on January 3, 1992. Radek later took a fellowship in Wichita, Kan., and at the University of Louisiana in New Orleans, where he finished interventional cardiology. He then joined Medcenter One Hospital in Bismarck, ND., as an interventional cardiologist.

In 1984, my mother developed throat cancer. It was hard for me not to be with her, but I was afraid to go to Poland, as I would probably not be allowed to return to the U.S. My brother tried to get permission for my mother to come to Columbia, but to no avail. I phoned Dr. Stawiński of the Laryngology Department at the Hospital for Miners to arrange her treatment, but despite his efforts, she passed away on January 7, 1985. It was heartbreaking not to be able to attend her funeral. Halina had to be there for both of us.

In the fall of 1984, my wife was with her best friend, Jola (Jolanta Ostrowska Jaźwiecka), at Busko Resort in Southern Poland. There they became acquainted with an important person who had connections to the Central Committee of the ruling communist party, the Polish United Workers' Party, and she arranged permission for my wife and younger son to join me in the U.S. The price for the "favor" was US$10,000,[1] a sum that I was then in a position to afford. Halina and Przemek, our younger son, were finally able to join me in Columbia on July 4, 1985, U.S. Independence Day, appropriately enough. I went to St. Louis Airport to pick them up in my Oldsmobile Delta 88. We were very happy to be together at last, but Halina's father had developed lung cancer and was in a critical condition back in Poland. He passed away not long after, on July 17, and Halina was unable to attend his funeral. Her mother was very supportive and calmed us with the assurance that her husband so strongly supported Halina's joining me in the U.S. that he would not have wished her to risk everything by returning to Kraków.

Dr. Moncrief organized a summer vacation for children on peritoneal dialysis and asked me to serve as a physician. I agreed and Przemek, Halina and I went to Colorado for two weeks. After my service ended we visited some places of interest in West Colorado (Mesa Verde, Sangre de Cristo Mountain) and traveled on the Durango and Silverton Railroad. We went to New Mexico, visited the Los Alamos Laboratory and Atomic Bomb Museum, stayed in Santa Fe, and then traveled through Amarillo, Tex., and Oklahoma, before heading back to Columbia. Przemek was not very keen on staying in the U.S., so he decided to return to Poland, completing his fourth year of medical school in Lublin. We were able to communicate with him by phone, but there was a good chance the calls would be monitored by the authorities, so we did not ask directly about his plans. In February 1986, Eugenia (Gena), Halina's mother, told us obliquely that there would be good news in the summer, and we figured that Przemek had probably decided to come to Columbia for good. That is indeed what happened. He arrived in New York with his friend from medical school, Wojciech (Wojtek) Poluha, on July 4, 1986 — once again, Independence Day — and we watched a very impressive fireworks display together. A few days later, we were back at the airport

---

1. In any totalitarian system, bribery can get many things done. Prominent party members did not receive high salaries, but their privileges were worth a lot of money. They could provide "tickets" to buy difficult to obtain, relatively inaccessible goods such as cars or TV sets, and they could grant favors in exchange for bribes. They were useful supplements to their salaries.

in our Delta 88 to pick up Dorota Nastaj, Wojtek's girlfriend and future wife whom he met in medical school. Przemek and Wojtek took jobs as farmhands for a while. Then Wojtek and Dorota left for New York in August. Przemek started to prepare for the MSKP and took some courses at Columbia College. In 1987 he went to Alaska to work on a fishing boat with his friend, Arkadiusz (Arek) Robert Krzyżanowski (no relation with Włodzimierz Krzyżanowski, the first administrator of Alaska; see below). By the summer of 1988 he had obtained a private pilot license for small planes. Around that time Gena visited us in Columbia. Like many a grandmother with her grandchild, she was very fond of Przemek, and when a plane flew overhead, she used to say, "It must be Przemek! The plane is flying so nicely, so straight!" Przemek would take me up in the plane, and Gena and Halina would always wave to us as we flew over the house.

Przemek passed the MSKP with excellent results and started the third year of medical school in 1988. Graduating *cum laude* in 1990, he was elected to the Alpha Omega Alpha Honor Medical Society in recognition of his academic achievements, and shortly after started a residency program at Northwestern University in Chicago. Przemek met his future wife, Katarzyna (Kasia) Wawszczak, in 1983, while training and taking part in competitions as a member of the swim team at the Lublin Medical Academy. After coming to Columbia, he kept in contact with her by mail and they arranged a canoeing trip with Wojtek and Dorota Poluha in Poland in 1989. Kasia visited Przemek in Chicago in 1990 and they got married on June 1, 1990. They had a Catholic wedding in Rzeszów, Poland, on February 21, 1991. After completing his three-year residency, Przemek was Chief Resident at Northwestern University for a year and then took a fellowship in hematology-oncology there. Meanwhile, Kasia took the ECFMG exam and began a residency program in internal medicine at Columbus Hospital in Chicago. By 1998 Przemek had moved to Pasadena, California, and taken a position in hematology-oncology at the City of Hope Hospital in Duarte. After finishing her residency in 1999, Kasia also moved to Pasadena and became a hospitalist.

In the late 1980s and 1990s, I traveled a great deal to give various presentations, a period I will describe in more detail later. My travels also took me to Europe and I was able to visit Poland. While in Kraków we stayed in Gena's apartment at 26 Wielopole, an apartment rented by Halina's parents since World War II. The rent was set by the communist government and was rather low, as the legitimate owner did not really own the house. After the collapse of communism in 1989, houses were slowly returned to their legitimate owners, who, naturally, wanted to increase the rents. Halina's younger sister, Joanna, lived with her mother. Gena was very afraid of rents rising and was especially concerned about Joanna's situation, as her income was not very high, so I promised to help her. On October 11, 1993, we celebrated our 35th wedding anniversary with the family in Kraków, but the following day Gena suffered a massive heart attack and was rushed to hospital, passing away the following day. Halina and I were both able to attend her funeral. By governmental decree, the rents were not supposed to be raised for a few years, but in 1996 we decided to buy a small apartment, Nr. 66 on Zakopiańska 2, to be used by Joanna in the event rents increased. Joanna was attached to Wielopole and wanted to stay there as long as she could, so we rented the apartment to students until she moved in during the fall of 2000. Unfortunately, the apartment was less than ideal, as the heating system frequently broke down in winter. We eventually bought a much nicer apartment, Nr. 2 at 7a Królowej Jadwigi, and Joanna moved there in August 2004. We sold the apartment on Zakopiańska 2 on July 21, 2005.

In March 1982, I started to work in the Outpatient Peritoneal Dialysis Program of the Division of Nephrology, located in Dialysis Clinic Inc. on Walnut Street. I followed peritoneal dialysis and hemodialysis patients. The peritoneal dialysis program grew very rapidly in the early 1980s, but later the greatest increase was noted in satellite hemodialysis patients as new satellite units were built. My main duties were patient care, teaching and research. I devoted about 40 percent of my time to patient care, 30 percent to teaching, and 30 percent to research, though I spent extra time conducting research in the evenings and over the weekends. Typically, about 20 peritoneal dialysis patients and 20 hemodialysis patients were under my direct care at any one time. Also, in a given year, I usually had two months as an attending physician on the general internal medicine ward and two months of consulting in nephrology. Most of my student teaching was done during these four months. The teaching of fellows was done during consulting services and weekly conferences. I also traveled extensively to give presentations on topics related to dialysis; I will say more about this later.

In 1983, there was another significant change at the Division of Nephrology. In October Fred C. Whittier, MD, left Columbia, and Ramesh Khanna accepted his faculty position. Dr. Khanna, who graduated from the Medical College in Parel, Bombay, India, undertook a fellowship at the Cleveland Clinic Foundation in Ohio from 1972 to 1975 and worked in Toronto with Dr. Dimitrios Oreopoulos from 1979. He was a tremendous addition to the division, especially with regard to peritoneal dialysis research, and our research accelerated markedly upon his arrival (Fig. 23). Dr. Nolph, Dr. Khanna and I cooperated very closely on patient care and we covered for one another when we traveled for presentations. At least one of us was usually in Columbia, but sometimes, typically when going to conferences regularly organized by the division, we had to ask other faculty members to cover for us. The time spent on presentation-related

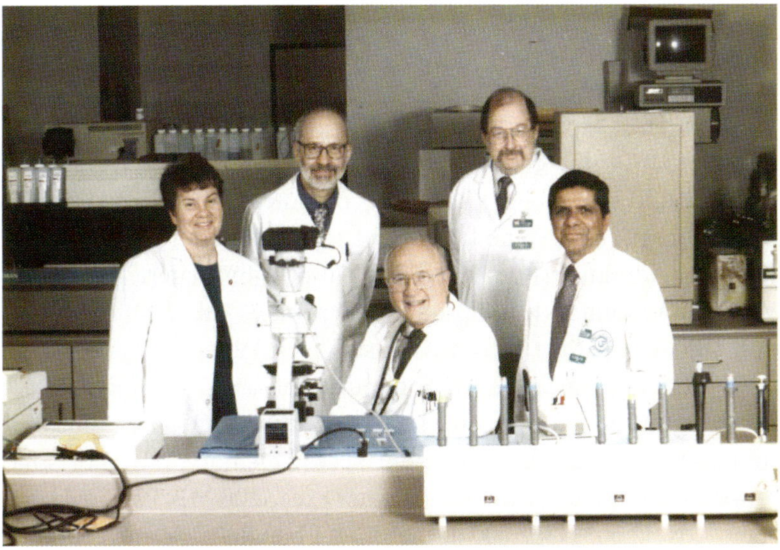

Figure 23. Group doing most of the peritoneal dialysis research. From left: Barbara ("Barb") F. Prowant, Karl D. Nolph, the author, Harold F. Moore, and Ramesh Khanna.

travel was substantial, but it was considered essential.[2] In fact, as the time away was often not exclusively for presentations but combined with visiting places of interest, I decided to take minimal vacation time for almost all the years before my retirement. Besides, the problem with taking a long vacation was that upon one's return, there was always a pile of mail and any number of pressing things to attend to.

My main office was in Dialysis Clinic Inc. (DCI) on Walnut Street, but I also had a small office in the hospital. I spent most of my time in DCI, as most of my work with patients and most of my research took place there. While progress notes were handwritten on charts, manuscripts were typed. At the time the division had three secretaries. Peggy Gray worked, for the most part, for Dr. Nolph, whose office was in the hospital. Another secretary, Jeanette Leroux, had an office at DCI, and I could initially dictate to her directly, and she would then retype the text after corrections. That changed in 1986, when she was moved to an office in the hospital. I then had to dictate manuscripts via telephone, and the text was subsequently mailed to DCI so that I could correct it and mail it back to the hospital. The text sometimes had to be corrected several times, as my heavy accent and illegible handwriting were undecipherable at times. It was frustrating for everyone involved, and it became clear that it would be better for me to type out manuscripts on a computer myself. I suggested to Dr. Nolph and Dr. Khanna that we buy three computers, arguing that for the cost of three computers we could have one less secretary and save money. Jag Gill, a computer whiz who could teach us some basics and some tricks, had replaced Susan Cooper as the division's Administrative Associate. We bought Generic computers with Texan monitors and Epson FX-85 printers, all of which worked with IBM-compatible software. I used WordPerfect 4.1 and 4.2 for word-processing tasks, Lotus for calculations, and 35 mm Express for preparing slides. The operating system used was DOS, programs were on 1.44 MB floppy disks, random access memory was very small (64 kB), and hard drive capacity did not exceed 20 MB. Personal computers cost about US$2,000 at the time. I bought the same computer for home use. Programs and data files were small, so it was a simple

---

2. The University of Missouri considered presentations given around the world by faculty members to be excellent public relations initiatives, so the time spent on trips to give presentations was not supposed to be taken from vacation time.

matter to transfer files on floppy disks from one computer to another. Since those early days I have always kept all my files on all my computers. With time the method of transferring files has changed; the thumb drive I now use for this purpose has a much higher capacity than the old floppies. There was similar progress in computing power and in software. There were new versions of WordPerfect, Quattro Pro replaced Lotus, Harvard Graphics superseded 35 mm Express, and Microsoft Windows supplanted DOS. With programs like Word, Excel and PowerPoint, Microsoft dominates the market these days, but I have to confess that I liked Harvard Graphics very much — and I still do. On my home computers in Columbia and Kraków, and on my Sony laptop, I still have a copy of Harvard Graphics 4 from 1996. It is difficult to give a presentation using the software nowadays, as PowerPoint is the only program available in conference rooms. Still, I like the colors in Harvard Graphics, so I frequently prepare slides using the program, copy, and then present them using PowerPoint.

It turned out that my prediction that we could make do with one less secretary did not materialize, as the total workload in the division increased. Peggy Gray left the division in 1992 and the Division hired Claire Oser, who, in addition to normal secretarial work, took on conference-related tasks, such as sending invitations to potential speakers and keeping track of their responses. She also helped with telephone calls from patients and paged us if needed, such as with renewing prescriptions or fixing appointments. Administrative Associates also changed. Jag Gill left the division for a higher position and was replaced by Ann Reeves, and then Alice Nichols, who remained for a few years. Joining in 1999, Carla Pudenz was originally the Administrative Associate for our division, but in 2003 there was a change in the organization of the Department of Medicine, and she became the Administrative Associate for several divisions, including nephrology.

In addition to publications related to our research, we wrote review papers. One has to review the literature for a particular topic as well as analyze the subject thoroughly. Such papers can be excellent teaching tools. In the early 1980s, various options were available for blood purification in acute renal failure. Andre Kaplan wrote a paper on continuous arteriovenous ultrafiltration and submitted it to the *Annals of Internal Medicine*. The editors asked Dr. Nolph and me to review the paper and write an editorial on the available methods, indications and contraindications for their use. We reviewed the available options — intermittent peritoneal dialysis, continuous peritoneal dialysis, hemodialysis, hemofiltration and continuous hemofiltration — and suggested choices depending on the cause of renal failure and concomitant diseases [Pu 75].

On March 21, 1989, I became a naturalized U.S. citizen and received a U.S. passport, which allowed me to travel to various countries without a visa. I kept my Polish citizenship, however, as did Halina, who was naturalized on May 22, 1992. As permitted by American and Polish law, we would begin the next chapter in our lives as citizens of both our homeland and our adopted country.

ized in the preceding section. The approach that gave the best result in the pre‑test is applied in the actual test.

CHAPTER 7

Cooperation with Fellows, Laboratory Visitors, Nurses and Technicians

Fellows

Every year, we had new fellows, many of them from abroad. Some achieved high positions after returning to their native countries. During the time I was a faculty member and before my retirement, there were 41 fellows. I undertook various studies and published many papers with them. In 1981 the fellows were Hans Gloor, MD, Garry Reams, MD, and Michael Young, DO. I knew Hans Gloor for only a few weeks, as he was preparing to leave when I arrived. After finishing his fellowship in 1983, Michael Young entered private practice in Jefferson City. Garry Reams was very interested in hypertension, so he collaborated mostly with John Bauer, MD, and Stephen Brooks, MD. He then became a faculty member and later a Deputy Director of Dialysis Clinic Inc. in Columbia, Missouri. Hans Gloor returned to Switzerland, where he worked in the Kantonsspital Schaffhausen in Geissberg. I prepared just one paper with Hans Gloor and Michael Young, and two with Garry Reams as coauthor [Pu 96, Pu 346]. In 1982 Sobha Sunderrajan, MD, became a fellow; as I already mentioned, it was her friend who sold us our present house on Devine Court. She was my coauthor for only one paper [Pu 78]. After completing the fellowship, she left to practice nephrology in Huntington Beach, California. Three physicians started fellowships in 1983: Perry Lovinggood, MD, Sunder Lal, MD, and Laust Nielsen, MD. While I did not coauthor a paper with Dr. Lovinggood, I published one paper with Laust Nielsen [Pu 114] and two with Sunder Lal [Pu 109, Pu 115]. Dr. Nielsen returned to Denmark to work at a hospital in Gentofte, a suburb of Copenhagen. Dr. Lal later became a faculty member at our division with a major interest in transplantation.

In 1984 three physicians from abroad began fellowships: Hannelore Hain, MD, Antonio Scalamogna, MD, and Erkki Lampainen, MD. Along with other coauthors, Dr. Hain and I coauthored three papers [Pu 94, Pu 110, Pu 115] before she returned to West Germany to work in nephrology in the Department of Internal Medicine, Klinikum Westendder Freien, Universität Berlin. I remember that Dr. Hain had never been to East Germany, but her views on the communist system were very positive; she called it a "system of social justice." Having lived in a communist system, I argued that I had never seen any social justice, only the majority living in poverty and affluence reserved for a tiny percentage of people in high posts of the ruling party. Discussing the topic on the sidelines of our dialysis conference, her point of view changed completely and she could finally appreciate the differences between East and West Germany in the early 1990s after Reunification. Dr. Scalamogna worked with me on the problem of intraabdominal pressure and we coauthored one paper [Pu 102] before his return to work in Italy as a nephrologist in Ospedale Policlinicadi Milano. Dr. Lampainen was the first author of a paper coauthored with me on the significance of the air under the diaphragm in CAPD patients [Pu 107]. After completing his fellowship, he went back to Finland to work in the Department of Medicine, Kuopio University Hospital, Kuopio. A member of the Finnish Registry for Kidney Diseases, Dr. Lampainen attends our dialysis conference almost every year.

In 1985, we had three new fellows, two of which were from abroad: Zeev Gluck, MD, from Switzerland, Robert Mactier, MD, MRCP, from the U.K., and James Frock, MD, from the U.S. Dr. Gluck coauthored one paper related to peritoneal clearances with various schedules [Pu 106]. After his year long fellowship ended, he became Chief of the Department of Nephrology in the Regional Hospital in Biel, Switzerland. Dr. Frock coauthored a paper on tidal peritoneal dialysis [Pu 166]. Dr. Mactier, despite a heavy clinical schedule, was very productive in the area of research. After we determined that there was a high absorption of polymers through lymphatics, he and Dr. Khanna embarked on a study of the problem (see below). Dr. Mactier coauthored several papers related to this and other problems, and he was the first author of most of them [Pu 108, Pu 113, Pu 116, Pu 117, Pu 123, Pu 124, Pu 126-128, Pu 133, Pu 135, Pu 161-163]. After completing a two-year fellowship, he assumed a position as a consultant in the Renal Unit of Stobhill General Hospital in Glasgow, Scotland.

We received three new fellows in 1986. Two of them were from the U.S., Kimberly Jamison, MD, and June Symens, MD, and they neither undertook research nor coauthored a paper with me. After finishing their fellowships, they both began practicing nephrology, Dr. Jamison in private practice in Columbia, Missouri, and Dr. Symens in Medford, Oregon. Three new internists started fellowships in 1987: Halina Krutak-Król, MD,

Salah Reyad, MD, and Fevzi Ersoy, MD. Dr. Krutak-Król graduated in Poland and was married to a cardiologist in the department. She was the first author of a paper on a mysterious case of accessory parathyroid gland, which we had difficulty of localizing [Pu 147]. She and her husband moved to New York after her one-year fellowship. While Dr. Reyad and I did not do any research together, Dr. Ersoy coauthored one paper with me on computerized tomography for the determination of intraabdominal fluid distribution and the diagnosis of complications in peritoneal dialysis patients [Pu 154], as well as coauthoring several presentations at various meetings [Pr 187, Pr 206, Pr 211, Pr 212, Pr 332, Pr 360]. Dr. Ersoy returned to the Department of Medicine, Akdeniz University Medical School Hospital in Antalya, Turkey, where he joined the faculty and later advanced to the rank of full professor.

In 1988, we had two new fellows from Bombay, India: NM Dedhia, MD, and Alan Fernandes Almeida, MD. Dr. Almeida and I did not collaborate on any papers or presentations, but Dr. Dedhia coauthored two papers, one on peritoneal membrane transport changes after incidental intraperitoneal infusion of sodium hypochlorite [Pu 148], and one already mentioned on computerized tomography for intraperitoneal fluid distribution, with Dr. Ersoy as another coauthor [Pu 154]. The following year we had three new fellows: Terry Ketchersid, MD, Mark Vaporean, MD, and Lakhan Saha, MD. Dr. Ketchersid gave two presentations as first author, with Dr. Ersoy and me as coauthors, on catheter position in pertioneal dialysis patients [Pr 332, Pr 360]. He moved to Des Moines, Iowa, after completing his fellowship. Neither Dr. Vaporean nor Dr. Saha did any research with me, and after their fellowships went into private practice in Columbia, Mo., and Columbus, Ohio, respectively.

Shahabul Arfeen, MD, and David Rosborough, MD, started their fellowships in 1990. Dr. Rosborough and I did not collaborate on research papers or presentations, though he coauthored one paper with Dr. Nolph, and Dr. Arfeen coauthored one presentation with me [Pr 385]. After their respective fellowships, Dr. Arfeen moved to Gary, Indiana, and Dr. Rosborough to Peoria, Ill.

Three new fellows, Nalini Vassa, MD, Robyn Jacobs, MD, and Todd Broome, MD, started in 1991. Dr. Vassa was the first author of a presentation [Pr 345] and a paper on hypebaric oxygen therapy in calciphylaxis-induced skin necrosis in peritoneal dialysis patients [Pu

204] as well as a paper on leucocyte kinetics in patients with peritonitis on long-term peritoneal dialysis [Pu 223]. I did not do research or publish with Dr. Jacobs or Dr. Broome, but Dr. Jacobs coauthored two papers with Dr. Nolph. She moved to Kansas City, Mo., Dr. Broome to Huntsville, Alabama, and Dr. Vassa to Medical Arts Clinic Inc. in Farmington, Missouri.

Richard A. Jensen, MD, and Hariprasad Trivedi began their fellowships in 1992. Dr. Jensen coauthored two papers on the association between patient weight, various exchange volumes, and urea clearances [Pu 199, Pu 212], and Dr. Trivedi coauthored a paper [Pu 211] and four presentations [Pr 371, Pr 376, Pr 377, Pr 385] Dr. Jensen moved to Sioux Falls, South Dakota, while Dr. Trivedi went into clinical nephrology in the VA hospital in Columbia, Missouri. He and I published a second paper, which was on the use of heparin locked in intravenous catheters post previous hemodialysis for loading heparin before the next hemodialysis [Pu 260].

In 1993, the new fellows were Brajesh Bhatla, MD, Pranay Kathuria, MD, and Oleg Georgiev, MD. While Dr. Georgiev did not coauthor any papers or presentations with me, Dr. Bhatla was the first author of a paper on pertitoneal access [Pu 234]. All three left in 1995, Dr. Bhatla to Harlingen, Texas, Dr. Georgiev to Lexington, Mississippi, and Dr. Kathuria to Bixby, Oklahoma. Dr. Kathuria was the first author of a presentation we gave on silver coated peritoneal catheters in rats [Pr 387], which was later published [Pu 248]. He also coauthored two papers on transport kinetics in peritoneal dialysis patients [Pu 254, Pu 258], and three chapters in a peritoneal dialysis handbook a few years after leaving our division [Pu 298, Pu 378, Pu 379].

Sharad Goel, MD, Rajnish Mehrotra, MD, and Rajiv Saran, MD, began fellowships in 1994. Dr. Goel coauthored three papers. One, as first author, was related to the influence of patient noncompliance on peritoneal transport of small solutes [Pu 229]; the second was on protein loss in peritoneal dialysis, with Dr. Kathuria as first author [Pu 258]; the third was in connection with the effect of antibiotic prophylaxis on the healing of catheter exit sites in rats [Pu 266]. Dr. Goel left our division in 1996 and moved to Cincinnati, Ohio. Dr. Mehrotra coauthored one presentation on silver coated peritoneal dialysis catheters in rats [Pr 387] and a paper on the same topic [Pu 248]. He was also the first author of two papers, one on the calculation of dialysate to plasma creatinine at 6 hours from the 4-hour peritoneal equilibration test [Pu 254], and one on targets for initiation of peritoneal dialysis [Pu 259]. Dr. Mehrotra moved to Philadelphia, Pennsylvania and later to Los Angeles, California. Dr. Saran spent three years as a fellow and then as a research associate. He then moved to the Division of Nephrology and Kidney Epidemiology and Cost Center at the University of Michigan in Ann Arbor, Michigan, where he remains very active in dialysis outcome practice pattern study (DOPPS). He coauthored five papers while in Columbia. Two were clinical papers: one, for which he was the first author, was about the use of urokinase infusion in hemodialysis patients [Pu 310]; the second was related to peritoneal dialysis, with Dr. Mehrotra as first author [Pu 259]. Other papers were on glycosylation end-products in diabetic rats on peritoneal dialysis [Pu 314, Pu 317] and on absorption of iron dextran from peritoneal dialysis solutions [Pu 318]. This latter study was also presented at the Annual Meeting of the American Society of Nephrology [Pr 457]. Later, when Dr. Saran continued to work in DOPPS, I asked him to look into the influence on mortality of longer hemodialysis and slower ultrafiltration. Published in 2006, with Dr. Saran as first author [Pu 363], that study confirmed my assumption that the mortality should be reduced with longer dialysis time.

In 1995, our fellows were Talha H. Imam, MD, Jones Samuel, MD, and Kumari Usha, MD. I neither did research nor work on papers or presentations with Drs. Imam and Samuel. Dr. Imam moved to Beckley, West Virginia, after a year long fellowship, and Dr. Samuel moved to Plaquemine, Louisiana, after two years. Dr. Usha was the first author of a paper on the repair of chronic peritoneal dialysis catheters [Pu 275], which I had taught her, and she also coauthored a paper on outpatient high dose urokinase [Pu 310]. Dr. Usha moved to Houston, Texas, after completing her two-year fellowship.

Katharina V. Meyer, MD, Sajjad Habid, MD, and Madhukar Misra, MD, started fellowships in 1996. Dr. Habid did not do research with me. Dr. Meyer was the first author of a paper on creatinine kinetics in peritoneal dialysis [Pu 268]; its second author was Vijaya Venkataraman, MD, who started a fellowship in 1998. Dr. Misra, who came from the U.K., coauthored several papers with me. The first concerned a case of green urine. We were called for consult on a patient with ulcerative colitis and several complications including renal insufficiency. Residents also noted that the color of the patient's urine was green. The patient was on an oral feeding tube with FD&C Blue No. 1,[1] a nonabsorbable food color that is routinely added to facilitate early diagnosis of aspiration. We determined that the green color was a result of this blue colorant being absorbed by the patient and mixed with the naturally yellow urine. The first two authors of the paper were students on consulting duty, with Dr. Misra as a fellow and me as an attending [Pu 280]. Dr. Misra coauthored three more papers with me [Pu 263, Pu 313, Pu 358]. He ultimately became a faculty member in our division and was involved in the hemodialysis part of our annual conference (which I will talk about later in the book). In 2010, we coauthored an editorial for the *New England Journal of Medicine* [Pu 383] (which I will also come back to later).

Laboratory Visitors

Every year we had visitors who worked in our laboratory in the VA and later in Dalton Research Center. In 1983 we had Charalambos Stathakis, MD, from Athens, Greece, and Mirosława Poskuta, a student from Poland who came to the U.S. with her father, a high-ranking party member, and who spent her summer vacation in our laboratory. They helped with some studies on polymers and we published a paper with them as coauthors [Pu 81]. Medical students worked in our laboratory during vacations. In 1990, Thomas W. Chen worked with me, published one paper as first author [Pu 179], and coauthored six presentations [Pr 238, Pr 243, Pr 253, Pr 254, Pr 266, Pr 267]. We also had some visitors from Poland. That same year, I helped Dr. hab. med. Alicja Grzegorzewska from the Department of Nephrolgy at the Medical Academy in Poznań to get a stipend for a year's work in the laboratory at Dalton Research Center. At the time I had suspended my work in the laboratory and was concentrating on clinical research, so she worked mostly with Dr. Nolph, Harold Morre

---

1. Aqueous solution of (a) disodium salt of ethyl [4-[p[ethyl(m-sulphobenzyl)amino]-α-(o-sulphophenyl)benzylidene]-2,5-cyclohexadien-1-ylidene], (b) propylene glycol, and (c) propylparaben (0.1%) and sulfites as preservatives.

and Thomas Chen. Her major area of study was carbon dioxide transport in pertitoneal dialysis in rats. This transport is markedly higher than urea transport, and carbon dioxide clearance is very close to the blood flow in peritoneal capillaries.[2] Dr. Grzegorzewska, now a full professor, regularly attends our Annual Dialysis Conference and gives presentations on interesting topics related mostly to peritoneal dialysis.

Katarzyna Wieczorowska, from the Department of Pathophysiology of the University Medical School in Poznań, visited the lab in 1994. She worked on the reproducibility of the peritoneal equilibration test in rats [Pu 209] and on peritoneal fibrosis [Pu 230, Pr 396]. Kazuyuki Suzuki visited from the Division of Nephrology at Sendai Shakaihoken Hospital in Miyagi, Japan. As my coauthor, he undertook several interesting studies, published various papers and gave several presentations, on the absorption of iron from the peritoneal cavity of rats [Pu 210, Pu 232, Pr 375, Pr 389], on white blood cell counts and differentials in a rat model of peritoneal dialysis [Pu 225, Pr 390], on peritonitis and peritoneal fibrosis in rats [Pu 231, Pr 388], on the effects of bicarbonate dialysis solution on peritoneal transport in rats [Pu 247], and on the peritoneal equilibration test in rats [Pr 402].

In 1996, Roberto F. S. Pecoits-Filho, MD, visited from the Department of Nephrology, Universidade Federal do Paraná, Curitiba, Paraná, Brazil, which was chaired by Dr. Miguel Carlos Riella. He coauthored two papers with me: one on antibiotic prophylaxis and the healing of catheter exit sites in rats [Pu 266], and another on the toxicity of intraperitoneal iron dextran in rats. We did not find any signs of toxicity [Pu 267].

Jeong H. Lee, from South Korea, visited the lab in 1997. He worked on glycosylation end-products and published two papers as first author [Pu 314, Pu 317]. He also worked on peritoneal dialysis in iron deficient rats with solutions containing iron dextran [Pu 318, Pr 457]. That same year, another South Korean visitor, Yong-Lim Kim, MD, PhD, coauthored two papers [Pu 266, Pu 267] and a presentation [Pr 435]. Now a professor of medicine, he is Director of the Division

---

2. Grzegorzewska AE, Moore HL, Chen TW, Nolph KD. (1992) Peritoneal clearances of carbon dioxide in the rat. *Adv Perit Dial* **8**: 26–29.

of Nephrology in the Department of Medicine at Kyungpook National University Hospital, in Jung-gu, Daegu, South Korea.

In 1998, Dr. Dheerendra Reddy visited from India, coauthoring four papers related to peritoneal dialysis in rats [Pu 282, Pu 314, Pu 317, Pu 318]. His real name is Kommala and he is now Medical Director and Division Head of Renal and Metabolics at Mitsubishi Tanabe Pharma Development America in Warren, New Jersey.

Nurses and Technicians

I have already mentioned my collaboration with "Barb" and I will describe that collaboration in detail later, but I have collaborated with many other nurses over the years — and published papers with them. These nurses worked at Dialysis Clinic Inc., initially located at Walnut Street and from January 1992 at 3300 LeMone Industrial Boulevard. Lois M. Schmidt coauthored eight papers, nine abstracts and nine presentations with me; Leonor (Ryan) Ponferrada, 15 abstracts, 12 presentations and 19 publications; Lavonne M. Burrows, five abstracts, three presentations and five publications; Barbara Pickett, four abstracts, three presentations and two publications; Roberta Satalowich, six abstracts, five presentations and eight publications; Michael S. Klusmeyer, one abstract, one presentation and one publication; Ron Usovsky, one publication; and J. M. Kennedy, one presentation and one publication.

Several technicians worked with me in the VA Hospital, Dalton Research Center, and the Dialysis Clinic laboratory. I worked with Carole A. Hopkins and Paul A. Brown in 1976 and 1977, and with Terry J. McGary and Harold L. Moore from 1981. Terry left the laboratory in 1986. Most of the laboratory papers, abstracts and presentations were coauthored by Harold. Jim Haynie performed various duties in Dialysis Clinic Inc., including providing computer services and some laboratory services. He worked with me on blood recirculation in intravenous catheters, dialyzer blood flow, and hemolysis in relation to negative inflow pressure before the pump in arterial tubing to the dialyzer.

CHAPTER 8

Major Research in the 1980s

Insulin Binding to Peritoneal Dialysis Bags

Peritoneal dialysis solutions in bags were introduced in the U.S. in 1978. Many patients with diabetes had already been treated with peritoneal dialysis. It was found that insulin was absorbed from the peritoneal cavity, so intraperitoneal delivery of insulin seemed to be very convenient. It was also found that the required dose of insulin delivered via peritoneal dialysis solution was about twice as high as it was when administered subcutaneously. There were several attempts at explanation. One was that the bags bound insulin by absorption or some other mechanism, but the amount of bound insulin was not precisely determined. In very precise experiments, using radioactive porcine insulin [Pu 67], we ascertained that the binding is mainly physical, according to surface phenomena. We found that a very large amount of insulin was trapped in foam.[1] This indicated that insulin behaved like a surfactant [Pu 68]. We determined some chemical binding (chemisorption) or diffusion of insulin into plastic, but it was minuscule and overall binding (adsorption plus absorption) did not exceed 10 percent of the injected amount [Pu 69].

Serositis in Renal Failure

Shortly after my arrival in Columbia, I started a study on serositis in renal failure. It has long been known that serositis (pericarditis, pleuritis and peritonitis) may occur in renal failure patients 1–3 weeks after bacterial or viral infection. For me, this situation resembled a sequence of events similar to that in immune complex-induced diseases. I hypothesized that serositis may be related to the presence of circulating immune complexes (CIC), which cannot be efficiently removed by dialysis or failing kidneys. The study was done in collaboration with the Division of Cardiology at the University of Missouri. CIC levels were measured by the Division of Rheumatic Diseases at the University of Colorado in Denver. The study in 71 patients confirmed my suspicions, as the levels of CIC were significantly higher in patients with serositis

---

1. Each system tends to minimize free energy. Substances decreasing surface tension like surfactants or detergents are preferentially adsorbed on air–liquid interfaces, particularly since the surface area of the foam is extremely large.

compared to those without evidence of serosal inflammation. In addition, immune complex-like materials were found in all of the four effusate samples (from pericardial or pleural fluid) and in 10 of 27 peritoneal dialysates. We suggested that immune complexes might be the "uremic toxins" responsible for the serositis in renal failure and may be secreted into serous effusions. Immune complex-like material can be removed in peritoneal dialysate, which may contribute to the lower CIC levels and lower incidence of serositis in CAPD patients. The results of this study were presented in part during a meeting of the European Society for Artificial Organs [Pr 43], published as an abstract in the proceedings [Ab 12], and later published in full [Pu 71].

Polymers as Osmotic Agents in Peritoneal Dialysis

One of my goals was to work on polymer solutions to achieve sustained ultrafiltration in long-dwell peritoneal dialysis exchanges. This was an extension of the studies we undertook in 1977, as discussed earlier, as well as being the impetus for Dr. Nolph's original suggestion that I come to work in his laboratory in Columbia. At the time all peritoneal dialysis solutions contained glucose as an osmotic agent. Glucose has several disadvantages. The absorption of glucose from the peritoneal cavity diminishes the osmotic gradient between the peritoneal dialysis solution and the plasma, and is sometimes associated with poor ultrafiltration, particularly in long-dwell exchanges. In addition, glucose is almost completely absorbed, so it contributes to obesity and hypertriglyceridemia in many patients.

To achieve our goal, we created a simulated peritoneal dialysis system (Fig. 24) to study polymer electrolyte solutions *in vitro* [Pu 74]. The system was composed of "peritoneal cavity" with capillary hemodialyzer and dialysis solution in a container, "plasma" space, and "extravascular" space. We did not know what would be an ideal electrolyte composition of the polymer solution, as part of the electrolytes would be bound to negatively charged polymer and would not be osmotically active. Therefore, after dissolving the poly(acrylic acid), we dialyzed it against a polyelectrolyte solution of desired composition in a hollow-fiber dialyzer with a hydrostatic pressure higher on the polymer side. After several hours, the composition of outflowing

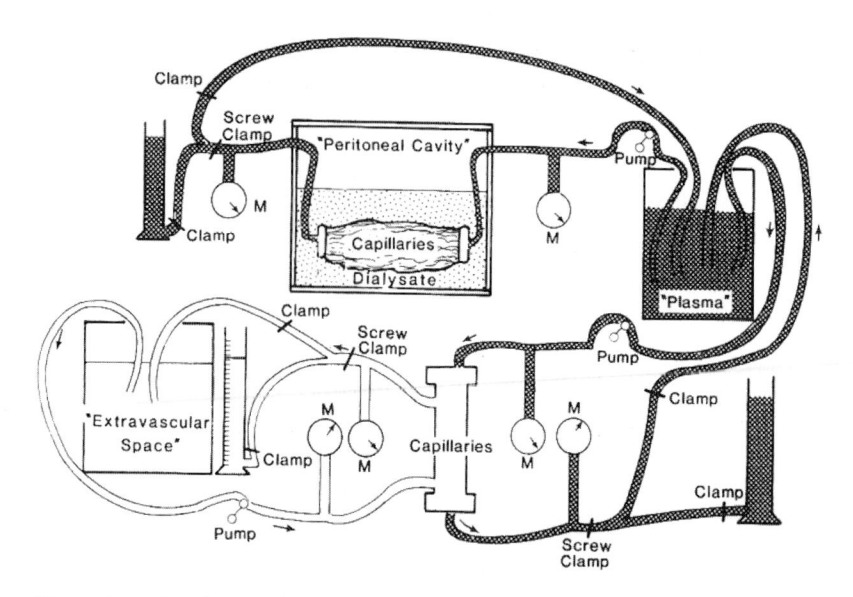

Figure 24. Simulation of a peritoneal dialysis system; diagram of the experimental set-up. (Reprinted from Pu 74.)

electrolyte solution was identical to the inflowing solution, so we assumed that the composition was exactly as desired. When this solution was used in the simulated peritoneal dialysis system, we obtained sustained ultrafiltration for 24 hours with a decrease in volume of "plasma" and "extravascular" space. This contrasted with the use of glucose based solution (Dianeal 4.25 percent), which gave only 3- to 6-hour dialysis, and a decrease in "plasma" and "extravascular" space, as glucose also moved between spaces. We started with poly(acrylic acid) as an inexpensive polymer. Then, after gaining some experience, we repeated the experiment with the more costly polymer, dextran sulfate, which gave results similar to that of poly(acrylic acid). This was very encouraging and we made plans to conduct animal studies.

Encouraged by *in vitro* studies, we began testing the solutions on rats and rabbits. We did not have a rabbit model of peritoneal dialysis, so I asked Dr. Przemysław Hirszel, who was then working in the Division of Nephrology at the Uniformed Services University of the Health Sciences in Bethesda, Md., to perform some peritoneal dialysis with polymers in rabbits. Dr. Hirszel agreed, and the studies commenced in 1983. We prepared the solutions as previously described and found that both poly(acrylate) sodium and dextran sulfate sodium gave sustained ultrafiltration, similar to that obtained *in vitro*, but damaged the peritoneum, causing bleeding. We also tested polyethylenamine, which turned out to be extremely toxic. The results were even worse in rabbits, which died of internal bleeding [Pu 81]. This was obviously a disappointment.

We began looking for less toxic solutions. I recalled that in the late 1940s surgeons from Harvard Medical School in Boston, Massachusetts, used gelatin as an osmotic agent.[2] They did not give details, but it was clear that gelatin was not toxic. We started experiments with crude Knox gelatin, preparing it using the method we employed in experiments with synthetic polymers. While 4.4 percent solution barely prevented adsorption of dialysate, 9 percent solution gave high and sustained ultrafiltration for up to 7 hours. The peritoneal membrane looked normal under light microscopy. The main problem with crude gelatin was its high viscosity, gelation at room temperature, and difficult sterilization. Thus, we decided to try gelatin derivatives, used previously as plasma substitutes: oxypolygelatin (Gelifundol), succinylated gelatin (Plasmagel), and gelatin isocyanate (Haemaccel). These derivatives were known to be nonimmunogenic, with molecular weights of 20–35 kDa, so we suspected that they would not be absorbed from the peritoneal cavity. The problem was that they were not available in the U.S. We presented our findings at the Travenol's headquarters [Pr 52, Pr 59], and they were very interested. They offered financial support for our Nephrology Research Fund, promised to buy Haemaccel from Hoechst (West Germany) and Gelifundol from Biotest (Dreieich, West Germany), and promised to pay for the patent application submitted though the University. We filed an application in June 1984 [Pa II-1], and presented and published our results [Pr 60, Pu 81, Pu 94]. We were very optimistic, of course, that we had found something of value and expressed our optimism in an editorial review published in 1986 [Pu 93], before conducting more studies.

In the meantime we continued our studies on rats using Haemaccel and Gelifundol. Sustained ultrafiltration was achieved, but

---

2. Frank HA, Seligman AM, Fine J, *et al.* (1948) Further experiences with peritoneal irrigation for acute renal failure. *Ann Surg* **128**(3): 561–608.

we found that absorption of gelatins ranged from 40–60 percent in 6 hours, which was a shocking discovery. It was clear that such big molecules were absorbed through lymphatics [Pr 70, Pu 110]. Initially, we speculated that lymphatic absorption in humans might be lower. But after discussions we came to the conclusion that the absorption would be too high anyway, and we decided to abandon the idea of studying gelatins in our patients. This was something of a disappointment, but the findings led to our later studies on lymphatic absorption in humans. These studies were continued mainly by Ramesh Khanna [Pu 108] and by Robert Mactier, a research fellow who had come from Glasgow, Scotland [Pu 122, Pu 124, Pu 128, Pu 133, Pr 90, Pr 102, Pr 103]. The limitations of the gelatin studies also stimulated me to work with glucose-containing dialysis solutions on dialysis techniques suitable for patients with various peritoneal transport characteristics. Ultimately, our patent [Pa II-1] was abandoned in 1989.

High Volume Exchange Peritoneal Dialysis

Studies on high volume exchanges were a continuation of ideas of mine already explored in Lublin, where we tried to use higher volume exchanges to decrease the number of exchanges per day. At that time we only used 2.5 L volumes. The availability of solutions in 3 L plastic bags was instrumental in facilitating measurements. They had already been used for continuous cyclic peritoneal dialysis (CCPD), developed by José Diaz-Buxo and colleagues in 1981.[3] Our study on high volume exchanges was mainly conducted by Barb and me, with the help of the Pulmonary Division of our Department of Medicine [Pu 66]. We performed anthropometry on 18 patients and measured intra-abdominal pressures and pulmonary functions in relation to intraperitoneal fluid volumes. We found that, similar to our studies in Lublin, pulmonary function was a very important determinant of the tolerance of increased volume in a patient. Intra-abdominal pressure was low in the supine position and increased by only 1.97 cm of water per liter of intraperitoneal volume (Fig. 25). Pressures were higher in the upright position and highest in the sitting position (2.72 and 2.80 cm of

---

3. Diaz-Buxo JA, Farmer CD, Walker PJ, *et al.* (1981) Continuous cyclic peritoneal dialysis — A preliminary report. *Artif Organs* **5**: 157–161.

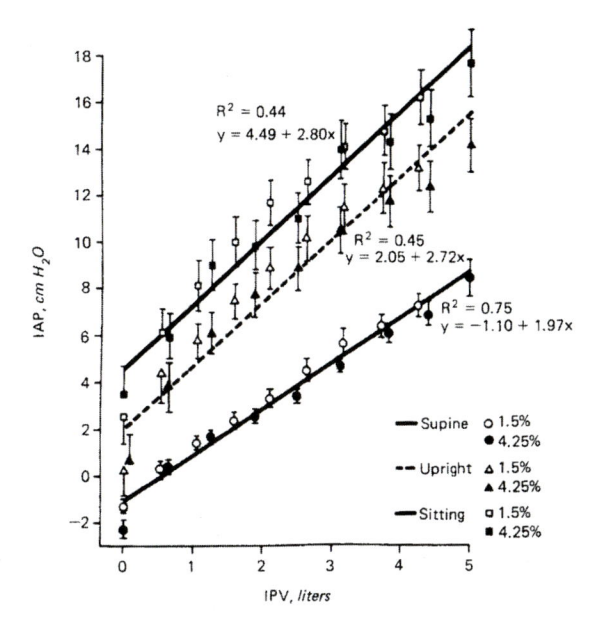

Figure 25. Intraperitoneal pressure related to calculated intraperitoneal volume at the umbilicus level. (Reprinted from Pu 66.)

water per liter, respectively). There was no correlation between the intra-abdominal pressure and the tolerance of higher volumes for routine dialysis. After the study we offered patients the possibility of using three 3 L volumes instead of four 2 L volumes. Nine patients decided to use this new schedule routinely, five patients could not tolerate 3 L volumes, and two of them had difficulty tolerating 2 L volumes at night. One of these patients (73-year-old female) had polycystic renal disease; the other (66-year-old male) had diabetes mellitus. The remaining four patients used 3 L volume for some exchanges. The patients who did not tolerate high volume exchanges had forced vital capacity in the supine position declining with intraperitoneal volume above 2 L (Fig. 26). As a result of our study we postulated that multiple bag volumes should be available, including 1.5 L and 2.5 L, in order to individualize exchange volumes. The efficiency of high volume, low frequency dialysis was another topic of study. We experimented with three 3 L exchange volumes and found that this technique is more efficient than the standard technique with regard to small and mid-sized molecule clearances, but protein losses were almost identical. The

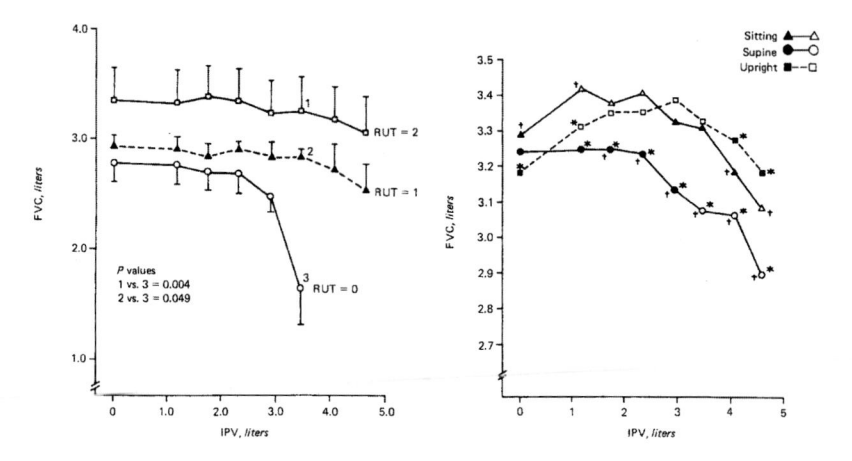

Figure 26. Left fig: Mean forced vital capacity in the supine position in relation to intraperitoneal volume. Patients designated as RUT = 0 did not routinely use 3 L volumes, RUT = 1 used 3 L volume for some exchanges, and RUT = 2 used 3 L volume for all exchanges. Right fig: Mean forced vital capacity in three positions in relation to intraperitoneal volume in 13 patients who tolerated up to 4 L intraperitoneal volume. (Reprinted from Pu 66.)

results were presented in part during a meeting of the American Society for Artificial Internal Organs [Pr 50] and published as an abstract [Ab 15] and in *ASAIO Transactions* in 1983 [Pu 73].

Intra-abdominal Pressure During Natural Activities in Patients with Intraperitoneal Fluid

At that time there were frequent reports of patients on CAPD developing dialysate leaks, hernias, cardiopulmonary compromise, and hemorrhoids. It was clear that these complications are related to the increased intra-abdominal pressure with the presence of dialysis solution. In our previous study we had already determined that in relaxed patients the intra-abdominal pressure increases, very little in the supine position and only slightly more in the sitting and standing positions. The pressures were measured with a pressure transducer secured at the level of the umbilicus (Fig. 27) in the supine, sitting and upright positions with 0–3 L of intraperitoneal fluid during talking, coughing, straining, changing position, walking, jogging, exercycling, jumping, and weightlifting. Coughing and straining generated the

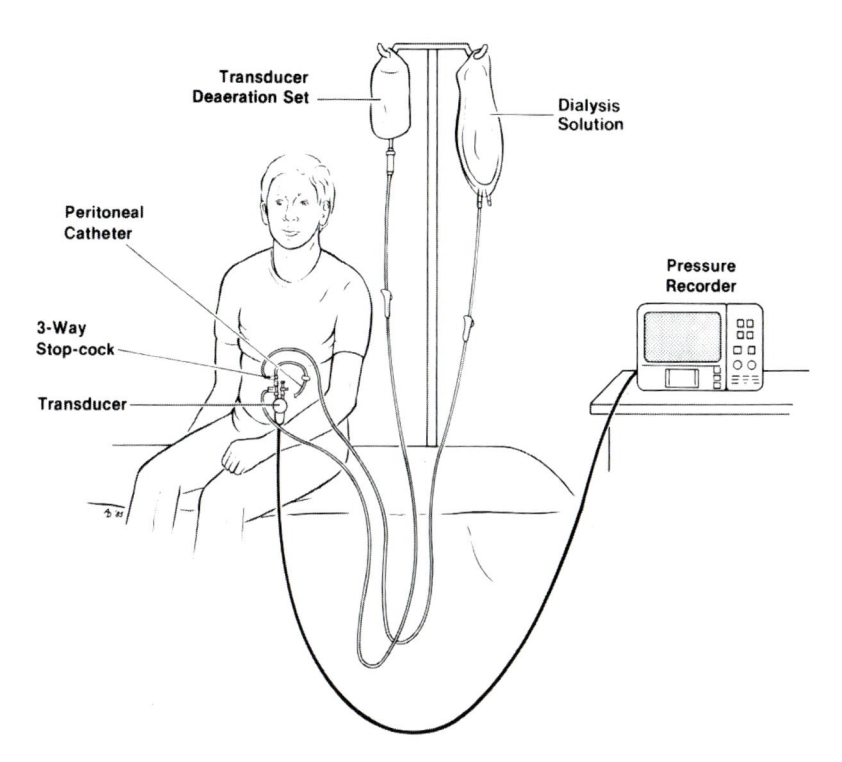

Figure 27. Experimental set-up for continuous intra-abdominal pressure monitoring. (Reprinted from Pu 102.)

highest intra-abdominal pressures in all positions (Fig. 28). The pressures associated with weightlifting were proportional to the magnitude of the weight lifted up to 50 lbs, but were lower than during coughing and straining. The pressures were generally higher with greater volumes of intra-abdominal fluid, especially with jumping and coughing. Exercycling was associated with lower intra-abdominal pressure than was jogging, and pressures were only minimally influenced by intraperitoneal volumes. The study indicated that from the intra-abdominal pressure point of view, exercycling is the most appropriate physical exercise for patients with intraperitoneal fluid [Pu 102].

Peritoneal Equilibration Test

When CAPD was introduced into clinical practice, it was assumed that patients had similar dialysis efficiencies, though it was observed

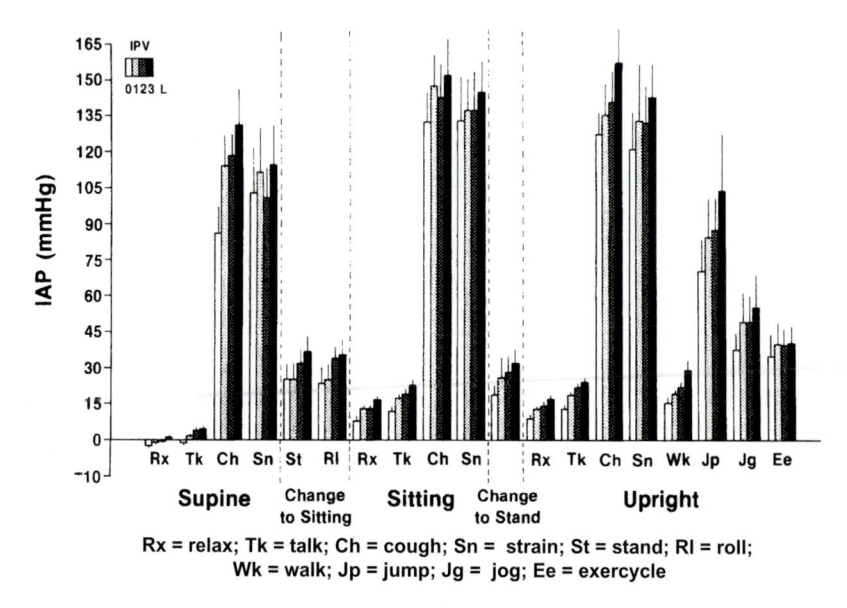

Figure 28. Intra-abdominal pressures (IAP) during natural activities with various intraperitoneal fluid volumes. (Reprinted from Pu 102.)

that ultrafiltration differed among patients. As mentioned above, in the late 1960s and early 1970s I studied protein losses during intermittent peritoneal dialysis in nine patients. Whereas remarkable differences in protein losses were found among patients, the losses were similar during consecutive dialyses in the same patients. I postulated that the wide "range of the protein loss is mainly due to the individual permeability of the peritoneum, which is characteristic of every patient; owing to individual differences in this permeability, each patient loses a different amount of protein under conditions which are considered identical" [Pu 12, Pu 12a].

The advent of continuous ambulatory peritoneal dialysis permitted us to study solute equilibration tests during long-dwell exchanges. We performed the first such studies in the original patient reported in 1978 [Pu 31] and later in five patients [Pu 35]. At the time we were interested in mean values, not individual patterns. Significant differences in ultrafiltration values among patients were noted during studies of peritoneal dialysis kinetics in the early 1980s [Pu 49]. While working on dialysis efficiency with high volume exchanges, we compared 12-hour ultrafiltration and equilibration curves with 2 L and 3 L volumes [Ab 15]. Though the variability was small, we again noted a striking interpatient variability in ultrafiltration values.

In 1984, I published the first paper presenting potential ranges of solute equilibrations among patients [Pu 77]. In this paper I stated that the individualization of dialysis prescription is absolutely necessary due to variations among patients in metabolic generation rate, residual renal function, intraperitoneal volume tolerance, and peritoneal mass transfer. At the time we were already in the process of developing a clinically useful peritoneal equilibration test (PET). Such a test would be useful if it were reproducible and stable, at least for a reasonable period of time. Unfortunately, it was frequently the case that a repeated test did not show similar results. Following the patients in the clinic, I observed remarkably stable serum chemistries in many patients. This indicated that peritoneal function must be stable and that the intrapatient variability in equilibration tests was due to a lack of standardization of the test.

Gradually I started to standardize the test. First of all there was the problem of selecting dextrose concentration. Solutions with dextrose concentrations of 1.5 percent, 2.5 percent and 4.25 percent were available in the early 1980s. We decided that the medium concentration was least likely to do any harm to patients. Since most of our patients were on CAPD, we decided that a long preceding exchange was most convenient. All other details of the technique were described in a paper published in 1987 [Pu 121]. A second paper on PET [Pu 119] was published that same year for the following reasons: the editors of the first paper wanted us to shorten it markedly (the first version was about twice as long as the final version) and we were forced to remove some crucial (in our opinion) information. The editors did not want us to include figures and tables based on the same values. We had figures in the first paper, as we considered them visually appealing and self-explanatory. The second paper contained tables with exact values, which we considered critical for the widespread acceptance of the test. In addition, the second paper contained information about the values of the test for diagnostic and dialysis modality planning purposes. An unabridged (or complete) test included dialysate to

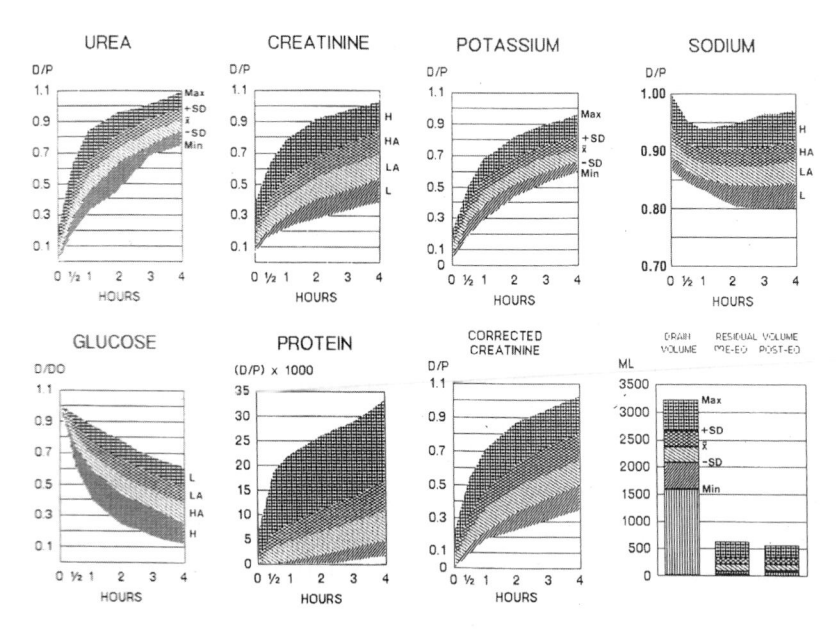

Figure 29. Peritoneal equilibration curves. (Reprinted from Pu 119.)

plasma concentration ratio (D/P) of urea, protein, creatinine, potassium, sodium and corrected creatinine,[4] as well as dialysate to dialysate at time zero[5] concentration ratio (D/D_0) of glucose, drain volume and residual volumes (Fig. 29). Prior to publication I wanted to present the test during the IVth Congress of the International Society for Peritoneal Dialysis in Venice and I submitted an abstract [Ab 51]. In fact, I submitted three abstracts as the first author and seven others as coauthor. Only two were not accepted for presentations. One of them was on peritoneal transport, an abstract I considered as describing a very important, original concept. I was in good company, as an abstract describing the concept of continuous peritoneal dialysis[6] was also not deemed suitable for presentation during the ASAIO meeting in 1976.

---

4. High glucose concentration in dialysate interferes with the Jaffe reaction, spuriously increasing creatinine concentration, so to obtain accurate creatinine concentration in dialysate the value has to be corrected.

5. Immediately after dialysis solution infusion.

6. Popovich RP, Moncrief JW, Decherd JB, et al. (1976) The definition of a novel portable/wearable equilibrium peritoneal dialysis technique. Abstracts, *Am Soc Artif Intern Organs* **5**: 64.

PET RESULTS

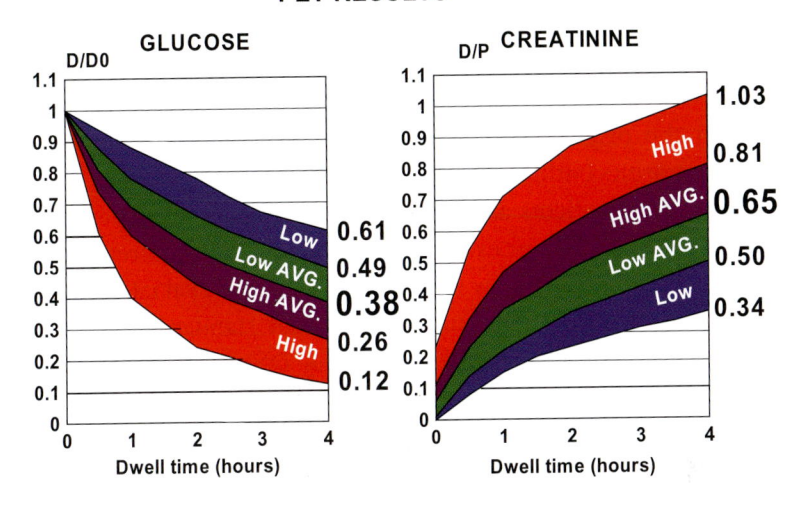

Figure 30. Transport categories designated as high, high average, low average and low.

PET is the most widely used peritoneal function test, because of its standardization and usefulness for diagnostic and prognostic purposes. An abridged test [Pu 144] looking only for D/D_0 glucose and D/P creatinine ratios, and drain volumes, is commonly used (Fig. 30). Based on PET, a computer model (PD Adequest, Baxter Healthcare Corporation, Round Lake, Ill.) has been developed that permits the prediction of small solute clearances and ultrafiltration for various alternative prescriptions of peritoneal dialysis. An excellent agreement between predicted and measured values has been validated in 111 patients.[7]

In the original PET, which established standard values for membrane categorization in 1987, glucose solution was used for the preceding exchange [Pu 119, Pu 121]. In recent years, many patients, particularly those with ultrafiltration problems, have used polyglucose solution for nightly exchanges. Lilaj et al.[8] found that polyglucose (icodextrin) containing solution used for the preceding exchange increases D/P ratios of creatinine, phosphate and sodium, as well as

---

7. Vonesh EF, Burkart J, McMurray SD, Williams PF. (1996) Peritoneal dialysis kinetic modeling: Validation in a multicenter clinical study. *Perit Dial Int* **16**(5): 471–481.
8. Lilaj T, Dittrich E, Puttinger H, *et al.* (2001) A preceding exchange with polyglucose versus glucose solution modifies peritoneal equilibration test results. *Am J Kidney Dis* **38**(1): 118–126.

glucose absorption, measured during the test. Therefore, they recommend that patients using icodextrin solution during the night should perform their night time exchange with conventional glucose solution before a scheduled PET. The preceding exchange dwell time was 8 hours in the original PET. This was convenient when almost all patients were on continuous ambulatory peritoneal dialysis. However, now that many patients are on some form of automated peritoneal dialysis (APD), an 8-hour exchange prior to the PET requires changes in the dialysis schedule. Our recent study [Pu 343] evaluated the differences in 2-hour equilibration curves with standard 8-hour and 3-hour preceding exchanges. The values for D/P creatinine and urea, as well as D/D_0 glucose, were almost identical throughout the 2-hour PET dwell after long and short exchanges. D/P protein values tended to be higher in the PET after the long exchange. We concluded that for creatinine and glucose equilibrations, any dwell time between 3 and 12 hours was acceptable for the preceding exchange, and the equilibration test may be performed with a 2- or 4-hour dwell, if the timing of sample taking is very accurate. The protein values obtained with a 3-hour prior dwell are different than with a long prior exchange [Pu 343]. This is not surprising, as our previous studies showed that protein transfer to the peritoneal cavity is steady and washout of protein in short preceding exchanges decreases protein concentration in dialysate during test exchanges.

For a full characterization of peritoneal membrane function, an unabridged test, as described in 1987 [Pu 119, Pu 121], should be used (Fig. 29). Although this test is extremely reliable and valuable for the characterization of peritoneal function, it is less frequently used than the abridged test because of the need for considerable nursing time. Nonetheless, it should be used in cases where full characterization of peritoneal function is necessary. An unabridged test should be performed shortly after the break-in period of peritoneal dialysis as a baseline for future comparisons.

Nightly Intermittent Peritoneal Dialysis

This kind of peritoneal dialysis was introduced in our center out of necessity in a patient who had suffered three failed kidney transplants and unsuccessful hemodialysis, CAPD, and twice weekly intermittent peritoneal dialysis (IPD) in 1983. The story of this patient, Mitzi Rosen, is described in detail later. It was already obvious that IPD was markedly less efficient compared to CAPD. Gradually we used nightly intermittent peritoneal dialysis (NIPD) in other patients with complications related to the constant presence of fluid in the peritoneal cavity, such as recurrent abdominal leaks and hernias, bladder prolapse, high peritoneal membrane permeability resulting in rapid glucose absorption and poor ultrafiltration, and abdominal discomfort with poor appetite. The major potential disadvantage of NIPD was insufficient clearance of solutes due to reduced dialysis time. At that time we had already had preliminary analysis of the PET in 82 patients, establishing four categories of solute transport rates: high, high average, low average, and low. In nine patients belonging to different transport categories, we compared clearances and ultrafiltration between CAPD and various NIPD schedules using inflow volumes of 14, 17, 20, 23 and 26 L per night on a PAC-X2 cycler [Pu 106]. The inflow, dwell and outflow times were varied to keep the total dialysis time close to 8 hours. It happened that the shortest inflow and outflow times and the longest total dwell time occurred with the 17 L inflow volume. The conclusions of the study were as follows: (i) NIPD at the maximum inflow of 26 L in 8 hours could not provide daily clearances comparable to CAPD except for urea and potassium in patients with above average peritoneal transport characteristics and for creatinine in patients with very high transport characteristics. (ii) Dialysis solution sodium concentration(s) should be lower than the currently available 132 mEq/L in order to compensate inadequate sodium removal. (iii) NIPD provided sufficient ultrafiltration at lower glucose concentration. (iv) Protein losses were similar to those on CAPD if NIPD was after 16 hours off dialysis; however, if NIPD immediately followed CAPD, protein losses were lower on NIPD. These results were similar to my previous results indicating that protein transport from the vascular to the extravascular space and thence to the peritoneal cavity proceeds at a steady rate independently of the presence or absence of the fluid in the peritoneal cavity. (v) With respect to dialysis efficiency, NIPD was superior to CAPD in patients with very high peritoneal membrane transport characteristics.

The efficiency of dialysis in NIPD was not linear in relation to the infusion volume. When analyzing data, I noted that dialysis clearances of small molecules with the schedule using 17 L of dialysis solution were slightly higher than those with schedules using 20 L and 23 L. This was a little puzzling, but it led me to the conclusion that there was some influence from the time of contact between the peritoneal membrane and the fluid, and it suggested the next study on tidal peritoneal dialysis.

Tidal Peritoneal Dialysis

In the 1960s, Boen observed that urea and creatinine clearances during rapid fluid exchange are higher with a solution inflow of 3 L/hour than 4 L/hour.[9] The findings were somewhat perplexing and not universally accepted. Our study on NIPD [Pu 106] strongly supported Boen's observations, suggesting that dialysis efficiency depends not only on the volume of solution used in a specified time, but also on the time of contact between the solution and the peritoneal membrane. These observations led to the idea of tidal peritoneal dialysis (TPD). In intermittent peritoneal dialysis the dialysate of each exchange is drained as completely as possible. With high dialysate flow, a high plasma-dialysate concentration gradient is maintained during dwell time, but at the beginning of inflow and at the end of outflow the area of contact between the peritoneal membrane and dialysate is not complete and solute diffusion is hampered (Fig. 31a). To eliminate this phenomenon, there were attempts to use so-called continuous flow peritoneal dialysis, where fluid was infused into the peritoneal cavity through one catheter and drained through another. This method had two disadvantages: firstly, two catheters were needed instead of one; secondly, the dialysis efficiency was not as high as expected because of the streaming of fluid from the inflow catheter to the outflow, leaving most of the fluid stagnant. The situation is akin to the wide river where most of the flow is through the middle and the water close to the banks is sluggish. TPD may be considered a hybrid of continuous and intermittent flow techniques, combining the

---

9. Boen ST. (1961) Kinetics of peritoneal dialysis: A comparison with the artificial kidney. *Medicine* **40**(3): 243–288.

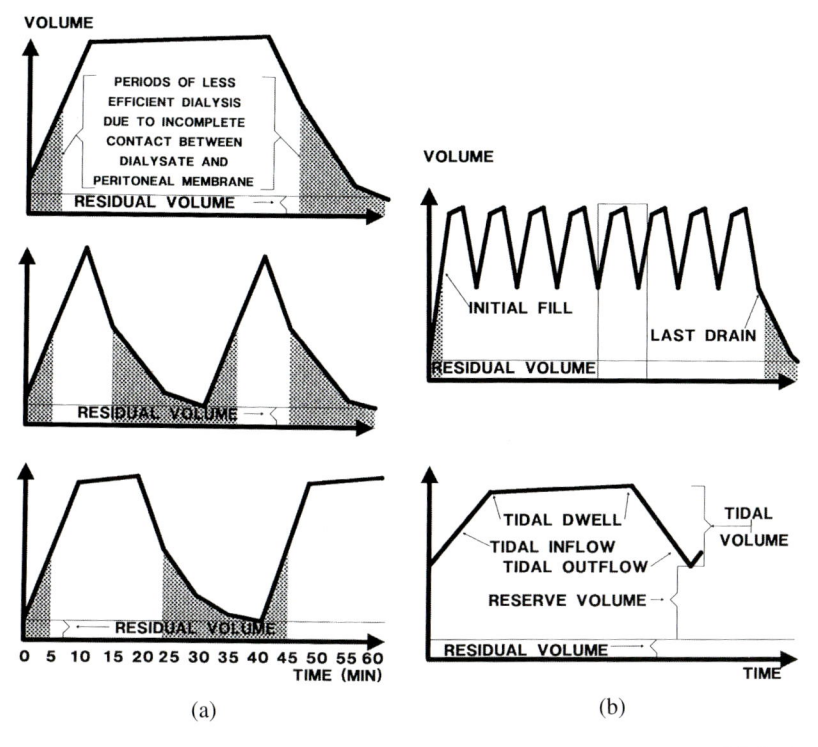

Figure 31. (a) Comparison of intraperitoneal volumes in regular peritoneal dialysis and tidal peritoneal dialysis. (b) Upper panel: intraperitoneal volumes during tidal peritoneal dialysis session; lower panel: terminology during single exchange. (Reprinted from Pu 142.)

advantages and eliminating the disadvantages of each. With tidal peritoneal dialysis, a bolus of fluid is infused into the peritoneal cavity at the beginning of treatment, but unlike a complete-volume drainage technique, only part of the fluid is drained. This leaves a reserve volume, on top of which a tidal volume of fresh solution is cycled (Fig. 31b). The idea was presented to Travenol [Pr 83] and the company decided to support the study. The term "tidal" was coined by Dr. James W. Dobbie, from the Research and Development Division at Baxter Travenol. He and others from Baxter participated in the study, including Rodney S. Kenley, with whom I cooperated on other projects later.

The study was performed on 12 patients, half with below mean peritoneal transport characteristics and half with above mean peritoneal transport characteristics. A comparison was made between 24-hour CAPD, 8-hour NIPD and 8-hour TPD. At the time we did not know how high intraperitoneal, tidal, total or reserve volumes ought to be. Using small tidal volumes would leave higher reserve volumes, which would be favorable for higher and longer contact between the fluid and the peritoneal membrane, but it would diminish mixing of the reserve volume with the tidal volume. We tried tidal volumes of 300 mL, 600 mL, 900 mL, 1200 mL and 1500 mL, with various reserve volumes. The highest efficiency turned out to be with 1500 mL tidal and reserve volumes, but schedules with 900 mL and 1200 mL tidal volumes were only slightly and insignificantly lower. Eight-hour TPD was about 20 percent more efficient than NIPD with regard to urea and creatinine clearance and may match CAPD in patients with above average peritoneal transport characteristics, but it was less efficient with respect to phosphate clearance. Protein losses were only slightly lower, but ultrafiltration volume was markedly higher per mass of absorbed glucose.

The results of the study were presented at several meetings in early 1987 [Pr 83, Pr 92, Pr 93, Pr 107], and published later [Pu 157, Pu 166, Pu 172]. After determining that TPD would be very successful if a large amount of dialysis solution were available, Baxter made the decision to develop a machine to manufacture peritoneal dialysis solution from concentrate and treated water. I was quite encouraged by the plans and in several papers I presented this idea as well as the principles of individualizing selection of the best peritoneal dialysis method for a patient [Pu 126, Pu 142, Pu 150]. I also contributed a comprehensive chapter on the topic [Pu 151] to a book I was co-editing at the time. Additionally, various peritoneal dialysis techniques and regimens were described in two papers on peritoneal dialysis glossary [Pu 130, Pu 153].

CHAPTER 9

Patients Who Inspired or Contributed to Progress

Alicja Balicka — Intrapericardial Corticosteroids for Uremic Pericarditis

Alicja Balicka, a 36-year-old white female office worker, apparently had no symptoms until a few days before admission to hospital. She was diagnosed with acute renal failure and referred to us in March 1966. The patient was anuric and semicomatose, and had pulmonary edema, a urea level of 285 mg/dL and creatinine of 13.4. After receiving peritoneal dialysis for a week, her condition improved and she regained consciousness. A history revealed that the patient had some symptoms for a few weeks before being admitted, X-ray showed small kidneys, and biopsy, chronic pyelonephritis with nephrocirrhosis, and nephrosclerosis.

This was our first patient with chronic renal failure on repeated hemodialysis. She had multiple complications, including severe neuropathy, pruritis, anemia, hypertension, heart failure and hyperparathyroidism. The patient also developed uremic pericarditis with a loud friction rub. There were no guidelines regarding treatment. The pericardial fluid was bloody, warning against the use of heparin. We did not have the capability to administer regional heparinization, so we decreased heparin as much as possible. Time and frequency of dialysis remained unchanged: 7-hour dialysis 10 times per month. On day 41 after admission the friction rub became softer, the heart sounds were muffled, blood pressure dropped, the jugular veins were markedly distended, pulsus paradoxus occurred, and the patient became comatose. It was clear to me that the patient had developed cardiac tamponade. I decided to perform pericardiocentesis through the substernal route. At that time no ultrasound was available to guide the needle. Using a long puncture needle on a 50 mL syringe, I located a fluid collection and aspirated the fluid, which appeared to be pure blood. I was scared that I had entered the right ventricle, but after aspiration of only 20 mL of fluid, Dr. Kłosowski, who was assisting me and checking her pulse, informed me that the pulse had strengthened. Ultimately I removed about 400 mL of fluid with a hematocrit of 2 percent. I was surprised how bloody the fluid looked with such a low hematocrit. The patient regained consciousness, blood pressure stabilized and pericardial friction rub recurred. The next day it appeared that the pericardial fluid was reaccumulating, and I asked

Dr. Kazimierz Łotkowski, Chairman of the Department of Surgery, to establish a continuous drainage of the pericardial sack through a polyethylene catheter. In addition to drainage, daily intrapericardial injections of hydrocortisone 125 mg via the catheter were instituted [Pu 8]. After 8 days there was no fluid drained and pericardial fiction rub disappeared after 13 days. In the paper we published relating the case, we claimed that we used the method of prolonged drainage with intrapericardial injections for the first time.[1] The patient continued to be treated with repeated hemodialyses with significant improvement not only in pericarditis, but also in other symptoms. As described earlier, the patient eventually received a kidney transplant from her father, but died due to graft rejection and sepsis.

Maria Zieleniec-Madejska — Constant Site (Buttonhole) Method of Needle Insertion

From 1969 until 1972, all needle insertions in our center in Bytom were done in different sites of the arterialized vein. Maria Zieleniec, daughter of a prominent official in the Ministry of Mining who helped us with the expansion of our dialysis facility in Bytom, married shortly after she started dialysis and added Madejska to her name. She had an arteriovenous fistula created on the left radial artery and cephalic vein, but before it developed she inadvertently hit the anastomosis with a Click Clack,[2] a popular toy at the time. The fistula clotted, but because she needed hemodialysis immediately, she was started, on April 4, 1971, on chronic hemodialysis with an

---

1. After many years I found confirmation that this was indeed the first case of uremic pericarditis treated with prolonged drainage and local injections of corticosteroids. Jerry C. Jacobs [Jacob JC. (1983) Adult Still's disease complicated by cardiac tamponade. *JAMA* **250**: 3282–3283] credited Buselmeier and colleagues with being the first to use this technique, but their publication appeared in 1973 [Buselmeier TJ, Simmons RL, Najarian JS, *et al.* (1973) Symptomatic pericardial effusion: Pericardial drainage and localized steroid instillations as definitive therapy. *Proc Clin Dial Transplant Forum* **3**: 55–61]. In 1984, in a letter to the editor, Dr. Jacobs admitted that our publication preceded that of Busemeier by four years and others followed our lead [Le 3; in reply: Jacobs JC. (1984) *JAMA* **252**(10): 1283].

2. A Click Clack was a toy comprising a pair of two-inch-diameter acrylic balls attached to either end of a 12–18-inch string. By holding the middle of the string and using an up-and-down hand motion, the objective was to make the balls "clack" against each other above and below your hand as many times as possible. They were sufficiently dangerous to receive a warning from the FDA, as they could result in injury, which is what happened with this patient.

arteriovenous shunt inserted originally into the right femoral artery and femoral vein and later into the left radial artery and the left cephalic vein. In February the following year an arteriovenous fistula was created on the right radial artery and hemodialysis was started on the fistula in March 1972.

The patient had very limited segments suitable for needle insertion. Only Sister Helena was sufficiently experienced to cannulate her fistula. Out of necessity, the insertion of needles was done repeatedly in the same spots. Within a few months the patient noted that needle insertions were not painful and requested not to use lignocaine. Hearing by word of mouth of the patient's positive experience, other patients requested constant site needle insertion. I agreed and Sister Helena started creating sites in other patients. By 1973 the method was being used in all patients. After at least a month of Sister Helena performing the technique, other nurses were in a position to cannulate fistulas. The overall results and our experience with the fistulas were published in 1977 [Pu 27]. In this paper we reported that we had seemingly paradoxical observations regarding improvement of fistulas with frequent dialysis up to six times weekly. As can be seen, the discovery of the constant site method was serendipitous. My role was positive in the sense that I did not reject out of hand the discovery made by a patient and nurse. At the same time, a manuscript describing our constant site method of needle insertion was sent to *Dialysis & Transplantation*.[3] In this paper we gave a detailed comparison of different site versus constant site needle insertion. A comparison of 4,060 hemodialyses using the different site method and 6,180 hemodialyses using the constant site method showed the tremendous advantages of the latter method, particularly with regard to hematoma formations, reinsertions, and patient and nurse preference.

We used needles manufactured by Fabryka Narzędzi Lekarskich i Dentystycznych in Milanówek, Poland, or Seattle Artificial Kidney Supply Company in Seattle, Washington. The needles produced in Poland were a little blunter and had a less smooth surface.

---

3. The publication of this manuscript was in limbo for some time. In the meantime I was on sabbatical in the U.S. and then moved from Bytom to Lublin. Having somewhat forgotten about it, I finally contacted the journal's editorial office in early 1979 and they told me that the paper had been misplaced and promised to publish it soon. It was finally published in October 1979 [Pu 41].

Our practice's policy at the time was to reuse needles for the same patients, so they were becoming even blunter over time. This seemed to be advantageous for the constant site method, as a blunter needle tended to follow the established path without cutting the insertion tunnel wall. We sometimes observed blood oozing alongside the needle when we used the American needles, so we stopped using them and only used the blunter and slightly rougher needles from Milanówek. Besides, as the U.S.-made needles were more expensive, the decision was meritorious from all points of view. The needles became blunter with reuse, so there was a smooth transition from sharper to blunter needles.

After my departure from Bytom, the constant site method continued to be used for Maria Zieleniec-Madejska. She gradually developed various complications, including arteriosclerosis and dialysis related amyloidosis.[4] When I was in Kraków in 1993, she visited me to ask for some advice. Given her amyloidosis I suggested transplantation,[5] but her candidacy was ultimately rejected because of very poor arteries. She lost her fistula in 1998, and it was impossible to create another one, so from 1998 she was dialyzed on intravenous catheters. Her nephrologist, Dr. Roman Rudka, told me that she received 6-hour three times weekly dialysis or sometimes 4 hours, four times weekly, and she never requested reduced dialysis. After almost 33 years of hemodialysis, she developed multiple myeloma and passed away in March 2004. I believe that she was the longest survivor exclusively on dialysis in Poland.

Mitzi Rosen — Nightly Intermittent Peritoneal Dialysis and Using Intraperitoneal Contrast to Diagnose Leak Sites

In December 1982, Mitzi Rosen, a 21-year-old white female patient, started on continuous ambulatory peritoneal dialysis. She had end-stage

---

4. Long-term dialysis patients develop amyloidosis related to elevated β_2-microglobulin, which has a molecular weight of 13 kDa and is not effectively removed by either peritoneal dialysis or hemodialysis. Deposition of amyloid (precipitated β_2-microglobulin) in joints is associated with inflammation and pain.

5. Transplanted kidney removes β-microglobulin and phosphorus very effectively; although deposited amyloid is not removed, new amyloid is not deposited.

renal failure due to polycystic kidney disease and Caroli disease.[6] She had started on chronic hemodialysis in 1979, but did not tolerate it well because of poor cardiac function, with left ventricular ejection fraction of only 17 percent (normal values are between 50 and 65 percent). With the short hemodialysis sessions practiced at the time, she had dyspnea (shortness of breath) before dialysis and hypotension during dialysis. In addition, she had difficulty in maintaining a functioning vascular access and had four blood access failures through December 1982. Three kidney transplants in May 1980, November 1980 and August 1982 were unsuccessful due to rejections. CAPD was initiated, but the clinical course was complicated by hospitalizations for the treatment of abdominal dialysate leaks and hernias. In 1983, she was hospitalized nine times for this purpose and lost two peritoneal accesses during surgical repairs of leaks and hernias. Two large polycystic kidneys and three failed allografts, none of which was removed, undoubtedly contributed to the high intra-abdominal pressure. A great challenge came in December 1983 when it proved difficult to localize a leak site. Because computed tomography (CT) of the abdomen did not reveal the site of the leak, we decided to infuse dialysis solution with diatrizoate meglumine (contrast material) into the peritoneal cavity, allow patient to walk for two hours and then repeat the CT scan. With this technique the leak site was revealed, located in the region where her previous peritoneal catheter was implanted [Pu 78] (Fig. 32).

This was the first use of computed tomography with intraperitoneal contrast to demonstrate leak sites. A previous study of ours [Pu 66] showed a large difference between intraperitoneal pressure in the supine and upright positions, so the patient was treated with intermittent peritoneal dialysis (20 hours twice per week) during 1983. This turned out to be inadequate, as the patient had no residual renal function and low transport characteristics as determined by the peritoneal equilibration test (D/P creatinine of 0.54), which was being developed at the time. After so many methods failed, I tried a new method, I believe used for the first time: nightly intermittent peritoneal dialysis (NIPD).

---

6. Caroli disease is a congenital dilatation of bile ducts in the liver. The anomaly was not associated with any problems in this patient and was incidentally discovered during abdominal imaging taken for her polycystic kidney disease. In fact, Caroli disease is relatively frequently associated with polycystic kidney disease.

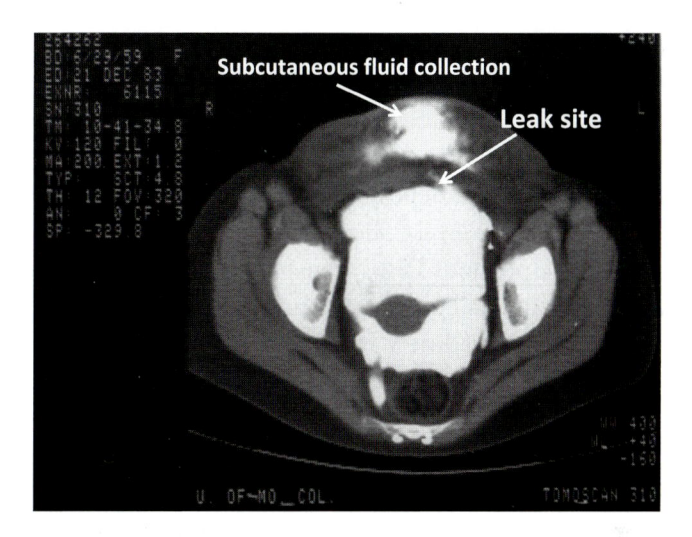

Figure 32. Computerized tomography with intraperitoneal contrast to detect a leak site. (Reprinted from Pu 78.)

The method required several modifications over the years, but the patient was clinically adequately dialyzed for over 10 years, without abdominal leaks or hernias [Pu 211]. Ultimately, the patient was being treated with 20.4 L of solution every night for 11 hours with a 1.57 L exchange volume and 14 min outflow time. The method allowed reasonable efficiency of dialysis with long contact time between the fluid and the peritoneal membrane. Overall, full contact of dialysis solution per day was 6 hours, so with the use of 20.4 L per day the full contact time of the dialysis solution volume was 20.4 L × 6 hours = 122.4 L × hours per day. In 1989, her weekly creatinine clearance increased from 33.6 to 40 L/week/1.73 m^2, and urea clearance from 71.4 to 76.3 L/week/1.73m^2. This was quasi-tidal peritoneal dialysis, a method I introduced to the armamentarium of peritoneal dialysis methods, as described above. Her peritoneal transport gradually increased (D/P creatinine of 0.74), such that her total weekly creatinine clearance had increased to 60 L/1.73 m^2 by 1994 [Pu 211], and urea clearance to 89 L/week/1.73 m^2. Her dialysis was clinically sufficient with respect to the control of anemia, hematocrit and nutritional status, in spite of lower than postulated creatinine clearance and urea clearance values. She was the longest surviving patient on peritoneal dialysis in our center [Pu 384].

Unfortunately, with no urine output and even with her low body surface area of 1.56 m², her calcium and phosphate were elevated, and she started to show metastatic calcifications and joint pains related to amyloidosis. In 1994 I advised her to undergo another kidney transplant to prevent further deposits of amyloid and normalization of calcium and phosphate levels. She was initially very reluctant, having already had three previous failed transplants. I explained to her that antirejection therapy had made tremendous progress during the previous decade and we had new medication (Tacrolimus) for chronic immune suppression as well as OKT3, an anti-T-cell monoclonal antibody for acute rejection not available 10 years previously. She agreed and underwent a cadaveric kidney transplant in 1994, had only one acute rejection treated with OKT3 and is otherwise doing very well. She paid me a visit in 1999 upon my retirement and gave me a token of appreciation (Fig. 33a); she, like almost all of my patients who had difficulties pronouncing my name, called me "Dr. T." She also showed me an award given to her for Outstanding Vocational

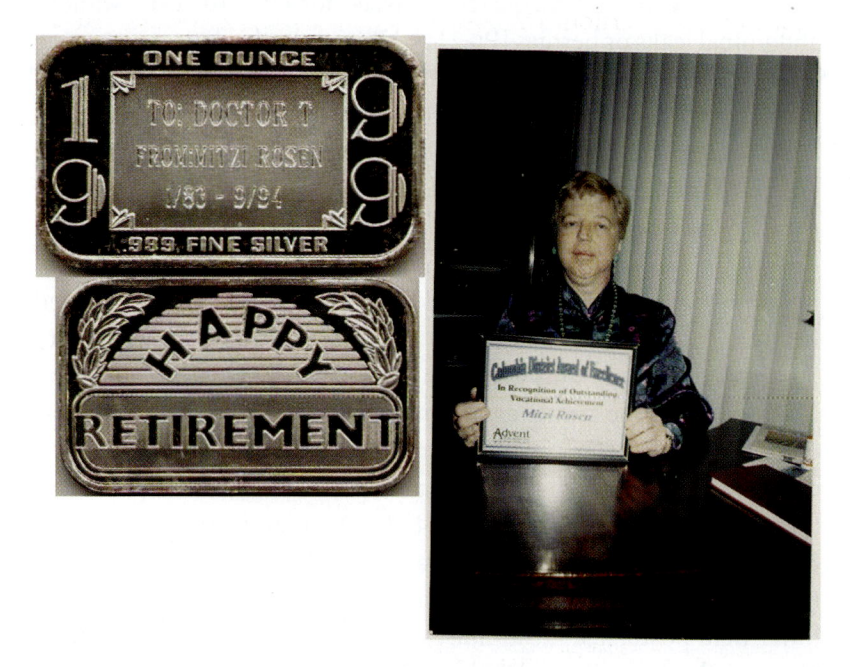

Figure 33. (a) Token of appreciation in 1999. (b) Columbia District Award of Excellence for Outstanding Vocational Achievement.

Achievement (Fig. 33b). She visited me again in 2005 and was in good spirits and excellent physical condition. I met her once more in March 2012. She continued to be in good spirit and doing well clinically. Without question she has stimulated tremendous progress in peritoneal dialysis therapy.

Joe Brodhacker — Swan Neck Catheter

A 28-year-old white male with a 17-year history of psoriasis had experienced clearing of his skin lesions with eight weeks of intermittent peritoneal dialysis in a controlled study in 1978.[7] Thereafter, a development of psoriatic plaques on his forearms, shins, feet, head, back, hands and palms, as well as psoriatic arthritis, without improvement over six months of conventional treatment, prompted him to ask for treatment with peritoneal dialysis. He was admitted to my clinic for psoriasis treatment on February 24, 1984. The same day, a Tenckhoff peritoneal catheter was inserted on the right side of the abdomen. The Koebner phenomenon[8] was apparent at the catheter exit site five days after catheter insertion. The patient responded well to therapy [Pu 88, Pu 99] (Fig. 34), but he became a significant patient for me, as it was when treating him that I came up with the idea for a new catheter for peritoneal dialysis. At the time a Tenckhoff catheter was implanted with its exit pointing in a different direction. Indeed, Tenckhoff recommended a downward direction for the exit,[9] but implantation of straight catheters with both tips pointing down caused an extrusion of the external cuff. As a result, many catheters were implanted with the exit pointing up, as was case in this patient.

The patient developed exit site infection. On April 2, 1984, when I saw the infected exit, it occurred to me that it would be difficult to cure the infection as the pus would not drain, but rather would penetrate deeper into the sinus. I also thought that the exit could easily be

---

7. Whittier FC, Evans DH, Anderson PC, Nolph KD. (1983) Peritoneal dialysis for psoriasis: A controlled study. *Ann Intern Med* **99**(2): 165–168.
8. After German dermatologist Heinrich Koebner (1838–1904), who discovered new lesions appearing on lines of trauma in psoriasis patients.
9. Tenckhoff H, Schechter H. (1968) A bacteriologically safe peritoneal access device. *Trans Am Soc Artif Intern Organs* **14**: 181–187.

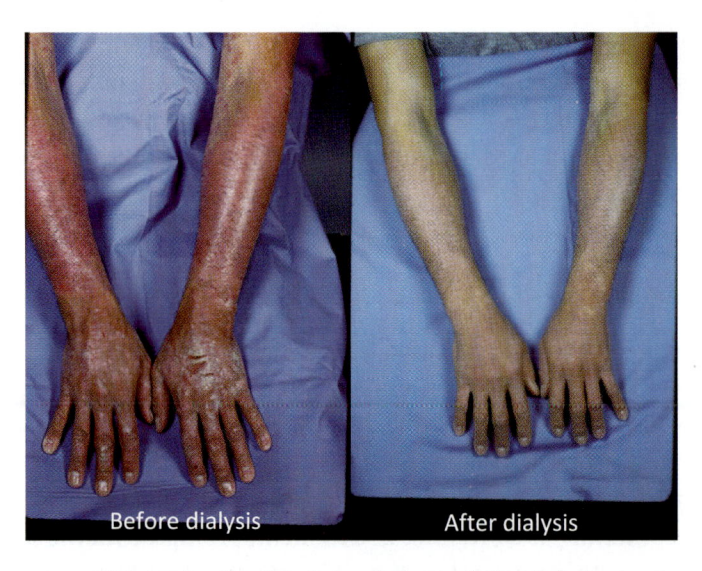

Figure 34. Psoriatic lesions before and after dialysis.

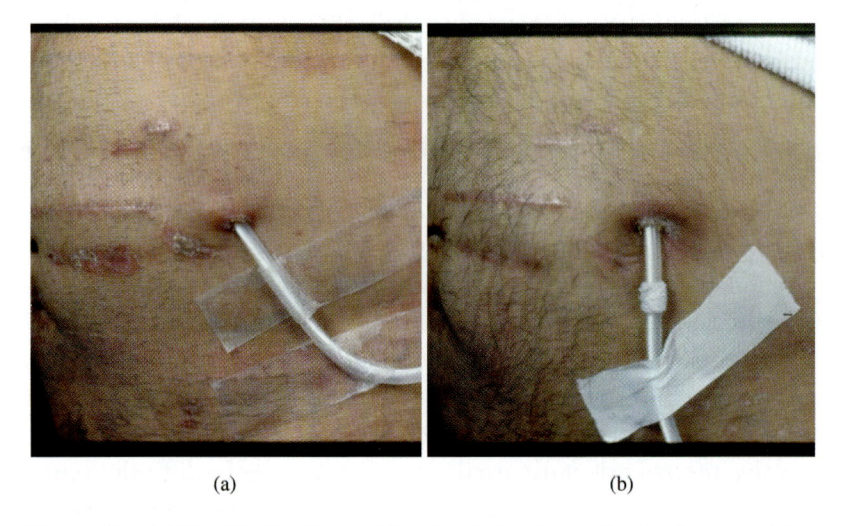

Figure 35. (a) Tenckhoff catheter with exit pointing down after implantation. Note Koebner phenomenon at sites of incisions. (b) Cuff extruded. Koebner phenomenon disappeared after dialysis.

contaminated if pointing up. The infection responded to antibiotics initially, but ultimately the catheter had to be removed. On June 27, 1985, a new Tenckhoff catheter was implanted on the left side with the exit pointing down (Fig. 35a). Unfortunately, the external cuff gradually extruded from the exit (Fig. 35b). These observations led me to work on a new catheter design, which I will describe in a separate chapter.

Hugh Blattner — Daytime Ambulatory Peritoneal Dialysis

A 62-year-old white male with renal failure due to nephrolithiasis came to Dialysis Clinic Inc. in Columbia on September 2, 1983. He was a CAPD patient of Kansas City Veterans Administration Hospital, but because of his noncompliance with peritoneal dialysis exchanges, they wanted him to transfer to hemodialysis and stopped providing him with supplies. He wanted to buy some from us and complained about his treatment in Kansas City. When I saw him for the first time, I thought that he was in a markedly elevated mood. In any event, he did not want to go for hemodialysis, so we provided him with peritoneal dialysis solutions. A subsequent psychiatric consultation revealed that he had bipolar disorder.

It was very difficult to regulate his fluid status, as he had low drainage volumes. I remember him telling me that he did not see any reason to keep fluid in his belly overnight as in the morning he could not drain more than half what he instilled, so on his own he decided to do four exchanges only during the daytime. At the time we were in the process of evaluating peritoneal transport characteristics in our patients, and he agreed to undergo a peritoneal equilibration test on October 22, 1983. The test showed very high transport characteristics, which explained the poor ultrafiltration with long-dwell exchanges. We agreed on the method he was using. It was known as the "Blattner Technique" in our center — it was a discovery that was clearly attributable to this patient — but officially we called it daytime ambulatory peritoneal dialysis (DAPD) [Pu 130]. Unfortunately, his bipolar disorder did not improve despite psychiatric treatment, and when he decided to stop dialysis after becoming depressed, he passed away.

Lucille Shirley — Daily Dialysis on a Personal Hemodialysis System

On January 25, 1996, I admitted Lucille Shirley, born November 25, 1939, to my service. A tiny lady weighing only 42 kg, she was referred to me from Barnes Hospital in St. Louis, Mo. Her medical history was extremely complicated and the diagnoses filled an entire page. The most remarkable were severe arteriosclerosis with peripheral vascular disease, coronary artery disease, cardiac arrhythmia, bilateral renal artery stenosis and chronic renal failure secondary to ischemic nephropathy. This last diagnosis was the reason why she was transferred. Due to severe hypertension, she had a left nephrectomy in 1985. There was some improvement in hypertension, but the stenosis of the right renal artery slowly progressed to the point of end-stage renal disease. In 1986 she had a quadruple coronary artery bypass graft performed and her right renal artery stenosis was repaired. After her cardiac surgery she had a separation (non-reunion) of the sternum. Other diseases included hypothyroidism after thyroidectomy for a goiter in 1962, partial gastrectomy for a bleeding peptic ulcer in 1970, stenosis of the papilla of Vater, and an appendectomy and hysterectomy in 1977. Typical for patients with end-stage renal disease, she had secondary hyperparathyroidism and was suffering from malnutrition. Chronic hemodialysis had already been started in Barnes Hospital on January 18, 1996, on an uncuffed (acute) catheter inserted into the right jugular vein. On January 29, an arteriovenous fistula was created on the left forearm and a left jugular PermCath was inserted.

After accepting her to our service she was dialyzed through the PermCath and gradually on an arteriovenous fistula in conjunction with the PermCath (catheter for inflow, fistula for outflow). She progressively developed steal syndrome, related to her peripheral vascular disease, and the fistula ultimately had to be closed in May 1997. The peripheral vascular disease involved the lower extremities with ischemic changes of the toes, which required surgical treatment. From May 1997 she had to be dialyzed only on intravenous catheters. We inserted an Opti-Flow catheter through the right jugular vein, but it was too long for her and the tip translocated from the right atrium to the right ventricle [Pu 320], and it had to be removed in June 1999. A Tesio twin catheter was inserted through the left jugular vein and, fortunately, functioned from then on.

Originally we tried to dialyze her three times weekly, as is routinely done, but her response was poor as she already had low residual renal function. Blood pressure control was poor, she was malnourished and she developed spontaneous morning hypoglycemic episodes, which were evaluated by an endocrinologist. She had normal insulin level, but low level of cortisone. George T. Griffin, MD, her endocrinologist, came to the conclusion that she had low gluconeogenic reserve from her single kidney, poor hepatic gluconeogenesis and insufficient food intake. She also had many problems unrelated to dialysis. She developed gastrointestinal bleeding from an arteriovenous malformation in the hepatic flexure of the large intestine and a right rotator cuff tear, which required surgery. Her *Kt/V*, the sacrosanct measure of dialysis efficiency as per National Kidney Foundation Kidney Disease Outcomes Quality Initiative guidelines, was very good because of her small body size (small *V*), but the dialysis was obviously inadequate on clinical grounds.[10]

She started home hemodialysis with the help of her husband, Robert, in April 1996 (Fig. 36). The frequency of dialysis had to be gradually increased to every other day in August 1996, with occasional increase to four or five times weekly. Eventually, in April 1999, I started her on daily home hemodialysis, which markedly improved her condition. Her blood pressure was better controlled; she started to eat better and did not have hypoglycemic episodes.

In spite of all these problems she had a great spirit. When she heard about the new personal hemodialysis system (PHD®) for daily home hemodialysis, manufactured by AKSYS Ltd., she immediately volunteered for the study. She told me that she wanted to contribute to scientific progress in hemodialysis treatment. She began a control period for the study in September 1999 and started using PHD® in February 2000, finishing the study in June 2000. Thereafter, AKSYS allowed her to continue on PHD®, which she did until her machine broke down on September 27, 2000. She felt much better on PHD®

---

10. In the *Kt/V* formula, *K* stands for urea clearance during dialysis, *t* is time of dialysis, and *V* is urea distribution in the body, or total body water. In several of my presentations and review papers I criticized this *Kt/V* index as useless because diffusion and dialysis of urea is faster than any other real uremic toxin, and because it does not take into account volume control by sodium removal as well as removal of real uremic toxins, which have bigger molecules and are slowly transported between body compartments during short dialysis [Pr 408, Pr 509, Pr 514, Pu 338, Pu 353, Pu 369]. The index is still considered a valid indicator of adequate dialysis. I hope that, during my lifetime, the nephrology community will reject it as an important measure of dialysis adequacy.

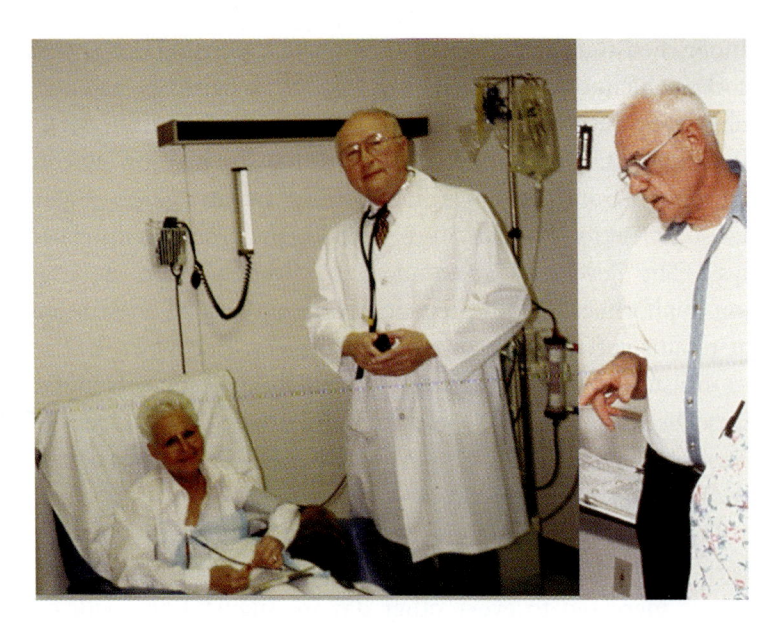

Figure 36. Lucille Shirley during training for home hemodialysis. Her husband was her helper.

Dr "T",
All I can say is Thank you for your tireless efforts to make things better for Lou.
Bob

Your thoughtfulness meant much more than any words can say.

Dr. Twardowski,

Five years ago when we left Barnes Hospital in St. Louis with instructions to report to D.C.I., Columbia, under the care of a "World Renowned Nephrologist" named Dr. Twardowski, little did I know that we would be treated by the most caring, compassionate, innovative and tireless professional I have ever encountered.

You were responsible for me having my little Lady five extra years and the priviledge of caring for her in our home. Lou's biggest thrill of accomplishment in the last half of her sixty years was to be a small part in the Clincal testing of the PHD. She felt she was helping in a small way to further your efforts to make things better for ESRD patients in the future.

Thank you so much for making all of this possible for her. Sincerely, Bob

Figure 37. Thank you letter from Bob Shirley.

and gained 3 kg of dry body weight. AKSYS decided not to fix the machine after it ceased to function, and she was switched to a regular machine with decreased frequency to five times, and then four times, weekly hemodialysis, as Medicare reimbursed patients for three or at most four times weekly dialysis with special justification. I was already retired from clinical service at that time, and after the study was completed, Dr. Ramesh Khanna became her primary physician. Gradually, her multiple diseases overcame her and she died on November 16, 2000. Her survival for such a long time with all her diseases can be attributed to her spirit and the unwavering help she received from her husband. I am certain that the more frequent dialysis also helped to prolong her survival and improve her quality of life. Her husband wrote to us showing his appreciation for our efforts (Fig. 37).

CHAPTER 10

Patents in Columbia

Peritoneal Dialysis Catheters

Swan Neck catheter

While dialyzing my patient Joe Brodhacker and observing his exit infection, I started thinking about a new catheter implanted according to Tenckhoff's recommendation that would prevent cuff extrusion. I recalled from my work on the capillary artificial kidney that plastics have so-called "shape memory," so if a straight catheter, even made of soft silicon rubber, is implanted in an arcuate tunnel then the external cuff is slowly pushed outside (Fig. 38). I came to the conclusion that the catheter should be precurved between both cuffs, and I began researching the literature to find some support for my theory before designing a new catheter. I found that periodontitis, an infection at the naturally occurring exit of the tooth through the epithelium, most frequently involves the lower incisors, i.e., sinuses pointing up. The influence of the exit position on the frequency and tenacity of paranasal sinuses infections was already noted in the 19th century, a fact that

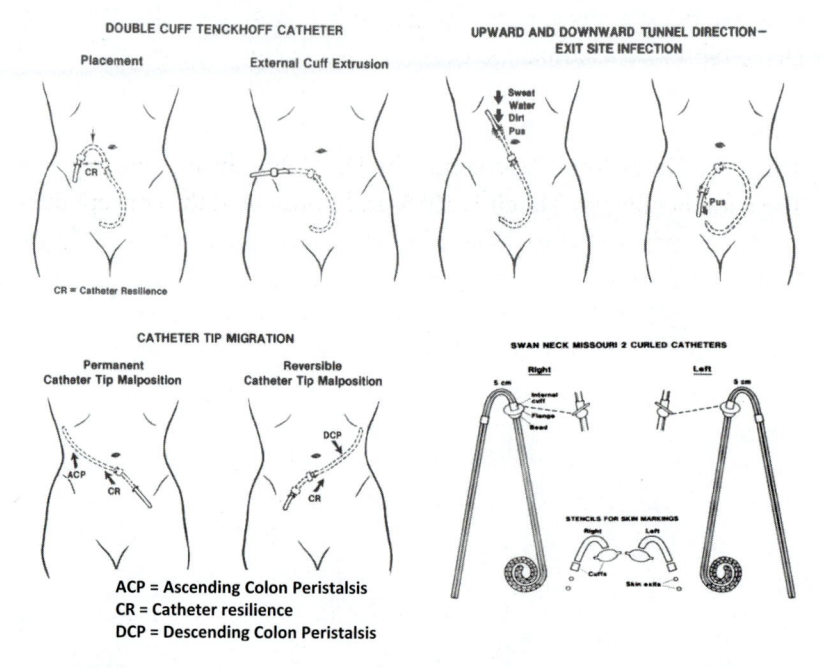

Figure 38. Complications related to the straight catheter and the design of the Swan Neck Missouri catheter. (Part of figure modified from Pu 92.)

was cited in one of our papers published later [Pu 111]. In addition to this, I started to work with Barb on the results of catheter complications in relation to the method of implantation in patients treated between October 1984 and January 1985. I was very confident that the idea was a good one, and even before completing the study I thought about contacting manufacturers of peritoneal catheters to cooperate with me in a new design. I knew about two companies: Quinton Instruments (Seattle, Washington) and Accurate Surgical Instruments (Toronto, ON, Canada). Dr. Khanna, who came from Toronto and joined our division in 1983, had cooperated with Mrs. Elisabeth Hoffman-Zellerman, President of Accurate Surgical Instruments, and he advised me to speak with her. It was a good advice: we talked about the idea and she agreed to cooperate.

Our study showed that more exit infections involved exits pointing upward and that there were more malpositions of the catheter tip if the exit was directed downward to the left (Fig. 38). These data confirmed my view that the best catheter should be precurved between the cuffs and implanted with both external and intraperitoneal segments directed downward. After some discussions with Drs. Nolph and Khanna, we came to the conclusion that there were enough data to patent the idea. We decided to call it the "Swan Neck" catheter, as the bent segment was rather similar to the neck of a swan. The term "Swan Neck" was coined by Dr. Nolph during our trip to a Travenol meeting on March 5, 1985, and I presented the concept during the meeting [Pr 66]. The idea was disclosed at the University Patent and Licensing Office on March 25, 1985.[1]

Travenol did not manufacture catheters but was interested in the improvement of peritoneal dialysis results in general, as they did manufacture peritoneal dialysis solutions. It was obviously a profitable business for them. As a consequence, Travenol provided patent attorneys to file a patent application with the U.S. Patent and Trademark Office on behalf of the University of Missouri. On May 1, 1985, the application (Ser. No. 729,185) was filed by Garretson Ellis with the rather broad claim of a catheter that may be "mounted in a tunnel formed through the abdominal wall in relatively unstressed

---

1. Twardowski ZJ, Nolph KD, Khanna R. Peritoneal dialysis catheter. UM Disclosure No. 85UMC101.

configuration with the proximal end portion extending outwardly from the abdominal wall and downwardly from the outer end of said tunnel and the distal end portion extending inwardly and downwardly from the end of said tunnel." A patent examiner rejected the claims as too broad and unpatentable over previous patents. Indeed, there were previous patents of catheters with a permanent bend of more than 90° arc angle.[2] Only after the patent was filed did we submit a paper with the results of our study on complications in relation to catheter implantation; the paper was published in October 1985 [Pu 92]. On February 6, 1986, and February 11, 1987, amended applications were submitted by Daniel D. Ryan, then Charles R. Matteson, lawyers for Baxter Travenol, with the specification that the arc angle should be in the range of (90°) 100°–180°, as a continuation of the application Ser. No. 729,185. Another feature was included in these applications. This was a modification of the Toronto Western Hospital catheter whereby a flange and bead are implanted at the entrance to the abdominal cavity. Unlike the Toronto Western Hospital catheter, in our design the flange was slanted at about 45° to better secure the downward direction of the intraperitoneal part of the catheter (Fig. 38). In time several U.S. and international patents were granted [Pa III-1, Pa III-2, Pa III-2a–e]. All the patents were assigned to the University of Missouri.

I did not know at the time that Mrs. Zellerman was manufacturing catheters with an 80° arc angle for a study by Dr. Dimitrios Oreopoulos from Toronto Western Hospital. He wanted to have the bent portion implanted in the peritoneal cavity in such a way that the tip of the catheter would be pointing downward. These catheters were never used clinically, but Accurate Surgical Instruments had slightly bent silicone rubber tubing, which were modified for my purposes by providing them with a cuff at each side of the arc. In fact, at the time, the tubing was manufactured by Sil-Med Corporation of Taunton, Massachusetts, and only provided with cuffs, sterilized and packed by Accurate Surgical Instruments. I considered these catheters to be Swan Neck prototypes and believed that they would be better than

---

2. Arc angle refers to a bent segment of tube forming an arc between 0° and 180°. The supplementary angle added to the arc angle produces an angle of 180°. A straight tube has an arc angle of 0° and a bent tube with both arms parallel has an arc angle of 180°.

straight Tenckhoff catheters, and I asked our surgeon, W. Kirt Nichols, MD, to start implanting them in August 1985. Unfortunately, cuff extrusions were not eliminated with this design [Pu 111], so we stopped using them in March 1986. After more discussions with Mrs. Zellerman, Accurate Surgical Instruments succeeded, in April 1986, in producing real Swan Neck catheters, as described in patents, with a 170° arc angle, slanted flange and bead, and 5 cm distance between cuffs. Only many years later did I learn that Mrs. Zellerman had some difficulty in obtaining properly bent[3] tubing from Sil-Med.

We received patents shortly thereafter, and I obviously thought that the University should license them to Accurate Surgical Instruments. However, there was an existing agreement between the University of Missouri and Austin Biomedical Corporation, founded by Jack W. Moncrief, MD, and Robert P. Popovich, PhD, the co-inventors of the peritoneal dialysis method, later called continuous ambulatory peritoneal dialysis by Dr. Karl D. Nolph [Pu 31]. According to this agreement, the university received royalties from Austin Biomedical related to peritoneal dialysis but was obliged to license all related patents to that corporation. As a result, the patents were licensed to Austin Biomedical, which in turn sublicensed them to Accurate Surgical Instruments.

In the mid-1980s Sil-Med developed permanently bent tubing with a variety of arc angles and supplied it to Accurate Surgical Instruments. However, Sil-Med wanted to sell catheters themselves and questioned the validity of the patents, providing prior arts with bent catheters in order for patent 4,772,269 to be reexamined. The challenge proved unsuccessful after a reexamination by the U.S. Patent Office confirmed the validity of all our claims and a certificate was issued on May 19, 1992. Despite this, Sil-Med continued to sell their catheters, infringing our patent for the bent (Swan Neck) peritoneal dialysis catheter. In 1994 Mrs. Zellerman sued the company in a U.S. District Court in Massachusetts over infringement of the patent, and the court ruled in favor of Accurate Surgical Instruments on June 25, 1995.

---

3. To obtain a permanently bent catheter, the silicone rubber tubing has to be properly cured by baking at 350°F for three hours in a desired shape after extrusion. This process, more difficult than obtaining straight tubing, was pioneered by Sil-Med.

Sil-Med was not Mrs. Zellerman's only problem. Moncrief and Popovich had developed a catheter, similar to the Swan Neck, only with a slightly longer superficial cuff, but with a different method of implantation whereby the external part remains under the skin until the ingrowth of the tissue into the cuff is strong; only after several weeks (three to six or more) is the external part exteriorized.[4] They did not receive a patent for the catheter design but rather for a new method of implantation. Austin Biomedical wanted Accurate Surgical Instruments to distribute these catheters separately from other Swan Neck catheters and ensure that other catheters would not be implanted using their technique. But with it being very difficult to police whether somebody was using the implantation technique, Mrs. Zellerman could not agree to the deal. Instead, she proposed to sell the catheters with longer subcutaneous cuff to Austin Biomedical for distribution. Unhappy with the deal, Austin Biomedical started legal action against Accurate Surgical Instruments for various claimed breaches of license agreement.

I wanted to put a stop to all litigation and concentrate on cooperation. Dr. Nolph arranged a meeting with the participation of Mrs. Zellerman, Dr. Moncrief, Dr. Khanna and myself in a St. Louis airport conference room, and we came to an agreement. According to that agreement achieved on November 6, 1993, Accurate Surgical Instrument would manufacture Swan Neck catheters with longer subcutaneous cuff and sell them to Austin Biomedical at half price; Austin Biomedical would, in turn, sell them to hospitals. I was rather skeptical about the possibility of policing the method of implantation, as I had experience with my method of dialyzer reuse patented in Poland and had never been able to determine who used my method.

Another problem arose with Vas-Cath Inc., a company from Mississauga, Ontario, Canada, which violated the patents and started to sell Swan Neck catheters in 1994. Accurate Surgical Instruments threatened to sue, and Vas-Cath agreed to stop infringing the patents on June 1, 1995. The sales of Swan Neck catheters were going extremely well until 1997, as shown in Fig. 39, but dipped with changes in patent

---

4. Moncrief JW, Popovich RP, Broadrick LJ, et al. (1993) The Moncrief–Popovich catheter: A new peritoneal access technique for patients on peritoneal dialysis. *ASAIO J* **39**(1): 62–65.

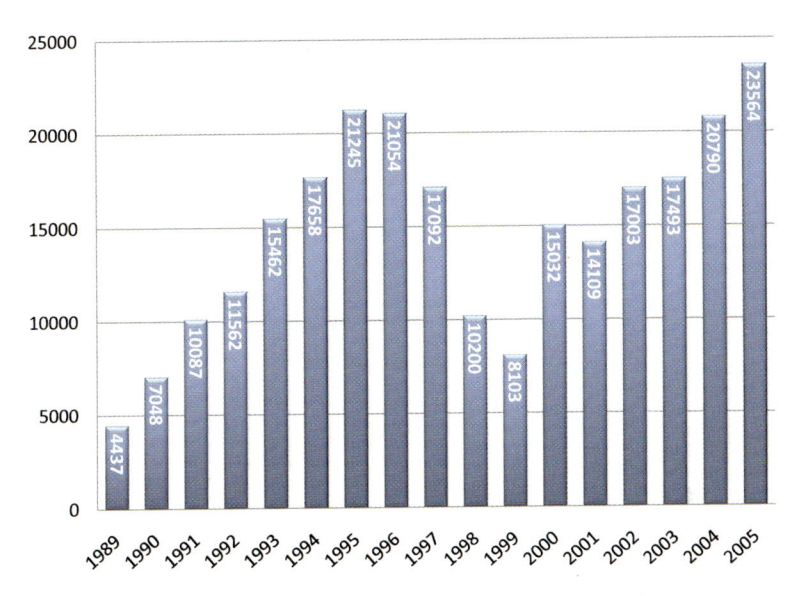

Figure 39. Worldwide use of Swan Neck abdominal catheters.

licensees and manufacturers.[5] To help with the implantation and care of Swan Neck catheters, we prepared several videos, which were widely used [Vi 1–Vi 5].

Swan Neck presternal catheter

In the early 1990s, I started thinking about new ways to improve the peritoneal catheter. I noted that some patients had problems with the catheter exit located in the abdomen, especially patients with ostomies, suprapubic catheters or even children with diapers, as the exit could be prone to contamination. Also, obese patients had increased rates of exit infections. I hypothesized that the Swan Neck catheter for peritoneal dialysis with the exit in the presternal area might be less likely to develop exit site infection. The chest is a sturdy structure with minimal wall motions; a catheter exit located on the chest wall is subject to minimal

---

5. In 1996 Mrs. Zellerman sold her company to Quinton Instruments, already part of A. H. Robins Company. In December 1995 that company was bought by Sherwood Davis & Geck, St. Louis, Mo., but was sold in 1998 to Kendall Company, Mansfield, Massachusetts, a part of Tyco Healthcare Group. In the fall of 2007 Healthcare Group left Tyco and formed Covidien, remaining headquartered at the same address.

Presternal catheter post implantation in relation to body structures

Deep cuff, flange, and bead in relation to abdominal wall

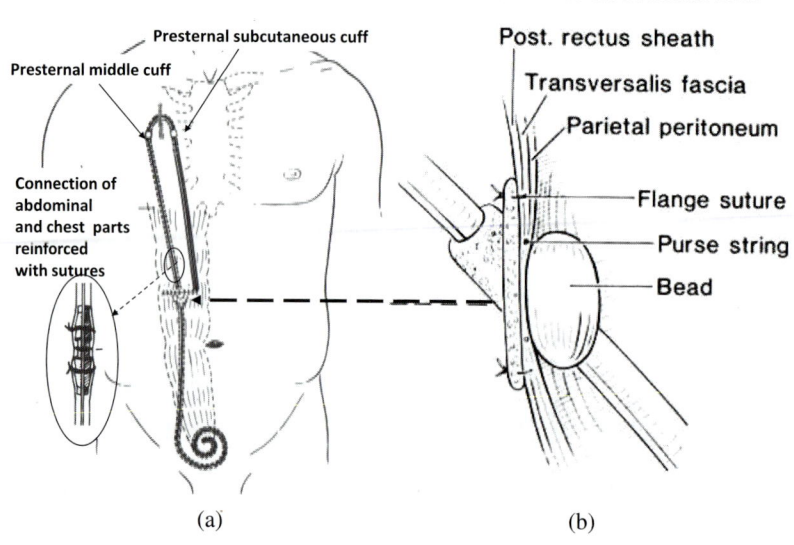

- Presternal subcutaneous cuff
- Presternal middle cuff
- Connection of abdominal and chest parts reinforced with sutures

- Post. rectus sheath
- Transversalis fascia
- Parietal peritoneum
- Flange suture
- Purse string
- Bead

(a) (b)

Figure 40. (a) Schematic drawing of presternal catheter after implantation. (Modified from Pu 235.) (b) Position of abdominal cuff, flange and bead in relation to abdominal wall. (Modified from Pu 182.)

movement, decreasing the chances of trauma and contamination. The subcutaneous tissue on the chest is markedly less thick than in the abdomen, so having an exit on the chest in obese patients would be preferable. After discussing the idea with Drs. Nichols, Khanna and Nolph, we decided to disclose our invention to the University Office of Patent and Licensing.[6] The catheter was to be composed of two silicon rubber tubes (distal and proximal) trimmed to the appropriate size for the patient and joined with a titanium connector in the subcutaneous tunnel at the time of implantation. The proximal tube was to be provided with two cuffs; the distal tube, with a bead, flange and cuff, similar to those of Swan Neck Missouri catheters. After implantation the tunnel (intramural) segment of the catheter was to be provided with three cuffs. The catheter required surgical implantation (Fig. 40).

---

6. Twardowski ZJ, Nichols WK, Khanna R, Nolph KD. Presternal peritoneal dialysis catheter. Disclosed in the University Patent and Licensing Office on December 21, 1990. Number 91-UMC-017.

I contacted Mrs. Zellerman, who agreed to cover the patent application expenses, license the patent (if granted) and manufacture the catheters in accordance with our specifications. We filed a patent application through Garretson Ellis. He advised us to change the name to *separable peritoneal dialysis catheter*, as it could also be implanted high in the abdomen; we agreed. This time we did not have issues with the patent examiner and received a patent shortly thereafter [Pa III-3, Pa III-3a–3e]. I had to help Mrs. Zellerman deal with the Food and Drug Administration (FDA), initially to receive investigational device exemption (IDE)[7] for a study comparing abdominal and presternal catheters. The FDA gave me an IDE for 10 patients. The first catheter was implanted on August 26, 1991. Our initial results in two patients who could not have abdominal catheters implanted were positive, and we presented them during the 12th Annual Conference on Peritoneal Dialysis in Seattle, Washington, in February 1992 [Pu 182]. Patients with a presternal catheter could use a bathtub or Jacuzzi without risk of exit contamination, so Dr. Nolph suggested dubbing it the "bathtub" catheter. Sometime later he presented the results with this catheter in Italy and mentioned that this catheter was suitable for bathtub lovers, which elicited peals of laughter — given the rather ambiguous meaning.

Our continuous study confirmed positive results [Pu 193]. After presenting the results to the FDA, Accurate Surgical Instruments received 510(k) Premarket Notification.[8] During discussions with the FDA I was posed an odd question: "How is it that the fluid can be drained from the abdomen by gravity if it would need to rise to the chest first." I was initially surprised by the question, but after a while I patiently explained that the catheter is filled with dialysis solution and drainage is possible because of siphoning, a principle discovered by the Ancient Greeks more than two millennia earlier. In our center

---

7. An IDE allows the investigational device to be used in a clinical study in order to collect safety and effectiveness data required to support a Premarket Approval (PMA) application or a 510(k) Premarket Notification submission to the FDA.

8. Any new device has to have the approval of the FDA, which certifies that its use in humans is not significantly more risky than any available devices. In order to be sold the new device does not need to be shown to be better but has to be considered "a substantial equivalent" of devices present on the market. A device requires the submission of a 510(k) Premarket Notification and cannot be commercially distributed until a letter is received of substantial equivalence from the FDA authorizing it.

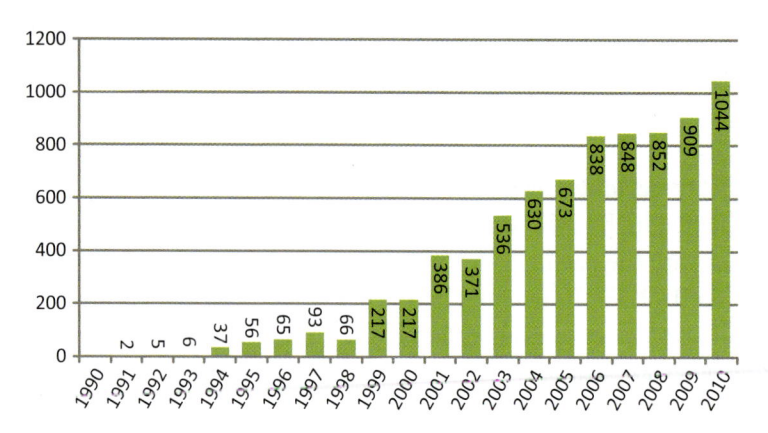

Figure 41. Worldwide use of presternal catheters.

the catheter became the preferred method of peritoneal access. In other centers it was used mainly in patients with specific problems like ostomies, obesity and multiple abdominal scars. The implantation of presternal catheter was a little more complicated than that of abdominal catheter, so we produced a video presenting the design, insertion and break-in of this catheter [Vi 6]. Sales increased year upon year (Fig. 41) [Pu 235, Pu 279]. It was also used in Poland at the Children's University Hospital in Warsaw. The first such catheter was implanted as early as December 15, 1991, in the Department of Pediatrics and Nephrology under the direction of Prof. Maria Sieniawska.[9] As well as being pleased with the success of the catheter, I was also impressed that no infringements of our patent rights were discovered until 2010. I learned that the Medigroup company of Oswego, Illinois, was manufacturing a similar design, which they called the ExxTended Catheter. I notified the University of Missouri's lawyers and Covidien about this fact. The University of Missouri did not take any action, as the patents were licensed to Covidien and it was supposed to defend them. Covidien decided against suing Medigroup, which was a business decision, as litigation would have been too costly. I saw the infringement for what it was — theft of intellectual property — and I expressed my displeasure to John Navis,

---

9. Sieniawska M, Roszkowska-Blaim M, Warchol S. (1993) Preliminary results with the Swan Neck presternal catheter for CAPD in children. *Adv Perit Dial* **9**: 321–324.

President of Medigroup. In any event, the patent expired in the U.S. on April 16, 2011, with foreign patents expiring in 2012.

Intravenous Catheters

Multiple lumen catheter for hemodialysis

Around the same time I was working on the Swan Neck peritoneal catheter, I started to theorize that a similar principle should be applied to intravenous catheters for hemodialysis. There were two companies manufacturing catheters for the treatment of acute renal failure at the time: Vas-Cath in Mississauga, Canada, and Quinton Instruments in Seattle, Washington. But there were no catheters that worked well for prolonged use in chronic renal failure. Quinton started making a silicone rubber, dual lumen catheter, but outcomes were less than ideal because of clotting and exit site infection. Both companies made straight catheters with two lumens side to side and with staggered lumens, the inflow being about 2.5 cm shorter than the outflow. This feature was used to prevent recirculation of blood in the catheter (outflow blood entering the inflow lumen). My idea was to shape a catheter in such way that it could be implanted into large veins in an unstressed condition and would be provided with one or two cuffs anchoring the catheter firmly in a tunnel. Also, I thought that the bore of the inflow tube should be away from the vein's internal wall, thereby preventing sucking of the wall and decrease the chances of injury to the intima. I discussed my ideas with John C. Van Stone, MD, Medical Director of Dialysis Clinic Inc., and W. Kirt Nichols, MD, a surgeon who did almost all insertions of various catheters for our dialysis patients. We disclosed our invention to the University Patent and Licensing Office on June 7, 1985.[10]

For three years I was busy with other projects and did not actively pursue the idea. In the meantime I gave presentations at the 34th Annual Meeting of the American Society for Artificial Internal Organs in Reno, Nevada, on May 3, 1988 [Pr 120]. After my presentation

---

10. Twardowski ZJ, Van Stone JC, Nichols WK. Multiple lumen catheter for hemodialysis. UM Disclosure 85-UMC-044.

Wayne Quinton[11] approached me and asked whether I had some new ideas that might be of interest to his company, Quinton Instruments. I mentioned to him that I had some ideas related to an intravenous catheter. Shortly after that meeting, on July 11, 1988, I submitted another disclosure of the invention to the University Patent and Licensing Office.[12] This version was called Swan Neck Pigtail Double Lumen Intravenous Catheter. The main changes in the design concerned the catheter tip. It was my deep conviction that many problems with blood flow and catheter clotting were related to the sucking of the inflow lumen into the vein wall. I proposed three solutions: Firstly, the outflow lumen extending beyond the inflow tip should assume a helical (pigtail) shape and thus prevent the inflow bore from touching the vein intima. Secondly, if this were technically difficult or impossible, we would provide a balloon on the outflow tubing, inflatable during dialysis. Thirdly, the inflow bore should be directed toward the outflow tubing (away from the vessel wall) (Fig. 42).

While the offer of cooperation with Quinton was very attractive, I felt some obligation towards Travenol and Mrs. Zellerman, thinking that one of them could be a sponsor in filing a patent application, developing a prototype and licensing the invention. Baxter-Travenol got first priority but was not interested. On July 13, 1988, I contacted Mrs. Zellerman, proposing that we cooperate, this time regarding intravenous catheters, but she informed me after a few days that she was not interested in the project. Four days later I notified Mr. Robert Killoren, Director of the University Patents and Licensing Office that Quinton Instruments had expressed an interest in our invention. He started negotiations and a confidentiality agreement was signed on August 15, 1988. I visited the company from January 15 to 18, 1989. At the time Quinton Instruments was part of A. H. Robins Company, and Wayne Quinton was not the president of the company but still advised engineers and the new board of directors. I met with Wayne

---

11. Wayne E. Quinton was working at the University of Washington in Seattle. To nephrologists he is best known as the inventor of an arteriovenous shunt made of inert materials (Teflon and silicone rubber). He founded Quinton Instruments Company in his basement and it later became a large company located at 2121 Terry Avenue, Seattle, WA 98121. He was honored by the University of Washington as the 2009 Alumnus Summa Laude Dignatus ("alumnus worthy of the highest praise").

12. Twardowski ZJ, Van Stone JC, Nichols WK. Swan neck pigtail double lumen intravenous catheters. UM Disclosure 89-UMC-003.

Pictures from disclosures of invention

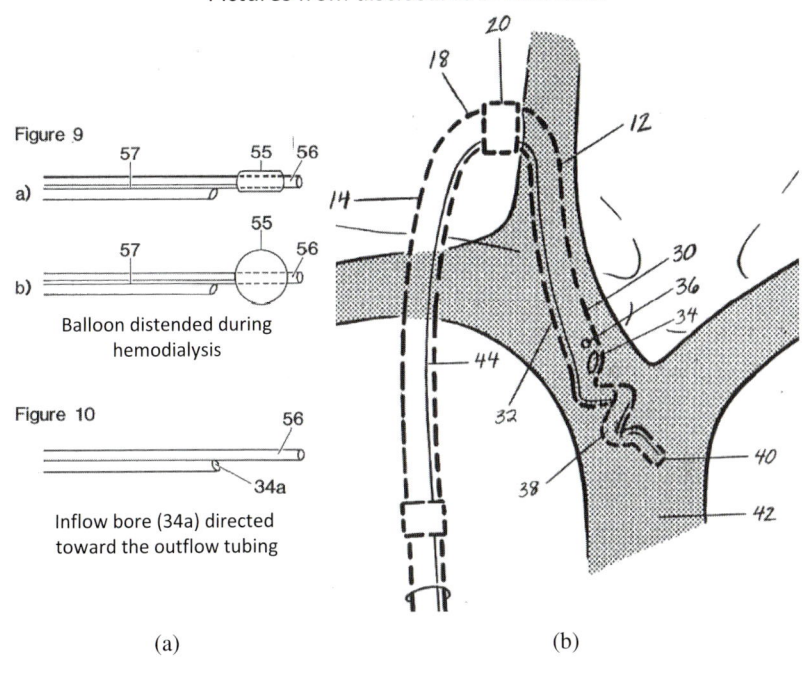

Figure 42. (a) Various methods to prevent sucking of the inflow lumen into the vein wall. (b) Jugular catheter with the pigtail outflow lumen in relation to thoracic veins.

Quinton; Toni Perri, President; Bruce Densmore, Manager for Medical Products; Lori Thompson, Product Manager; and Brad Fowler, a biomedical engineer. I presented my ideas and showed them prototype wire models of subclavian and right jugular vein pigtail catheters (Fig. 43). To mark the occasion of our meeting, a picture of the three of us (Brad Fowler, Wayne Quinton and myself) was taken with the pigtail models (Fig. 44). Negotiations between the company and the university began, the license agreement being signed on October 12, 1989. Connie Armentraut, Coordinator of the University Patent and Licensing Office, asked Garrettson Ellis, who had already left Baxter and co-founded the Gerstman and Ellis law firm, to submit a patent application.[13] Quinton Instruments covered the cost of application.

---

13. Twardowski ZJ, Van Stone JC, Nichols WK. Multiple lumen catheter for hemodialysis. Application No. 461,684, filed on January 8, 1990. Contributions: Twardowski 70 percent, Van Stone 20 percent, Nichols 10 percent.

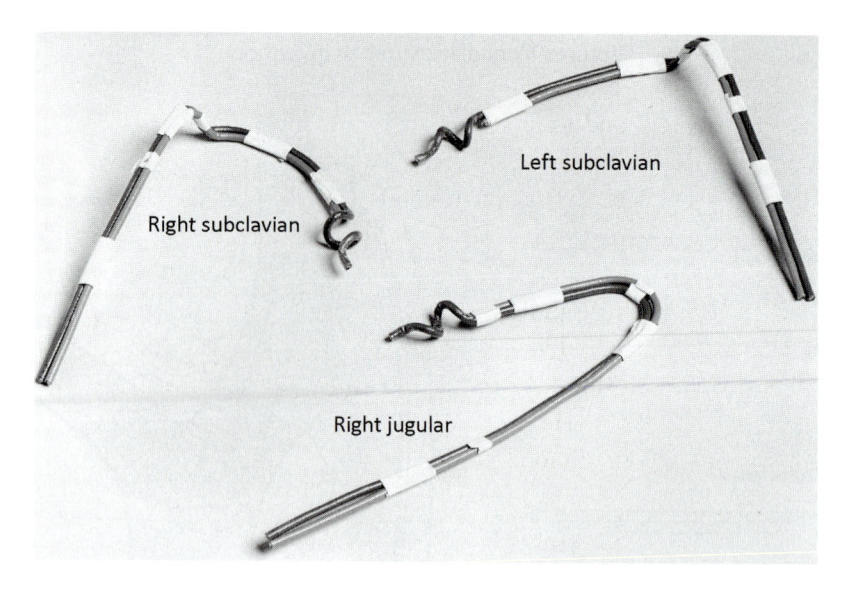

Figure 43. Wire models of pigtail intravenous catheters.

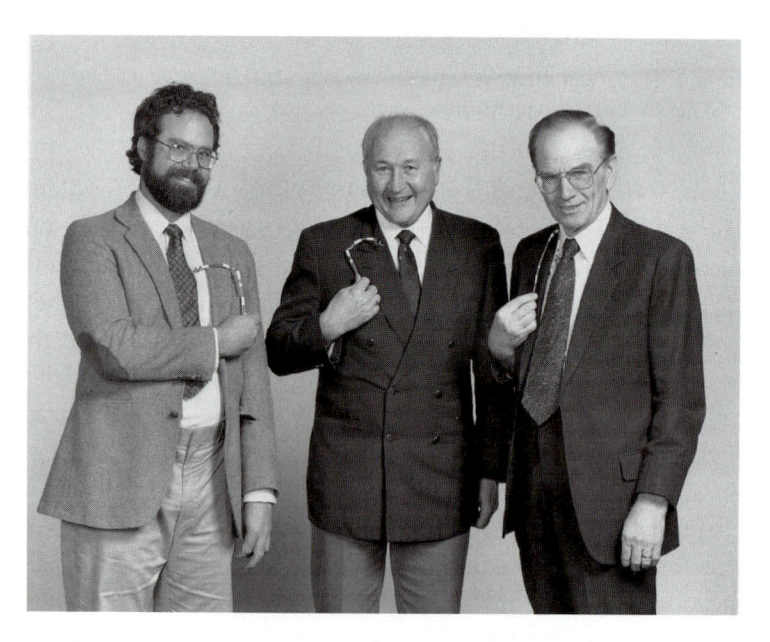

Figure 44. Brad Fowler, the author and Wayne Quinton with the pigtail models.

In the meantime I worked with Brad Fowler on the dimensions and shapes of various catheters. Brad was able to get an FDA IDE for new catheter designs, and an intensive period of cooperation commenced shortly thereafter. First of all we decided to start with catheters that were easier to manufacture. The pigtail feature was rather challenging, so we agreed to start with the third feature, the inflow bore directed toward the outflow tubing (away from the vessel wall). I prepared a study protocol entitled "Prospective randomized evaluation of double lumen intravenous catheters as blood access for hemodialysis." The goal of the study was to compare the results of our design with Quinton-made PermCath, the best dual lumen catheter on the market at the time. The protocol was approved by the Institutional Review Board, and we started using these catheters in April 1991. By 1992 we had determined that the third feature was less prone to clotting than the regular PermCath, but was still not satisfactory. There was another problem related to production of the staggered catheter tips. This was done by grinding the tip of the outflow lumen. Additionally, there were two holes made on the side of the inflow lumen to ensure blood inflow in case the inflow bore was occluded by clot. While removing failed catheters, we found a clot "sitting" on the outflow lumen, blocking the inflow lumen and firmly anchored to the inflow side holes [Pu 319] (Fig. 45, upper part). It was my opinion that the grinding of the catheter left a rough surface (Fig. 45, lower part), which was known, even in the 19th century, to lead to clot formation.

The cooperation with Brad Fowler was extremely productive. We gradually received various prototypes. We came to the conclusion that to reduce the chances of clot formation it would be better to decrease the distance between the inflow and outflow lumens and only cut, not grind, the outflow lumen. We received such a catheter, which we called SNIJ 3 (Swan Neck Internal Jugular Catheter Model 3), in the middle of 1992 (Fig. 46). With its permanent bend and a tip protected from sucking to the vein intima, the catheter performed better than PermCath, but I was still not satisfied with the results. Still, one of the catheters implanted in 1992 functioned until 1997, which was the longest catheter survival in our center. We had also started measuring recirculation, and we presented our studies at a meeting in Baltimore [Ab 101, Pr 340] and published them in 1993 [Pu 191]. In a letter to Brad on June 2, 1992, I suggested "that the inflow and outflow lumens

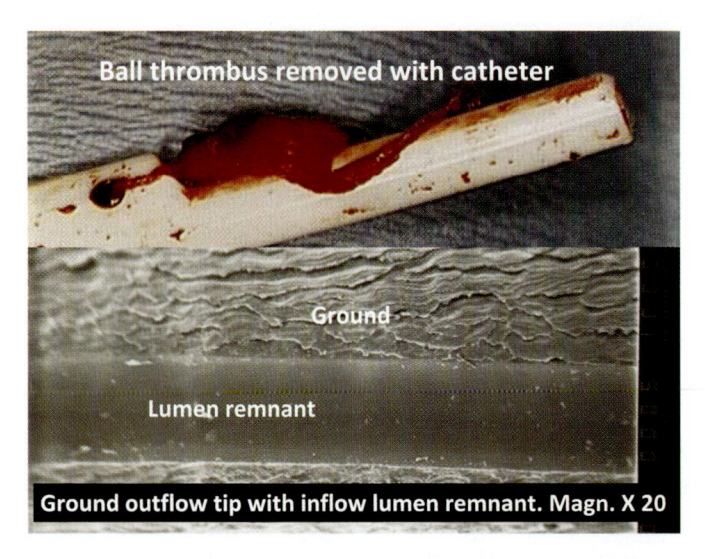

Figure 45. Upper part: ball thrombus anchored to the hole; lower part: rough surface of the outflow tip of PermCath. (Modified from Pu 319.)

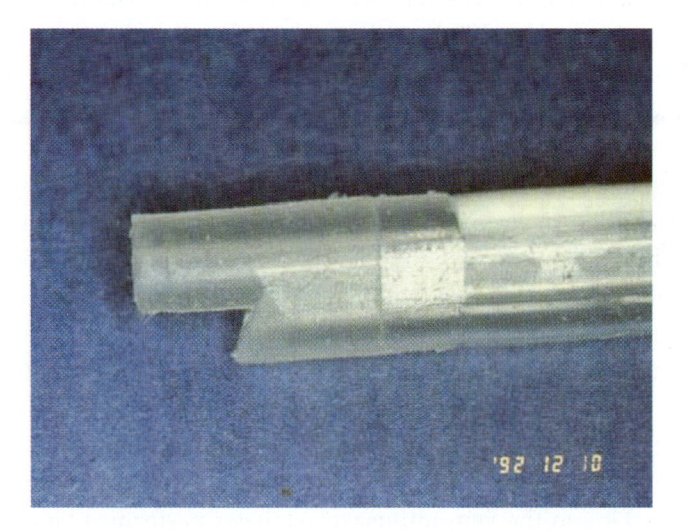

Figure 46. Catheter with the inflow bore directed toward the outflow tubing.

may be at the same level (just flat tip) without significant recirculation," predicting that such a catheter would be less prone to clotting.

Meanwhile, we were also battling with an examiner at the patent office regarding claims. Although it was not unusual, we had tremendous difficulties having all the features allowed. The first objection was that we were claiming too many features. It was suggested that our patent claims be split up, so we submitted applications in three parts as a continuation of the original application filed on January 8, 1990. Another major objection of the examiners (primary: John D. Yasko; assistant: Anthony Gutowski) was our claim that the intravenous catheter shape in its unstressed condition conformed to the site of the venous system of the patient where the catheter was to be implanted. The examiners' objection was that the claimed shapes were indefinite, as "the venous system has an infinite number of shapes." At the time we were in the process of determining vein dimensions in a number of volunteers, but we had to agree that the examiners were correct. After many changes we ultimately received three patents with claims related to the catheter tip [Pa IV-1, Pa IV-2] and the method of catheter implantation using so-called reverse or retrograde tunneling (Fig. 47) [Pa IV-4]. However, as the examiners found that a similar feature had already been patented, the most important feature, the U-shaped precurved catheter, was not allowed. I was extremely surprised at this outcome after learning that the

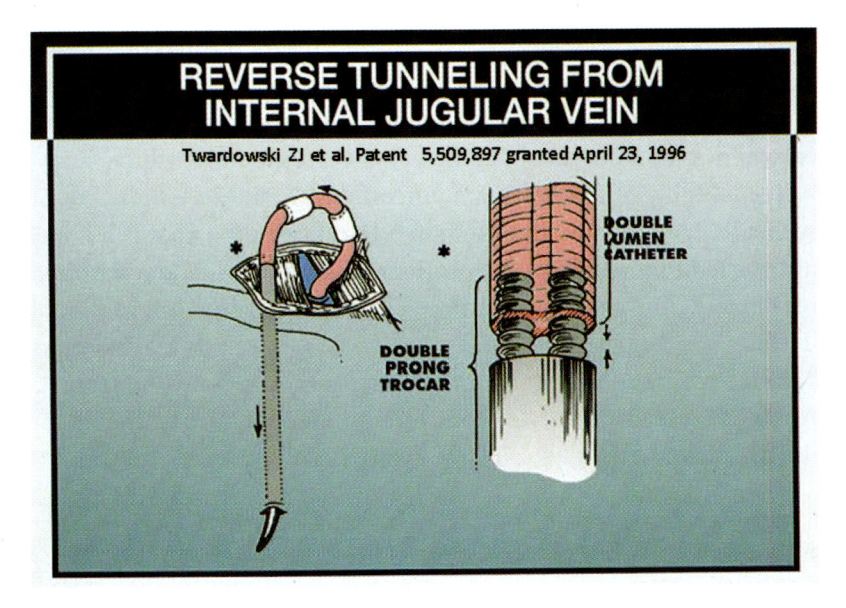

Figure 47. Reverse tunneling of the jugular catheter.

application for the rival patent had been submitted almost three months after ours. It is a very interesting story and I will return to it later in a separate subchapter.

Following Brad Fowler's departure from the company in 1993, I cooperated with Pauline Young, and then with Gretchen Solberg and Lori Thomson. Unfortunately, the Quinton company was already winding down its operations, as it was to be taken over by Sherwood-Davis & Geck, which was less inclined to make products than to sell Quinton Instruments' intellectual property (licensed patents) to another company (Kendall) to make profit. Indubitably, my best cooperation with regard to intravenous catheters was with Quinton Instruments, particularly with Brad Fowler.

Our catheter with the retrograde tunneling feature has a story of its own. Many years after the patent was issued, licensees of the patent (Quinton, then Sherwood-Davis & Geck, then Kendall) were not interested in manufacturing such catheters. In 2005 I found a paper in the *Journal of Vascular Access*[14] describing results with a catheter manufactured by Arrow International Inc., Reading, Pennsylvania, that was clearly based on our patent 5,509,897 [Pa IV-4]. I notified Covidien and the university's Office of Technology Management and Industry Relations, which at the time assumed some responsibilities previously covered by the Office of Patents and Licensing. I asked for two things: first, to force Arrow to stop infringing the patent licensed to them, and second, for Covidien to commence manufacture of catheters with this feature, which I considered highly valuable. I am uncertain about the rules, but it seems that a company like Covidien that licensed a patent but has not started to manufacture a product based on this patent within a reasonable time cannot sue another company, Arrow International in this case, for patent infringement. In fact, it was about five years before Covidien started manufacturing catheters with the feature. As far as I am aware, Arrow continues to manufacture catheters for retrograde tunneling.

---

14. Davanzo WJ. (2005) Efficacy and safety of a retrograde tunneled hemodialysis catheter: 6-month clinical experience with the Cannon Catheter™ chronic hemodialysis catheter, *J Vasc Access* **6**: 38–44.

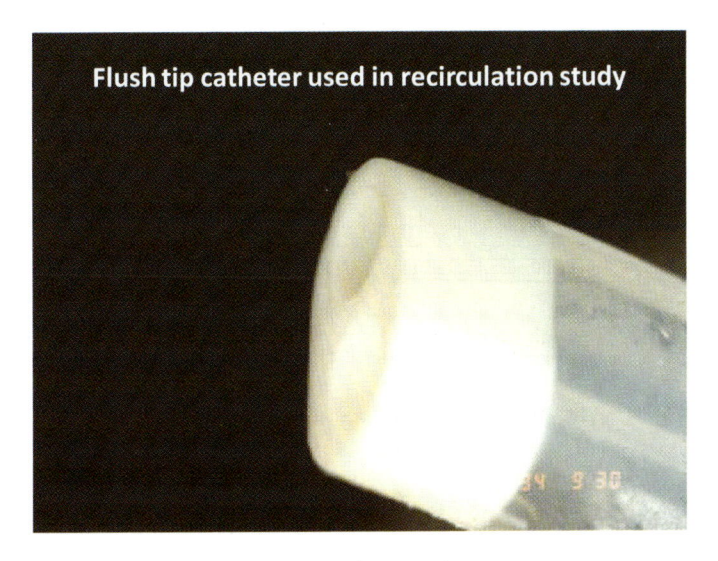

Figure 48. Flat tip catheter.

Clot resistant multiple lumen catheter

As I mentioned previously, I speculated in my letter to Brad Fowler of June 2, 1992, that there would not be much recirculation with a flat tip (both inflow and outflow bores at the same level). It happened that one of the catheters manufactured by Quinton for our study was too long for one of our patients, so I asked Dr. Nichols to simply cut the tip of the catheter and make it flat (Fig. 48). We had already done some electron microscopy studies of various catheters and knew that all catheter tips had a rough surface, which obviously predisposed them to engender clot formation. But we also knew that a surface created by cutting was not as rough as that made by grinding, so the idea was that a catheter with a flat tip fashioned by cutting would be less likely to form a clot at the tip.

We started a more sophisticated recirculation study almost immediately after our previous study was published in 1993 [Pu 191]. Firstly of all, in the previous study we used a chemical method, which was not very accurate. In the new study we compared several methods and came to the conclusion that the most accurate was the ultrasound dilution method. We confirmed our previous results that recirculation with the staggered catheter is minimal with the proper direction of lines and

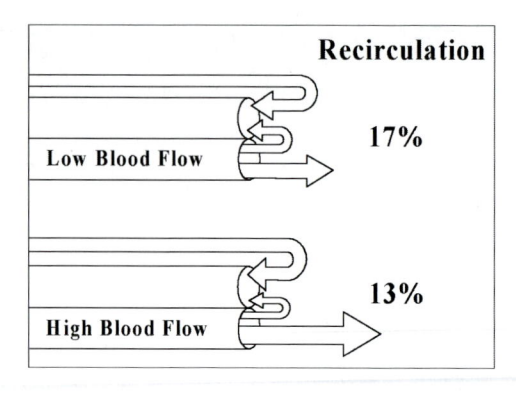

Figure 49. Recirculation with flat tip catheters.

substantial with the reversed direction of lines. The study confirmed our assumption that recirculation should not be high with flush catheters regardless of the direction of flow, especially with high blood flow (Fig. 49). The preliminary results were presented in 1995 [Pr 395], with the final paper appearing in 1998 [Pu 277]. However, before the presentation and publication we submitted a disclosure of invention with the University of Missouri,[15] and our patent application was submitted on February 9, 1995, six days before the presentation in Baltimore, Md. It is important not to publicly reveal any new idea before the patent application, as this may preclude obtaining the patent. Ultimately several patents [Pa IV-5a–IV-5f, Pa IV-6, Pa IV-7] were granted for this invention, with many claims, but the most important feature of this new double lumen catheter was a flat tip (not staggered, without longitudinal spacing). To prevent the possibility of recirculation even more strongly, the lumens were to be separated by a wall projecting distally beyond distal lumen ends (Fig. 50). At the time when the patents were granted, Kendall Healthcare Company acquired licenses from the University of Missouri, the owner of the patents, and started working on the project. Michael G. Tal, an interventional radiologist from Yale University School of Medicine, New Haven, Connecticut, helped the company with animal experiments and designing the final shape of the tip (Fig. 51), so

---

15. Twardowski ZJ, Nichols WK, Van Stone JC. Multiple lumen catheter for hemodialysis: New tip design of intravenous catheter for hemodialysis. UM Disclosure 94-UMC-036, disclosed on May 20, 1994. Contributions: Twardowski 70 percent, Nichols 20 percent, Van Stone 10 percent.

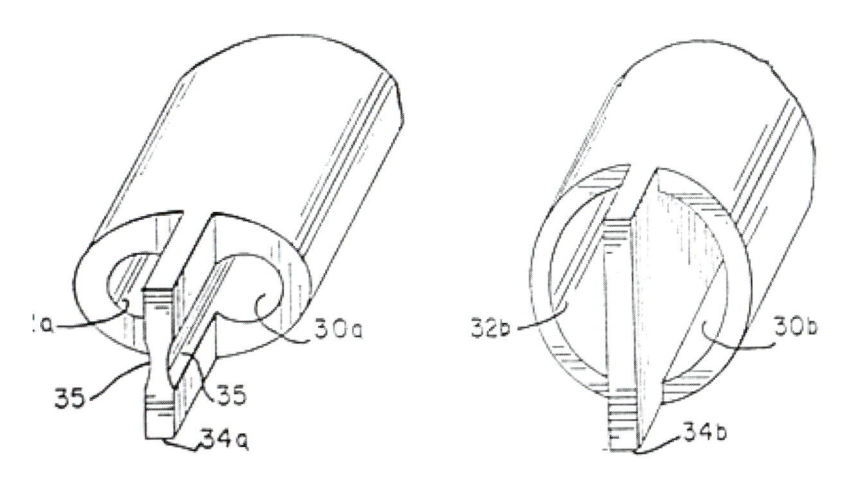

Figure 50. Flat tip with extended septum.

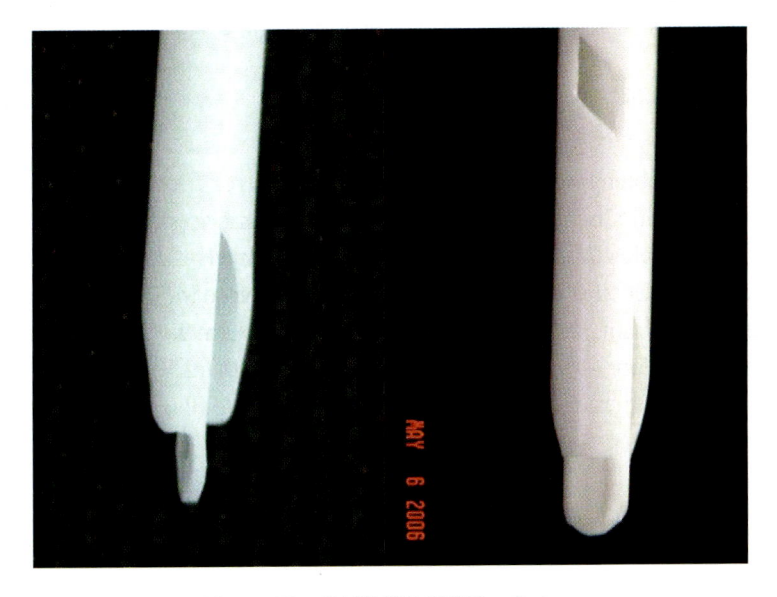

Figure 51. PALINDROME™ catheters.

the company named the catheter Tal PALINDROME™. The name "palindrome" reflects the most important feature of the catheter: no recirculation regardless of the direction of blood flow. Because of changes in the ownership of the patents, it took quite some time to start manufacturing and selling these catheters. However, from the second quarter of 2004, the worldwide use of these catheters rapidly increased (Fig. 52). There

Patents in Columbia 205

Palindrome catheter sales in the world

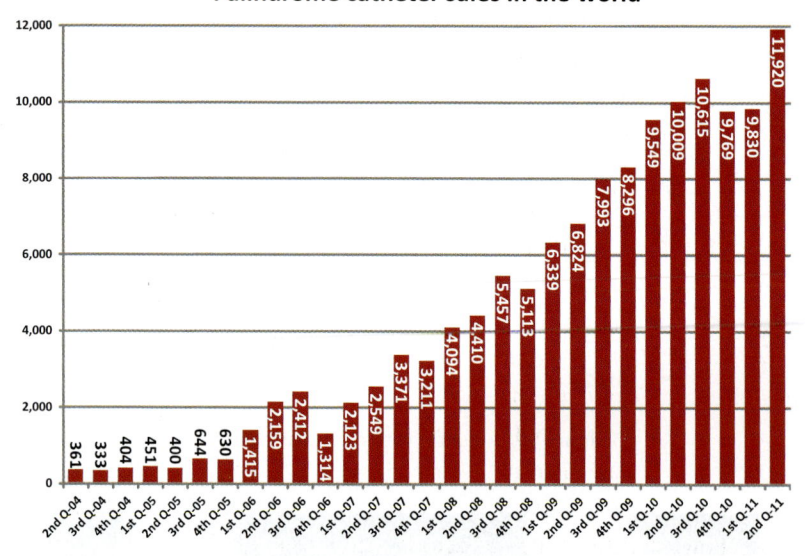

Quarter	Sales
2nd Q-04	361
3rd Q-04	333
4th Q-04	404
1st Q-05	451
2nd Q-05	400
3rd Q-05	644
4th Q-05	630
1st Q-06	1,415
2nd Q-06	2,159
3rd Q-06	2,412
4th Q-06	1,314
1st Q-07	2,123
2nd Q-07	2,549
3rd Q-07	3,371
4th Q-07	3,211
1st Q-08	4,094
2nd Q-08	4,410
3rd Q-08	5,457
4th Q-08	5,113
1st Q-09	6,339
2nd Q-09	6,824
3rd Q-09	7,993
4th Q-09	8,296
1st Q-10	9,549
2nd Q-10	10,009
3rd Q-10	10,615
4th Q-10	9,769
1st Q-11	9,830
2nd Q-11	11,920

Figure 52. Worldwide use of PALINDROME™ catheters by quarter.

were no problems with these patents: no major rejections of claims by examiners and no interferences to date. The University of Missouri Office of Intellectual Property Administration[16] receives 4 percent royalties from sales and distributes them among inventors (1/3), inventors' departments (or divisions) (2/9), the Office of Intellectual Property Administration (2/9), and the Office of Research (2/9). Ultimately I receive 0.93 percent of sales, and the Division of Nephrology, 0.59 percent.

Interference

Interference is a proceeding to determine the priority of inventorship between two patent applications, or between a patent and a pending patent application.

As described earlier, Drs. Van Stone and Nichols and I submitted an application for a "multiple lumen catheter for hemodialysis" on January 8, 1990 (Application number 461,684). The examiners,

---

16. Formerly Office of Patents and Licensing of the University of Missouri.

John D. Yasko and Anthony Gutowski, objected to there being too many inventions within one patent application, so following the advice of our patent attorney, Garrettson Ellis, we abandoned the application and submitted continuations, for which we ultimately obtained three patents [Pa IV-1, Pa IV-2, Pa IV-4]. This last patent was mainly regarding the method of implantation. For us the most important feature was the precured U-shape. However, in April 1994, Garretson Ellis notified me of the examiners' decision regarding Application No. 08/045,016, namely that this feature could not be allowed, citing as a prior art the patent of Geoffrey S. Martin and Jonathan E. Last (5,156,592) issued October 20, 1992. I was flabbergasted, as their patent application was filed on April 4, 1991, one year after their Canadian application of April 4, 1990, while ours was filed three months earlier, on January 8, 1990. In my letter of April 13, 1994, I notified Mr. Ellis, Richard D. Allison, Esq. (a Quinton lawyer), Brad Fowler (Quinton), Bruce Densmore (Quinton) and Connie Armentraut from the University Patent and Licensing Office that the examiners had committed a serious error in citing Martin and Last's patent as a prior art. That patent had already been issued and was licensed to Vas-Cath, which was already manufacturing and selling catheters based on the patent.

In 1994 the Quinton company decided to fight for the rights to the invention, as they had already paid for the patent application and cooperation with the University of Missouri. They hired Barbara Clarke McCurdy, Esq., and Lara C. Kelly, Esq., from Finnegan, Henderson, Farabow, Garrett & Dunner LLP, a law firm from Washington, D.C. They continued to work on the case when the license was transferred to Sherwood-Davis & Geck, then to Kendall, and then to Covidien. Finnegan initiated the interference by filing a new continuation application 08/412,114 in the Patent and Trademark Office (PTO), on March 28, 1995. This application was based on Application No. 08/045,016, April 8, 1993, Patent No. 5,405,320, granted on April 11, 1995. The prior application was a continuation-in-part of Ser. No. 07/772,613, filed October 8, 1991 (Patent No. 5,209,723, granted on May 11, 1993), which was a continuation of Ser. No. 07/461,684, filed January 8, 1990, and then abandoned. The 08/412,114 application was filed with the primary claim directed to a catheter being "generally U-shape in its natural, unstressed condition" and with additional claims directed to a catheter as claimed in the Martin and Last 5,156,592 patent. Additionally, Finnegan filed a request for interference to be declared between the 08/412,114 application and Martin and Last's 5,156,592 patent. After the examiners found all claims to be allowable, the Board of Patent Appeals and Interferences of the PTO declared Interference No. 103,988 between our 08/412,114 application and Martin and Last's 5,156,592 patent on August 19, 1997.

It is worth stressing that Vas-Cath was manufacturing catheters with the U-shape feature, which they called Opti-Flow™, and earning money from the sales. Vas-Cath was taken over by Bard from Salt Lake City, Utah, and continued to manufacture Opti-Flow catheters in three sizes. It was for this reason that they had decided to fight as hard as possible. Quinton had also made the decision to fight, as sales from the catheters were substantial and they could not manufacture them without our patent. During the first phase of the interference, Vas-Cath sought a judgment that most claims were not patentable to us. The Administrative Patent Judge (APJ) did not agree with Vas-Cath and rendered a decision in our favor on January 8, 2001. In the second phase, Vas-Cath sought to prove, based on an unrelated Canadian patent owned by Martin and associated products sold in the 1980s, that it was first to invent the new catheter. This new strategy was calculated to show that neither Martin's claims nor our claims were patentable. A protracted legal battle ensued. Barbara McCurdy and Lara Kelly visited me in Columbia to discuss our evidence of prior invention, as well as evidence that Martin's earlier catheter was not U-shaped and therefore not related to the subject matter of the interference. I loaned them copies of my journal collection from the 1980s containing advertisements that showed Vas-Cath's earlier catheters were not U-shaped, which they used as evidence against Martin and Last's priority case in the PTO. They cited my disclosure of the invention in March 1985, diligence beginning in March 1985, and reduction to practice in March 1989, but all these prior ideas and attempts were unimportant, as our opponents never proved that they conceived or reduced to practice the U-shape idea before filing the Canadian application three months after our patent application. In any event, the Board of Patent Appeals and Interferences rendered a decision in our favor on July 30, 2003, after a long battle (1997–2003) and no real happy ending.

Vas-Cath appealed the board's decision by suing the Curators of the University of Missouri, the assignee of the 08/412,114 application, in the U.S. District Court for the District of Columbia on September 23, 2003. As it was an inappropriate venue, the court decided to transfer the matter to the U.S. District Court for the Western District of Missouri, on April 15, 2005, which dismissed the case on August 11, 2005. Vas-Cath in turn appealed that dismissal to the Court of Appeals for the Federal Circuit, which reversed the district court's action on January 29, 2007. The district court then dismissed the case a second time on December 6, 2007. Vas-Cath filed a second appeal to the Federal Court.

I was a little concerned that with the speed of the proceedings the matter might go to the Supreme Court before a final verdict would be rendered. I even joked with my lawyers, Barbara and Lara, that the speed of the interference teaches us that any invention ought to be made early in life so that one can live long enough to hear the final outcome. Eventually, Vas-Cath determined that their efforts were futile, with their legal expenses being higher than their possible earnings, so the second appeal was dismissed on March 17, 2008 on Vas-Cath's motion. Jurisdiction for the 08/412,114 application was then transferred back to the PTO examiners. Barbara McCurdy and Lara Kelly filed for a patent with additional claims prepared in cooperation with Covidien lawyers Betsy O'Brien and Douglas Denninger, on December 23, 2008. The claims were allowed on July 6, 2009. The patent was issued on April 13, 2010, as U.S. Patent No. 7,695,450, more than 20 years after the application on January 8, 1990 — and I lived to see the day.

Since we submitted the application before June 8, 1995, our patent will expire on April 12, 2027. Prior to June 8, 1995, the rule was that a patent expires 17 years after the date of issuance or 20 years after the date of an application submission, whichever is later. After 1995, it was ruled that patents expire 20 years after the date of application. However, there was another very important new rule: the priority of the patent is based on the date of application and nothing else.

Before 1995, inventors could claim that they had some idea before the patent application and witnesses and notes could be taken into account during the interference procedure, as it was in our case. If our legal battle had started after 1995, we would have won quickly but received the patent with an expiration date of 2015 or later, and the company could have manufactured and sold the catheters earlier.

In addition to the lesson that it is preferable to file a patent application at a young age, our interference saga taught us that it is insufficient to have a good idea to get a patent. It does not mean that the inventor gets royalties. It is also extremely important to have good patent lawyers, such as Barbara McCurdy and Lara Kelly, and license the patent to a wealthy company, which can pay costly legal expenses.

The company fought very hard for the patent and won, but during the interference process, several competitors launched products incorporating the precurved shaft, the subject matter of the interference. Covidien made the decision to launch a competing product using the design, but with multiple competitors sales are always limited. The company also decided to combine features of palindrome catheters with the precurved feature in the latest version of their catheter (Fig. 53). It has the option of filing various legal proceedings

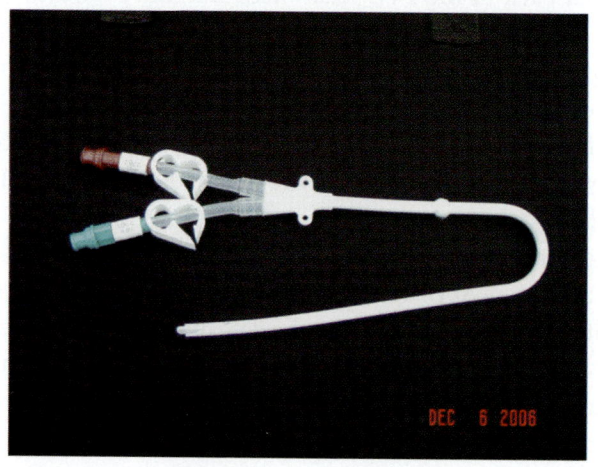

Figure 53. Prototype of precurved palindrome catheter.

against competitors selling catheters incorporating the design. With those proceedings potentially costing large sums of money, Covidien is currently weighing its options and determining the value of going forward with legal proceedings, but it has not yet reached a final decision. Ultimately, it will be a business decision based on U.S. sales of products with that design and numerous other factors. Ideally, legal action should be taken against all infringers, but the cost–benefit analysis may say otherwise.

Patient tailored catheter

For the best performance the tip of a central vein catheter for hemodialysis should be located in the upper third of the right atrium (Fig. 54). In this position there is no structure to hinder its function. The tip should not be higher while the patient is supine, so it will move no higher than to the lower superior vena cava while the patient is upright. Both excessively high and excessively low positions of the

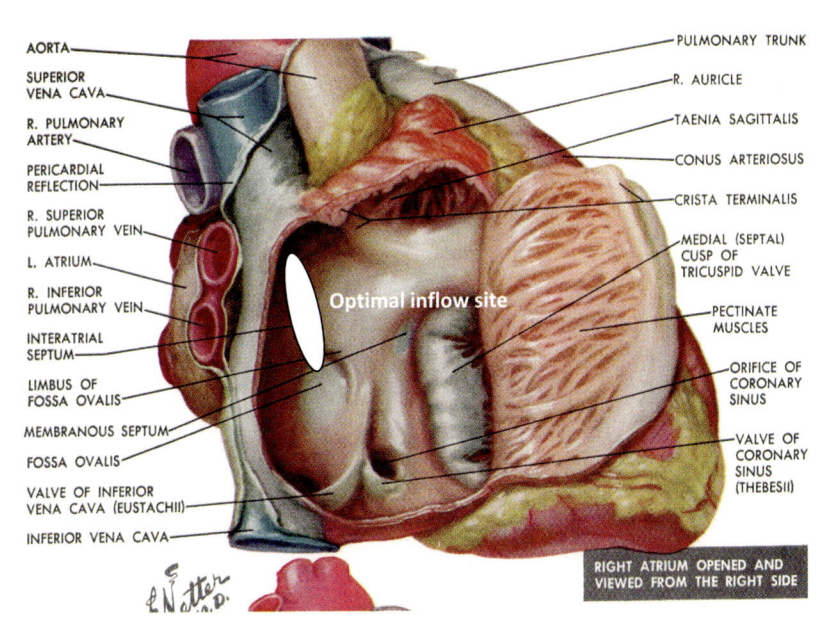

Figure 54. Optimal inflow site in the upper right atrium without structures to interfere with blood flow. [Heart structure according to Netter FH. (2010) *Atlas of Human Anatomy*, 5th ed. Saunders, an imprint of Elsevier Inc.]

catheter tip are unfavorable. The heart moves down in the upright position and up in the supine position. Because the catheter length is fixed, the catheter moves deeper into the right atrium, while the patient is supine, and closer to the brachial veins, while the patient is upright. Breathing also influences the catheter position. During deep inspiration the diaphragm and the heart move down, so the catheter tip moves up; during expiration the movements are in opposite directions. Finally, the chest wall subcutaneous tissue moves down when the supine person assumes the erect posture. The catheter cuff, which is anchored in this tissue, pulls the catheter tip upward. If the catheter tip is located high in the superior vena cava, it may translocate to one of the brachiocephalic veins where the blood flow is insufficient to secure adequate blood flow through the dialyzer. However, if the catheter goes too low, its tip may be stuck in one of the valves (thebesian or eustachian) and the tip may be occluded.[17] In the majority of people both thebesian (coronary sinus) and eustachian (inferior vena cava) valves are small and constitute what is called the crista terminalis. These structures are located low in the medial aspect of the right atrium. There is a large variability in size, shape, thickness and texture of the persistent eustachian valve. At one end of the spectrum, the embryonic eustachian valve disappears completely or is represented only by a thin ridge. Most commonly, it is a crescentic fold of endocardium arising from the anterior rim of the inferior vena cava orifice. At the other extreme, it persists as a mobile, elongated structure projecting several centimeters into the right atrial cavity. Finally, if the catheter tip is too low, it may migrate to the inferior vena cava, as in a study on recirculation where we noted this event in one of our patients [Pu 277], or to the right ventricle [Pu 320].

While working with Brad Fowler we thought about manufacturing catheters tailored to patients' vein dimensions. This would be particularly important for catheters with permanent bends, as the tip position is determined by the length of the catheter from the bend to the tip. He was willing to manufacture catheters in several sizes. I started cooperating with Dr. Richard M. Seger from the Radiology

---

17. These structures were described in the 16th (Bartolomeo Eustachio, 1524–1574) and 18th (Adam Christan Thebesius, 1686–1732) centuries, but only recently, with increased cardiac catheterizations, has their variability been appreciated.

Department of the University of Missouri. Using magnetic resonance imaging (MRI), we studied 31 volunteers to determine the dimensions of upper body veins in relation to anthropometric measurements. In order to determine the best way to do the study, I became the first volunteer. All measurements were performed from March 1992 to May 1993, and in November 1993 I received coordinates of appropriate points in the veins so that I could determine the lengths of veins and correlate them with the anthropometrics of volunteers. However, with Brad Fowler leaving Quinton, the study was not finished before we ended our cooperation with Quinton, as the company was sold and all our patent licenses were transferred to Sherwood-Davis & Geck, then to Kendall, and ultimately to Covidien. My cooperation with Quinton was excellent, almost nonexistent with Sherwood-Davis & Geck, and rather limited with Kendall.

Kendall was not interested in the project, as they were concentrating on the palindrome catheter (see above). The idea of tailoring the catheter length to the dimensions of the patient's upper body veins would be more important for the permanently bent catheter than for the palindrome catheter. Besides, the situation with regard to the interference did not look too good at the time and Kendall did not have an incentive to pursue this other idea. I continued to work on the dimensions of upper body veins from 1994 to 1999, as I thought that it would be possible to use this to choose an appropriate catheter length for a particular patient regardless of who manufactures bent catheters. The study was done on volunteers from the Division of Nephrology and Dialysis Clinic Inc. in Columbia. The heights and weights of all volunteers were taken on the day of study. Skin marks were made at the points indicating the optimal insertion sites to the large upper body veins: in the right and left Sédillot triangle (between the sternal and clavicular heads of the sternocleidomastoid muscle) and just below the clavicle in the right and left midclavicular lines. All volunteers had MRIs without enhancement taken in the supine position during maximal inspiration in three planes, horizontal, frontal (coronal) and sagittal, according to the standard method. The MRI scanner was a Siemens Magnetom Vision, which uses a 1.5 T superconducting magnet. Selected points as shown in Fig. 55 were localized in a three-dimensional coordinate system: lateral, side to side (x);

The distance between the catheter entrance to the vein and the upper right atrium was a summation of distances between the adjacent points.

URA = Upper right atrium

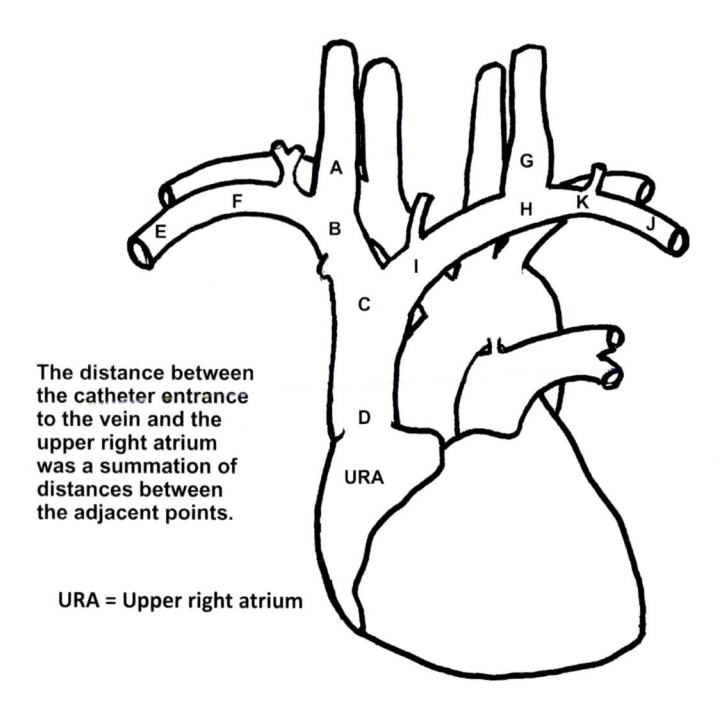

Figure 55. Selected points in the venous system of the chest and neck. (Modified from Pu 335.)

perpendicular, anterior to posterior (y); vertical, cranial to caudal (z). In addition to the points shown in the figure, both acromions were localized.

The coordinates were taken from a computer workstation, each point having three coordinates $P(x, y, z)$ as shown in Fig. 56. The distance (d) between two adjacent points P_1 and P_2 (e.g., A and B) was calculated according to an analytic geometry formula (Fig. 56); the distance between acromions was calculated using the same formula. The distance between the catheter entrance to the vein and the upper right atrium was a simple summation of distances between the adjacent points. For instance, the distance from A to D is a sum of distances from A to B, B to C, and C to D. Taking into account that the images were taken during deep inspiration, the catheter tip located in this position at this point will move to the mid atrium during normal breathing in the supine position and to the superior vena cava/right atrium junction in the upright position. I did all of the calculations

Three-dimensional coordinates were taken from a workstation computer program in the machine

$P_1(x_1, y_1, z_1)$
$P_2(x_2, y_2, z_2)$

x = lateral (r-l)
y = perpendicular (a-p)
z = vertical (c-c)

Analytic geometry formula

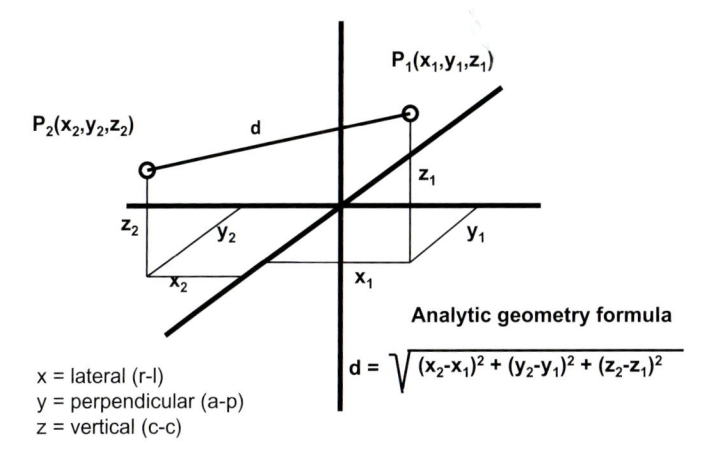

$$d = \sqrt{(x_2-x_1)^2 + (y_2-y_1)^2 + (z_2-z_1)^2}$$

Figure 56. Analytical geometry formula to measure distances between points. (Modified from Pu 335.)

using Quattro Pro. I was happy that this spreadsheet program was available, as using a calculator — not to mention an abacus, slide ruler or arithmometer — would have been painstakingly slow. Descriptive statistics, correlations and regressions were performed using the software Sigma Stat (SPSS Inc., Chicago, Illinois). In spite of the help I got from the computer, it took me some time to finish the calculations and determine that the best correlation of the desired lengths of the catheters and body anthropometrics was with the body surface area. In the 1990s, I was preoccupied with other studies in addition to my regular patient care and teaching, so it took me quite a long time to finish a manuscript discussing the calculations.

Before publishing the data, I disclosed my invention to the University Patent and Licensing Office on August 12, 1998 (disclosure number 99UMC009). I asked the university to submit an application and pay for the patent, but I was informed that the university's policy was only to pay for patents when there was industry interest in licensing the invention. So the next day I asked Connie Armentraut to waive the right to the patent and I would pay for it myself. I received the waiver on August 25, 1998. The waiver stated that: "The inventor has committed a return to the University of 5 percent of any future money he receives from any source based on the invention." I submitted a patent application to my patent attorney, Garrettson Ellis of Gerstman & Ellis Ltd., on December 30, 2000. He submitted a patent application on April 26, 2001 and the patent was granted in 2003 [Pa VII-1]. Only after submission of patent application to the patent office did I submit the manuscript for publication in the *International Journal for Artificial Organs* [Pu 335]. The *Journal of Vascular Access* asked for permission to republish it and I agreed [Pu 335a].

I prepared a special nomogram for selection of catheters according to patient anthropometrics and approached Covidien again on April 11, 2008, but the company was not interested. I also approached the Bard company with my suggestion to license my patent in December 2007, but they too were not interested, as they had probably already contemplated dismissing the interference appeal early in 2008. After Covidien won the interference I again tried to convince them of the value of the patent but to no avail, and I decided to abandon the patent and stop paying the maintenance fees. This story proves that not all "great ideas" buttressed with hard work are rewarded.

Home Hemodialysis Machine

The idea of quotidian[18] hemodialysis came to mind while working on my habilitation thesis when considering the adequacy of hemodialysis in relation to the frequency and duration of sessions in Bytom, Poland, from March 1969 through May 1973 [Pu 21–Pu 23]. I concluded the last paper in this series with the statement: "It seems that daily short-lasting dialyses will in the near future be the basic form of treatment of uraemia" [Pu 23]. At the time I had also reviewed the

---

18. Hemodialysis performed every day is frequently called "daily." I have been trying to convince people that this is inappropriate, since "daily" in English has two meanings: (i) of or occurring during the daytime, and (ii) happening or done every day. To avoid such awkward expressions as "daily nocturnal" or "daily nightly" I have proposed introducing new terminology for dialysis performed every day or every night. Everyday dialysis would be referred to as "quotidian" (from Latin *quotidie*, each day), dialysis performed during the daytime would be called "hemeral" (from Greek *hemera*, daytime as opposed to nighttime), and dialysis performed nightly would be called "nocturnal" (from Latin *nox*, night). To my chagrin this terminology is not widely used; even in our recent editorial published in the *New England Journal of Medicine*, the term "quotidian" was changed by the editors to "daily" [Pu 383].

available machines for hemodialysis and summarized their advantages and disadvantages [Pu 24]. My feeling was that for quotidian home hemodialysis a new machine would be necessary. Such a machine should have several important features. First of all, it should reuse dialyzers and lines to decrease the cost. This was based on my experience with the reuse of the coil dialyzer with a cuprophane membrane [Pu 16] and the RP-6 dialyzer with a polyacrylonitrile membrane [Pu 64]. Secondly, it should prepare dialysis solution from dry chemicals. Lastly, to save time for patients, the machine should make its preparations for dialysis automatically. The first two features would markedly decrease storage space requirements and reduce waste, thus making it environmentally friendly. The third would make the machine user-friendly — easy to learn and operate — and could obviate the need for a helper.

Two elements that I wanted to include in the overall concept was a tank system, somewhat similar to the Travenol RSP machine, and direct measurement of ultrafiltration taken from the Rhodial 75 system. For adequate removal of uremic toxins I reasoned that the tank should have a capacity somewhere between 60 and 100 L. I disclosed my invention to the University Office for Patents and Licensing on May 18, 1983, which started looking for a potential licensee, sending an abstract to several companies, including Baxter Travenol. On May 20, 1983, I sent a letter to Donald W. Joseph, the company's vice president, suggesting potential cooperation in developing the machine. I was invited to visit them in September 1983 and presented my concept to the group, including engineer Thomas E. Muller. I felt that Mr. Muller and others in the engineering department were in favor of working on the project, but after about a year the Baxter Travenol higher-ups informed me that they were not interested in pursuing the idea. I was not given any reasons at that time. With no enthusiasm from other companies, the University Office of Patents and Licensing remained reluctant to submit an application.

The University Office for Patent and Licensing was typically rather inept at finding a company interested in a project. I learned later that the office was absolutely of no help in this respect, at least for me. At the time I was busy with other projects, so I temporarily suspended my efforts to find a company that would be interested in the project. My other projects included work on tidal peritoneal dialysis (described earlier) with Baxter Travenol, which was renamed Baxter International Inc., in 1988. I worked very closely on tidal peritoneal dialysis with the highly innovative Rodney S. Kenley, Advanced Systems Development Manager at Baxter. After determining that tidal peritoneal dialysis would be very successful if a large amount of dialysis solution were available, Baxter decided to develop a machine for manufacturing peritoneal dialysis solution from concentrate and treated water. The project was later abandoned by Baxter for no clear reason, and Rod was very upset, as it was his favorite project. In December 1988, at the 21st Annual Meeting of the American Society of Nephrology in San Antonio, Texas, Rod and I met again, and I took the opportunity to talk to him about the feasibility of a machine for daily home hemodialysis. We spent perhaps 10 hours talking about it, and Rod was firmly behind the idea, promising to try to convince Baxter to take the project on.

On January 25, 1989, I had a presentation on tidal peritoneal dialysis at Baxter Healthcare Corporation Headquarters in Round Lake, Illinois [Pr 148]. After the presentation we had a meeting with Donald W. Joseph (Corporate Vice President), Lee W. Henderson,[19] MD (Vice President for Medical Affairs), Arthur Holden (Marketing Vice President) and others from Baxter. Rod Kenley was also there. We tried to sell them the idea of a daily home hemodialysis machine, but they were adamant that they were not interested in the venture. I was given two reasons. Firstly, it was uncertain whether the project would be successful and they would have to spend a great deal of money with no guarantee of a return. Secondly, if the project were successful, they would cannibalize their very successful business in peritoneal dialysis. I tried to argue that it would be better to cannibalize a business than to be devoured by another company that develops the system, but they remained unconvinced.

Rod and I tried again in 1989, but to no avail. Ultimately, Rod decided to leave Baxter and found a new company. Before he left, he

---

19. Lee W. Henderson is a very innovative researcher in the field of dialysis who, with Karl D. Nolph, developed a kinetic model for mass transport in peritoneal dialysis in 1969. In 1975 he developed a new method of blood purification, hemofiltration, which is more efficient than hemodialysis at removing uremic toxins of higher molecular weight.

decided to provide funds he had at his disposal for a study on daily hemodialysis in DCI in our center in Columbia. In a letter I sent to him on December 19, 1989, I presented our protocol, "Clinical and laboratory comparisons of routine and daily hemodialysis," which was approved by our Institutional Review Board two days later. We received funds on January 24, 1990. We originally planned to have 12 patients, but with the available funds we started with four patients (James Coleman, Raymond Cooper, Michael Kelleher and Pearlie Warren), hoping to secure more funds at a later date. The study was planned for (A) three months as a control period with three times weekly regular hemodialysis, and then (B) six months of daily dialysis with exactly the same total dialysis time per week. With the available funds we were able to finish periods A and B on only four patients. The results were, as expected, much better in period B than in period A, with lower swings in blood chemistries, fewer hypotensive episodes, better blood pressure control, and tremendous subjective improvement in all patients. With such a small number of patients, we did not publish our findings, but the results were included in a paper published many years later as part of a larger number of patients (21 individuals). The results confirmed previous observations of better tolerance of dialysis, fewer hypotensive episodes, no detrimental effect on blood access, and overall improvement in subjective assessment by patients [Pu 350].

Rod left Baxter before we completed the study on our four patients. He advised me to ask for a waiver of the university's right to my invention disclosed in UM Disclosure No. 83-UMC-027 and submit the patent application privately. I received a waiver on June 13, 1989. I was a consultant for Baxter at the time, so I decided to terminate my relationship with the company to avoid any claims to the patent ownership. I started to work on the submission, consulting with Rod regarding some details, and submitted the draft to my patent attorney, Garrettson Ellis, on May 22, 1991. The application was filed in the U.S. Patent Office on August 21, 1991, and the patent was issued on August 9, 1994 [Pa V-1]. Based on the initial submission, three more divisional patents were granted [Pa V-2, Pa V-3, Pa V-5]. A very important fifth patent was filed on November 7, 1994, as a division of the previous application but with a new claim related to the method of filling the blood compartment in the dialyzer. This claim was discussed with Rod before I submitted my first patent application, so the patent was issued with both of us as inventors [Pa V-4]. This last feature was very important to decrease the storage space, as no saline was needed for the initiation and termination of dialysis as well as saline boluses if the patient became hypotensive during dialysis. The feature also accomplished some cost saving.

In the meantime, Rod founded Aksys Ltd. on January 4, 1991, finalizing the incorporation papers on January 20. He recruited a very innovative lady called Dawn Matthews, who left Baxter for a new challenge. They rented a small office and laboratory space on Industrial Drive in Libertyville, Illinois. When the one-year lease was up and they had not raised any capital, they moved into Dawn's basement in Grayslake to save money. On July 12, 1991, Rod asked Baxter to agree not to bring litigation against him and me, based upon restrictive covenants in our respective contracts, in exchange for the right of first offer for the daily hemodialysis system that we might develop. Baxter agreed.

Aksys was established on January 1, 1992 (Fig. 57), with Rod (President), Dawn (Secretary) and myself (Treasurer) as its three

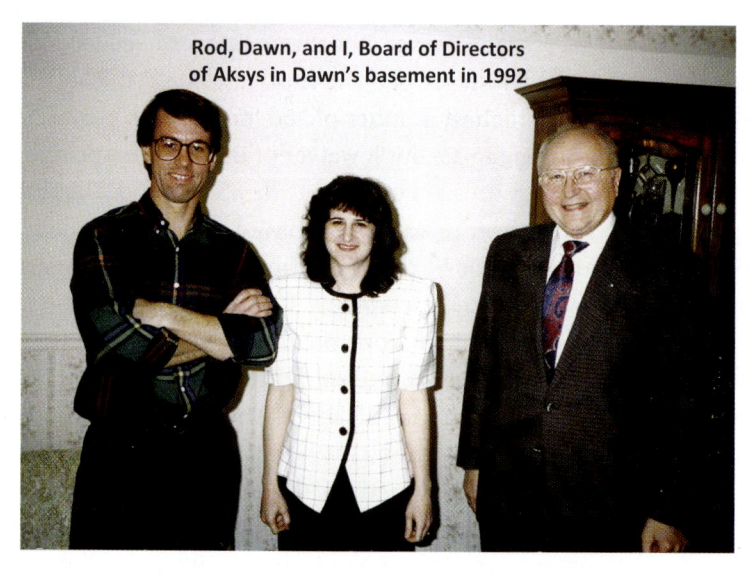

Figure 57. First Board of Directors of Aksys. (Picture taken in Dawn Matthews' basement.)

directors. Early in 1993 William J. Schnell was co-opted to the Board of Directors. Rod tried to raise funds. First of all, Baxter, Rod and Dawn's former employer and the company I provided consulting services to for many years, was given right of first offer (according to the previous agreement) to provide funds for Aksys and distribute the daily home hemodialysis system. Baxter again declined. Rod found several other candidates, including David S. Utterberg, President of Medisystems Corporation in San Francisco, California, Jack K. Arhens from Pathfinder Venture Capital Funds, and Peter H. McNerney from another venture capital group. Utterberg and Ahrens were not convinced about the prospects of daily home hemodialysis and declined to support the new company, but we were more successful with Pete. I spent a day with him presenting my take on the potential for the company, and he decided to join the venture, signing an agreement on April 2, 1993. On February 13, 1993, I had signed a license agreement with Aksys on all my patents related to the artificial kidney for frequent (daily) hemodialysis with a 3 percent royalty on all income, with an understanding that minimum royalties would be paid starting in 1996 and increasing each year until a 3 percent royalty exceeded the minimum. Rod signed the license agreement with me on April 1, 1993, when it was certain that the deal with Pete was close to completion. Five days later we agreed that I would receive 2.4 percent, Rod 0.5 percent and Dawn 0.1 percent royalties, but that Rod would be eligible to buy the highest number of "preferred stock" at US$0.01 per share, Dawn lower, and I the lowest. Funds for company operations and preferred stock were provided in 1993, 1994 and 1995.

After hiring engineers, work on the prototype machine began. I resigned from my post on the Board of Directors, and Peter H. McNerney, Dekle Rountree, Lawrence Kinet and Rodney Kenley were elected to a new board. I signed a consulting agreement with Aksys and became Chairman of the Scientific Advisory Board, which included Eli A. Friedman, MD,[20] John Daugirdas, MD,[21] A. Peter

---

20. Distinguished Teaching Professor and Chief, Division of Renal Disease, Health Science Center, State University of New York; editor: *Journal of the American Society of Artificial Internal Organs*.

21. Professor of Medicine, Department of Nephrology, University of Illinois; co-editor: *Handbook of Dialysis*.

Lundin, MD,[22] James Binkley (daily home hemodialysis patient), Karl D. Nolph, MD, Richard Sherman,[23] and Ann Compton (home hemodialysis nurse). Our first meeting was held on November 2, 1993, and was devoted to the overall direction of the company. I presented the medical and general technical requirements of the system; Rod presented its detailed technical, fiscal and logistical requirements. We discussed problems with teaching health professionals and pondered whether the annual peritoneal dialysis conference could include a daily home hemodialysis symposium.

In August 1994, Rod started to think about constructing a machine giving results not worse than three times weekly dialysis in centers but performed at home six or seven times weekly. He was extremely impressed with the results of Umberto Buoncristiani, MD,[24] which were achieved with a relatively small amount of dialysis solution of 25 L. This would decrease the capacity of the tank and make construction of the machine much easier. In my letter to Rod on August 15, 1994, I strongly encouraged him to go with a higher capacity tank of at least 50 L, calculating that for the removal of various uremic toxins this would be the necessary minimum. He eventually agreed with my argumentation and the tank capacity was set at 50 L. My calculations were supported later by the experience with NxStage system for daily home hemodialysis that used only 15–25 L of dialysis solution. Patients treated with both systems immediately felt the difference in favor of the Aksys machine.

---

22. Andrew Peter Lundin was an undergraduate student when his kidneys failed in 1966. He learned home hemodialysis, graduated from the Stanford University and was accepted to medical school at Downstate Medical Center in Brooklyn, New York (now SUNY Health Science Center at Brooklyn) and later trained under Dr. Eli Friedman. While dialyzing himself three times weekly at night, he ultimately became a professor of medicine with a specialty in nephrology. He had the same arteriovenous fistula for 30 years and used the constant site (buttonhole) method for hemodialysis blood access with the exception of five years while his kidney transplant worked.

23. Professor of Medicine, Robert Wood Johnson Medical School, University of Medicine and Dentistry of New Jersey; editor: *Seminars in Dialysis*.

24. Umberto Buoncristiani, from Azienda Ospedaliera di Perugia, Uniti Organica di Nefrologia-Dialisi Ospedale Silvestrini, Perugia, Italy, started a chronic daily home hemodialysis program in 1982. He had excellent results: Low mortality, good blood pressure control, and excellent subjective assessment of the value of this type therapy by patients [Buoncristiani U, Quintaliani G, Cozzari M, et al. (1988). Daily dialysis: Long-term clinical metabolic results. *Kidney Int* **33**(Suppl 24): S137–S140].

The next Scientific Advisory Board Meeting was held immediately after the 1st Home Hemodialysis Symposium in Baltimore on February 13, 1995, and also included Umberto Buoncristiani, MD, Todd S. Ing, MD,[25] Christopher R. Blagg, MD,[26] and Allen R. Nissenson, MD.[27] The Scientific Advisory Board was in favor of a higher tank capacity. In 1995 a new Board of Directors was elected, with Lawrence H. N. Kinet as Chairman and Chief Executive Officer (CEO). On March 18, 1996, he submitted a so-called S-1 Registration Statement to the Securities and Exchange Commission to obtain the rights to sell shares to the public as soon as possible, achieving the goal with the initial public offering on May 17, 1996. The first prototype of the kidney "Version A," or simply PHD®i, was built shortly afterwards and was demonstrated during the next Scientific Advisory Board Meeting on February 23, 1996, following the 2nd Home Hemodialysis Symposium in Seattle (Fig. 58). Progress was slow over the next few years due to various technical difficulties. In 1997 Carl M. Kjellstrand, MD,[28] was appointed Vice President for Medical Affairs; he became responsible for conducting animal studies, which he did on goats, and creating the clinical trial protocol for PHD®i.

When it became clear that a clinical study would be done in the near future, I was asked for an interview by Sue Salzer from *Missouri Medical Review* to describe how I came up with the idea of a machine for daily home hemodialysis and why I thought that the method would be better for patients. I briefly described my studies in Bytom, Poland, that led me to believe in the merits of daily home dialysis, and that a machine doing most of the chores for patients would make it practical.

---

25. Professor of Medicine, Loyola University, Hines VA Hospital, Renal and Hypertension Section; co-editor of numerous books related to dialysis.

26. Professor of Medicine, University of Washington, and Executive Director, Northwest Kidney Centers, Seattle, Washington, involved in home hemodialysis for over 40 years; current Chief Editor of *Hemodialysis International*.

27. Professor of Medicine, UCLA School of Medicine, Director of Dialysis Program.

28. Carl M. Kjellstrand was the creator of the concept of the "unphysiology" of hemodialysis, which was characterized by "peaks and valleys" of various substances during short, efficient dialysis performed three times weekly [Kjellstrand CM, Evans RL, Petersen RJ, *et al.* (1975) The "unphysiology" of dialysis. A major cause of dialysis side effects? *Kidney Int* 7(Suppl 3): S30–S34]. He was the recipient of an Award for Lifetime Achievements at our Annual Dialysis Conference [Pr 451, Pu 307]. Dr. Kjellstrand started working in hemodialysis as a medical student under the direction of Nils Alwall in Lund, Sweden.

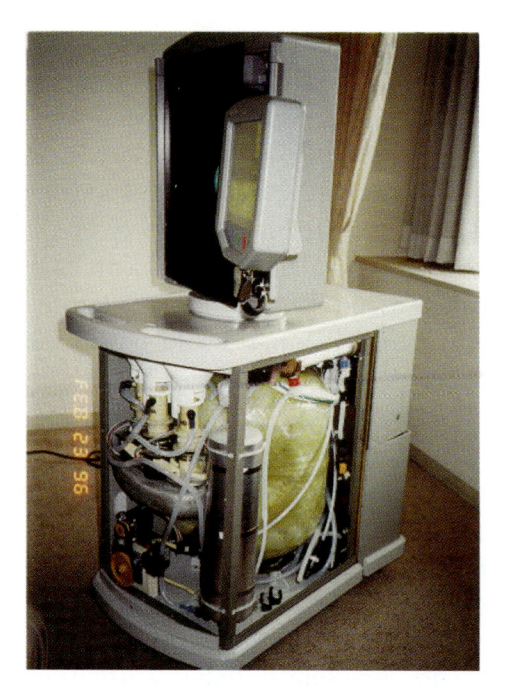

Figure 58. PHD®i: The first version of Aksys machine.

The interview appeared in the summer of 1998. I concluded the interview with the statement, "I am grateful to have had the chance to do something useful." And indeed, to this day, I believe that this is one of my most important contributions to the development of dialysis treatment in patients with renal failure.[29]

In the summer of 1999, Aksys obtained an investigational device exemption (IDE) from the FDA and the recruiting of patients began. The control period on regular machines started in September 1999. Laurence Kinet resigned as the CEO of Aksys, and William C. Dow joined the company as its new CEO in October 1999. His goal of expediting the clinical trial, necessary for obtaining a 510(k), proved successful. Beginning in February 2000 and finishing in October 2000, the study had 23 patients, 13 of which were from the Northwest Kidney Center in Seattle, Washington, with four patients from our center in Columbia and six from the University of Mississippi in

---

29. Sue Salzer. (1998) Home hemo redux. Experts say: There's no place like home. *Missouri Med Rev* Summer: 3–7.

Jackson, Mississippi. Barbara Pickett, RN, took care of our patients' nursing problems in Columbia. The patients liked the system very much, as they felt much better than on three times weekly dialysis and on daily dialysis with other machines.

Three of my four patients (Lucille Shirley, Sandra Hampton and Robert Burton), who were already anuric when switched to daily dialysis on PHD®i, claimed that they felt much better within a few days after the change. An additional advantage was that the machine did all the chores related to preparation for dialysis and tear-down after dialysis, so the total dialysis time was close to the effective dialysis time. Robert Burton, a very experienced dialysis patient who had been treated with three times weekly hemodialysis and peritoneal dialysis, told me that after switching for the first time in many years he felt like his thinking was clearer, not hazy like before (Fig. 59). Lucille, a patient with numerous problems who felt ill on three times weekly dialysis, markedly improved clinically after switching to more frequent dialysis on PHD®i (see above). All three patients requested continuation of the treatment on PHD®i, after the study ended, and the company agreed on a compassionate basis. One patient

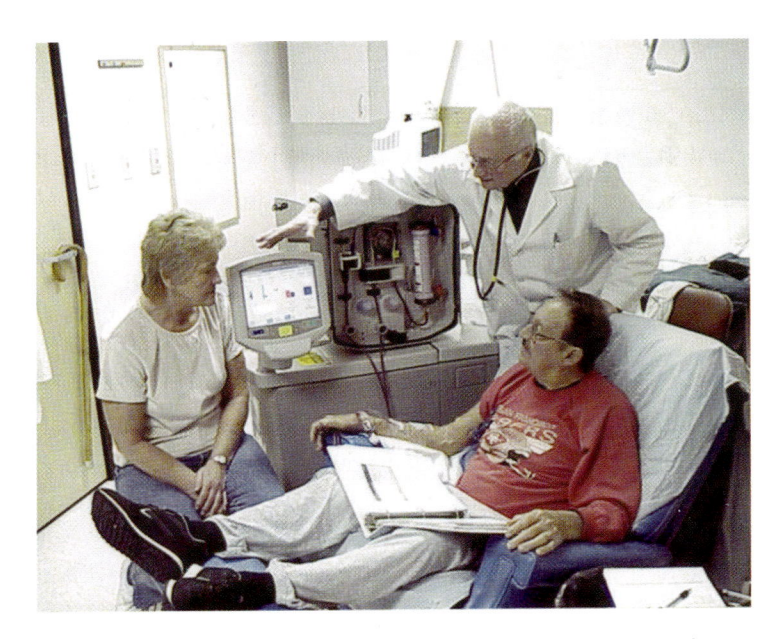

Figure 59. Robert Burton and his wife during training on PHD®i.

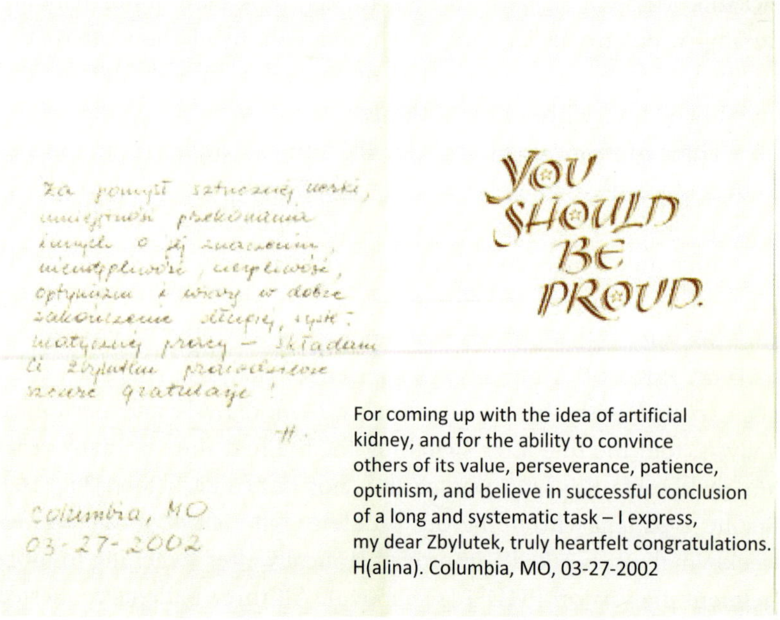
YOU SHOULD BE PROUD.
Columbia, MO
03-27-2002
For coming up with the idea of artificial kidney, and for the ability to convince others of its value, perseverance, patience, optimism, and believe in successful conclusion of a long and systematic task – I express, my dear Zbylutek, truly heartfelt congratulations. H(alina). Columbia, MO, 03-27-2002

Figure 60. A congratulatory card from Halinka.

(George Plybon), who was not anuric, did not notice that much difference; however, his chemistries showed substantial improvement.

After the clinical trial was completed, the application was submitted to the FDA on January 16, 2001, and Aksys received the go-ahead to market the PHD® system on March 18, 2002. The very next day I received a wonderful congratulatory card from my wife (Fig. 60). On April 13, 2002, the company organized an event to celebrate the approval by FDA; during the dinner a second version of the PHD® machine was shown for the first time (Fig. 61). Rod, Dawn and I met again, and a photo of the three of us was taken (Fig. 62).

The PHD® machine was composed of a dialyzer module, dialysis solution module, water treatment module, control module, and graphical user interface (Fig. 63). The dialyzer module contained a dialyzer, an arterial line with blood pump, and a venous line with air trap (Fig. 64). The arterial and venous lines were provided with pressure gauges. Between dialyses, the arterial and venous lines were connected to the fluid lines of the dialysis solution module. The water

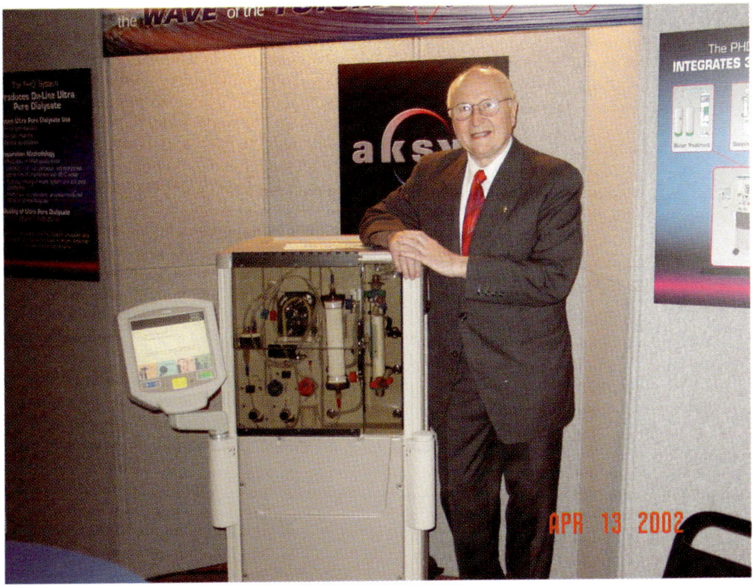

Figure 61. A second version of PHD® machine shown during the FDA approval dinner.

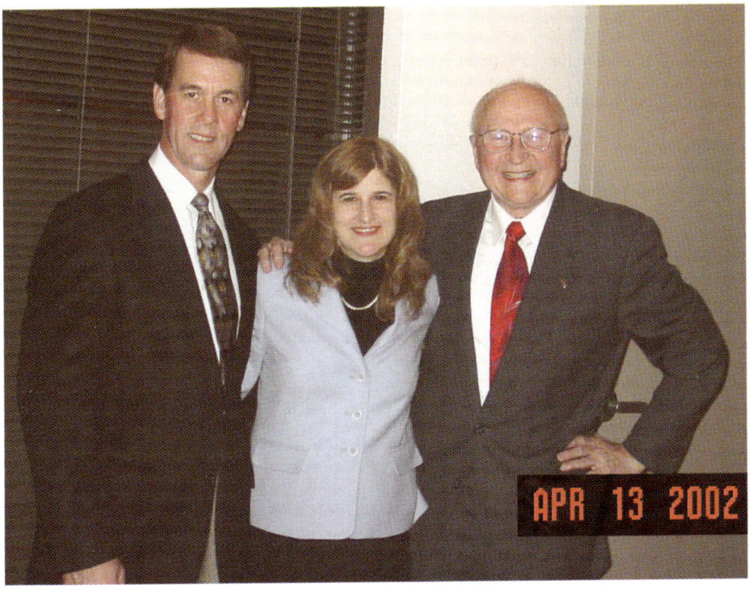

Figure 62. Rod, Dawn and the author, eleven years older but still young.

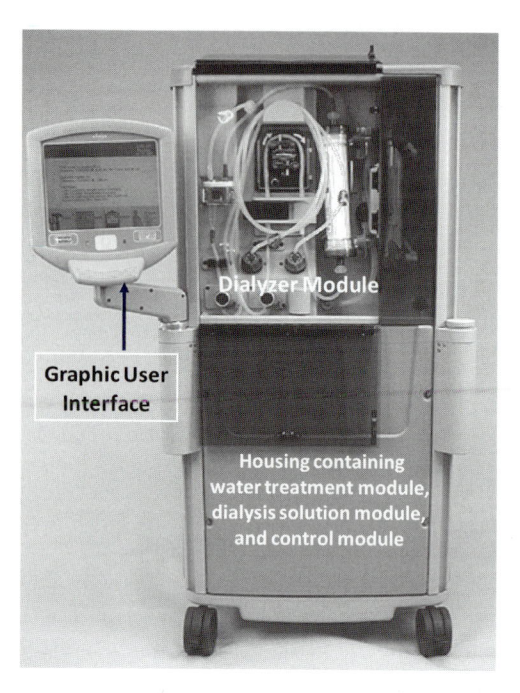

Figure 63. General view of the "Phase 2" PHD®. (Reprinted from Pu 335, Chap. 5Q.)

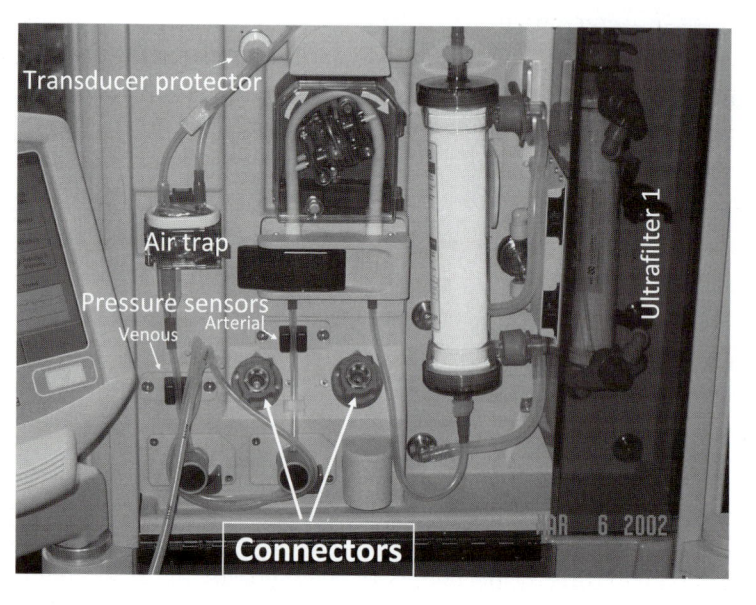

Figure 64. Dialyzer module. (Modified from Pu 335, Chap. 5Q.)

228　Around the World with Nephrology

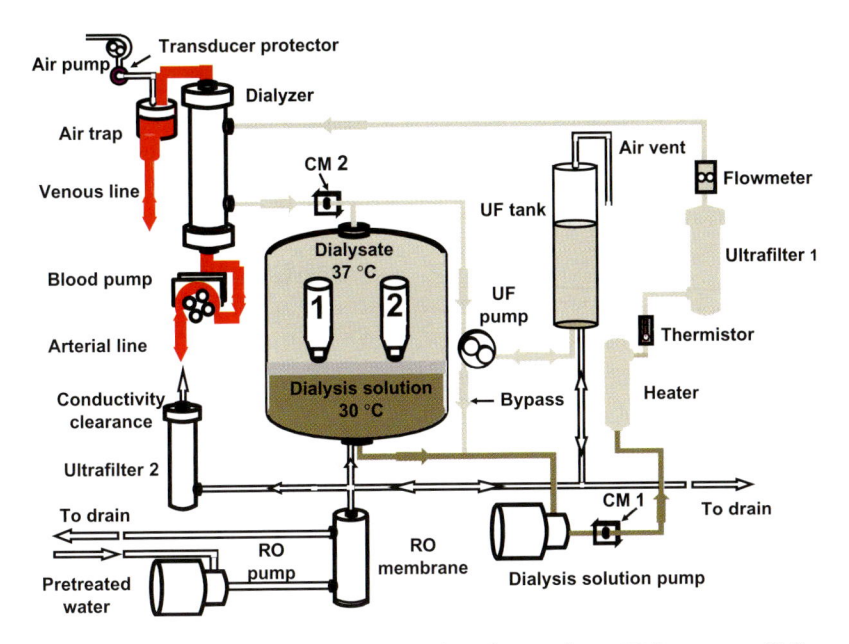

Figure 65. Simplified diagram of fluid paths in the PHD® system. CM1–conductometer 1; CM2–conductometer 2. (Modified from Pu 340.)

treatment module (Fig. 65) consisted of a pump and the reverse osmosis (RO) membrane. The machine was connected to a water supply, pretreated by a series of filters. The central feature of the dialysis solution module (Fig. 65) was a 50 L main tank with two receptacles for bottles with the chemicals necessary to produce dialysis solution. Bottle #1 (acid concentrate) contained an aqueous solution of sodium chloride, potassium chloride, calcium chloride, magnesium chloride, acetic acid and dextrose. Bottle #2 contained powdered sodium bicarbonate and sodium chloride. The machine prepared ultrapure dialysis solution from the dry chemicals, the concentrate, and RO water warmed to 30°C. Dialysis solution, taken from the bottom of the tank, was warmed to about 37°C and delivered through the dialysis solution line to the dialysate compartment of the dialyzer via an inline ultrafilter 1. Dialysate was returned through the dialysate line to the top of the tank. The dialysate solution circuit was connected to the 4 L ultrafiltration (UF) tank and excess fluid was transferred to the UF tank and measured directly. Because of the temperature difference between fresh dialysis solution and spent dialysate, the mixing of the two in the main tank was limited, as depicted in Fig. 65 by the shaded area between the dialysis solution and dialysate. Almost the entire tank volume may be used as a single pass dialysis solution delivery system for short dialysis. All operations were guided by a computer in the control module and by commands from the graphic user interface module.

The PHD® system combined four machines in one: a dialysis machine, a reuse apparatus, a water treatment appliance, and a device manufacturing ultrapure infusion-quality solution. Hence, there was no need for the delivery of solutions for infusion. The machine was based on the tank dialysis solution system. Eliminating the proportioning system simplified the machine design, and the use of positive pressure ultrafiltration eliminated the need for a deaeration pump. Finally, the closed system allowed direct measurement of the ultrafiltrate. By setting up for dialysis and tearing down after dialysis, the machine saved the patient (or helper) time, and saved money by reusing supplies, decreasing transportation costs and minimizing storage space. In addition, a very important feature was the almost complete recovery of blood after dialysis using so-called backfiltration, the transfer of dialysate through the membrane and thereby pushing blood from the dialyzer to the patient through both arterial and venous lines [Pu 340].

There was no question of the superiority of frequent (five to seven times weekly) hemodialysis over routine (three times weekly) dialysis, not only on the basis of the clinical trial of PHD® for FDA approval, but also on the basis of numerous other trials. Unfortunately, more frequent dialysis was more expensive, so those involved in daily (frequent) dialysis wanted increased reimbursement from Medicare. Before a decision with regard to increased reimbursement could be made, the National Institutes of Health summoned a Task Force on Daily Dialysis in Washington, DC., on April 11, 2001 (Order #342, Conference ID 108). Despite the arguments of those who had personally observed excellent clinical and laboratory results of more frequent dialysis, the conference decided that observational studies were unreliable and a randomized controlled trial (RCT) would be needed to justify higher reimbursement. Those of us involved in daily dialysis (among others, Carl Kjellstrand, Robert Lockridge, Christopher Blagg,

John Bower and myself), being aware of the tremendous advantages, considered the decision to be an unjustified delay tactic to postpone reimbursement for better therapy. It was our opinion that the probability of hundreds of observational studies showing improved results with more frequent hemodialysis being wrong was close to zero. Regardless, the prospective randomized trial was started, lasted almost 10 years, cost millions of dollars, and the outcome was published in December 2010.[30]

As expected, the study showed that the results with frequent dialysis were better than with routine dialysis. I expressed my feelings about the need for the study in an invited editorial written with Dr. Misra and published in the same issue of the *New England Journal of Medicine* [Pu 383]. In my opinion such a study to find out which frequency of dialysis was better for a particular patient was absolutely unnecessary and inappropriate. My major problem was the selection of patients for daily home dialysis, as not everybody is a good candidate for it. Only paired observations used in the same patients may provide the correct answer (A–B). The criticism of such studies (A–B) is that mortality cannot be compared and this is the ultimate criterion of the superiority of one method over the other. However, there is more to life than the absence of death; hematocrit, blood pressure control, nutritional indices and quality of life would be the most important criteria. These results predict mortality in dialysis patients very well and correlate closely with the subjective assessment of quality of life. In fact, mortality was not used to evaluate the value of frequent hemodialysis in this RCT study, as it would "require over 1,500 subjects per trial and several years of accrual and follow-up."[31] Another criticism is that patients may be biased and report better subjective health (the so-called Hawthorne effect)[32] than is actually the case. However, it is impossible to influence

---

30. Chertow GM, et al. for the Frequent Hemodialysis Network (FHN) Trial Group. (2010) In-center hemodialysis six times per week versus three times per week. *N Engl J Med* **363**(24): 287–300.

31. Suri RS, Garg AX, Chertow GM, et al. (2007) Frequent Hemodialysis Network (FHN) randomized trial: Study design. *Kidney Int* **72**(4): 249–359.

32. The Hawthorne effect refers to the tendency of some people to perform better when they are participants in an experiment. Individuals may change their behavior due to the attention they are receiving from researchers rather than because of any manipulation of independent variables. They also tend to want to please researchers.

hematocrit, blood pressure control and nutritional indices in this way. When I talked about the Hawthorne effect during presentations, I cited my personal experience participating in John Bauer and Steve Brooks' study on the 7000-J diet in 1977. Despite my desire to do so, I was unable to please the investigators and keep my potassium level in the normal range; such objective changes are independent of the will of the study subject.

How did the idea of randomized prospective studies come into being? In 1923 randomization in experimental studies was established by Sir Ronald Aylmer Fisher, a statistician at the Rothamsted Agricultural Experimental Station.[33] The problem was to compare the effect of different fertilizers on potato yield. The old method was to apply each fertilizer to an entire field and compare yields between fields. However, some fields (and certain parts of each field) are more fertile than others. Fisher divided fields into rows and small plots within rows, randomly assigned fertilizers to plots and assessed the results for each fertilizer. With regard to the best kind fertilizer for potatoes, it is a sound method, but used in medicine it is less likely to provide reliable results. This is particularly true when studying therapeutic methods or devices, because there are tremendous differences between Fisher's original design and RCTs in medicine, particularly in the study of methods. Potatoes and plots are different than patients. Nobody asks potatoes and plots to agree to be assigned to a particular row, there are no exclusions, they are not asked to do anything, they are always compliant, they do not withdraw from a trial, comparison is always fair, and no special equipment is needed for different plots. Extrapolating the need for randomization to all clinical hypothesis testing (or else the clinical equipoise would be violated) can create problems.

Sir Austin Bradford Hill is credited with introducing RCTs in medicine, but he himself warned that, "Any belief that the controlled trial is the only way would mean not that the pendulum had swung too far but that it had come right off its hook."[34] Patient recruitment is

---

33. Fisher RA. (1926) The arrangement of field experiments. *J Ministry Agriculture* **33**: 503–513.

34. Hill AB. (1965) Heberden Oration 1965: Reflections on the controlled trial. *Ann Rheum Dis* **25**: 107–113.

one such oft-encountered problem. There is an important difference between the studies of pharmaceuticals and of therapeutic methods. In the study of pharmaceuticals, one group takes one medication and the other takes a placebo or another medication. In the study of therapeutic methods, patients are asked to perform procedures, and frequently the equipment or venue should be different. Not everybody with end stage renal disease is a good candidate for frequent home hemodialysis. This is the reason that the value of CAPD in comparison to hemodialysis has never been proven in an RCT. An RCT study designed to compare outcomes on peritoneal dialysis versus hemodialysis as the initial dialysis therapy had to be terminated because it was not possible to find volunteers for randomization.[35] It is worth remembering that hemodialysis itself has never been tested in randomized clinical trials. The proof of how difficult it is to select patients for the randomized study of therapeutic methods is the fact that an NIH frequent study project could, after 10 years, have the agreement of only a minuscule number of patients potentially eligible for the study. As a result, it was impossible to compare mortality, which was one of the important arguments to undertake the study.

I would like to mention that in assessing the significance of difference we have to be aware of what kind of difference we consider. This was nicely presented by Alvan R. Feinstein in his discussion on statistical significance versus clinical importance.[36] Quantitative difference is a large difference and fulfills the criterion of the Traumatic Interocular Test (T.I.T.). If the difference is impressive, the distinction hits you between the eyes and you do not need fancy "p" values or other statistical measures to say, "Yes, that's a real difference." Many extremely valuable discoveries have never been compared in RCTs. To mention only a few: thyroxine for myxedema (1891); insulin for diabetic ketoacidosis (1922); vitamin B_{12} for pernicious anemia (1926); penicillin for G+ cocci sepsis (1941); N-acetylcysteine for paracetamol (1979); imatinib for chronic myeloid leukemia (2002); imatinib

---

35. Korevaar JC, Feith GW, Dekker FW, *et al.* (NECOSAD Study Group). (2003) Effect of starting with hemodialysis compared with peritoneal dialysis in patients new on dialysis treatment: A randomized controlled trial. *Kidney Int* **64**(6): 2222–2228.

36. Feinstein AR. (1988) Statistical significance versus clinical importance. *Quality Life Cardiovasc Care* Autumn: 99–102.

(Gleevec) for gastrointestinal stromal tumors (GIST) (2005). According to Belding H. Scribner, the father of chronic hemodialysis, "Successful treatment of Clyde Shields represents one of the few instances in medicine where a single success was all that was required to validate a new therapy." Whenever I undertook studies on less frequent and more frequent dialysis, the results, for me, belonged to the T.I.T. category. Subjectively, patients saw the difference within a few days after switching to more frequent sessions; objectively, positive differences were seen within a few weeks or months. In summary, the NIH's decision to defer increased reimbursement for better therapy was clearly a delay tactic to save money, and it was to the detriment of many patients.

Returning to the story of PHD®, the commercial products were launched in the second half of 2002, initially in Seattle, Washington, Lincoln, Nebraska, and New York City. One center was opened in Oxford, England, in November 2002. For commercial use an improved "Phase 2" version of the machine was launched (Figs. 61, 63 and 64). Our center in Columbia was offered the opportunity to use the machine, but our administration declined because it was too expensive. The limiting to just a few centers was dictated by the lack of a sufficient number of technicians qualified to repair machines in the event of malfunctions. Having a smaller number of centers reduced travel costs and guaranteed quicker repairs. The machines were initially unreliable and required repairs every 20 treatments on average, though some were very reliable and had no problems for many months. The number of patients grew steadily but very slowly. By 2004 over 100 patients were on the PHD® system. William Peckham, a very experienced hemodialysis patient, during a presentation in San Antonio in 2004, said this about his treatment on PHD®: "I'm able to feel more like myself and be at peace on dialysis. To me, the difference between dialyzing in the clinic and self-treating at home is like taking a trip ... you can get there on a bus full of strangers or drive yourself. You decide which experience you want." Another PHD® patient, Nelson Snowball, during a presentation in San Francisco in 2006, compared his previous experience using NxStage and expressed a definitive opinion that PHD® gave him a tremendous subjective advantage. Since starting dialysis on PHD® five months earlier, he had not experienced any machine malfunctions. Regular three times weekly dialysis was markedly worse from both daily schedules.

The most extensive experience with treatment on PHD® was at the Northwest Kidney Center in Seattle.[37] By 2004 more centers had begun using the PHD® system, and 35 centers were using PHD® in 308 patients by 2006. Unfortunately, the growth of the number of patients was insufficient to make the company financially viable. In 2004, together with Dr. Kjellstrand, we tried to convince the Board of Directors to expand the use of the machine for the treatment of acute renal failure. The argument against this was that the machine needed a long period of preparation (about 12 hours) to be ready for use. I argued that in my experience I was usually aware of the need for acute dialysis in a given patient about 24 hours in advance. In any case, if the treatment were needed immediately, the initial dialysis could be done on another machine with the following treatments on PHD®. Regrettably, our arguments were not heeded. On March 4, 2006, I again urged Bill Dow to reconsider using PHD® for the treatment of acute renal failure. The following day Bill responded that, "Rich Bowman, the ex-head of Baxter's renal acute business, ... after a couple months of working on the project, concluded it was not possible with the PHD® system for a variety of reasons including but not limited to the weight of the machine, the necessity for hard plumbing the unit, and the need to have dialysate prepared about 12 hours before the treatment." The decision was against expanding the program to acute dialysis. I was really surprised as very heavy X-ray machines are transported all over hospitals and this machine could be prepared in a special room. Our scientific advisory board was never asked about this issue.

In 2006 it was clear that the company was in financial difficulty, as it did not support our Annual Dialysis Conference as it had done in previous years. The price of shares had also dropped below US$0.20. In December that year we exchanged e-mail with Dr. Kjellstrand concerning the situation at Aksys; it was obvious that the company could not survive. For his part, Dr. Kjellstrand, who was seeing many patients on PHD® in Seattle, considered the PHD® system to be "the best dialysis machine." That the reimbursement was

---

37. Blagg CR, Hutton J, Hynes J, et al. (2006) The Northwest Kidney Centers' experience with the Aksys PHD system. *Nephrol News Issues* **20**(11): 56–57, 59–61.

inadequate for more frequent dialysis was just one hurdle. The company also made many mistakes, the most important being, in our opinion, the slow improvement in reliability. Increasing the reliability faster would have decreased costs and increased the number of centers and patients using the machine.

In early January 2007, I received a call from Rod that Aksys was in dire financial straits, would go bankrupt, and would have to take all patients off PHD®. The patients were very unhappy as they had to go to the less desirable NxStage system or use the regular machines for three times weekly dialysis. He also advised me to terminate my license, which I had the right to do as I had not received royalties for the second half of 2006. With the help of my lawyer, Garry Ellis, I sent a letter to Howard Lewin, the new CEO, advising him of the immediate termination of our License Agreement. Rod also sent me a long letter with a recommendation about the best strategy to follow with respect to my patent portfolio. It was only then that I learned that my last patent (U.S. Patent No. 6,146,536) filed with Rod as coauthor was actually co-owned by Aksys and could be sold or licensed on a non-exclusive basis without my permission. In any case, I could license or sell all other patents, giving the buyer or licensee exclusive rights. Rod also warned me that some companies might try to buy or license my patents without involving him. In fact, at the end of January 2007, during a meeting in which I debated with Dr. Frank Gotch[38] about what was most important in dialysis prescription [Pr 503], I got a phone call from Richard Moss, Vice President, Business Development and Strategy at Baxter Renal, Baxter Healthcare Corporation, asking me to sell my patents to Baxter. I was a little surprised, recalling my futile negotiations with Baxter some 25 years earlier; however, there were different people at Baxter at that time. I declined. Not only was the offer too low, but I was a little concerned that without licensing patents, only buying them, Baxter may not work on the project, again considering it competition to peritoneal dialysis. After some negotiations Richard doubled the offer for the purchase (not license) of my five patents on February 15, 2007. Baxter were adamant that they did not want to negotiate with Rod, but Rod and I wanted him to be

---

38. One of the creators of the *Kt/V* concept as the most important measure of dialysis adequacy.

involved in work on the project. I rejected the offer, and Rod and I started looking at other possibilities.

Rod had already had some talks with Dean Kamen, President of DEKA, about working on the next generation of PHD®, the so-called G2, or Pluto. The new machine would have most of the important features of PHD® — automatic set-up for dialysis and tear-down after dialysis, graphical user interface, reuse of dialyzers and lines, manufacturing of infusion-quality solution, and backfiltration for complete reinfusion of blood to the patient after dialysis — but would use a proportioning system with only a small tank for mixing and reuse. Rod also thought about using the machine for peritoneal dialysis, a concept that we had already considered 20 years earlier. DEKA had good engineers and were already manufacturing Homechoice PD machines for Baxter. Rod's idea was to create a new company (NewCo) with funds from Pete McNerney and his venture capital group, and enlist DEKA as the provider of engineering capability. Another possibility was to negotiate with Gambro or Fresenius, very strong companies involved in the dialysis business. Fresenius was not interested, so we decided to pursue the project with DEKA and Gambro.

Our Annual Dialysis Conference was taking place in Denver between February 18 and 20, 2007, so we decided to negotiate with the companies present at the conference. I talked with Dean Kamen, but it was a short meeting without details. Rod and I had a long discussion with Gambro representatives, including Martin Danielson, Juan P. Bosch, MD, and Jerry McIntyre. We continued our discussion with Dean Kamen and Robert M. Tuttle from DEKA, Pete McNerney, and Martin Danielson from Gambro. All parties were aware that I had exclusive rights to four patents but that U.S. Patent No. 6,146,536 was co-owned by Aksys, so I could not offer exclusive rights for that patent. On March 27, 2007, Gambro came up with an offer of a down payment, lower than that of Baxter, but for license, not purchase, and minimum royalties or 1.5 percent royalty on sales (whichever was greater) until the expiration of the last patent on October 17, 2017. They were not prepared to employ Rod and only offered him a consulting agreement. I was to get 5/6 of the royalties and Rod 1/6, an adequate offer from my point of view but a great disappointment for Rod. I informed Martin Danielson that although the offer from another company was slightly worse, I had some moral obligations to Rod and did not feel good about his lack of involvement in product development. However, I also told him that if a deal with another company were not to materialize, I would accept his offer. Martin agreed, saying, "I understand your decision to pursue this path in the continued discussions and I hope that you find a good solution."

On May 4, I got an e-mail offer from Hazim Ansari from Patentmetrix LLC in Irvine, California, for an acquisition or license of my patents 5,336,165; 5,484,397; and 5,902,476. He told me that the inquiry was on behalf of a "public company that is financially capable of providing a lucrative offer." I informed him that I had already received offers from other companies, revealed their ballpark figures, and asked him the name of the company. However, he never provided a name and the e-mail correspondence ended.

At the time I was at an advanced stage of negotiations with DEKA and Pete McNerney regarding the foundation of NewCo. I was not sure as to the nature of any obstacles, but the finalization of the agreement was not forthcoming for some time. I imagine that there were negotiations about the composition of the board of directors, the CEO, preferred stocks, and so on. It may appear trivial, but negotiators also took issue with the name of the new company. After NewCo was decisively rejected, Rod suggested Renigen (Latin/Greek root). I preferred Nephrogen (Greek root), or Renessence, from *ren* (kidney) and *essence* (crucial ingredient). Pete suggested Renesense. In the end, we agreed on Renigen. I asked Garrettson Ellis to help me with the license agreement and I signed it with Renigen on May 4, 2007. One of the articles stipulated that Rod and I would each receive 50 percent of common stock equal to 1.5 percent of fully diluted equity of the licensee. Rod and I were to receive down payment and royalties, and Rod was to be employed by Renigen.

In the meantime, I was invited to Istanbul to give some lectures at a conference organized by Ege University (Izmir) and Fresenius [Pr 506]. Afterwards, I went to Kraków, Poland, for my regular stay in Poland during the summer months, and I was surprised that I had not yet received the agreement signed by Renigen. I assumed that they were having problems with financing and securing the other half of patent 6,146,536.

In early June I received a phone call from Pete explaining that the creation of Renigen had not materialized for many reasons, which I did not insist on knowing. I learned that instead of financing by venture capitalists, Baxter would support DEKA in their efforts to make the new machine and use for home, outpatient and hospital dialysis. The new company was created with the name HHD LLC. With the help of Garry Ellis, I continued negotiations during June. Robert M. Tuttle, Vice President of DEKA and HHD LLC, and I signed the License Agreement on July 12, 2007. According to the agreement Rod and I would receive down payments as well as minimum quarterly royalty payments until the expiration of the last patent in 2017. The financial conditions were only slightly less favorable than with Gambro, but Rod was promised employment.

After signing the agreement with HHD LLC, I received an e-mail from Rod that he had not been employed. I sent several e-mails to Dean Kamen and Bob Tuttle reminding them that one of the conditions of signing the agreement with them was their promise to employ Rod. Without Rod's employment, I would have had a better deal with Gambro. It took some time, but on September 23, 2007, Rod finally began work. In July 2011, Baxter acquired all the assets and obligations of HHD under the License Agreement of July 2007. At the time of writing (August 2011), the G2 machine is ready, an investigational device exemption (IDE) from the FDA has been obtained, and patient recruitments have started. The new version of the machine will be presented during the Annual Dialysis Conference in Seattle in March 2013.

One thing is certain. Without Rod Kenley's passionate pursuit of the idea of a machine for daily home hemodialysis, without his determination to take a risk, the method itself would have developed much later, if at all. It is worth remembering that the NxStage machine was developed after the PHD® system had already demonstrated the value of frequent home hemodialysis. Now that the next generation of machine is finally ready, Rod has embraced another challenge, becoming President of Aethlon Medical, the company that manufactures the Hemopurifier®, an extracorporeal purification device capable of removing from the blood certain viruses and exosomes, virus-sized particles shed by tumors that protect them from a host's defense mechanisms in the blood.

CHAPTER 11

Major Research in the 1990s

Constant Site (Buttonhole) Method of Needle Insertion into Arteriovenous Fistula

Following the success of the constant site method of needle insertion in Bytom and Lublin, I tried to introduce the method after starting my clinical duties in the Hemodialysis Center at Dialysis Clinic Inc. in 1982. However, there was some skepticism among the nursing staff about the possibility of having a single sticker establish the site, as there was a good deal of staff rotation. Blunter needles were not available, and the nurses told me that the needles did not go through the same needle tunnel but cut the adjacent tissue. I knew that the method was being used in the U.S. by Dr. Belding H. Scribner,[1] because he had published two papers mentioning this fact[2] and I knew about the paper by Gerhard Krönung[3] on the method, which he had renamed "the buttonhole method," but I was so preoccupied with peritoneal dialysis research, hemodialysis catheters and our machine for home hemodialysis that I had abandoned my efforts to disseminate the method more broadly. Scribner taught the method to one of his home hemodialysis patients, A. Peter Lundin [I have mentioned about his interesting history earlier (page 222)], who informed Georg Harper, another home hemodialysis patient from Rome, Georgia, about the advantages of the method. Both Peter Lundin and George Harper only used sharp needles and cannulated themselves. Mr. Harper was very interested in new hemodialysis machines; he contacted Rod Kenley and told him about the buttonhole method of needle insertion. In 1994, Rod called me asking whether I was aware of this method apparently suitable for home hemodialysis, and I told him that I was certainly aware, as I was the first who described it, but that I was not successful in introducing it in our center in Columbia. He prodded me to work on the problem, as it might be important for our home hemodialysis program.

---

1. Belding H. Scribner, MD (January 18, 1921–June 19, 2003) introduced chronic hemodialysis on March 9, 1960. He received an Award for Lifetime Achievements from our Annual Dialysis Conference [Pu 337].

2. Scribner BH. (1982) Circulatory access — Still a major concern. *Proc Europ Dial Transplant Assoc* **19**: 95–98; Scribner BH. (1984) The overriding importance of vascular access. *Dial Transplant* **13**: 625.

3. Krönung G. (1984) Plastic deformation of Cimino fistula by repeated puncture. *Dial Transplant* **13**: 635–638.

First of all I decided to invite George Harper to the 1st International Symposium on Home Hemodialysis to present his experience with the method (see below in the section on our Annual Dialysis Conference). Secondly I decided to write another paper on the method, as my paper from 15 years earlier was not readily available. In the new paper [Pu 226] I presented a history of the method and speculated why the method had not been popular in spite of excellent initial results. I blamed several factors, including the predominance of graft fistulas in the U.S. that were not tested to determine whether the method was suitable for this kind of access. I also suggested that the currently used needles were too sharp; in Bytom we had serendipitously used blunt needles. Finally I blamed the organization of the fistula puncture technique in a busy hemodialysis center, the so-called "multiple sticker" practice. As I mentioned previously, in Bytom, and later in Lublin, only one nurse was initially sufficiently experienced to establish the puncture site. Only after several weeks did other nurses become qualified to cannulate the fistula in the established site. In the majority of centers, stickers were different for each dialysis. The "single sticker" practice was used for home dialysis, and the results were better as a consequence.

In January 1992, Dialysis Clinic Inc. moved from Walnut Street to LeMone Industrial Boulevard; there were changes in the hemodialysis nursing staff in our center in Columbia. I talked again with the nurses and provided copies of our paper published in 1979 [Pu 41] with a table showing the tremendous advantages of the constant site method over the different site method (Fig. 66), and the appearance of constant sites (Fig. 67). Some nurses were interested in studying the buttonhole method. On August 29, 1996, I received a letter from Fred Peter, Director, Ex Vivo Development, Aksys Ltd., stating that they had some discussions regarding blood access. One of the top questions that people ask about daily hemodialysis, he wrote, was, "What about access?" I was not particularly concerned, as in my paper in 1977 [Pu 27] we noted that frequent dialysis did not deteriorate the fistula — to my surprise, frequent dialysis was even beneficial to the fistula. Incidentally, the beneficial effects of frequent use on fistula condition was also observed by Buoncristiani. I presented his experience and that of others during the 5th International Symposium on Hemodialysis in Charlotte, N.C., in 1999, and published a related

	Different sites	Constant sites
Number of fistulas	22	25
Number of dialyses	4060	6180
Time of setting up dialysis (min)	15–25	5–15
Reinsertion (%)	9.91	0.96
Hematoma formation (%)	12.5	0.1
Fistula limb failure	3	1
Fistula failure	1	1
Infection requiring ABX	1	3
Patients' preference	No	Yes
Nurses' preference	No	Yes

Twardowski Z, Kubara H: Dial Transplant 1979; 8: 978–980.

Figure 66. Comparison of two methods of needle insertion. (Data taken from Pu 41.)

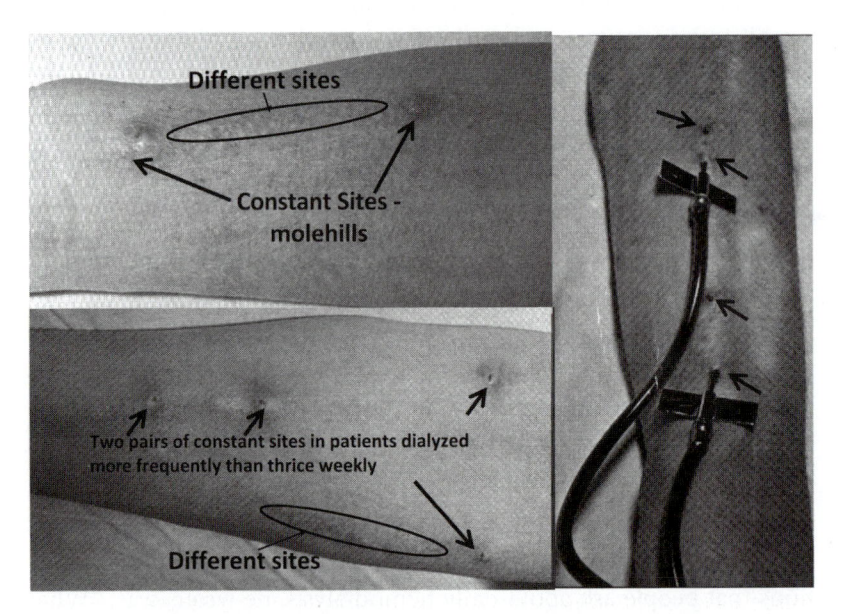

Figure 67. Appearance of constant sites and different sites in original patients. (Modified from Pu 41.)

paper in the proceedings of the symposium [Pu 289]. In the years that followed, I published reviews of various experiences with frequent fistula use, all of which indicated that blood access was not a problem in daily dialysis [Pu 295, Pu 351].

I was a little puzzled that people were concerned about the frequent use of fistulas but not about using high flow dialysis, which was never proven not to be detrimental to fistulas. In any event, Fred Peter put me in contact with William J. Schnell, an engineer in Medisystems Research Corporation, Lakemoor, Illinois, and already on the Board of Directors of Aksys, and we began our cooperation in September 1996. Bill used electropolishing to prepare several needles with varying degrees of bluntness and asked me which one would be appropriate. To remove spikes or burrs, some electropolishing was always done for regular needles, but prolonged electropolishing made the needle blunter. The longer the electropolishing, the blunter the needle — ultimately dissolving the needle entirely. I did not have any objective method of measuring bluntness, so I tested them by touching the tip with my index finger, not knowing how a particular needle had been prepared. We eventually decided upon two kinds of blunt needles, one with a 45° bevel and the other with a 20° bevel. The nurses established the puncture sites and then started using the blunt needles. I first started to work with Mike E. Klusmeyer, RN, with whom I had already worked on blood recirculation in hemodialysis catheters [Pu 191], and Jerry Evans, RN. After a few months we established that the best needle was the one with the 45° bevel and moderate bluntness. I notified Bill Schnell about our choice, and Medisystems provided us the needles for a study. From 1996 to 1998 we studied 16 patients, with good results, which were presented by Jerry Wells, RN, CNN, during the 5th International Symposium on Home Hemodialysis in Charlotte, N.C., in February 1999. In 1997 we produced a video with George Harper on the technique of buttonhole needle insertion [Vi 7], which was shown for the first time during the 3rd International Symposium on Home Hemodialysis in Denver, Colorado, on February 17, 1997 [Pr 425, Pu 316]. Medisystems also made a video showing details of the buttonhole technique.

After some time Medisystems stopped manufacturing the blunt needles in accordance with our request. Instead they started manufacturing very blunt needles that did not require needle guards and were used mostly for subcutaneous catheters, such as Dialock™, manufactured by Biolink Corporation in Middleborough, Massachusetts, and LifeSite®, manufactured by VascA in Topsfield, Massachusetts. The needles are called ButtonHole™ Needle Sets with Anti-Stick Dull Bevel. The subcutaneous catheters provided poor results and were ultimately taken off of the market. Needles that were too blunt were not suitable for the buttonhole method in many patients. I received e-mails from nurses and home patients saying that they could not use the blunt needles as they were too blunt. Out of necessity I advised them to use sharp needles. I contacted David Utterberg of Medisystems to ask him to manufacture needles with intermediate bluntness, so that there would be four types of needles: sharp for the creation of the tunnel, and three kinds of needles with different degrees of bluntness. I suggested grading them by the force needed to puncture the skin (or synthetic material with a resistance similar to skin). He promised to work on the problem but encountered some difficulties. I also asked the same of Tim Dillon of Nipro, U.S. Division, but he was also unable to do it. Nevertheless, Nipro began manufacturing blunt needles, which they called the BioHole™ Needle "for established access sites only." These needles are duller than sharp needles but less dull than the Medisystems ButtonHole Needle. JMS North America Corporation in Hayward, California, was a third company making dull needles, which they called Harmony™. I asked Dennis O'Neill, the company's Sr. Vice President for Sales and Marketing, to consider needles of a different degree of bluntness. No such needles have yet emerged.

Many nurses pushing for the use of the constant site method got the go-ahead from nephrologists. Several centers in Seattle, Toronto, Louvain, Maastricht, Brazil and New Zealand started to use the buttonhole method, particularly in home hemodialysis patients, with positive results. In Japan, Shigeki Toma, MD, developed a faster method of creating a buttonhole tunnel. After needle removal "a dull-tipped, thumbtack-shaped, 5-mm long, polycarbonate peg (BH Stick®, Nipro Corporation, Osaka, Japan), which does not quite reach the access vessel when entering from the skin, is thrust toward the access vessel along the path previously taken by the just-removed dialysis needle." The tunnel is usually ready after two weeks, and a BioHole needle can then be used. In the realm of research on buttonhole needle insertion, Stewart Mott, RN, a blood access nurse in our center in Columbia, Tony Goovaerts, a nurse from Louvain, Belgium, and Dr. Emma Vaux, consultant nephrologist from Reading, UK, are very active. Recently, Magda van Loon from Maastricht, the Netherlands, successfully defended a PhD thesis on blood access with a large part related to the buttonhole method of needle insertion (see below). I also received an e-mail from Rosa Marticorena, a nurse at St Michael's Hospital, Toronto, ON, Canada, describing her plans to write a PhD thesis on the buttonhole method. One of the most active researchers of the buttonhole method was Lynda Ball, RN, BSN, CNN, from the Northwest Kidney Center in Seattle where many daily dialysis patients were being treated. In an e-mail sent to me in August 2007, she remarked that the "buttonhole has caught on like wildfire." And indeed numerous papers on the method are being published, all stressing lower pain, lower hematoma formation, fewer missed needle insertions and better fistula preservation. The only concern is a slightly higher rate of infectious complication — already noted in my original papers — compared to the traditional method. Recently introduced stricter antiseptic precautions, avoiding insertion of the needle too deeply ("hubbing"[4]) and the use of antibiotic ointment on the puncture sites have markedly ameliorated this problem.

My paper published in *Dialysis & Transplantation* in 1995 [Pu 226] has been one of the most frequently cited articles in the 40-year history of the journal. On August 12, 2011, Samara Kuehne, an editor at Wiley-Blackwell, sent me an e-mail with the following: "This year marks the 40th anniversary of *Dialysis & Transplantation*, and to commemorate the occasion, we are putting together a special issue of some of the highest-cited and landmark articles we've published over the past four decades. We're only highlighting 6 of our highest-impact papers in this special issue, and we are delighted to inform you that your wonderful 1995 article "Constant site (buttonhole) method for needle insertion for hemodialysis" has made the list! What we'd like to do is publish your original article with some contemporary text to accompany it, and we would be honored if you would write a brief commentary on the article." In the October 2011 issue of the journal my 1995 article was republished together with my

---

4. "Hubbing" means that the hub of the needle enters the buttonhole track and causes its enlargement (dimple instead of molehill), which jeopardizes the proper sterilization of the site before needle insertion.

commentary under the title given by the editors, "The buttonhole method spreads 'like wildfire'" [Pu 385].

Catheter Tunnel Morphology

In the late 1980s, I was interested in the morphology of the peritoneal dialysis catheter tunnel in humans, as very little was known about it and most studies on the tunnel had been done on animals. In animals it was found that the epidermis lined the whole sinus tract, i.e., the part of the tunnel between the skin exit and the external cuff. It was presumed that the spreading of the epidermis is inhibited by the collagen ingrown into the external cuff. Similar observations were reported in one study in humans; however, while inspecting the sinus tract in patients several months or years after catheter implantation during the exit site study (see below), it was my impression that the epidermis extended only a few millimeters and the deeper part of the sinus was covered with a glistening surface that did not look like the epidermis. I was interested in this problem as it was very important how far the external cuff should be located from the exit. A long sinus tract is predisposed to exit infection by a large range of catheter motion out of the skin. Such motion tends to collect contaminants and infect the exit after retraction. This would indicate that the cuff should be located just beneath the exit; however, this location is predisposed to cuff extrusion, contamination and infection. At the time we were already using Swan Neck catheters, but the problem was how deep the external cuff should be located. A preliminary study of catheter tunnels with healthy exits, removed because patients stopped peritoneal dialysis, confirmed my impression by showing that the epidermis spread only a few millimeters from the exit and that the rest of the sinus was covered with granulation and fibrous tissue, with scattered foreign body giant cells, plasma cells, lymphocytes and macrophages [Pu 137]. From 1987 to 1990 we evaluated five catheter tunnels removed because of infection as well as 13 catheter tunnels removed because patients were transferred to hemodialysis or received kidney transplants [Pu 176].

Dr. Nichols removed all of the catheters. During surgery the catheters were removed with a 2–5 mm cylinder of tissue surrounding the catheter, from the exit to the internal cuff with the flange.

Immediately after removal, the specimen was placed into 2 percent glutaraldehyde and 2 percent paraformaldehyde in 0.1 M cacodylate buffer at pH 7.4. The tissue cylinder was then cut longitudinally and the catheter cuffs were separated from the catheter with the scalpel. Harold Moore took macro photographs with a Yashica Dental Eye camera and handled the specimens. Half of the catheter tunnel tissue was used for light microscopy and divided into four specimens as shown in Fig. 68: (1) The exit hole, the sinus tract with epidermis (E) and granulation tissue (G), and the outer half of the external cuff (EC); (2) The inner half of the external cuff with adjacent 5 mm of the intercuff segment (IS); (3) Intercuff segment (IS) excluding cuffs; (4) Internal cuff (IC) and flange (F) with 5 mm of the intercuff segment. The specimens were embedded in paraffin and cut on AO (American Optical) microtome into 6 µm sections and stained with multiple stains. All histology specimens were read by Harold and myself and verified by Dr. Dobbie, Dr. Andersen and Dr. Loy. The final version of the manuscript was discussed with all coauthors.

A well-healed tunnel of a double cuff Swan Neck Missouri catheter removed electively (Fig. 68) consists of tissue ingrown to the flange and internal cuff, tissue surrounding the intercuff segment, and

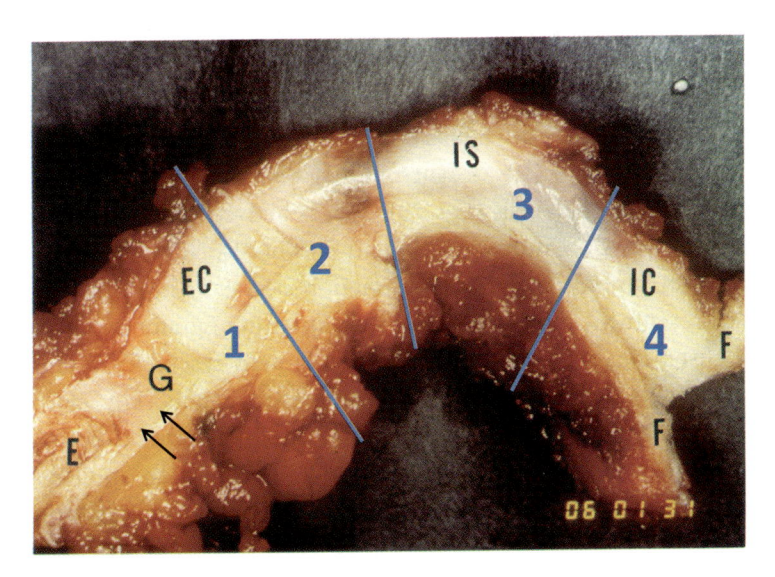

Figure 68. Half tissue cylinder of the tunnel cut longitudinally; see text for explanation. (Modified from Pu 176.)

tissue ingrown into the external cuff and the sinus tract. The most external part (0.5–1 cm) of the sinus tract and the skin surrounding the skin exit of the tunnel constitute the exit site. In the majority of humans the epidermal cells penetrate only a few millimeters from the skin exit and may reach the cuff located less than 15 mm from the exit. Close to the exit, the surface of the sinus tract is covered with the wrinkled epidermis (E) (Fig. 68), containing all the layers of the epidermis including the horny layer. Deeper in the sinus, the epidermis loses the horny layer and becomes similar to the mucosal epithelium; hence the surface becomes glistening and white (Fig. 68, between the black arrows). The rest of the sinus tract is covered with the granulation tissue that is yellowish in appearance (Fig. 68; G, from the black arrow to the external cuff, EC). A thick layer of collagen fibers surrounds the sinus. The granulation tissue contains numerous multinucleated giant cells, capillaries, cellular infiltrate composed mostly of mononuclear cells, and scant collagen fibers. The collagen fibers do not attach to the smooth surface of the silicone rubber, the material from which most peritoneal dialysis catheters are made. The epithelium of uninfected sinus tracts forms three kinds of junctions with the granulation tissue (Fig. 69): (a) mortise and tenon,[5] (b) overlapping, and (c) underlapping. In the same sinus all three junctions could be seen, but one type was usually dominant, and overlapping was most common.

The junction between the granulation tissue in the sinus and the cuff is well defined. The cuff is surrounded by a dense fibrous capsule that contains numerous capillaries (C) (Fig. 70). About 80 percent of the polyester fibers (P) are surrounded completely or partially by multinucleated giant cells (Fig. 70). Spaces between the polyester fibers are filled with mature collagen and fibroblasts. No neutrophils are seen in an uninfected cuff. The junction between the cuff and the intercuff segment shows a smooth surface without granulation tissue. The glistening, shiny intercuff tunnel segment resembles a tendon sheath (Fig. 68, IS) and contains numerous micropits (Fig. 71). The absence of any cellular reaction indicates that bacteria do not reach this part of the tunnel. The surface is covered with an amorphous, mucinous substance on top of a modified layer of fibroblasts forming

---

5. A term borrowed from carpentry; a mortise is a notch cut in wood or other material to receive a corresponding projecting piece called a tenon.

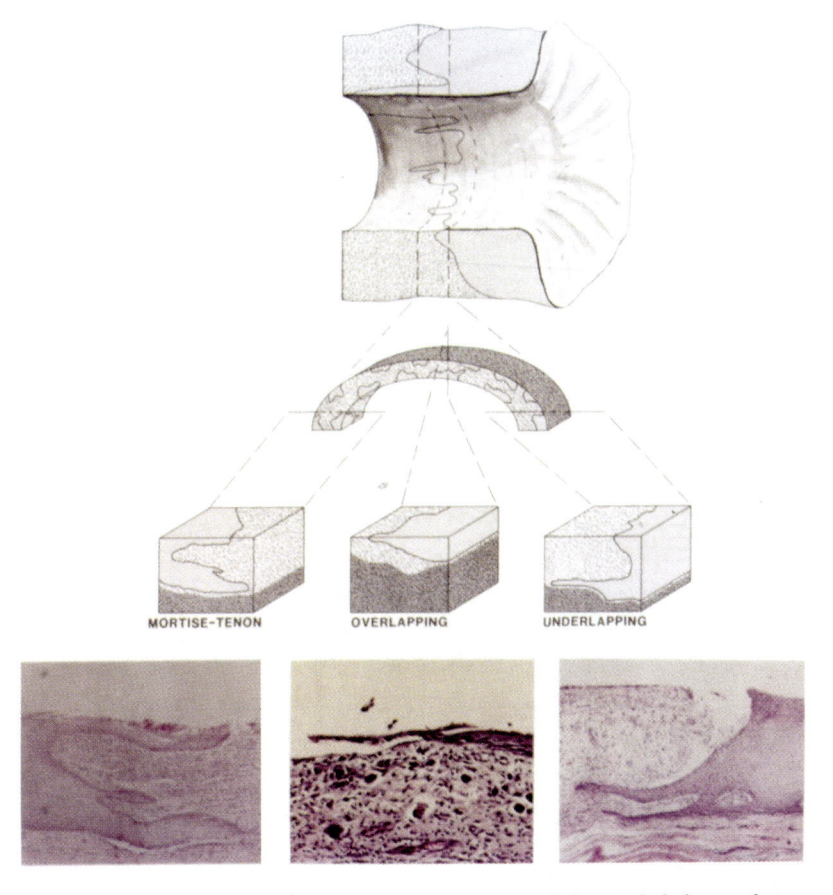

Figure 69. Probable three-dimensional appearance of the epithelial-granulation tissue junction types; see text for explanation. (A black and white version of this picture is published in Pu 176.)

pseudo-synovium. There are no giant cells in this segment because silicone rubber *per se* does not induce giant cell formation. The transition between the intercuff segment and the deep cuff is abrupt due to the change from an avascular, acellular, fibrous sheath to a highly vascular, cellular tissue ingrown into the cuff. If the deep cuff is implanted into the muscle, the fibrous capsule surrounding the cuff and the cuff tissue itself are highly vascularized, otherwise the tissue ingrown into the cuff is similar to that of the external cuff.

Infected exits and tunnels contain inflammatory infiltrate with numerous granulocytes. The surface of intercuff segment is dull and

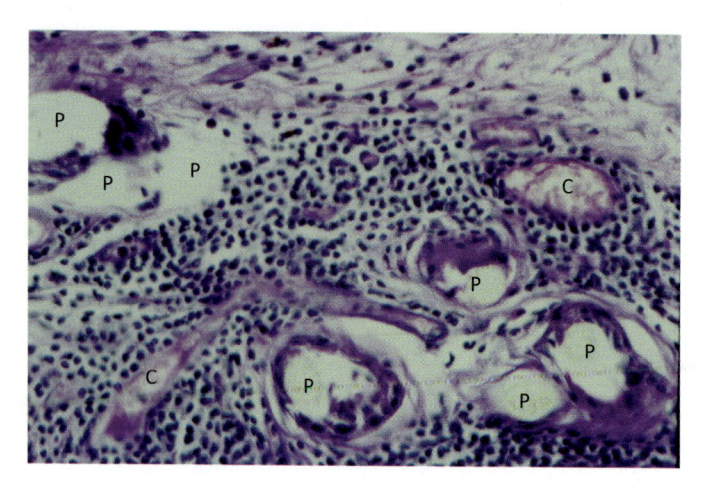

Figure 70. External cuff under light microscopy. C: capillaries; P: polyester fibers of the cuff.

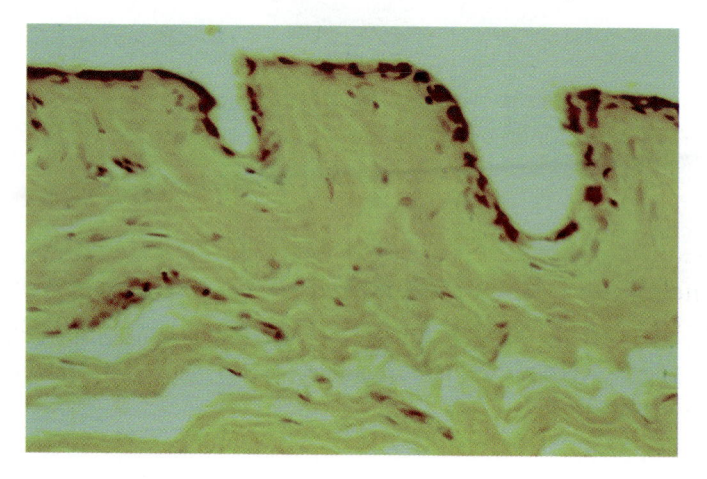

Figure 71. Intercuff segment of the uninfected tunnel under light microscopy. A dense fibrous capsule is covered with mucin. Multiple micropits are seen on the surface.

yellow and may contain ulcers (Fig. 72A, arrow). The cuff may be partly or completely separated from the tunnel due to abscess formation (Fig. 72B, arrow).

I concluded from this study that the optimum distance between the exit and the external cuff is 2 cm, and all catheters in our institution were implanted in this way. This pioneering study has not been

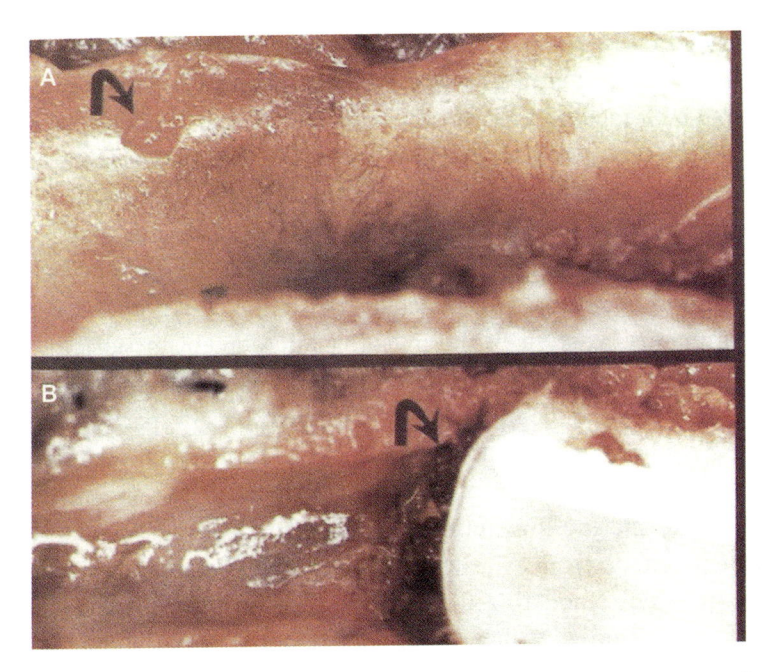

Figure 72. (A) Infected intercuff segment. The arrow points to an ulcer. (B) Infected tunnel close to the internal cuff with visible necrotic tissue. (Modified from Pu 176.)

widely cited in the literature, but I hope that it will be rediscovered in the future. Two of our recommendations are typically followed: the external cuff is predominantly located 2 cm from the exit, and the exit is mostly directed downwards.

Exit Site Study

Starting in July 1988 and continuing until August 1993, this longitudinal study evaluated 61 exit sites after they were healed and 43 exits during the healing process after implantation. The analysis of the results continued up until 1996 and was published in Supplement 3, Volume 16 of *Peritoneal Dialysis International* [Pu 237–Pu 244].

Healed exits [Pu 237, Pu 238]

Prior to this study there was no classification of exit status; exits were usually classified as infected or not. The most widely accepted was that published by Pierratos in 1984,[6] which was agreed upon by the vast majority of *Peritoneal Dialysis Bulletin* editorial board members. Pierratos defined an exit site infection as follows: "Redness or skin induration or purulent discharge from the exit. Formation of the crust around the exit may not indicate infection. Positive cultures from the exit in the absence of inflammation do not indicate infection." Our study stemmed from our disappointment with the lack of satisfactory description of normal and infected exit sites. We hypothesized that inflammatory reaction to the invading microorganism starts in the sinus, because, as we already knew from our tunnel morphology study, the sinus is rarely completely epithelialized, usually partly covered with granulation tissue, and usually colonized with microorganisms.

The study was approved by the University of Missouri and Dialysis Clinic Inc. Institutional Review Boards. The patients were instructed to perform exit site care 10–16 hours before the exit evaluation to assure standardized comparisons of various exits and visible sinus tract features. Histories were documented of preceding events, such as trauma, contamination, excessive sweating, and presence of pain, tenderness or soreness. Next, the external exit and visible sinus were inspected using a Zeiss prism loupe (Fig. 73). The "external exit" was defined as the visible exit without lifting the catheter. The term

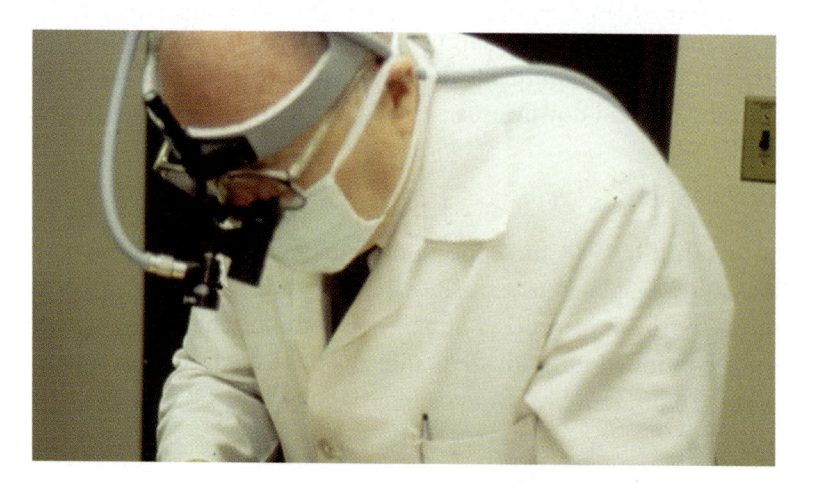

Figure 73. Zeiss prism loupe.

---

6. Pierratos A. (1984) Peritoneal dialysis glossary. *Perit Dial Bull* **4**: 2–4.

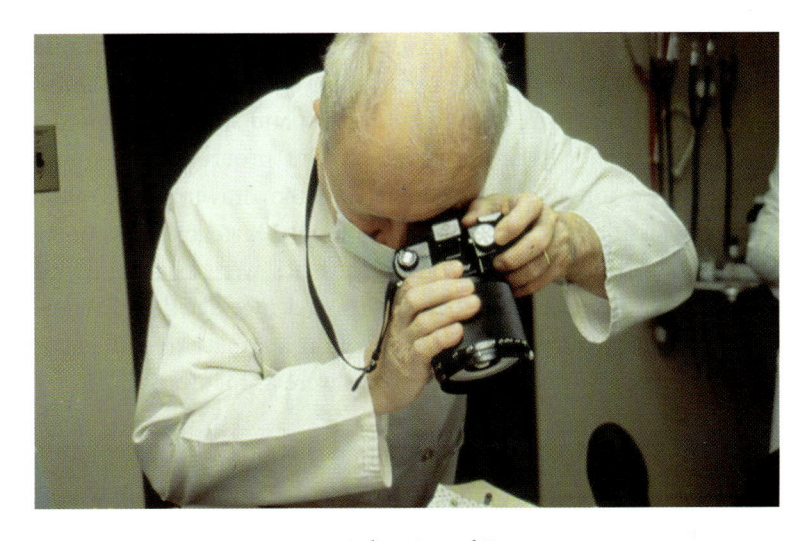

Figure 74. Yashica Dental Eye camera.

"visible sinus" was used to indicate the outermost part of the sinus tract (inside the sinus rim) visible after lifting the catheter or moving it laterally. Thereafter, pictures of the external exit and the visible sinus tract were drawn, and photographs were taken with a Yashica Dental Eye camera (Fig. 74). Finally, the photographs of the right, central and left parts of the sinus were taken. All visual attributes discerned by the loupe inspection and drawn in pictures were confirmed by a review of photographs. I made all the evaluations and later reviewed the photographs with Barb. There were 565 evaluations of 61 exits, and over 6,200 pictures were taken. Cultures from the exit sinus were taken with each evaluation.

After about 100 initial evaluations it became apparent that using only two categories (infected versus uninfected) for exit classification was insufficient. Additional categories were added as multiple comparisons were made between the exit appearance and treatment outcomes in the next 200 evaluations. Ultimately, the classification relied on the four cardinal signs of inflammation as proposed by Aulus Cornelius Celsus in his treatise *De Medicina*, written in the first century AD. These are well known: *calor* (heat), *rubor* (redness), *tumor* (swelling) and dolor (pain). In the second century AD, in his treatise *De tumoribus praeter naturam*, Claudius Galen added the fifth cardinal sign, *Functio laesa* (impaired function). Additional features of inflammation, specific for an exit of any skin-penetrating foreign body, are drainage, regression of epidermis, and slight exuberance of granulation tissue or its profuse overgrowth ("proud flesh").

When we initially started reviewing the drawings and photographs, we classified exit appearance into about 30 categories. Distinctive exit site and visible sinus tract characteristics were established after approximately 300 exit evaluations. Ultimately, we decided that seven categories could be distinguished and that the approach to each of them should be different. The seven categories were as follows:

- *Acutely infected exit*: Purulent and/or bloody drainage from the exit site, spontaneous or after pressure on the sinus; and/or swelling; and/or erythema with diameter 13 mm or more from border to border; and regression of epithelium in the sinus. Acute catheter exit inflammation lasts less than four weeks and may be accompanied by pain, exuberant granulation tissue around the exit or in the sinus, and the presence of a scab or crust (Figs. 75 and 76). Exit culture may be negative in patients receiving antibiotics.
- *Chronic catheter exit site infection*: Purulent and/or bloody drainage from the exit site, spontaneous or after pressure on the sinus; and/or exuberant granulation tissue around the exit and/or in the

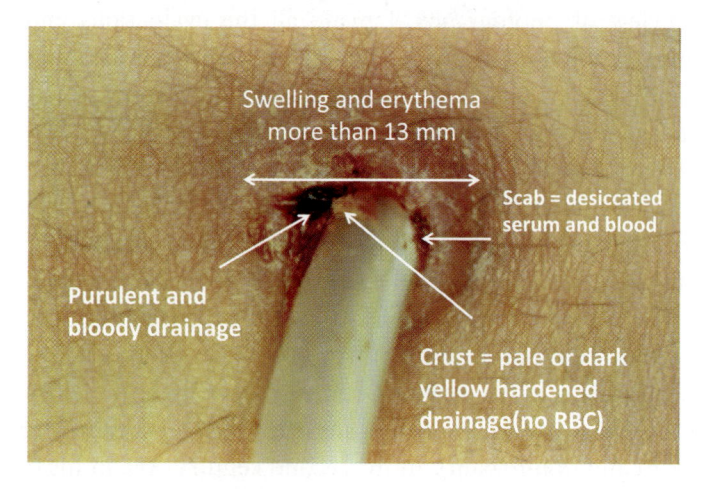

Figure 75. Acutely infected exit outside. (Modified from Pu 238.)

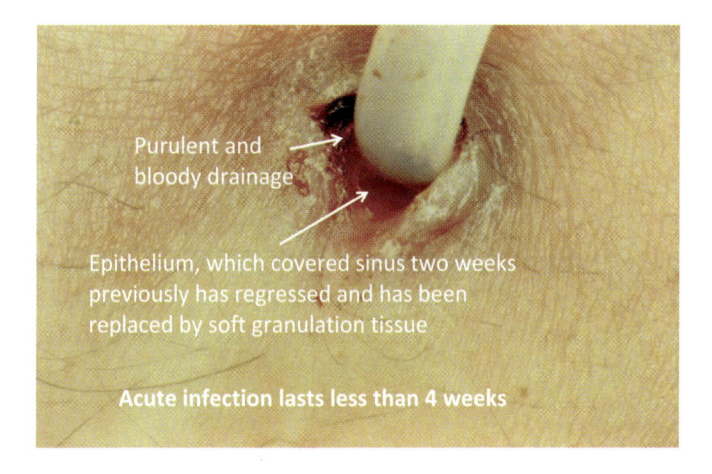

Figure 76. Sinus of acutely infected exit. (Modified from Pu 238.)

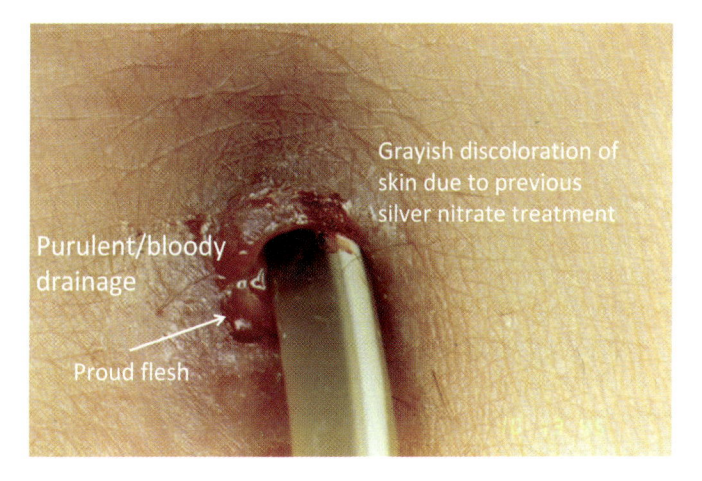

Figure 77. Chronically infected exit. (Modified from Pu 238.)

sinus; and regression of epithelium in the sinus. Chronic infection persists for more than four weeks and crust or scab is frequently present. Swelling, erythema and/or pain indicate exacerbation, otherwise are absent (Figs. 77 and 78). Exit culture may be negative in patients receiving antibiotics.
- *Equivocally infected catheter exit site*: Purulent and/or bloody drainage that cannot be expressed outside the sinus, accompanied by the regression of epithelium, and occurrence of slightly

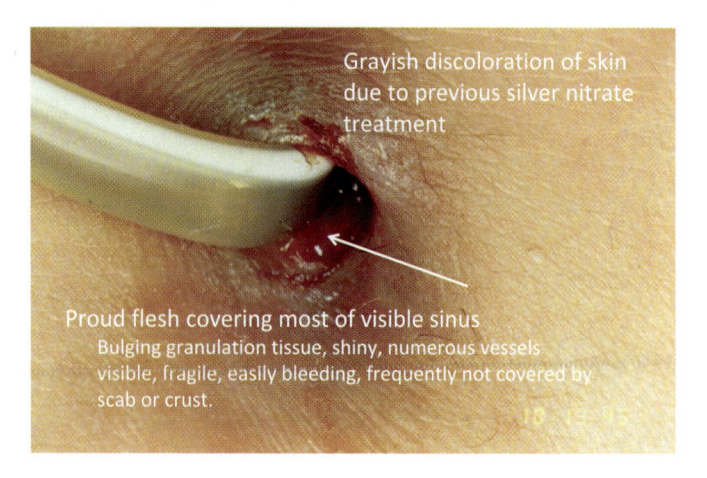

Figure 78. Sinus of chronically infected exit. (Modified from Pu 238.)

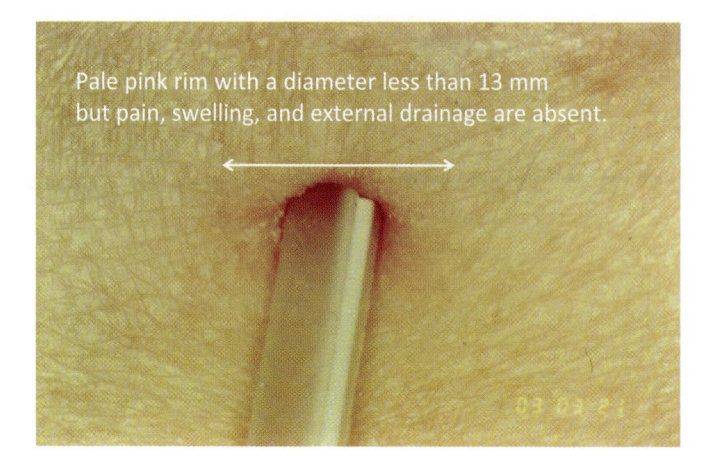

Figure 79. Equivocally infected exit. (Modified from Pu 238.)

exuberant granulation tissue around the exit and/or in the sinus. Erythema with a diameter less than 13 mm from border to border may be present, but pain, swelling and external drainage are absent. Exit culture may be negative in patients receiving antibiotics (Figs. 79 and 80).
- *Good catheter exit*: Exit color is natural, pale pink, purplish or dark and there is no purulent or bloody drainage. Clear or thick exudate may be visible in the sinus. Mature epithelium covers only part of

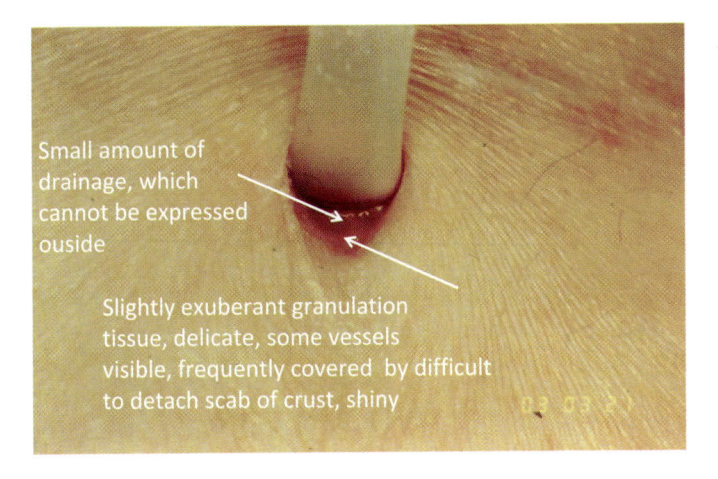

Figure 80. Sinus of equivocally infected exit. (Modified from Pu 238.)

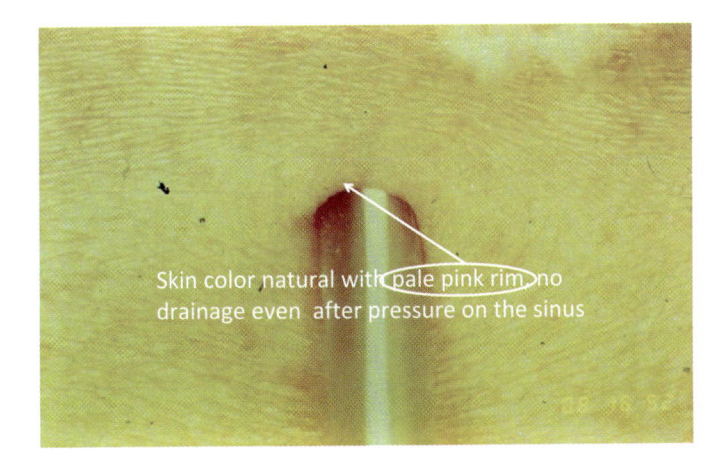

Figure 81. Good exit. (Modified from Pu 238.)

the sinus; the rest is covered by fragile epithelium or plain granulation tissue. Pain, swelling and erythema are absent. Positive peri-exit smear culture, if present, indicates colonization not infection. (Figs. 81 and 82).

- *Perfect catheter exit*: At least six months old with its entire visible length of sinus tract covered with the keratinized (mature) epithelium. Exit color is natural or dark and there is no drainage. A small, easily detachable crust may be present in the sinus or

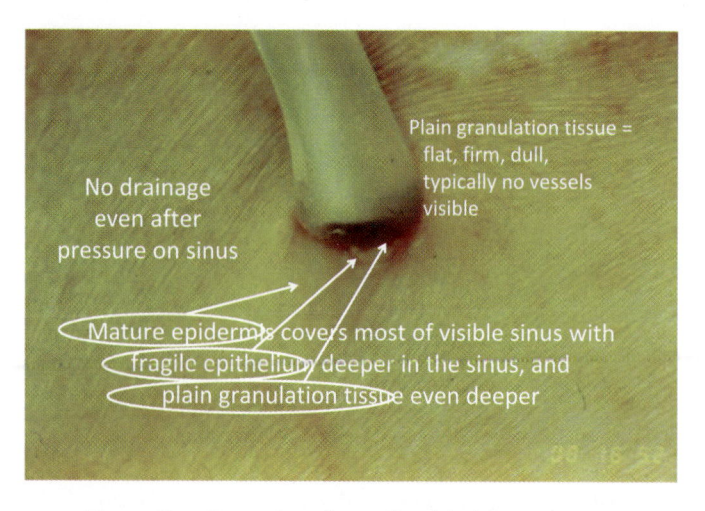

Figure 82. Sinus of good exit. (Modified from Pu 238.)

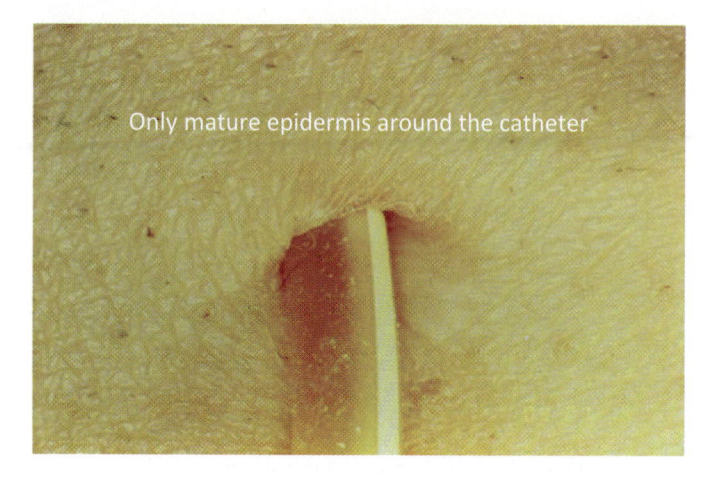

Figure 83. Perfect exit. (Modified from Pu 238.)

around the exit. Positive peri-exit smear culture, if present, indicates colonization not infection (Figs. 83 and 84).
- *External cuff infection without exit infection*: Intermittent or chronic, purulent, bloody or gooey drainage, spontaneous or after pressure on the cuff and induration of the tissue around the cuff. Exuberant granulation tissue may be seen deep in the sinus; sinus epithelium may be chronically or intermittently macerated. Exit

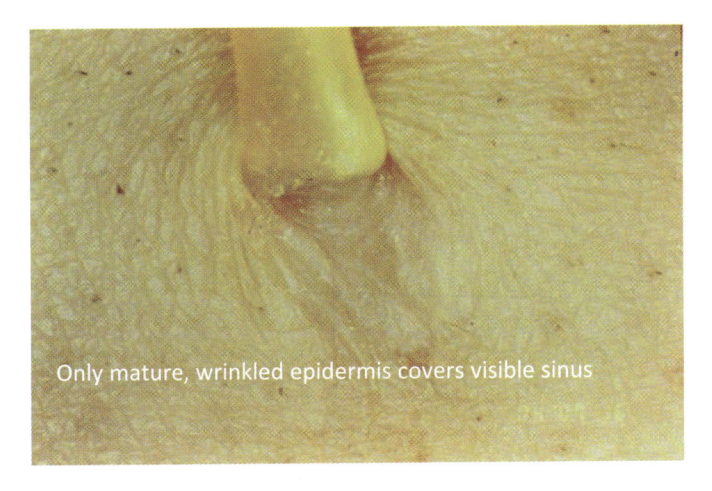

Figure 84. Sinus of perfect exit. (Modified from Pu 238.)

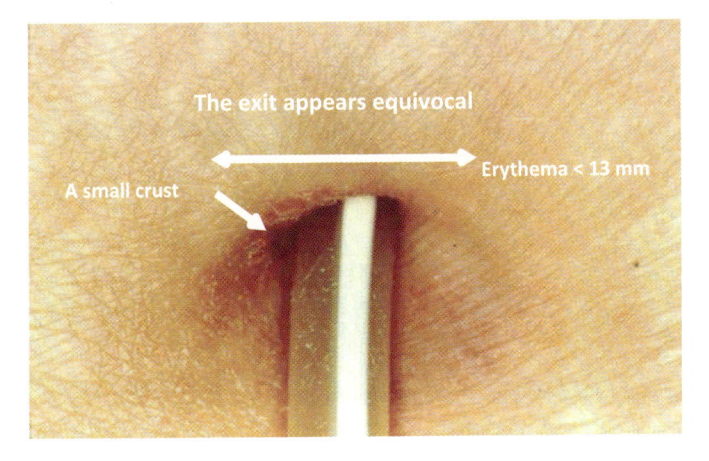

Figure 85. External cuff infection without exit infection. (Modified from Pu 238.)

site may look normal on external examination (Figs. 85–87). Ultrasound may show fluid collection around the cuff, but negative ultrasound does not rule out cuff infection. Exit culture may be negative in patients receiving antibiotics.

- *Traumatized exit*: Features of the traumatized exit depend on the intensity of trauma and time interval until examination. Common features of trauma are: pain, bleeding, scab and deterioration of exit appearance (e.g., perfect exit transforms to good or equivocal or acutely infected) (Figs. 88 and 89).

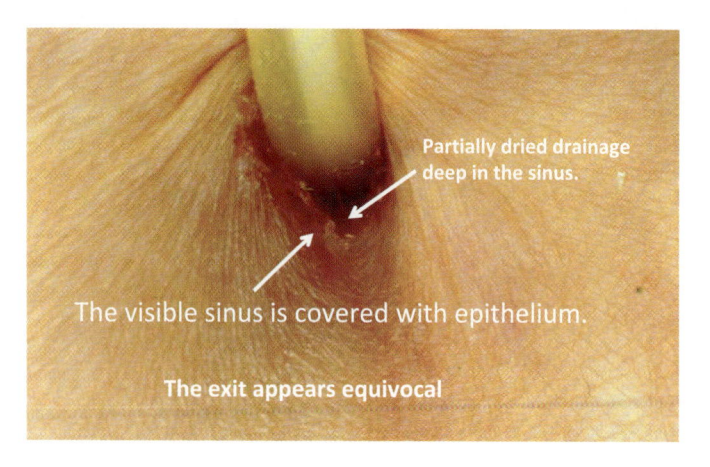

Figure 86. Sinus of cuff infection without exit infection. (Modified from Pu 238.)

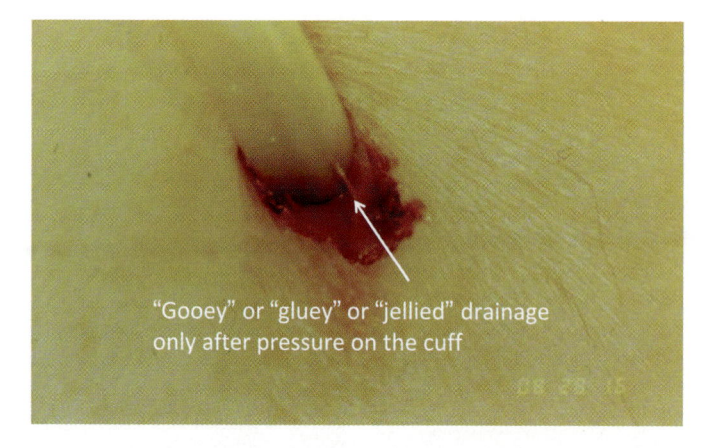

Figure 87. Another example of external cuff infection without exit infection. Drainage only after pressure on the cuff. (Modified from Pu 237.)

Care and treatment recommendations

Based on our classification system, and on experience, we developed specific recommendations for the prevention and treatment of exit infection, publishing the work in several papers [Pu 183, Pu 240–Pu 242, Pu 252, Pu 255]. Prevention is very important, particularly avoidance of trauma and exit contamination.

In acute exit site infection, a culture of the exit site should be taken immediately, but antibiotics against Gram-positive organisms

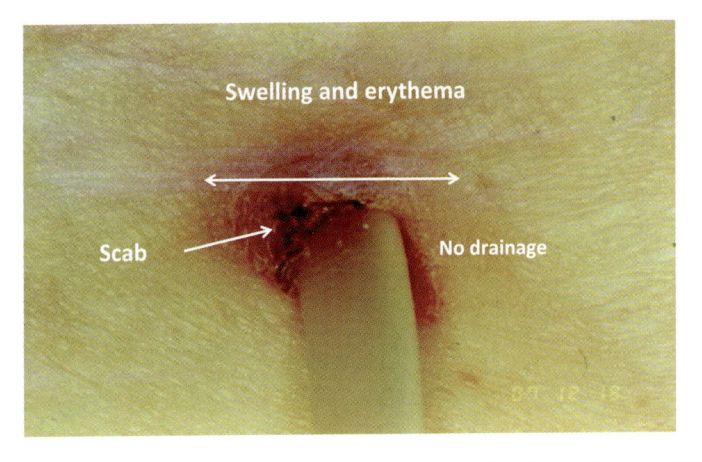

Figure 88. External appearance of traumatized exit. (Modified from Pu 238.)

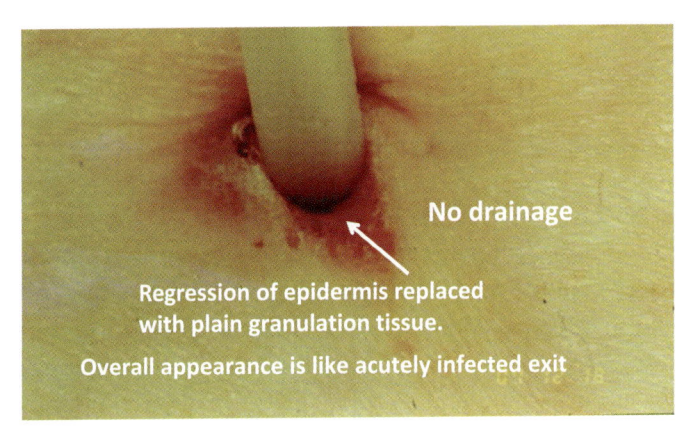

Figure 89. Sinus appearance of traumatized exit. (Modified from Pu 238.)

should be started before culture results are known. Antibiotics may be changed, if indicated, after culture results are known. Treatment should continue for 7 to 10 days after the exit acquires a good appearance. Exuberant granulation tissue (proud flesh) should be cauterized with a silver nitrate stick. No more than one or two applications may be necessary in acute infection (Fig. 90). This procedure speeds up the healing process and facilitates epithelialization. Cauterization should be restricted to granulation tissue only, and accidental touching of the adjacent epithelium should be avoided. Use of a magnifying glass aids in precise cauterization.

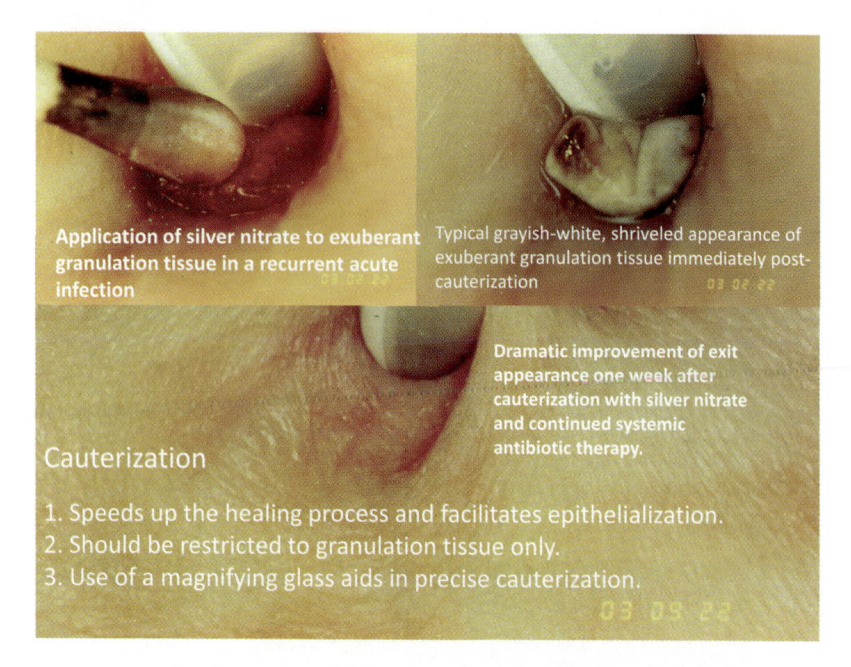

Figure 90. Cauterization of proud flesh. (Modified from Pu 237.)

For chronic infection prolonged treatment with antibiotics according to culture and sensitivity results is needed. Our experience indicated that topical antibiotics were useless in copious drainage, as antibiotics were washed away. Local antibiotics or nonirritating bactericidal solutions were useful only in equivocal exits, as this kind of exit indicates a low grade or subclinical form of infection.

In cuff infection, removal of the catheter is usually needed. In our experience, cuff shaving and deroofing prolonged catheter life for approximately 6 to 12 months. These temporary measures may be suitable for patients who are expected to remain on therapy for a short period, e.g., patients awaiting transplants; however, cuff infection is a strong indicator for catheter removal in long-term peritoneal dialysis patients. Our experience indicated that cuff shaving may provide better results in presternal catheters. This may be related to the presence of three cuffs and a long tunnel in the presternal catheter. Shaving of the subcutaneous cuff leaves two cuffs as a double barrier against periluminal bacterial penetration.

One interesting observation in our studies, which was contrary to some others, was that the culture from the sinus indicated different a microorganism than cultured from the nares but very similar to that from the surrounding skin. I remember having a discussion during a controversial presentation about the incidence of exit infections in relation to nasal carrier status of *Staphylococcus aureus* in peritoneal dialysis patients [Pr 252]. Mary Luzar, a Baxter Europe employee at the time, insisted that the organism from the exit and nares was the same, while our studies indicated that the sensitivity and strain was frequently different. I suggested that the difference between our study and other studies was related to the different behavior of patients in our region. I insisted that "in our region it is socially unacceptable to pick one's nose and then fondle the catheter." I did not say that the opposite sequence was acceptable.

For good and perfect exit-only catheter immobilization, protection from trauma, use of liquid soap and water for daily care, and use of Shur-Clens® to remove large, irritating crust are appropriate measures to prevent infection. In our experience a perfect exit is unlikely to become infected unless severely traumatized or grossly contaminated after submersion in water loaded with bacteria.

Bleeding is a common sequela of trauma. Extravasated blood is a good medium for bacterial growth. Bacteria that have colonized the exit multiply rapidly in the presence of decomposing blood and infect the disrupted tissue. Infection may occur as early as 24 to 48 hours after trauma. The prompt administration of an antibiotic, chosen based on the past history of skin colonization, may prevent acute infection. In the absence of information about previous skin colonies, an antimicrobial agent sensitive to Gram-positive organisms, such as a cephalosporin or a quinolone, may be chosen. Therapy may have to be continued for about seven days after achieving a good appearance. Aggressive treatment is necessary in every instance of trauma reported by the patient. Local care requires gentle cleansing of all blood from the exit site.

Exit site healing [Pu 239]

The goals of this study were (1) to describe the natural healing process after peritoneal catheter implantation, (2) to discern factors that

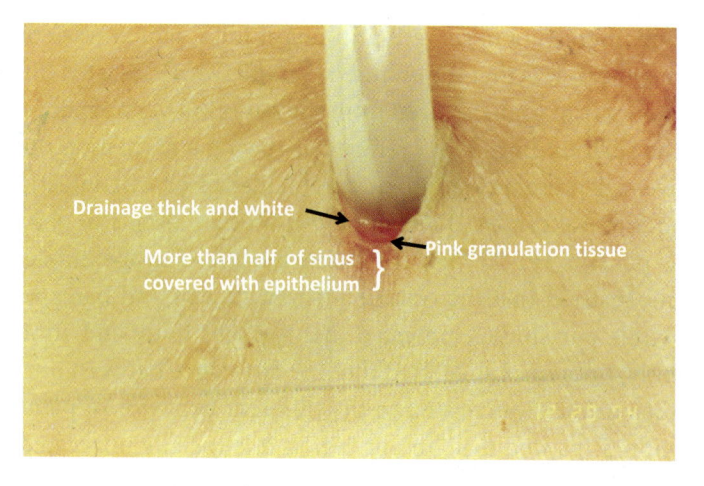

Figure 91. Fast healing exit. (Modified from Pu 239.)

predispose to exit infection, and (3) to recognize early signs of exit site infection. We performed 226 evaluations of 43 exits, 32 in the abdomen and 11 in the parasternal area. The evaluations were similar to those of healed exits, with culture taken from exit, nares, careful descriptions and almost 2,500 photos.

After reviewing the evaluations the exit sites were categorized into four types: (1) fast-healing exits had no drainage or minimal moisture deep inside by the third week; the epidermis started to enter into the sinus within 2 to 3 weeks, progressed steadily, and covered at least half of the visible sinus tract within 4 to 6 weeks after implantation (Fig. 91); (2) in slow-healing exits without infection, the epidermis started to enter into the sinus after 3 weeks or progressed slowly and did not cover half of the visible sinus by 5 weeks (Fig. 92); (3) healing interrupted by infection initially looked identical to a fast-healing exit, but within 6 weeks acquired the features of an acutely infected exit (Fig. 93); (4) in slow-healing exits due to early infection, granulation tissue became soft or fleshy and drainage became purulent by 2 to 3 weeks (Fig. 94).

Compared with patients with fast-healing exits, patients with early-infected exits were more likely to be diabetics, to have an abdominal not presternal catheter, wound hematoma, higher body mass index, and higher percentage of positive cultures for *Staphylococcus aureus* in the nares. Early colonization of the exit was

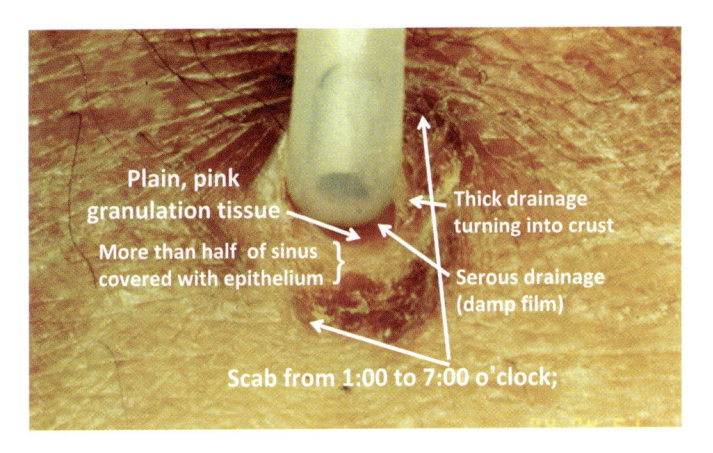

Figure 92. Slow healing exit. (Modified from Pu 239.)

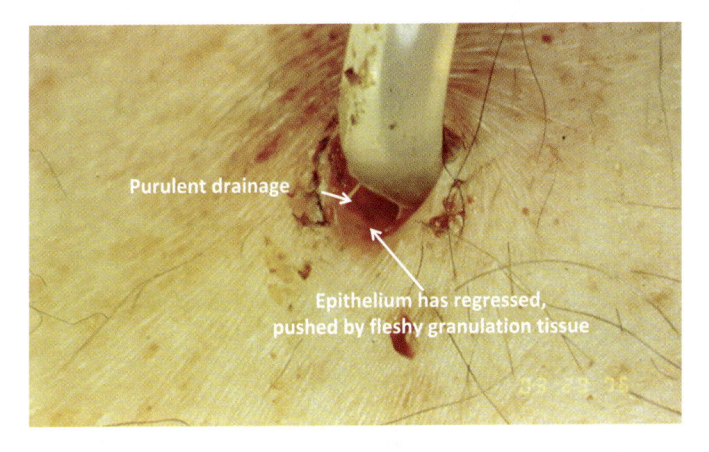

Figure 93. Interrupted healing. (Modified from Pu 239.)

the most significant factor in determining the healing pattern: the later the colonization the better the healing. We postulated that exit infections and peritonitis rates might be decreased by delaying exit colonization using prophylactic antibiotics for at least 2 weeks after implantation and sterile exit dressing procedures for the entire healing time of approximately 6 weeks.

This study was one of my most involved, as it was carried out over almost eight years, with hundreds of evaluations, cultures and thousands of pictures taken and analyzed with Barb. Our classification has

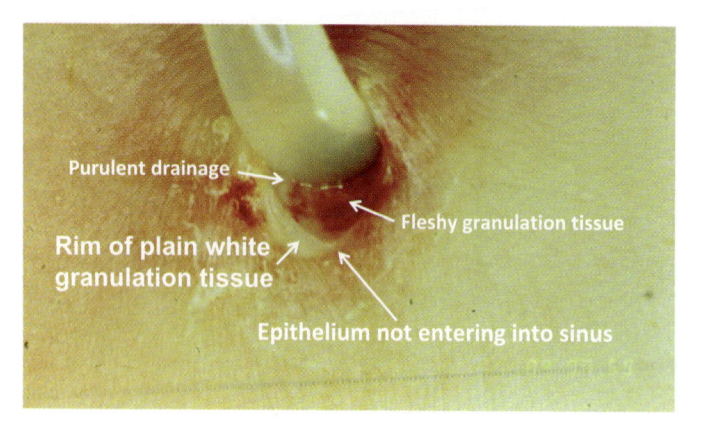

Figure 94. Early infected exit. (Modified from Pu 239.)

been followed by several centers, and some of them consider it to be the most accurate. However, most centers do not follow our classification and some of our recommendations. My explanation is that our evaluation is very time-consuming and requires the use of a magnifier, and most centers are reluctant to do that. In many centers a local antibiotic is given regardless of whether it is really needed or not (e.g., in the case of a good or perfect exit); systemic antibiotics are given indiscriminately. Although this study has not been received as well as I hoped it would be, I am still convinced that it was valuable work that may be rediscovered in the future.

CHAPTER 12

Teaching and Consulting

Annual Dialysis Conference

Our Annual Dialysis Conference started as the CAPD conference in February 1981. It was organized by Dr. Nolph with administrative help from Barry Kling, Director of the Continuous Medical Education (CME) at the University of Missouri. Travenol provided some financial support, as the conference professed to spread knowledge about this relatively new dialysis method. The first conference was held at the Crown Center Hotel in Kansas City, Mssouri, and there were 330 attendees. My attendance began the following year, when it was also held in Kansas City. I gave three presentations for that conference [Pr 36–Pr 38]. I also joined the organizing committee of the conference. The next six conferences were also organized in Kansas City, but the number of attendees had begun to grow rapidly so, in 1986, Elaine Rogers became our Special Conference Coordinator, helping Barry Kling with administrative issues. The Crown Center Hotel became too small and the conferences were organized in Dallas, Texas, in 1989 and 1990. In the years that followed we decided to start changing the conference location annually.

In 1990, for the very first time, the pediatric group, under the chairmanship of Steven Alexander, MD, organized the Annual Symposium on Pediatric Dialysis. Proceedings were first published in 1985, for the fifth conference, under the name, "Advances in Continuous Ambulatory Peritoneal Dialysis." Containing articles from presentations given during the conference, the proceedings were edited by Ramesh Khanna, MD, Karl D. Nolph, MD, Barbara Prowant, RN, Dimitrios G. Oreopoulos, MD, and myself. Beginning in 1986, abstracts were accepted and those of high quality were presented in the slide or poster forums. In 1992 I organized the Peritoneal Dialysis Case Forum, a two-hour session considering a case that was interesting but lacked a crucial study or test necessary for final diagnosis. One of two experts was invited to discuss the case and try to establish a diagnosis. The final diagnostic procedure was then presented, the outcome of the case was given and a broad discussion was initiated. I edited the Case Forum in a special section of *Peritoneal Dialysis International*, with Martin J. Schreiber, MD, and John M. Burkart, MD, serving as associate editors. The last case I organized and edited was in 1998, as I was becoming less involved in the peritoneal dialysis part of the conference and markedly more in the hemodialysis part.

1993 National Torchbearer Award Dinner
March 8, 1993
San Diego, California

honoring

Zbylut J. Twardowski, M.D.

7:00 p.m.   Cocktails
8:00 p.m.   Dinner
            Presentation of Award
            Speakers:
                Steven Alexander, M.D.
                Ram Gokal, M.D.
                Hiroshi Hayashidera
                Prakash Keshaviah, M.D.
                Ramesh Khanna, M.D.
                Kimihiko Matsuzaki
                Susan D. Molumphy, Ph.D.
                Jack Moncrief, M.D.
                Karl Nolph, M.D.
                Dimitrios Oreopoulos, M.D.
                Barbara Prowant, R.N.
                Wayne Quinton
                Miguel Riella, M.D.
                Larry Rohrer
                Martin Schreiber, M.D.
                Maria Sieniawska, M.D.
                John Van Stone, M.D.
                James Winchester, M.D.

Mary Rathburn, Harpist

AMERICAN KIDNEY FUND

1993 National

Torchbearer Award Dinner

honoring

Zbylut J. Twardowski, M.D.

March 8, 1993

Hyatt Regency San Diego
San Diego, California

Figure 95. Torchbearer Award Dinner Program.

The annual conference went from strength to strength. Attendance grew consistently each year until 1993, when the conference in San Diego, California, had 2,401 attendees. On March 8 the 1993 National Torchbearer Award Dinner was held in conjunction with the conference to honor my achievements in dialysis research, teaching and patient care (Fig. 95). There were 18 speakers and Steven Alexander was the Master of Ceremonies (Fig. 96). All of the speakers poked fun at me in a very pleasant way, so we were laughing frequently (Fig. 97). Ram Gokal, from the Manchester Royal Infirmary, reminded the audience of our trip to Seoul, where my luggage was lost and I did not have a tie with me so I needed to buy one. He had imagined that given the very colorful slides I was known for using in my presentations, I would be leaving the shop with a multicolored tie, but to his surprise, I had bought a very plain one. So, as compensation, he presented me with a nice, colorful tie at the dinner (Fig. 98). Barbara F. Prowant ("Barb") reminisced about the difficulties I had communicating with patients in the early 1980s. She recalled one funny situation when one of the nurses had notified me that a patient had come to the clinic for

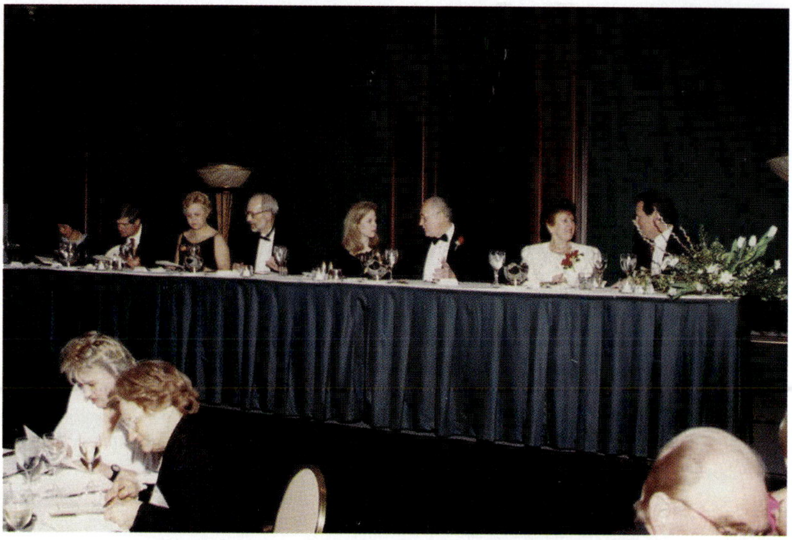

Figure 96. Front table: (from left) Leonor Ponferrada, John C. Van Stone, Georgia and Karl Nolph, Susan D. Molumphy, the author, Halina, and Steven Alexander. Left table: Alicja Grzegorzewska and Maria Sieniawska. Right lower corner: Wayne Quinton.

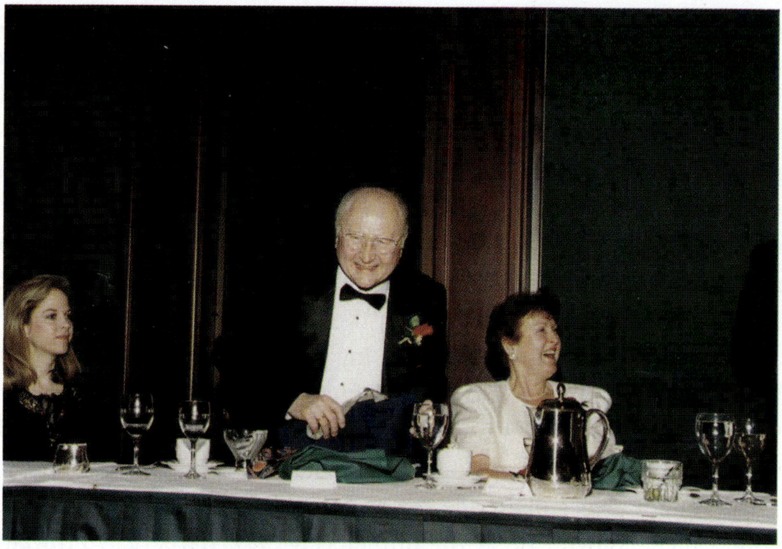

Figure 97. Speakers poke fun at the author.

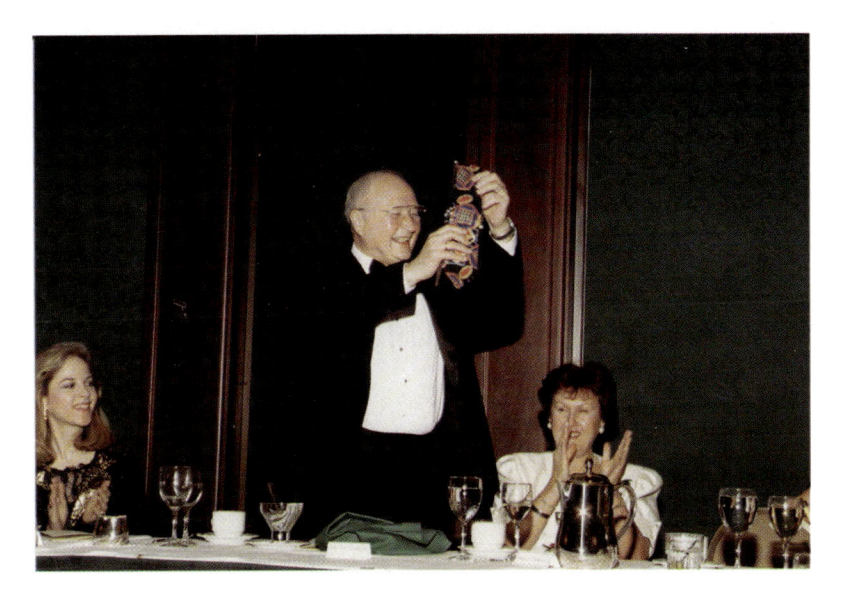

Figure 98. Colorful tie: a present from Ram Gokal.

a checkup after momentarily passing out that morning. I had gone to the patient's room and after greeting him and his wife, I had said, "I heard that you passed away this morning, is that right?" The patient and his wife had been shocked and the nurse had been forced to intervene and explain what I had meant. In spite of such mishaps, the nurses decided to crown me King of Peritoneal Dialysis (Fig. 99). After all the amusing anecdotes — and congratulatory messages from senators, the president of the University and the U.S. President (Fig. 100) — Susan Molumphy from the American Kidney Fund presented me with the Torchbearer Award (Fig. 101), and the post-award dinner could start. My sons came for the ceremony. At the end of the dinner a commemorative photograph of former and current awardees was taken (Fig. 102).

Attendance dropped slightly to 2,353 for our 1994 conference in Orlando, Florida. At the same time there was a drop in the number of patients on peritoneal dialysis in our center, and in the U.S. generally, so I was worried that the number of attendees might continue to decline. I expressed my concerns to Dr. Nolph and suggested expanding the conference by including a home hemodialysis session. Dr. Nolph

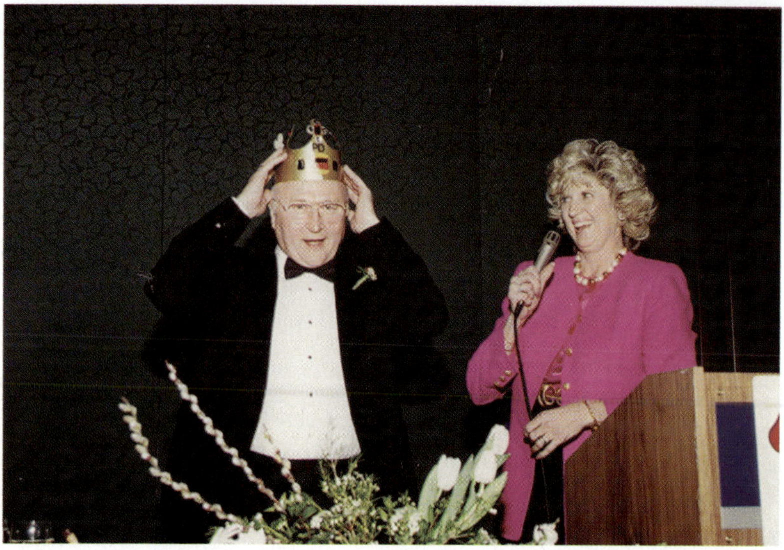

Figure 99. Roberta Satalowich crowning the author King of Peritoneal Dialysis.

THE WHITE HOUSE
WASHINGTON

March 8, 1993

Zbylut J. Twardowski, M.D.
304 Devine Court
Columbia, Missouri 65203

Dear Dr. Twardowski:

Congratulations as you are presented with the National Torchbearer Award from the American Kidney Fund.

Kidney disease kills tens of thousands of people in America every year. Your numerous contributions to the field of nephrology have improved lives and have given hope to many. The National Torchbearer Award symbolizes the high regard in which you are held by your colleagues around the world for your long-standing dedication to ending kidney disease.

I commend your commitment to helping others. Hillary and I send our best wishes for an enjoyable evening.

Sincerely,

Bill Clinton

Figure 100. Letter of congratulations from President Clinton.

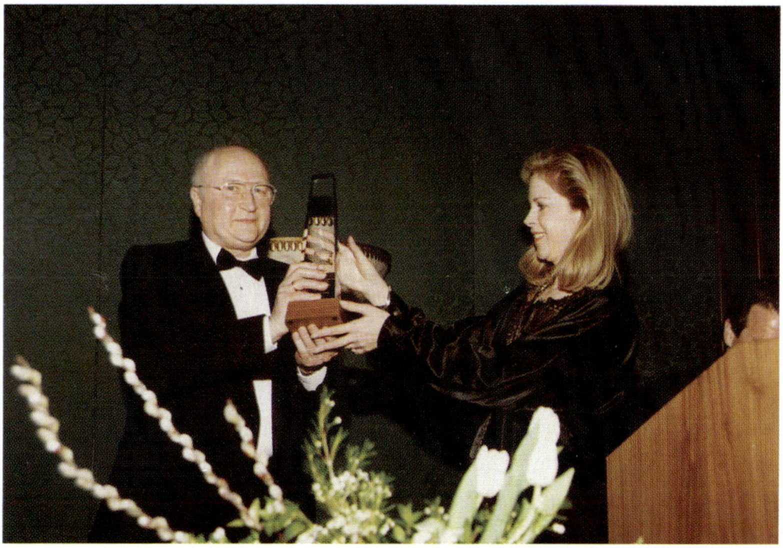

Figure 101. Susan Molumphy from the American Kidney Fund presents the Torchbearer Award to the author.

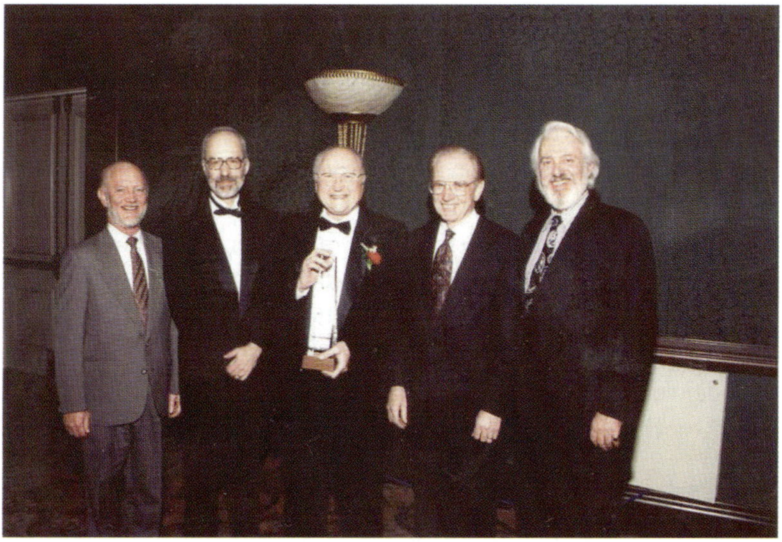

Figure 102. Former and current awardees: Jack Moncrief, MD, Karl D. Nolph, MD. Current awardees: Wayne Quinton, PhD, and Robert Popovich, PhD.

and the rest of the organizing committee accepted the suggestion, and the first session was to take place during the Baltimore conference in 1995. We were a little afraid that peritoneal dialysis enthusiasts might feel betrayed and abandon the conference, so we decided to go very slow and see what would happen. That first year, the part of the conference related to hemodialysis was called the 1st International Symposium on Daily Home Hemodialysis and was held on Monday afternoon, February 13, 1995. I presided over the symposium with Eli Friedman, MD. I made the introductory presentation entitled, "DHHD — A hybrid of HD and CAPD" [Pr 394], where I argued that daily home hemodialysis combines the best features of hemodialysis and peritoneal dialysis. A major feature from hemodialysis was the very high efficiency of dialysis, and a major feature from peritoneal dialysis was frequent dialysis sessions, avoiding the ups and downs typical for three times weekly hemodialysis. The presentation was published the following year [Pu 245].

Umberto Buoncristiani, MD, from Perugia, Italy, participated in the symposium and presented his 13-year experience with daily home hemodialysis. Robert Uldall, MD,[1] from Toronto, presented his experience with slow nocturnal hemodialysis in an initial five patients. George Harper, a long-term home hemodialysis patient, presented his experience with the buttonhole method of needle insertion. For my part, I presented the concept of the Swan Neck internal jugular (SNIJ) catheter [Pr 395], which at the time was the subject of an interference proceeding, as described previously. Rodney S. Kenley presented our concept for a machine for daily home hemodialysis (DHHD), and Eli Friedman closed the symposium with the presentation, "Daily home hemodialysis: The ultimate dialysis modality?"

It turned out that there was significant interest in the symposium, and the number of conference attendees increased to 2,540. Attendence increased further over the ensuing years, reaching a peak of 3,293 at the San Francisco conference in 2000. The numbers started

---

1. Robert Uldall, MD, an extremely innovative researcher, died suddenly four months after the conference. The nocturnal hemodialysis program in Toronto was taken over by Andreas Pierratos, MD, who would present the results many times at our conferences. Dr. Pierratos received our award for lifetime achievements in hemodialysis at our Phoenix conference in 2011.

to drop after that; the most dramatic decline was after the terrorist attacks on the World Trade Center on September 11, 2001, but also in 2006 owing to the global financial crisis, and due to incidental events like a blizzard in Denver in 2007. After 1995 the Home Hemodialysis Symposium started to grow, and the name was changed to Hemodialysis Symposium to reflect the inclusion of all forms of hemodialysis. I became the chairman of this part of the conference. The name of the conference had also changed — to encompass all forms of peritoneal dialysis, hemodialysis and pediatric dialysis — to the Annual Dialysis Conference. The second symposium in Seattle in 1996 had three sessions. A. Peter Lundin gave a very interesting presentation entitled, "Why I chose home hemodialysis for myself." Aksys demonstrated PHD®i for the first time (Fig. 58).

With a growing workload related to the organization of the Hemodialysis Symposium, Ellen Steltzer was hired as a secretary to help Barb, Harold Moore and me with administrative issues. Her office was in the DCI Laboratory. Initially, in 1994, she was working part-time, but she was given a full-time position from 1995 onwards. In 1997 I started editing the proceedings of the 3rd International Daily Home Hemodialysis Symposium, initially as Home Hemodialysis International, then from 2000 as Hemodialysis International. The publisher was Multimed Inc., from Milton, Ontario, Canada. Barbara F. Prowant, RN, MS ("Barb") became the deputy editor in 1998. She was extremely good at editing and I cannot imagine being able to edit the volume without her help. The associate editors were Christopher Blagg, MD, Eli A. Friedman, Ramesh Khanna, MD, Karl D. Nolph, and Dimitrios G. Oreopoulos, MD. Belding H. Scribner became consulting editor in 1999. Ellen Steltzer was an excellent secretary, helping Barb and me with editing journals and other jobs.

In 1999 we began publishing *Home Hemodialysis Today*. I was the editor and Barb was the deputy editor. It was a news-style publication meant to provide rapid information with highlights of the symposium to all the participants. The publisher was again Multimed Inc. and the publication was supported by a grant from Aksys Ltd. It was mailed out within two months after the symposium. Two further issues in this format were published under the name *Hemodialysis Today* in 2000 and 2001. Ellen was with us until 2000, and she was replaced by Julie Helgerson, who worked with us until we transferred the editorial office to Allen Nissenson, MD, in 2003. After the transfer we did not need that much secretarial help, so Julie was transferred to another division in the Department of Medicine. In later years we had some help from secretaries employed in the main nephrology office: Lindsay Hammond in 2003, Judy McDowell in 2006, and Maggie Nichols from 2008. Claire Oser was also always very helpful in more complicated matters.

Published by Blackwell Publishing, *Hemodialysis International* became the official publication of the International Society of Hemodialysis in 2003. The number of issues was increased to four per year, and Allen Nissenson became the second deputy editor of the journal. One issue was devoted to the Proceedings of the Hemodialysis Symposium. In 2004 I resigned from the post of editor and Allen Nissenson, MD, became the new editor, with Dr. Madhukar Misra becoming the editor of the proceedings. Allen Nissenson resigned from editorial duties in 2008 and Christopher R. Blagg replaced him. In 2002 Barry Kling resigned from his post and Allison Rentfro became the Director of CME. In 2003, Madhukar Misra, MD, became co-chair of the Hemodialysis Symposium and in 2004 he became the editor of the proceedings. Since 2008, with my diminishing contribution, he has gradually been assuming the duties of the chairman of the Hemodialysis Symposium. The number of submitted hemodialysis abstracts gradually increased and in 2010 exceeded the number of peritoneal dialysis abstracts, whose numbers gradually decreased.

Until 1999 the conference lasted two-and-a-half days, usually from Sunday to Tuesday. In 2000 the Pediatric Group decided to organize the Fundamentals of Dialysis in Children one day before the main conference. The Fundamentals of Extracorporeal Therapies started in 2004; in 2008 it changed its name to Comprehensive Course in Hemodialysis. In 2007, in cooperation with the International Society of Hemodialysis, a special one-day symposium on home hemodialysis, the day before the main conference, was organized by Leonor Ponferrada and Christopher Blagg. This special symposium continued in the years that followed. In 2010 the conference was held in Seattle from March 5 to 9. The last day of the conference was on the 50th anniversary of the first chronic hemodialysis, when surgeon David Dillard created the first arteriovenous shunt and Clyde Shields, a Boeing mechanic and patient of Belding H. Scribner, received hemodialysis. On the anniversary a half-day session was held with recollections of the early days of hemodialysis by those still living who had participated in its development. I co-presided over the session with Dr. Carl Kjellstrand. In a 7-minute presentation I recalled my 10-year experience with dialysis from 1962 to 1972 [Pr 516]. After the conference in Seattle, Elaine Rogers retired and Natalie Carter became the Special Conference Coordinator. In 2011 our conference was held in Phoenix, Arizona from February 19 to 22. We again had a slightly lower number of attendees. In the conference in San Antonio in 2012, there was a slight increase in the number of attendees.

Presentations on Dialysis Related Topics all over the World — Many Combined with Visiting Places of Interest

1981–1986

As mentioned previously, as the division had limited funds, my university salary was rather modest. In 1981, Dr Nolph, who was a consultant for Travenol, wanted me to present some of our studies at the company's headquarters in Deerfield. I presented studies on new osmotic agents [Pr 31], high volume exchanges [Pr 32] and cell count in dialysate in relation to time [Pr 33]. During the presentations I became acquainted with many prominent company employees. We also presented our study on polymer during the meeting of the American Society on Nephrology on November 23, 1981 [Pr 34]. In 1982, on the recommendation of Dr. Nolph, I became a consultant initially for Travenol, and later for Baxter, which significantly improved my financial situation.

As a Travenol consultant I traveled to give various presentations related to peritoneal dialysis [Pr 40, Pr 41, Pr 44]. I was once asked to give a seminar on peritoneal dialysis in Denver, Colorado [Pr 48]. I flew to Denver Airport and took a taxi to my hotel. I remember that the taxi driver immediately recognized my foreign accent and asked me where I was from. I told him I was from Poland and worked in Lublin. He said, "Lublin, Lublin… the Union of Lublin on July 1, 1569." I was stunned that an American taxi driver would know such a detail about Polish history and I asked him how he knew. It turned out that he had studied European history but could not find a job, so he had decided to become a taxi driver. After the seminar, held on Thursday, March 17, 1983, I rented a car and went skiing over that weekend in Winter Park, Colorado. I had been warned that the sunshine in Colorado was very deceptive and could burn one's skin, even in cloudy weather. I found it hard to believe, as I had never been at such an altitude and latitude before. I decided not to apply sunscreen and was duly sunburned.

In later years I became a consultant for Accurate Surgical Instruments, Quinton, Sherwood–Davis & Geck, Kendall Healthcare and Aksys. My consulting services mostly involved conducting studies, advising on new devices, and traveling and giving lectures on topics related to peritoneal dialysis and hemodialysis. In the 1980s and early 1990s most of my lecture travels were for Baxter, which was very interested in spreading the word about peritoneal dialysis therapy. Initially, my presentations were solely in the U.S., but after obtaining a "green card" in 1983, I was able to give presentations abroad. My first overseas travel was to the Netherlands, where I gave a presentation at the 4th Benelux Symposium on Continuous Ambulatory Peritoneal Dialysis in Rotterdam [Pr 62]. I called Halina from there and learned that she had been making progress in her efforts to join me in the U.S. During my stay in the Netherlands I visited Rotterdam and then The Hague, the seat of the Dutch government (though not the capital of the Netherlands). I visited the miniature city Madurodam, which offers the highlights of the Netherlands on a 1:25 scale, including a selection of Dutch architecture, ranging from Amsterdam's canals and Utrecht's church spires to Rotterdam's modern architecture. Madurodam also has a mini-sized airport, seaport and beaches — and little cars and trains running through the entire town.

Between 1982 and 1985 I had roughly 10 presentations per year. The number doubled in 1986 and 1987. In September 1985 I obtained a consular Polish passport issued by the Consulate General in Chicago, and I could travel to Poland and other countries. Most countries still required an entry visa, but it was relatively easy to obtain, having permanent residency in the U.S.

1987

In June 1987 Prof. Stig Bengmark, Chairman of the Department of Surgery, University of Lund, organized an international conference related to the peritoneum, including peritoneal dialysis and peritoneal access. Our group from Columbia, Missouri, was invited to participate. It was my first trip to Lund, Sweden. For me, Lund was associated with Nils Alwall and his struggle to improve hemodialysis and ultrafiltration and his spiral dialyzer, which was the first dialyzer in my clinical practice; regrettably, Alwall did not participate in the meeting, as he died a year earlier. I participated in two panel discussions [Pr 99, Pr 101] and gave a lecture on recent advances in peritoneal catheters [Pr 100]. Prof. Bengmark edited the proceedings from the conference and I contributed a chapter on continuous cyclic peritoneal dialysis [Pu 141]. At the conclusion of the conference, the University of Lund organized a gala dinner with speeches and performances from folk choir from southern Sweden.

We were back in Columbia for a week, but then returned to Europe to participate in the 4th Congress of the International Society for Peritoneal Dialysis in Venice, Italy. Two events stick in my mind from the congress. I have already mentioned one of them in the section on the peritoneal equilibration test, when what I considered to be my best and most important abstract on the PET was not accepted for presentation. However, that an abstract with a very new concept should not be accepted for presentation was a really relatively frequent occurrence. Nowadays congresses are more generous in accepting abstracts for presentations, as it is sometimes difficult to determine the value of a study based on the abstract. If reviewers are uncertain, they give a score suitable for a poster presentation instead of a slide presentation, rather than reject an abstract out of hand. The other issue that sticks in my mind was the extremely high temperature in the Palazzo del Cinema; there was no such thing as air conditioning at that time. I presented a poster on Swan Neck peritoneal catheters [Pr 106] and remember being completely soaked with sweat as the poster was situated close to the window and the June sun was extremely strong. Immediately after the Congress I was invited to give presentations in Poland at the Monument Hospital Children's Health Center, Warsaw, and in Poznań on the advances in peritoneal dialysis [Pr 110, Pr 111].

As I mentioned, the congress was held in the Palazzo del Cinema on Lido. As I had my presentations in Warsaw and Poznań in the middle of July, and Halina was with me, we decided to spend two extra days in Venice to see places of interest and three days visiting Rome, the Vatican in particular. From Lido we took a water taxi to Venice and visited the Piazza San Marco and the Biblioteca Marciana. We saw the famous Campanile di San Marco (the bell tower of St. Mark's Basilica) as well as the Triumphal Quadriga of St. Mark's Basilica. A fourth-century sculpture that was originally displayed at the Hippodrome in Constantinople, it was looted by Venetian forces during the Fourth Crusade and later installed on the terrace of the façade of St. Mark's Basilica in 1254. We were told that it was a replica on the terrace and the original was inside the Basilica. Finally, we walked over to the Ponte di Rialto. One thing I remember very clearly was buying a US$7 bottle of Coca-Cola on Piazza San Marco — the most expensive Coke I have ever bought!

We arrived in Rome on July 4 and stayed in the convent of the Parrocchia Santo Sergio e Bacco in Piazza della Madonna dei Monti. The sojourn was organized by our older son, Radek, who was acquainted with Rev. Jan Piotrowski, a priest staying in Rome temporarily who had recommended the convent to us. Rev. Piotrowski also arranged a "private visit" with the Pope in the Vatican on July 5, a visit that was, in fact, not quite private since there were about 300 people in the room. On the same day we visited the Vatican Library, Saint Peter's Basilica, and the Vatican Museum. St. Peter's Basilica was originally founded by Constantine in 324 on the traditional site where the first Pope, St. Peter, was crucified and buried. St. Peter's tomb is under the main altar and many other popes are buried in the basilica as well. The Basilica was rebuilt in the 16th century by Renaissance masters including Bramante, Michelangelo and Bernini. The dome was designed by Michelangelo, who became chief architect in 1546. In 1987 the basilica was the largest in the world. There is an enormous number of wonderful paintings in the Vatican Museum, but I can recall only a few: *The School of Athens* by Raphael, *The Battle of the Milvian Bridge* by Raphael's assistants from his original drawing, and a painting depicting Polish King Jan III Sobieski's victory over Kara Mustafa in Vienna, which was painted by Jan Matejko in 1883, 200 years after the Battle of Vienna. We then went to the Sistine Chapel. The chapel takes its name from Pope Sixtus IV, who restored the old Cappella Magna between 1477 and 1480. In 1508 Michelangelo was commissioned by Pope Julius II to repaint the vault, or ceiling, of the chapel. It was originally painted as golden stars on a blue sky. The work was completed between 1508 and 1512. Michelangelo is known to have dissected numerous cadavers, starting in his teenage years, and these anatomic studies aided him in creating extremely accurate depictions of human figures in his paintings of God and other figures from the Book of Genesis in the Sistine Chapel. When we visited in 1987, perhaps 70 percent of the ceiling and the top part of the wall had been renovated. We could see part of the aged ceiling, the rolling platform, and the beautifully restored ceiling of the chapel — brightly colored and in amazing detail. We did not see the fully restored ceiling, as it was completed in 1999.

The next morning we visited Piazza Navona. It is built on the ruins of the first-century Stadium of Domition, and this is the reason the Piazza has an elongated shape, like an ancient stadium. In the center is Gian Lorenzo Bernini's most spectacular fountain, La Fontana dei Quattro Fiumi (Fountain of the Four Rivers), representing the rivers Nile, Danube, Ganges and Rio de la Plata. Later we went to the Colosseum, originally Amphitheatrum Flavium (the Flavian Amphitheater), the largest ever built in the Roman Empire. Its construction started in 72 AD under the emperor Vespasian and was completed in 80 AD under his son Titus of the Flavius family, hence the name of the amphitheater. Next were the Forum Romanum, the Trevi Fountain, and the Spanish Steps. We stopped at the stairway of the Barcaccia, a fountain built by Pietro Bernini in the form of a boat below road level. On July 7 we visited the Papal Archbasilica of St. John Lateran. We learned then that this is the official ecclesiastical seat of the Bishop of Rome — the Pope — and not St. Peter's Basilica. We then went on foot to the Chiesa di Santa Maria delle Piante (Church of St. Mary in Palmis), better known as Chiesa del Domine Quo Vadis, located where the Via Ardeatina branches with the Via Appia Antica. This church takes its name from the legend that the Apostle Peter, fleeing from Rome to escape crucifixion, met Christ here and, recognizing him, asked, *Domine, quo vadis?* ("Lord, where are you going?"), whereupon Christ replied *Ego Romam iterum crucifigi* ("I'm going to Rome to be crucified anew.") Peter was then stricken with shame and returned to Rome. The little church of Santa Maria in

Palmis was built in the ninth century and became known as the *Domine Quo Vadis* Church; it was rebuilt in the 17th century. Within the church is a reproduction of the footprint of Christ and a bust of Henryk Sienkiewicz, author of the novel *Quo Vadis?* The novel, which won Sienkiewicz one of the first Nobel Prizes in Literature, describes this event among other stories from first-century Christianity in Rome. The walk on Via Appia Attica was very testing, as there was a lot of dust with each passing car and the road was rather narrow, but we made it and were happy to have seen this church. On July 8 we went to spend a few days in Kraków, Poland. While there we invited our friends to the famous Wierzynek Restaurant[2] for dinner. At the time the Polish złoty was very weak and we paid just US$20 for dinner with wine for 12 people. It remains the least expensive fine dining meal I have ever had.

1988

In 1988 I had 33 presentations in the U.S., Europe and Japan. In the section on intravenous catheters, I have already mentioned my presentation at the 34th Annual Meeting of American Society for Artificial Internal Organs in Reno, Nevada, on the subject of peritoneal catheter development [Pr 120]. It was after this I was approached by Wayne Quinton, who asked me whether I had some new ideas that might be of interest to his company, and I later cooperated with him in designing intravenous catheters for hemodialysis. At the same meeting I held a tutorial [Pr 119], and I felt that the style of my presentations had improved markedly.

My first overseas trip was to Poland, where I had a presentation at the IVth Conference of the Polish Society of Nephrology in Poznań, Poland. The trip was not without its complications, however. I was supposed to fly from Columbia Regional Airport through St. Louis, and from there to London, and then to Warsaw. At the check-in counter in Columbia they issued me boarding passes on Trans World

---

2. A very highly regarded establishment in Kraków, Wierzynek Restaurant was established by an innkeeper called Mikołaj Wierzynek in the 14th century. In 1364 he put on a splendid feast for the Great Conference of the Monarchs convened by the Polish King Casimir the Great. Among those in attendance were the German Emperor Charles IV and King Louis of Hungary.

Express (TWE) to St. Louis and Trans World Airlines (TWA) to London, but they did not ask to see my passport. During my flight to St. Louis I realized that I had forgotten it. In St. Louis I called Jag Gill, the Administrative Associate of the Division of Nephrology, and asked him to have my passport delivered to me in St. Louis, as I needed to be in Poznań the next day. He said that it would be possible to do that through the next Trans World Express flight, but he needed my passport as soon as possible. I called Halina and asked her to give it to Jag Gill. There were no cell phones at that time, so I was calling from the AT&T telephones at the airport and had to occupy one phone so that I could accept return calls from Columbia. I also realized I did not have the phone number of the conference organizers in Poznań; it was on my home computer, but Halina did not know how to operate a computer at that time. Besides, she was busy looking for my passport and preparing to drive to meet Jag Gill. Fortunately, my wife's best friend, Jola, was visiting us in Columbia at the time, and although she was not familiar with computers either, she managed to find the phone number on my PC by following my instructions through the phone. When I knew that my passport was on its way, I rescheduled my travel to Warsaw through Chicago O'Hare and let the organizers know that I would arrive in Poznań in the afternoon. I arrived in Warsaw early that morning and took the train to Poznań, since there were no flights at the time. Fortunately, my talk was scheduled for the afternoon, so I managed to make it in time [Pr 124]. During my stay in Poland I also visited my relatives: my brother's family in Chorzów and my mother-in-law in Kraków. I also visited the Medical Academy in Lublin, where I met my former assistants, visited my former dialysis patients, and delivered a grand round [Pr 125].

Later that year Halina and I visited Japan at the invitation of the Hayashidera Medinol Company, with its headquarters in Kanazawa, Ishikawa Prefecture. The company was distributing peritoneal dialysis catheters, including Swan Neck catheters manufactured by Accurate Surgical Instruments. Mrs. Zellerman, the president of the company, had been asked by Mr. Kimihiko Matsuzaki, a representative of Hayashidera Medinol, whom she would recommend to give presentations related to peritoneal dialysis, and particularly peritoneal access. She recommended me. The original plan was to spend two weeks in

Japan, give three or four lectures and spend the rest of the time sightseeing. Baxter had learned about my planned visit to Japan and had asked me to give some more lectures. At the time Baxter was distributing in Japan a full range of supplies for peritoneal dialysis except for peritoneal access. It was convenient for Baxter as the travel expenses were covered by Hayashidera Medinol. The ultimate plan was to give 14 lectures in eight Japanese cities. Planning was very fast and efficient as we used faxes, which had recently come into use, and our university had acquired one that year. Both companies had arranged visas to Japan (we needed visas as we were traveling on Polish passports) and first class tickets for the whole trip. As Halina was traveling with me, she could make sure that I did not forget my passport.

We started at 8 am on Thursday, October 13, 1988, from Columbia Regional Airport by TWE to St. Louis, then by TWA to Los Angeles, and then by Japan Airlines (JAL) to Narita Airport. Our flights were only during the day, but we landed at Narita on Friday, October 14, at 4:20 pm, as we crossed the Date Line during the flight. We were greeted by Mr. Hiroshi Hayashidera, the founder of the company, and Mr. Kimihiko Matsuzaki, with typical Japanese *ojiji* (bowing). Mr. Hayashidera only spoke a little English; Mr. Matsuzaki's was excellent and he also knew several other European languages. The travel to Hotel Okura took about 90 minutes; Japan's population density of over 330 people per square kilometer means the traffic on the country's roads is rarely light. In 1988 there were 125 million Japanese living in a country about the size of California.

The next day, we went to Sendai, in the northern part of Honshu Island. We traveled by Bullet Train — the Shinkansen, which literally means "New Trunk Line." All Bullet Trains have names; the train from Tokyo to Sendai is called Yamabiko (*yama*: mountain; *biko*: echo). Trains in Japan do indeed go very fast — well over 125 mph — but it was a surprisingly smooth ride. The railroad tracks are excellent, particularly in northern Japan. In Sendai we stayed in Tokyu Hotel, which has wonderful views of the Japanese Alps. In the evening I gave two lectures for the Sendai Medical School organized by Baxter at the Hotel Plaza [Pr 128, Pr 129]. The lectures were in English without interpreters, but the discussion was with an interpreter. Many Japanese doctors understand English but have difficulties speaking

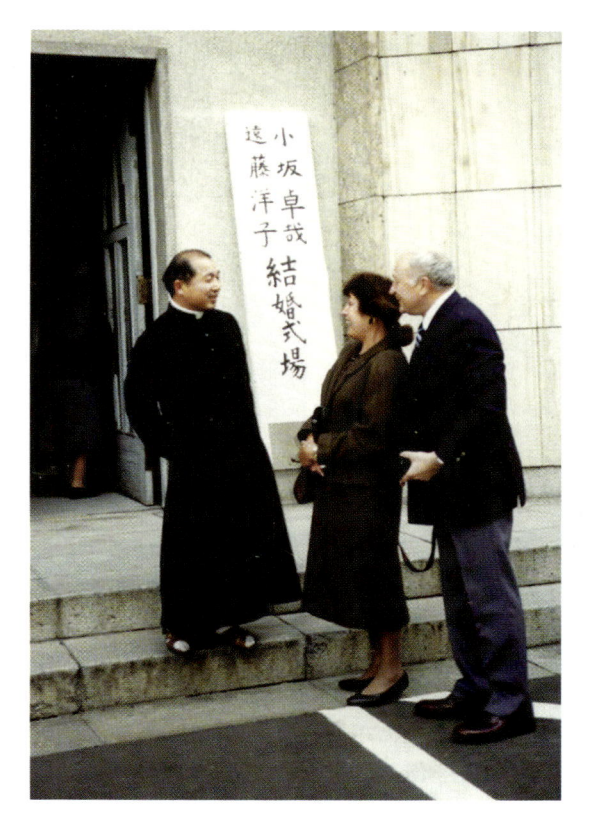

Figure 103.   Motokoji Church in Sendai, Japan.

the language, so interpreters are typically used for discussion sessions. Interpreters are usually young ladies who have spent time in the U.S.

The next morning our hosts took us to St. Peter's Catholic Church in the Motodora Koji District of Sendai (Fig. 103). Mass was held in Japanese, though a Mexican choir was in attendance and sang *Ave Maria* in Spanish. In Japan there are only about a million Catholics, less than one percent of the population, but each large city has a Catholic church. The two main religions are Shintoism and Buddhism, each with a great many shrines and temples, respectively. The vast majority of Japanese people who take part in Shinto rituals also practice Buddhist ancestor worship. Most "life" events are handled by Shintoism, while "death" or "afterlife" events are associated with Buddhism. For example,

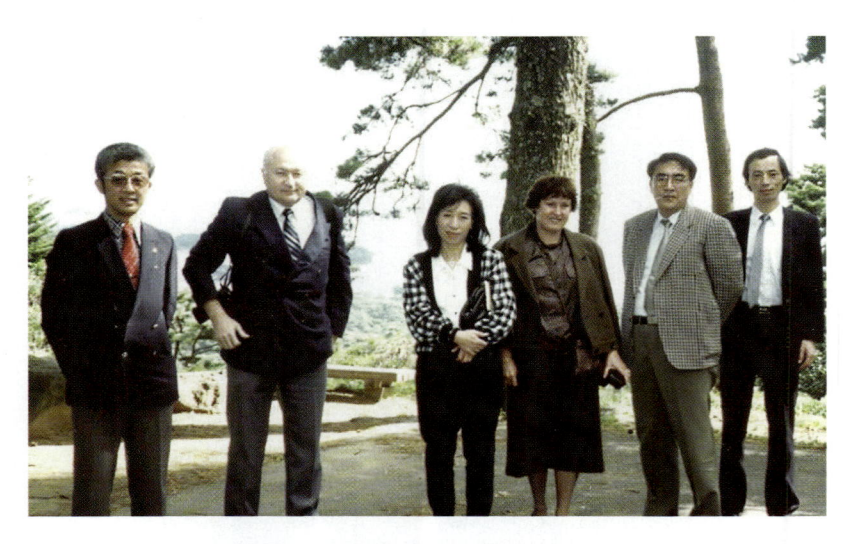

Figure 104. National park at Matsushima, Japan. From left: Dr. Ishizaki, the author, Mrs. Ishizaki, Halina, Hayashidera and Matsuzaki.

it is typical in Japan to register or celebrate a birth at a Shinto shrine, while funeral arrangements are generally dictated by Buddhist tradition. Mr. Matsuzaki told us that the majority of Japanese are not religious. After the Mass we went to the national park at Matsushima (*matsu*: pine; *shima*: island) with our hosts, Dr. Ishizaki[3] and his wife (Fig. 104). Matsushima is in Sendai *wan* (bay), which joins with the Pacific Ocean. Dr. Makoto Ishizaki, an advocate of the Swan Neck catheter, designed the slightly modifed "Sendai catheter" manufactured by Accurate Surgical Instruments and distributed by Hayashidera Medinol in Japan. In the evening we returned to Tokyo on the Yamabiko and stayed another night in Okura Hotel.

I did not have any lectures the next day (Monday, October 17), so we visited some places of interest in Tokyo. In the morning we went to the Akihabara shopping district, with its huge number of shops selling electronic gadgets, many of which are not available in the U.S. In the afternoon we went on a bus tour with our guide, Yumi. (She told us that her name is easy to remember as it sounds like "you me.") We visited the Imperial Palace Plaza and took pictures at Nijubashi

---

3. We met Mr Hayashidera at our Annual Dialysis Conference in Phoenix and he told us that Dr. Ishizaki had passed away in 2010.

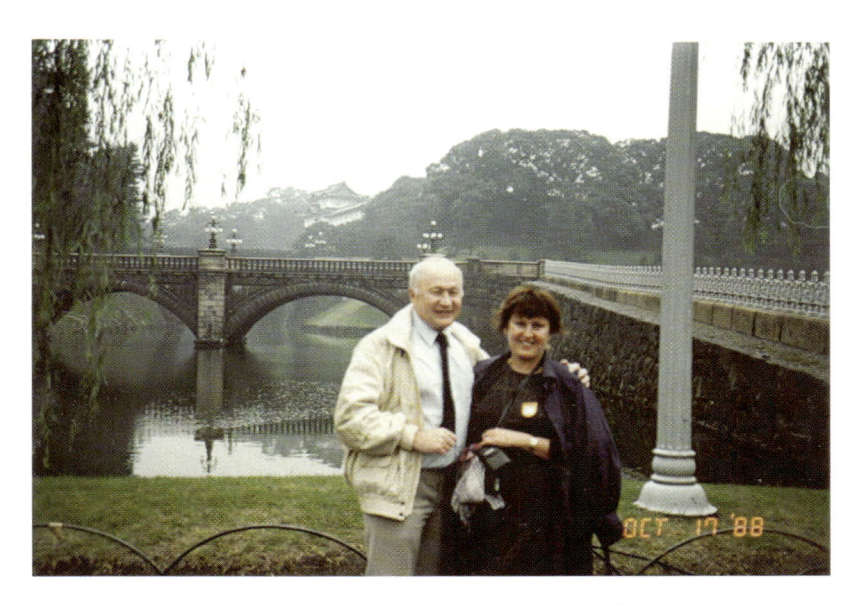

Figure 105. Nijubashi double-arch bridge, Japan.

(*ni*: two; *ju*: arch; *bashi*: bridge) leading to the palace (Fig. 105). The Emperor of Japan, already over 90 years old, was very ill at the time. Later we visited the Meiji Jingu Shrine, built in 1920 in divine honor of the Emperor Meiji and his wife Shoken, grandparents of the incumbent emperor. The Meiji era took the country out of isolation and created the basis for modern Japan. Interestingly, shrines do not have sculptures or paintings. We then visited Tasaki Shinju Pearl Gallery, where we observed a tea ceremony and a demonstration of pearl production. We were told that to produce a pearl, a tiny piece of mantle tissue of a donor shell is transplanted into a recipient shell and covered with *nacre* (mother-of-pearl). After four years the perfect pearl can be harvested. But without covering the mantle tissue with nacre this tissue is expelled and the pearl does not form. Later in the afternoon we visited Ginza and its huge department stores, even larger than those in Akihabara. We stopped at the Zakuro Restaurant, where we tried some very tasty *shabu-shabu*.[4]

---

4. *Shabu-shabu* consists of very thin slices of raw beef (about 1 mm) dipped for a few seconds in boiling broth and usually served with various dipping sauces.

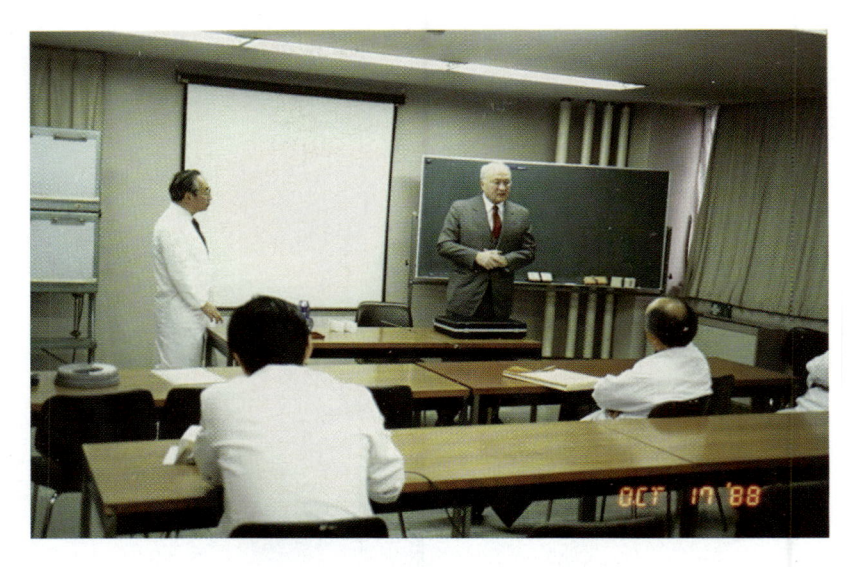

Figure 106. Tokyo Women School lecture; Professor Ota presiding.

The next day Halina went on another tour of Tokyo with another guide, Harumi (*Harumi* means "beautiful spring"). Among other places, she visited Asakusa Kannon Temple and the Nezu Institute of Fine Arts. I went to the Tokyo Women's Medical College, where I met Prof. Kazuo Ota and gave a lecture on peritoneal access [Pr 130]. Prof. Kazuo Ota[5] (Fig. 106), Chairman of the Institute of Kidney Diseases, a famous surgeon who was known for performing living related kidney transplants, was unhappy with the transplant situation in Japan, where cadaveric transplants were not performed because the definition of brain death had not yet been established.[6] He worked hard to convince authorities to accept the internationally recognized definition of brain death. The institute had 140 physicians and treated over 1,000 patients with renal failure, mostly on hemodialysis. Because of Japan's high population density and the loaded network of

---

5. Prof. Ota died in 2010 and his obituary by Karl D. Nolph appeared in *Peritoneal Dialysis International* that year.

6. The situation changed later and kidney transplants from non-heart-beating donors became socially acceptable. On October 16, 1997, Japan altered its definition of "brain death" and cadaveric kidney transplants became more frequent, but they not match the frequency of cadaveric transplants in Europe and the U.S.

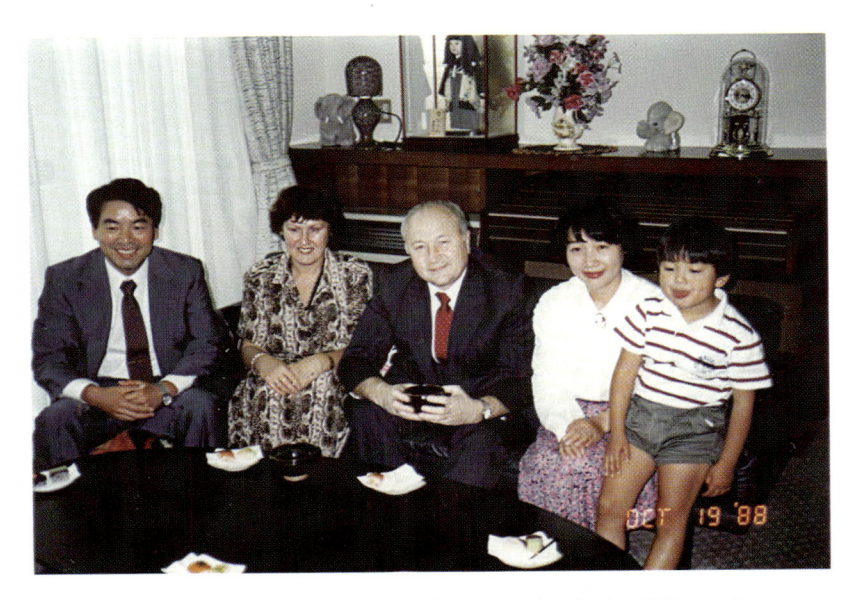

Figure 107. Visit to Dr. Shinji Sakai's home in a suburb of Niigata, Japan.

hemodialysis centers, patients did not have a great deal of incentive to undertake therapy at home. Only 60 patients were on peritoneal dialysis in the Institute of Kidney Disease. One of the goals of my visit organized by Baxter and Hayashidera Medinol was to familiarize doctors with the new techniques of peritoneal dialysis and to encourage them to increase the number of patients on this valuable therapy. In the afternoon we went to the little town of Omiya, where Baxter organized a meeting for the Saitama Medical School in the Sonic City Building. I was greeted by Prof. Kazuo Isoda, Chairman of the Department of Internal Medicine. I had two lectures on tidal peritoneal dialysis [Pr 131] and the Swan Neck catheter [Pr 132].

The following day we traveled by Shinkansen Asahi 309 (*asahi*: rising sun) to Niigata, on the coast of the Sea of Japan. We first went to a suburb to visit Dr. Shinji Sakai, an interventional nephrologist who inserted Swan Neck catheters. He had a 10-room house furnished in a Japanese-Western style (Fig. 107). Later we went to Shinrakuen Hospital, Niigata University, where I was greeted by Dr. Yoshihei Hirasawa, the vice president of the university. Before the seminar a Japanese version of my video (Fig. 108) on the Swan Neck

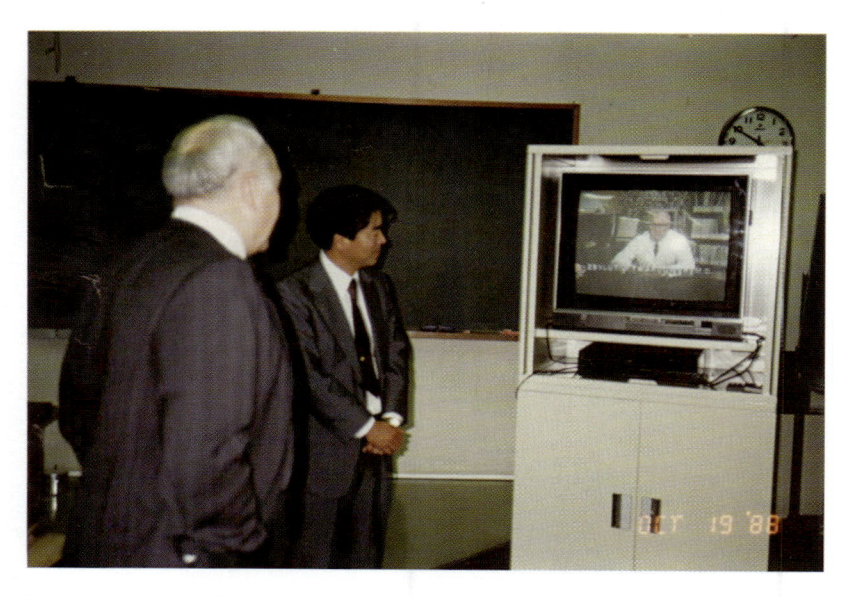

Figure 108. Dr. Sakai and the author watch the Japanese version of the Swan Neck catheter video.

catheter was shown [Vi 2a]. After the video I had a grand round on the history of peritoneal dialysis access [Pr 133] with following discussion translated by Mr. Matsuzaki. I noted that my short answers were followed by markedly longer answers in Japanese, something I had noticed with other interpreters as well. The reason Mr. Matsuzaki gave was that the Japanese language requires some extra courtesy phrases. In the evening we went to the Ikinaritei Niigata Restaurant, where Shinrakuen Hospital had organized a Japanese-style reception for us. As usual there were 12 dishes, including sushi, sake, tea, and excellent Japanese Asahi beer. Geisha (*gei*: art; *sha*: person or doer) girls (Fig. 109) served us and performed Japanese dances with accompanying music on the shamisen.[7]

The day after, Thursday, October 20, we took an express train, Raicho 16, to Kanazawa in Ishikawa (*Ishi*: rock; *kawa*: river) Prefecture to visit Hayashidera Medinol headquarters. We checked into Kanazawa Miyako Hotel, located by the railway station. Early that afternoon

---

7. *Shamisen* is a Japanese three-stringed instrument similar to the banjo, which has four or five strings.

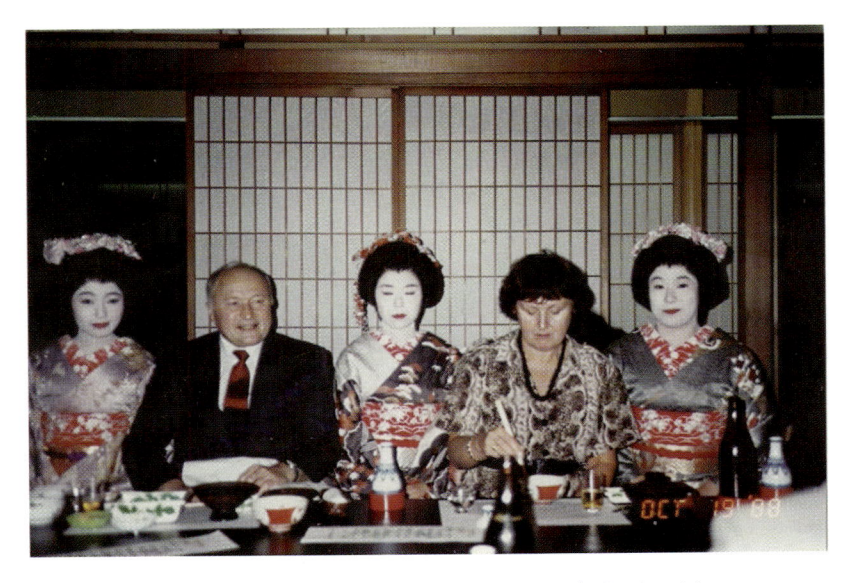

Figure 109. In the Ikinaritei Restaurant with Geisha girls.

I met Prof. Akira Shinoda (Fig. 110), Director of the Department of Nephrology, Kanazawa Medical University, and had a grand round on peritoneal catheters [Pr 134]. Having spent several years in the U.S., Prof. Shinoda served as an interpreter. At 6 pm I gave another lecture at a seminar organized by Baxter and Hayashidera Medinol at Kanazawa Miyako Hotel. The seminar was opened by Prof. Shinoda, who stressed my education and training in Poland. The interpreter was Mrs. Ayako Saito, who had come from Sapporo, Hokkaido Prefecture. (The organizers had a hard time hiring interpreters, so they had to import them from afar.) I gave two lectures similar to those in Omiya [Pr 135, Pr 136]. After the seminar there was another Japanese-style reception.

On Friday morning we visited a 350-year-old Samurai home called the *Ninja*[8] *Derra*. The house was built to fulfill a defensive role and permitted escape if the situation turned hopeless. In the same district we visited a 100-year-old house, *Saihitsu-an*, which belonged

---

8. A *ninja* was a covert agent or mercenary of feudal Japan specializing in unorthodox arts of war. The functions of the ninja included espionage, sabotage, infiltration and assassination, as well as open combat in certain situations.

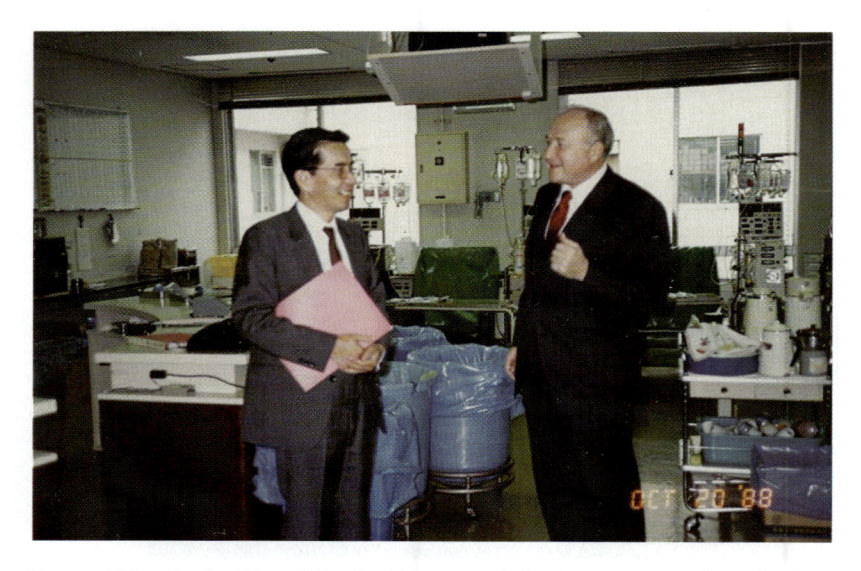

Figure 110. Prof. Akira Shinoda, Director of the Department of Nephrology, Kanazawa Medical University, showing the author a hemodialysis unit.

to an artist fond of drinking tea. One room was still devoted to the tea ceremony, but the rest of the house was used to display the craft of Kaga Yuzen, a hand dying method of creating kimonos. Kaga is one of the 11 cities that make up Ishikawa Prefecture. The method is extremely elaborate, so the price of a kimono dyed in this way can reach 1,000,000 yen (about US$13,000). In the afternoon we went to the Toyama Pharmaceutical University and visited the dialysis center, where we were greeted by Associate Professor Hiroyuki Iida. In the evening I gave a lecture on new advances in automated peritoneal dialysis [Pr 137] at a seminar organized by Baxter and Hayashidera Medinol at Meitetsu Toyama Hotel. The discussion was interpreted by Keiko Suzuki from Tokyo. A reception with speeches and toasts was held after the seminar. Dr. Tatsuhiko Touyama (Fig. 111) gave a toast in Polish, "*na zdrowie*" (to your health), and I raised a toast in Japanese, "*kampai*" (cheers).

The next day, October 22, we went to Kenrokuen (*ken*: combining; *roku*: six; *en*: garden), a garden developed from 1620 to 1840 by the Maeda clan that possesses six attributes of a perfect garden: spaciousness, quietness, art, stateliness, abundance of water and rocks, and

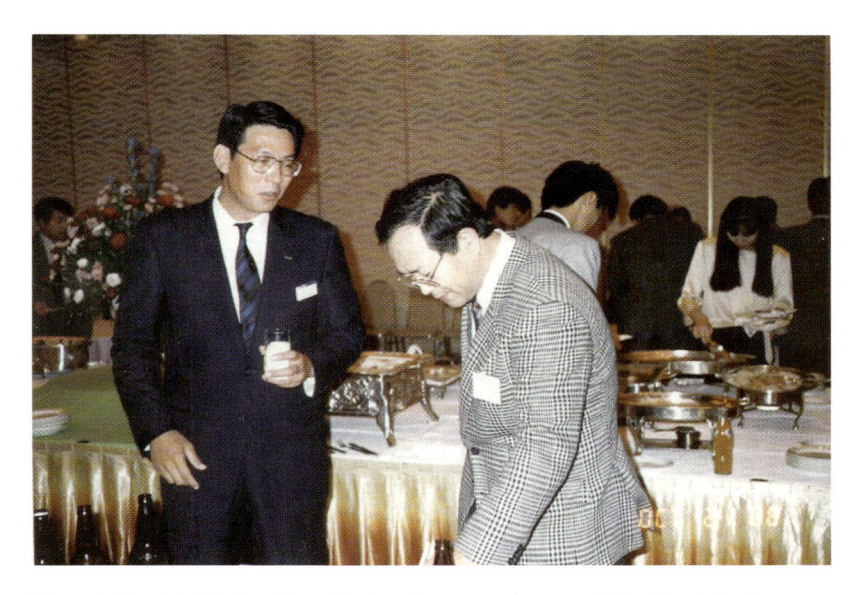

Figure 111.   Mr. Kakitani from Baxter, Kanazawa, Japan, and Dr. Tatsuhiko Touyama.

beautiful views. The oldest fountain in Japan can be found there, operating by natural water pressure from a lake situated above it (Fig. 112). In the early afternoon we visited Dr. Touyama, who lived in Tanaka. We had a single dish lunch there, *nabe*, which is a special soup made with vegetables, crab, octopus, snails and fish, all of which are boiled in a large pot using a gas burner. Mr. Izumi, one of the founders of Hayashidera Medinol and something of an expert in making *nabe*, prepared it for us — though we had only a few bites, despite his expertise. Later in the afternoon we visited Dr. Isao Ishikawa, whose main interest at the time was uremia-induced polycystic kidney disease.[9] He lived in a very nice home with a *kotatsu*[10] at its center. In the evening we went to the Yamanoo Restaurant in Kanazawa.

---

9. This disease develops in patients with long-standing renal failure on dialysis and predisposes sufferers to the development of renal cell carcinoma. Dr. Ishikawa authored many papers on this topic and summarized his experience in a book published by Springer in 2007, *Acquired Cystic Disease of the Kidney and Renal Cell Carcinoma: Complication of Long-Term Dialysis*.

10. A *kotatsu* is a small table with an electric heater underneath below the level of the floor. A futon is placed over the frame of the *kotatsu* to keep the heat in. It is often the center of domestic life during the winter months. In the evening, family members sit around the *kotatsu* to enjoy food, television and conversation, and play games — keeping their lower half warm.

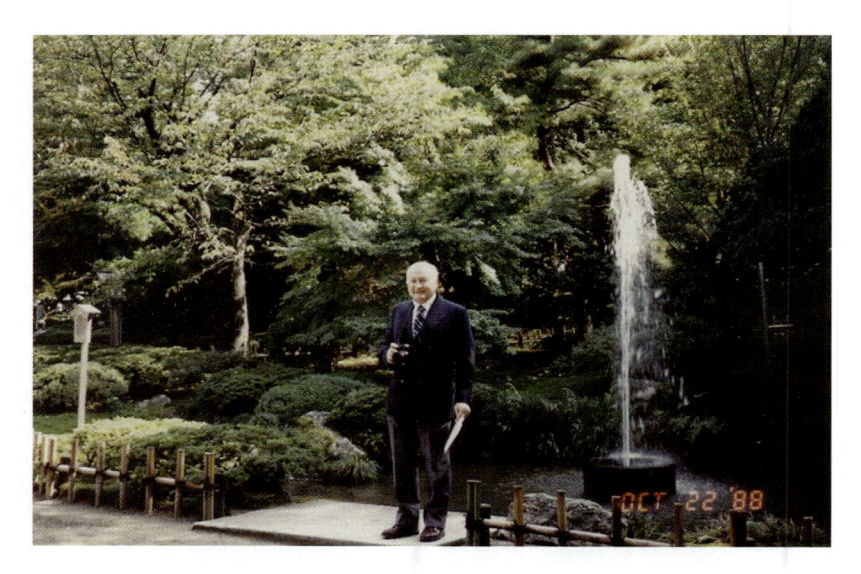

Figure 112. Kenrokuen: the oldest fountain in Japan.

Joining us were Dr. Ishikawa and his wife, Mr. Matsuzaki, and Mr. Hayashidera with his wife Kazuo (Fig. 113). It was again a dinner with 12 courses delivered on small plates and in dainty bowls decorated with leaves and flowers, and served by waitresses dressed in traditional kimonos. Fortunately for those of us unaccustomed to Japanese food, the portions were rather small and it is not impolite to leave dishes uneaten. We were surprised to learn that it is considered very polite to slurp soup as an indication of appreciation, something contrary to the French savoir-vivre.

The next day we went to the Carmelite Church in Hirosaka District, Kanazawa (Fig. 114). After the Mass we visited the home of the Hayashidera family and met their son, Takashi, and daughters, Maya and Yumi. The home was spacious and every member of the family had his or her own room. One room was a chapel with the Buddhist altar, and inside were various personal items associated with their son who had tragically died 12 years before. In the afternoon we visited Edo Mura Heritage Park, which reproduces the appearance of a town from the early 17th to mid-18th centuries, the days of the Samurai. It is one of the heritage parks honoring Japan during one of its most prosperous periods. In the evening we went with Mr. Hayashidera and

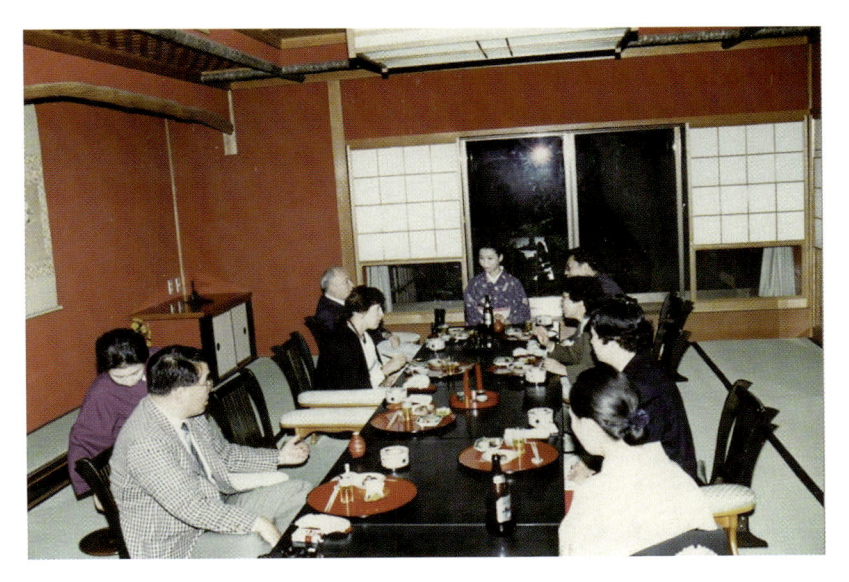

Figure 113. Dinner in Yamanoo Restaurant, Kanazawa.

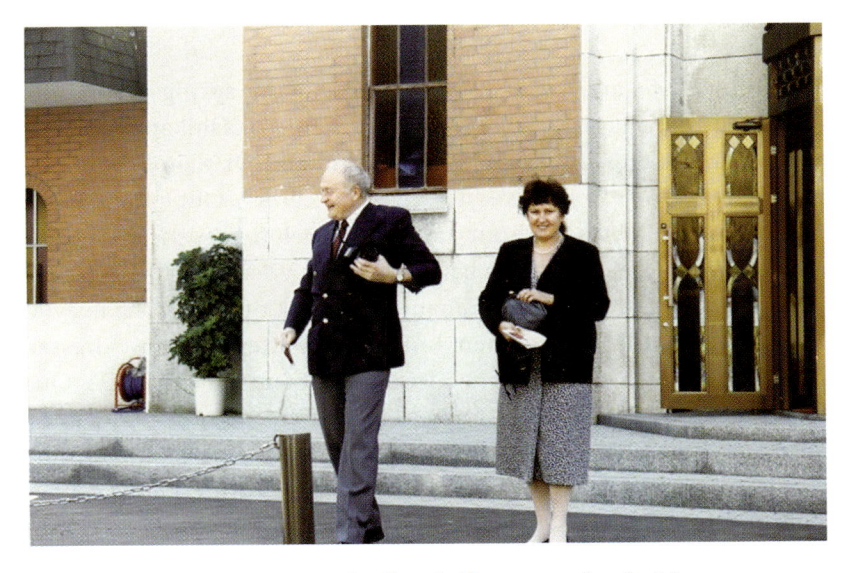

Figure 114. Hirosaka Church, Kanazawa, after the Mass.

Mr. Matsuzaki to the Noto Peninsula, which is located north of Kanazawa. We drove along the western coast of the Sea of Japan, and it was possible to drive on the beach as the sand was so hard. Late in

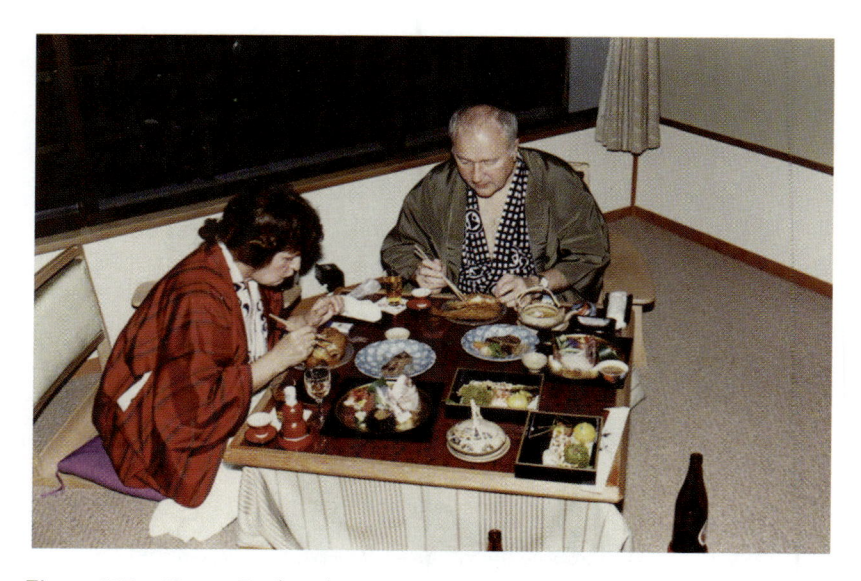

Figure 115. Kagaya Ryokan (Japanese inn), dressed accordingly and sitting at the *kotatsu*.

the evening we arrived at Wakura Onsen hot spring resort and sojourned in Kagaya Ryokan (*Kaga*: old name of Ishikawa; *ya*: inn; *ryokan*: hotel). Our group joined Mr. Izumi and Dr. Saitoh, who had received a kidney from his sister 12 years earlier. Our group of six stayed in three suites, and our suite had three rooms including one with a *kotatsu* (Fig. 115) and a bathroom with a deep hot tub. We were served by *jochu* (hostess; *jo*: woman), who took our bags; the heavier luggage was handled by bellmen. Immediately after arrival we dressed in a *yukata* (loose robe), fastened with a sash, and *haori* (jacket). One suite cost US$1,500 and had to be booked eight months in advance. Breakfast, lunch, dinner, public bathing in a hot spring, and admission to a cabaret were all included in the price. A three-hour dinner there entailed 15 courses, including *matsutake* (*matsu*: pine; *take*: mushroom). These "mushrooms growing under pines" are highly prized and very expensive: a pound costs about US$500. The service was excellent and could be summed up by the expression, *age-zen sue-zen* — serving tasty meals and taking away the empty dinnerware without guests having to say anything or trouble themselves at all. After dinner we were treated to an Australian cabaret performance. In true traditional

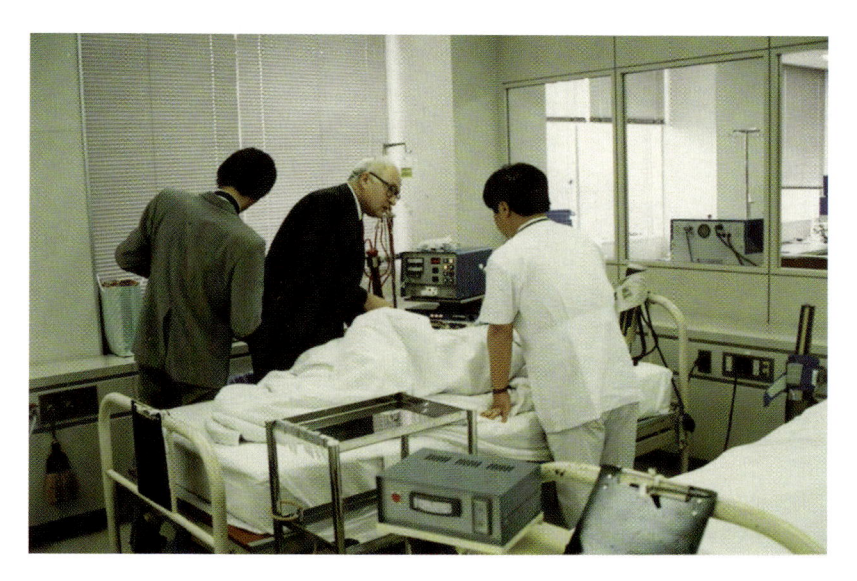

Figure 116. Dr. Takashi Sato showing the author the hemodialysis unit. Note that patients in Japan are dialyzed in beds.

Japanese style, we slept on futons (*fu*: sleep; *ton*: pillow; a cushion for sitting is called a *zabuton*, as *zabu* means to sit). The following day we had a normal Western-style breakfast, which we liked much more as we were obviously used to having such things as toast, ham and fruits. There was a beautiful view across Nanao Bay from the hotel. Despite the high room prices, the hotel was under development, as the long advance booking period evidently meant that there were many more potential guests than there was space to accommodate.

Later we went back to Kanazawa, where I paid a courtesy visit to the Ishikawa Prefectural Hospital. The president of the hospital, Dr. Tasuku Noto, greeted me, and Dr. Takashi Sato showed me the hemodialysis unit (Fig. 116). I noted that contrary to hemodialysis in the U.S., where most patients are dialyzed while sitting in chairs, in Japan patients were dialyzed in beds, similar to the practice in Europe. In the evening we visited the headquarters of Hayashidera Medinol, an impressive four-story building. I noticed there was a picture of me in Mr. Hayashidera's office that was taken at the Accurate Surgical Instruments booth during our conference in Kansas City in February

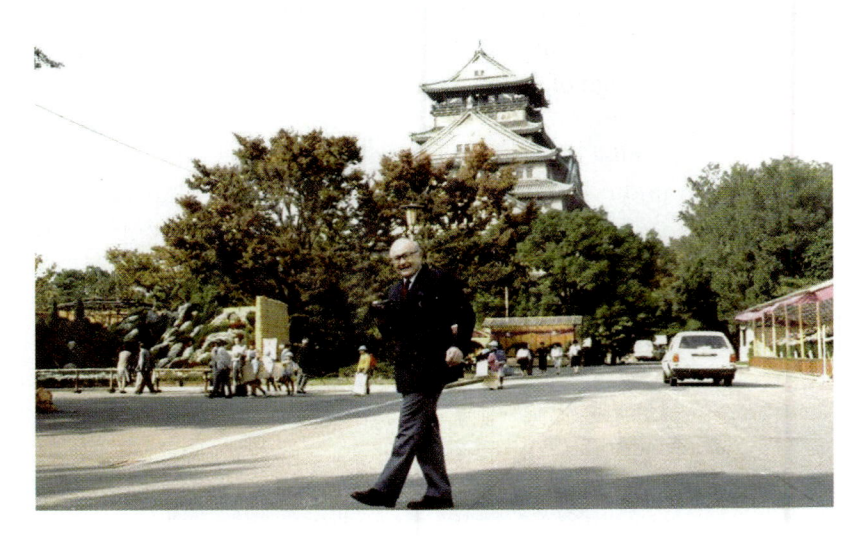

Figure 117. Osaka Castle, Japan.

1988. Later in the afternoon various doctors came from Kanazawa University, including Prof. Hiroshi Kida. I gave a presentation [Pr 138], and we had a free discussion on the complications of peritoneal dialysis. Afterwards, as previously, a wonderful reception had been laid on for us.

On Tuesday, October 25, we took a 9:10 am express train, Raicho, to Osaka, arriving at exactly 12:08 pm. I was impressed, as always, with the punctuality of the Japanese trains. We stayed in a two-room suite at the Royal Hotel, a very nice place with two TV sets, one in each room, providing several channels in English. A one-night stay cost about US$350. Shortly after arriving, we visited Osaka Castle, the oldest of its kind in Japan (Fig. 117). The history of the castle is very complicated and not entirely clear. From my understanding, in 1496 where the castle would later stand was a small cloister rebuilt into the Ishiyama Hongan-ji shrine. In 1580 the shrine was conquered by the powerful territorial lord Oda Nobunaga, but two years later it was taken over by his traitorous general Akechi Mitsuhide. Nobunaga committed suicide when he was betrayed by the general, who set fire to the temple in Kyoto where he was lodging. Ishiyama Hongan-ji eventually fell to Toyotomi Hideyoshi, a daimyo warrior and politician who started to unite the political factions of Japan. Hideyoshi built a formidable castle on the site, but in 1615 the building was burned down during the *Natsu no Jin*, the summer campaign of the pivotal Siege of Osaka. Shogun Tokugawa Hidetada subsequently rebuilt the castle, completing it in 1629, and it stood until the mid-19th century when it was burned during the civil conflicts surrounding the Meiji Restoration. The castle was damaged once more during World War II, was rebuilt again and finally opened to the public in 1948. Today the castle and the surrounding gardens cover an area of 15 acres and *Tenshukaku*, the main donjon that was destroyed and rebuilt so many times, has eight floors. On the fifth floor there is a display showing the life of Hideyoshi in pictures with explanations in Japanese and English. There are also flower exhibitions held at the castle, with competitions for the best chrysanthemums, Japan's national flower. In the afternoon I paid a visit to Osaka Koseinenkin Hospital (*koseinenkin*: insurance), where I was greeted by Dr. Dairoku Shirai, Director of the Nephrology Department. That evening I had a grand round on peritoneal catheters [Pr 139], and afterwards there was a reception at a Chinese restaurant in the Hilton Hotel.

We took the 10:02 am Shinkansen (Hikari 83; *hikari*: ray of light) to Hiroshima the following day. My impression was that about half of the track was located in tunnels. The railroad tracks in southern Japan were built about 20 years before — and were worse, in my opinion, than — those in northern Japan; there was some shaking as the train approached higher speeds. On arrival we checked into the ANA Hotel Hiroshima, operated by All Nippon Airways, and we had beautiful views of Hiroshima, which is surrounded by mountains on three sides. In the afternoon we went to visit the city, starting with the Genbaku Domu (Atomic Bomb Dome), the only building that was not completely destroyed during the explosion on August 6, 1945 (Fig. 118), and the Hiroshima Peace Memorial Museum, which describes in detail the history of the A-bomb explosion and its consequences. We also spent some time in the city itself, rebuilt from scratch after World War II, and went to a department store. It was surprising to see streetcars in Hiroshima, as we had not seen them in other Japanese cities.

In the evening I gave a lecture at a seminar organized by Baxter at the ANA Hotel. I was greeted by Prof. Kiyohiko Dohi, Chairman of the Second Department of Surgery of the Hiroshima University

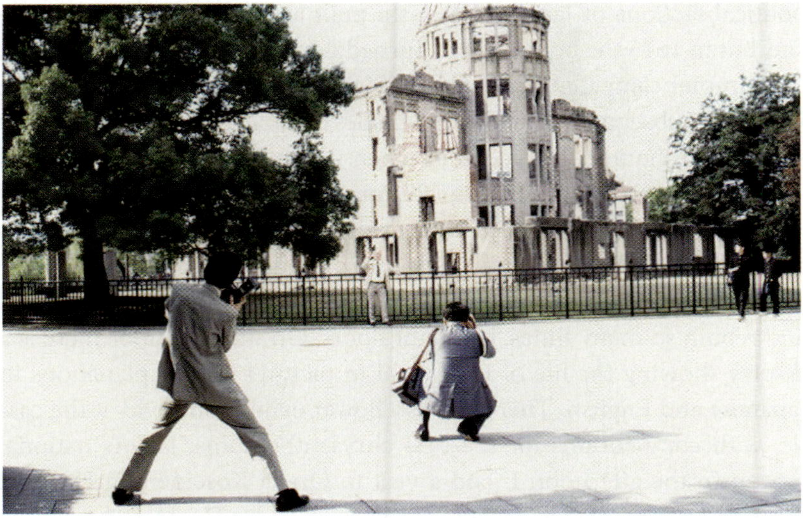

Figure 118. The author pictured in front of Genbaku Domu (Atomic Bomb Dome), with Mr. Matsuzaki and Mr. Hayashidera taking photos. (Note the classic photographer's pose.)

School of Medicine. My two lectures were on advances in automated peritoneal dialysis [Pr 140] and the Swan Neck peritoneal catheter [Pr 141] (Fig. 119), and there was a lively discussion afterwards — with the expected lengthy translations in Japanese of my rather shorter answers. After the seminar was a dinner with speeches and toasts, and we were given some very nice presents: a neckerchief for Halina and a Maneki Neko for me. The ceramic "Beckoning Cat" (otherwise known as a Welcoming Cat, Lucky Cat, Money Cat or Fortune Cat) is supposed to bring its owner good luck (Fig. 120).

At 10 am on October 27 we took ANA flight 674 to Tokyo, landing at 11:15 am; ninety percent or more of the passengers were men. We checked in again at Okura Hotel. That afternoon we went to a Shinjuku department store, which seemed even bigger than Akihabara's or Ginza's. Shinjuku is really huge; we surely would have gotten lost were it not for our savvy hosts. The next morning we visited Tokyo Tower, a communications and observation tower in Shiba Park, Minato. Built in 1958, the structure is an Eiffel Tower-inspired lattice tower painted white and orange in accordance with aviation safety

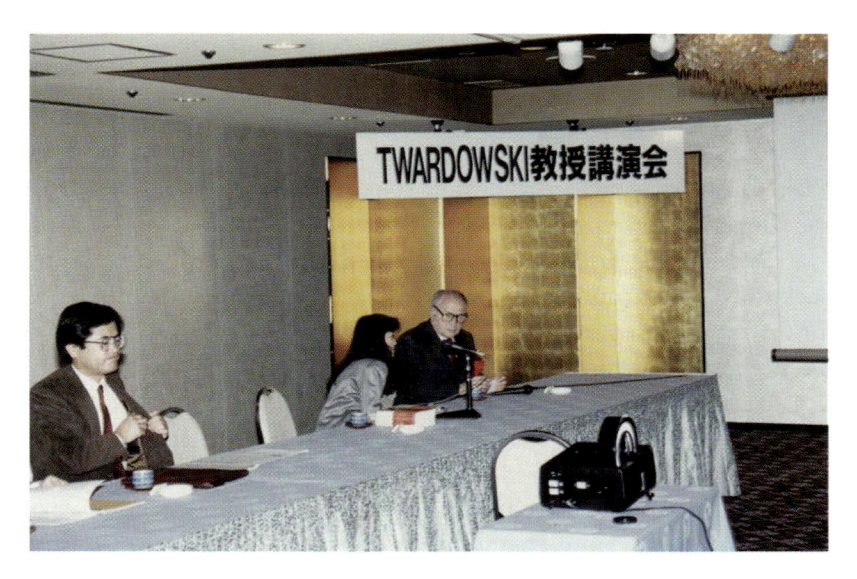

Figure 119. Hiroshima lecture in the ANA Hotel. (Note the slide projector and interpreter, Mrs. Yukari Asahina, from Tokyo, at author's side.)

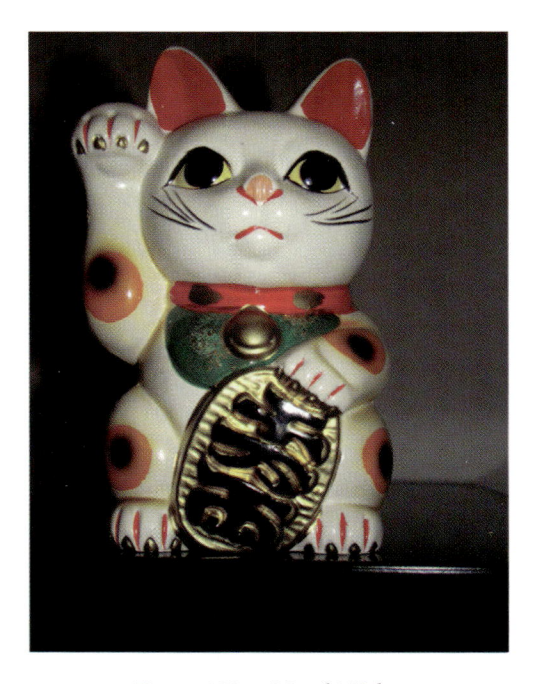

Figure 120. Maneki Neko.

Teaching and Consulting

regulations. From the Special Observatory, located at a height of 820 feet, we could see our hotel room as well as the embassies of the U.S. and the Soviet Union. The weather happened to be excellent and we could see Mount Fuji (Fujiyama; *yama*: mountain) and the double-peaked Tsukubayama. At the time Tokyo Tower was the tallest free-standing steel tower in the world.

By 1 pm that Friday, October 28, 1988, we were finally on our way back to Narita Airport at the end our visit to Japan, boarding JAL 066 for the 4:25 pm departure. I was very tired and slept all the way — and did not notice the turbulence that was bothering Halina. We arrived in Los Angeles at 10:10 am on Friday, the same day we had left. It was amazing to me: we had started in Tokyo on Friday afternoon, flown mostly at night and arrived in Los Angeles in the morning on the same day, as we had crossed the International Date Line heading east. It was a very interesting, though tiring, journey for me. Our hosts had spent a lot of money on us. Apparently, they considered it a good investment to popularize peritoneal dialysis in the country. In spite of such efforts, however, peritoneal dialysis has never caught on there: no more than 6 percent of its dialysis patients are on peritoneal dialysis. Still, over the years, the Swan Neck catheter has become very popular in Japan.

In the meantime I was invited to participate in the 6th Benelux CAPD Symposium in Amsterdam in early December. I gave two presentations there, the first on the best selection of peritoneal dialysis methods based on the peritoneal equilibration test [Pr 142], and the second being our video describing details of design, insertion and care of Swan Neck peritoneal dialysis catheters [Pr 143, Vi 2]. Halina accompanied me and after the meeting we had a sightseeing tour through Amsterdam. On Saturday, December 3, we went for an evening Mass in a chapel. There were few attendees and we were surprised that we seemed to be the youngest among them. Ten days later I went for the 21st Annual Meeting of the American Society of Nephrology in San Antonio. I had only two poster presentations and I was not the first author in either one [Pr 144, Pr 145]. The most productive encounter I had there was my discussion with Rod Kenley about a machine for daily home hemodialysis, as described earlier. I had no further presentations to give that year.

1989

I again delivered 33 presentations in 1989, beginning at the Baxter Healthcare Corporation Peritoneal Dialysis Consultant Meeting in Naples, Florida, in early January [Pr 146, Pr 147]. Thereafter, I was at Baxter's headquarters to update the company on our studies on tidal peritoneal dialysis [Pr 148]. After eight years of holding our Annual Conference on Peritoneal Dialysis in Kansas City, for the first time it was held in Dallas, Texas, because the number of attendees had outgrown the capacity of Kansas City's Crown Center Hotel. I gave only two presentations in Dallas. One was in the so-called "Quiz the Experts" session [Pr 149]; in the other lecture, I presented for the first time our study on peritoneal catheter tunnel morphology [Pr 150]. I went on to give six more presentations in the U.S.: two at the University of Missouri [Pr 152, Pr 157] and four more in various cities [Pr 151, Pr 155, Pr 156, Pr 158]. They were all short trips for one or two days just to give the presentation before returning to Columbia. Most of the seminars were organized by Baxter, but I was often also invited by local nephrologists or urologists to give presentations. For instance, Dr. William B. Baker, MD, from Danville Urologic Clinic in Danville, Virginia, invited me to present my results with the Swan Neck catheter [Pr 153] and new cycler techniques [Pr 154].

Later, in June, I traveled overseas to give nine more presentations in Sweden, Denmark, England and Switzerland. The trip started with the Cruise Symposium on automated peritoneal dialysis organized by Baxter Sweden in conjunction with the XXVIth Congress of the European Dialysis and Transplant Association. This symposium was in a very interesting place, the Gothenburg Archipelago, a collection of numerous islands at the mouth of Göta Älv, the river running through Gothenburg into the Kattegat Strait. I had only one presentation [Pr 159], and a whole free day before the congress, so I took a coastline cruise among the islands. I had three more presentations at the symposium in conjunction with the congress [Pr 160–Pr 162]. Having a couple more days to spare before going to Denmark, I took a tour through the city. Gothenburg is similar in some respects to Amsterdam, which is not surprising as Dutch city planners were contracted to build the city with canals similar to those in Amsterdam. I was particularly impressed by the Poseidon statue erected on Götaplatsen, the central square in the city that was inaugurated for Gothenburg's 300th anniversary in 1923. Over the next few days I had grand rounds, arranged by Baxter, in Copenhagen [Pr 163], Aarhus (Denmark) [Pr 164], Nottingham (U.K.) [Pr 165], Geneva [Pr 166] and Lausanne (Switzerland) [Pr 167].

Returning from Europe I had nine presentations organized mostly by Baxter and the University of Missouri's Office of Continuing Education, but I was also invited by a number of universities to give grand rounds in various American cities [Pr 168–Pr 176]. One presentation was simply a matter of sending our video to Videomed '89 without the necessity of being there [Pr 177]. The year concluded with a coauthored poster shown at the 22nd Annual Meeting of the American Society of Nephrology that was presented by Dr. Nolph [Pr 178].

1990

My travel engagements intensified in 1990, with a total of 58 presentations around the world mostly based on my research related to peritoneal dialysis. In addition, eight poster presentations where I was not the first author were shown by other coauthors. I gave five presentations during the 10th Annual Conference on Peritoneal Dialysis in Dallas, Texas, in February [Pr 179–Pr 183]. In early April I was invited to give a lecture at the Annual Meeting of the California Dialysis Council [Pr 184], and at the end of April the 36th Annual Meeting of the American Society for Artificial Internal Organs was held in Washington, D.C., where I had two slide presentations [Pr 185, Pr 186]. In one presentation I showed the results of our study on the value of computerized tomographic peritoneography in the assessment of intraabdominal fluid distribution and diagnosis of complications in peritoneal dialysis patients [Pr 187]; another was on the results of chronic tidal nightly peritoneal dialysis [Pr 188]. In May I made several short trips for presentations in several cities in the U.S. It started with Minneapolis, where I was invited by Thomas Pence, MD, Assistant Professor of Medicine at the University of Minnesota and Executive Director of the Interstate Dialysis Division of the Regional Kidney Disease Program at Hennepin County Medical Center, to give presentations at the Minnesota Kidney Club [Pr 189] and Hennepin County Medical Center [Pr 190]. Jim Hasbargen, MD, Chief of Nephrology at the Fitzsimons Army Medical Center in Aurora, Colorado, invited me to give lectures in Denver [Pr 191, Pr 192] and Aurora [Pr 193]. The Tri-State Renal Network invited me to give a presentation on automated and tidal peritoneal dialysis in Indianapolis, Indiana [Pr 194]. At the end of May Lois Schmidt, RN, a nurse from our center, and I were invited by Mrinal Dasgupta, MD, to attend the 1st Western Canada Conference on Peritoneal Dialysis. We talked about peritoneal dialysis prescription based on PET [Pr 195, Pr 196], and about diagnosis and treatment of exit site infection [Pr 197, Pr 198]. Our presentations were held on a single day, Thursday, May 24. Halina came with me, so we decided to stay two more days to visit West Edmonton Mall, at the time the largest shopping center in the world, which included Fantasyland and World Waterpark, the largest indoor water park in the world. I decided to take a ride on a high-speed water slide called the Sky Screamer, which is the park's fastest but at 79 feet tall, not the tallest. The highest slide in the park is the Twister, which is 83 feet high, but it is slower as well as being longer. Halina did not want me to go on the rides as she thought they were risky, but I survived without any major injuries. I do not think that I was the oldest rider there, but I might have been having the most fun. On Saturday, May 26, we were invited to visit Dr. Dasgupta and his wife, Shibani, and their daughters, Bonnie and Tina. In June I had only two quick trips to Phoenix, Arizona, for a talk at a Kidney Club Meeting [Pr 199], and to Crystal Lake, Illinois, for the Science and Technology Conference organized by Baxter [Pr 200, Pr 201].

In the second half of the year my presentations were mostly abroad. In July there were two important congresses in Japan: the XIth International Congress of Nephrology, and the Vth Congress of the International Society for Peritoneal Dialysis. I sent seven abstracts for the first and ten for the second. I had originally thought that the selection of abstracts would be very stringent, so I sent plenty of abstracts in order to have a high probability of acceptance. However, it turned out that they were all accepted, so I had to prepare a lot of posters. Having also decided to go to Japan, Dr. Khanna prepared some of the posters and we both presented them in the poster forums in Tokyo [Pr 202–Pr 208] and in Kyoto [Pr 209–Pr 218]. We were asked to give

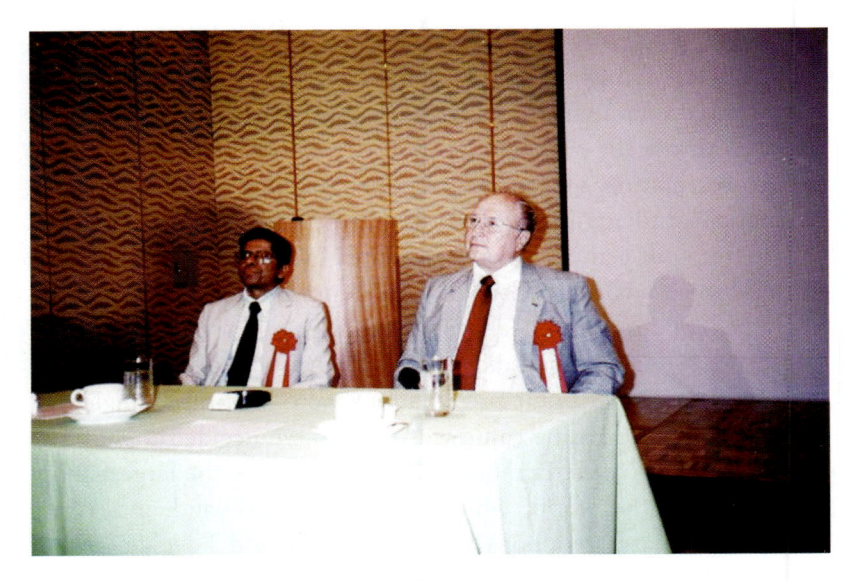

Figure 121. Ramesh Khanna and the author at a lecture in Toyama, Japan.

some presentations after the congresses, so our travel expenses were covered by Hayashidera Medinol and Baxter Japan. Immediately after the congress in Kyoto we went to Toyama, where we gave various lectures (Fig. 121). I talked about the value of PET in the selection of the best peritoneal dialysis method [Pr 219]. The next day we went to Kanazawa, where we again visited the Kenrokuen garden and Kanazawa Castle (Fig. 122). In the evening Dr. Khanna and I gave grand rounds (Fig. 123), mine being on the same topic as in Toyama [Pr 220]. As usual, a reception was organized after the lecture (Fig. 124).

The next day, Friday, July 26, we went to Matto, a sister city of Columbia, Missouri. Mr. Hayashidera notified Mr. Kumeo Kosakawa, the city mayor, of my visit to Ishikawa Prefecture, where Matto is located, and the mayor declared me a friendly citizen of Matto (Figs. 125 and 126). In the afternoon we traveled to Kyushu, which is southwest of Honshu. It was our first trip out of Honshu island, as we had never been to Hokkaido to the north, Shikoku in the southeast or Okinawa in the far southwest. In the morning we visited Kumamoto Castle, the third largest after those in Osaka and Nagoya. This castle, built in the 15th

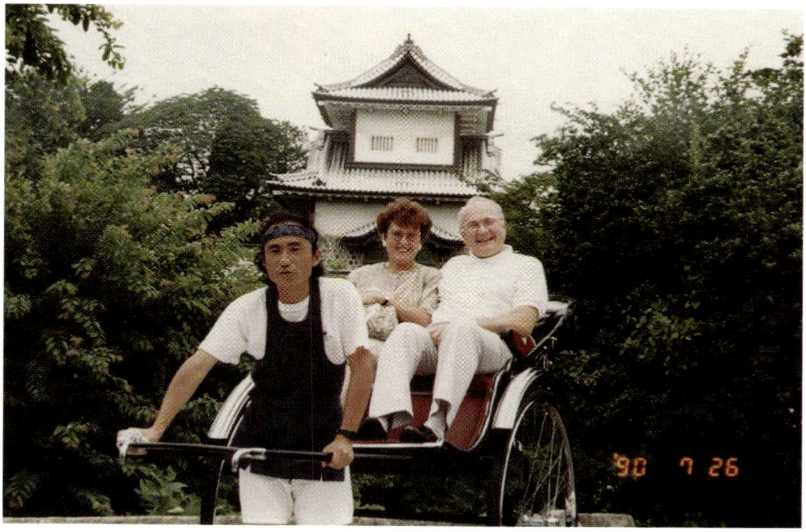

Figure 122. Halina and the author on *jinrikisha* at Kanazawa Castle.

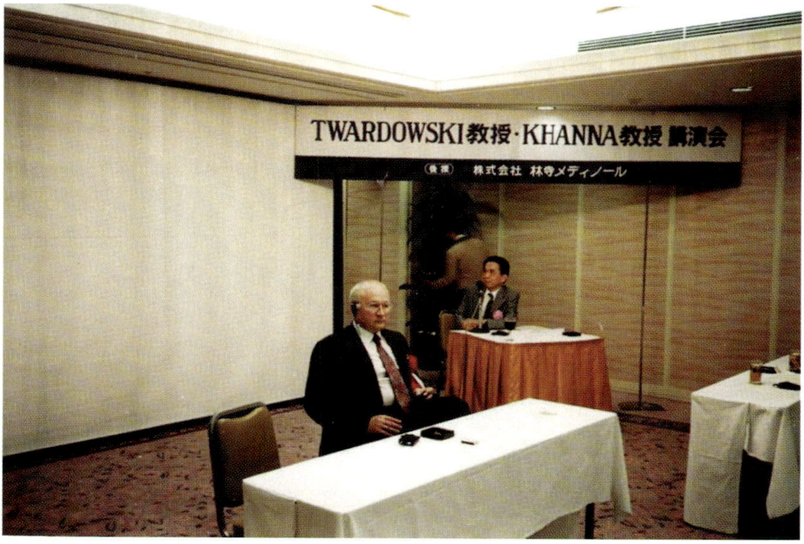

Figure 123. Lecture in Kanazawa: poster with name of lecturers; Prof. Shinoda presiding.

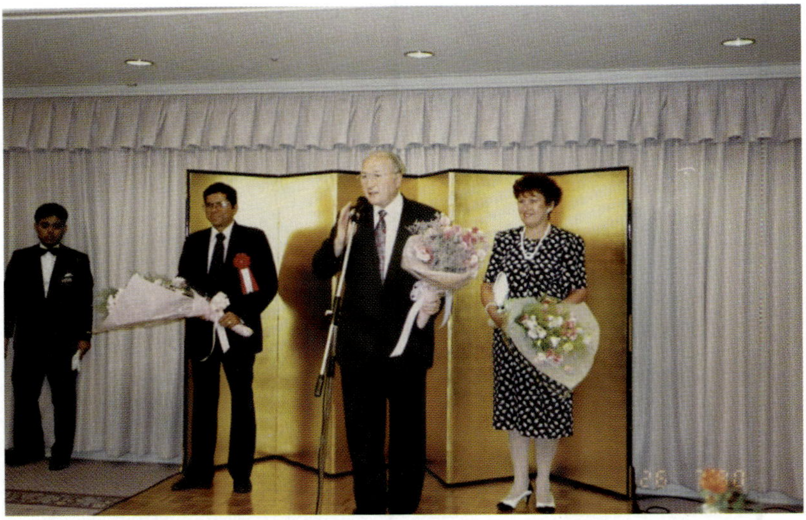

Figure 124. Ramesh, the author and Halina at the reception after Kanazawa lecture.

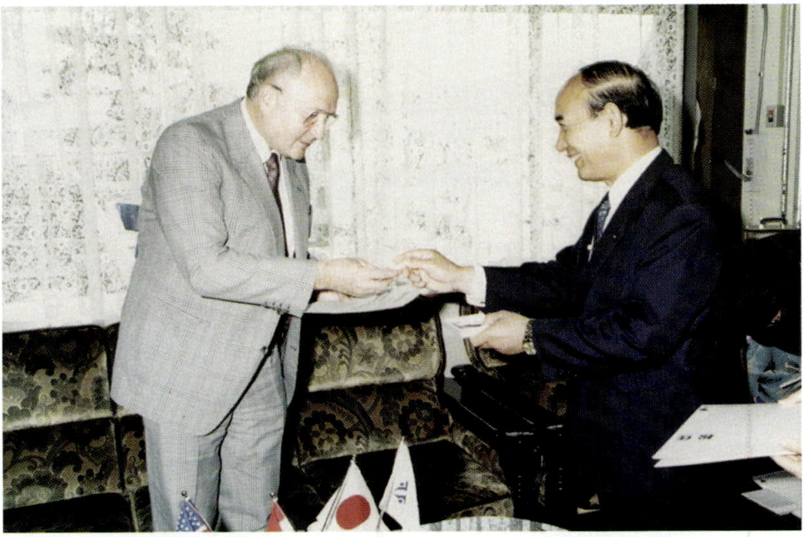

Figure 125. Mayor of Matto, Kumeo Hosakawa, presents a certificate of recognition to the author.

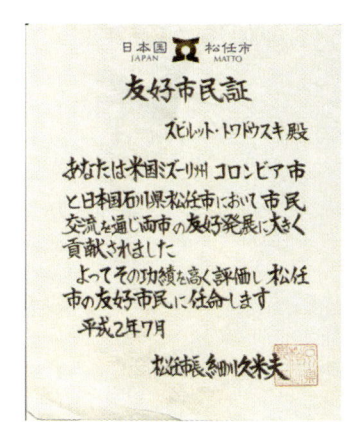

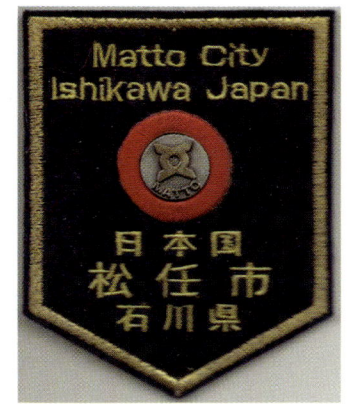

By virtue of the authority vested in the office of the Mayor

I do declare DR. ZBYLUT J. TWARDOWSKI a Friendly Citizen of City of Matto
Ishikawa Prefecture, Japan

in recognition of

his dedication in promoting medical cooperation between
the United States and Japan and his continued efforts in promoting
good will between the City of Columbia and the City of Matto.

Given at the City of Matto, Ishikawa, Japan
On this twenty-seventh Day of July, 1990

KUMEO HOSOKAWA

MAYOR OF MATTO CITY
1 Furushiro-machi, Matto-shi
Ishikawa-ken 924 Japan

Figure 126. Certificate of recognition from the mayor of Matto.

century by the Ideta clan, went through various clans until it was taken by the Hosokawa clan at the beginning of 17th century and held until 1871. We spent a few hours visiting the castle and its impressive donjon, turrets and gates (Fig. 127). In the evening I had a lecture in a Fukuoka seminar [Pr 221] organized by Ms. Kay Kurokawa, Dialysis Business, Baxter Limited, Tokyo, who cooperated closely with Hayashidera Medinol.

We were supposed to go to Taiwan with Halina, but we received word that her mother, Eugenia, had developed jaundice. Halina decided to go to Kraków immediately and help with her care, and

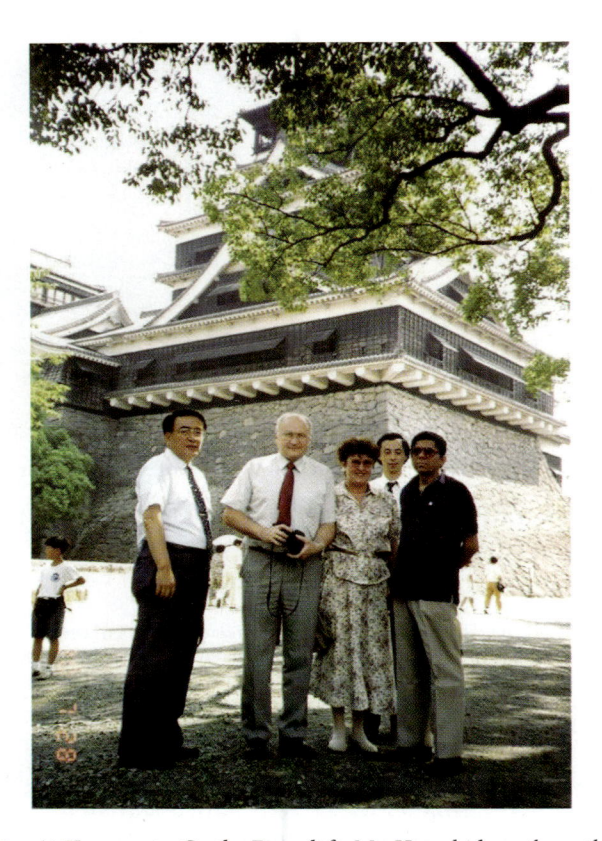

Figure 127. At Kumamoto Castle. From left: Mr. Hayashidera, the author, Halina, Mr. Matsuzaki and Dr. Khanna.

Mr. Matsuzaki rescheduled her flight through Zurich to Kraków. Her mother was admitted to the Gastroenterology Department under the care of my former colleague Doc. Józef Bogdał, who had changed his specialty from nephrology to gastroenterology and became chairman of the department. It turned out that she had obstructive jaundice despite having had a cholecystectomy about 40 years earlier. Ultimately, she was operated on by Prof. Tadeusz Popiela and recovered.

Dr. Khanna and I took a Northwest flight to Taipei in the evening of July 29. As our presentations were scheduled for July 31 and August 1, we had one free day the day after our arrival. First we decided to visit an amusement park with exactly reproduced miniatures of Chinese and Taiwanese wonders including the Great Wall and the Forbidden

City in Beijing. Then we visited the National Palace Museum, which contains an enormous number of artifacts taken from the Palace Museum in the Forbidden City. When the Kuomintang's National Army soldiers were losing to the Communist forces and retreated to Taiwan, they took many valuable exhibits. We were really enchanted by the ivory and jade sculptures, including the most famous jade grasshopper on white cabbage. The next day I gave three presentations at the Taiwan Peritoneal Dialysis Symposium [Pr 222–Pr 224], and the day after, I gave my last presentation in Taiwan [Pr 225], returning to Columbia on August 3. Within a few days I went to Naples, Florida, to give a presentation at a seminar organized by Baxter Healthcare [Pr 226].

In the meantime I was invited by Miguel Carlos Riella, President of the Latin American Federation for Peritoneal Dialysis, to participate in the 10th Anniversary Workshop on CAPD in Curitiba, Parana, Brazil. Dr. Allen Nissenson went with me, but Halina did not want to go for the short trip to Brazil. On the way Dr. Nissenson and I stayed for a day in Rio de Janeiro and took a half-day tour. Naturally, I had to see Christ the Redeemer at the top Corcovado Mountain and the Maracanã Soccer Stadium, which had seated almost 200,000 people for the final game of the 1950 FIFA World Cup. I also went to the Hans Stern jeweler shop on Rua Visconde de Pirajá to buy a coral ring for Halina, which she still treasures to this day. We arrived in Curitiba on August 23, and the next day I had four presentations, including two workshops given with Dr. Nissenson [Pr 227–Pr 230]. The day after, I had three presentations, including one with Dr. Nissenson [Pr 231–Pr 233], and in the afternoon I had some free time. Marila Zaguelb Vidal, the wife of Dr. Riella, was very kind to show me Curitiba, including Bosque do Papa (Pope's Park) and the Polish Immigration Memorial, created in honor of Pope John Paul II and the Polish community in Curitiba. The seven original log houses in the center of the forest illustrate the architecture and way of living of Curitiba's Polish immigrants.

My next trip was in October to Scottsdale, Arizona, to participate in a seminar organized by Baxter Healthcare [Pr 234, Pr 235]. Later that month I participated in an Expert Meeting in Miyazaki, on Kyushu Island, Japan, organized by Kay Kurokawa from Baxter Japan

[Pr 236, Pr 237]. I returned to Columbia for only a few weeks, and then I went to Poland to give a lecture in Kraków [Pr 239]. I was also invited by surgeon Jan H. M. Tordoir, Chairman of the Second International Congress of Access Surgery, to give a presentation in Maastricht later in November [Pr 241]. In addition, I had an invitation to Vienna, but I could not make it, so Dr. Nolph gave the presentation on my behalf [Pr 240]. The final presentation of the year was in Washington [Pr 242], and another given by the first author [Pr 243].

1991

With 51 presentations internationally, the intensity of my travel engagements continued in 1991. Again, most of these presentations were based on my research related to peritoneal dialysis. In addition to this, four poster presentations where I was not the first author were shown by other coauthors. In January I had a local presentation on the Swan Neck Missouri catheter [Pr 244], followed by seminars arranged by Baxter Healthcare in Palm Springs, California [Pr 245–Pr 247], the last one being organized by Kay Kurokawa for Japanese nephrologists. I remember Ms. Kurokawa asking me for slides in advance in order to make some summary slides in Japanese. Our annual conference that year was held in Nashville, Tennessee, and I gave several presentations there as I usually did [Pr 248–Pr 250]. The following presentation was the controversial discussion with Dr. Prakash Keshaviah where I argued that *Kt/V* was an inappropriate indicator of dialysis adequacy [Pr 251]. As mentioned earlier, I argued against this index in publications, and I later argued against it in many presentations. My final presentation at the conference, on culture results from nares and catheter exits [Pr 252], was also controversial. Our studies showed that the results were different, whereas the results from the exit and surrounding skin on the abdomen were usually similar. My opponent's results indicated that the results from nares and exits were usually identical. In the section on exit site care I have already mentioned that I had this debate with Mary Luzar on the differences in culture results. I concluded my talk with the suggestion that the difference may be related to the fact that "in our region it is socially unacceptable to pick a nose and then fondle the catheter." After the meeting Halina and I went to

Poland for the Catholic wedding of our younger son, Przemek, to Kasia in Rzeszów on February 21. We spent only a few days in Poland.

In the first half of 1991 I traveled mostly in the U.S., including Hawaii. My next trips were for a meeting organized by the National Kidney Foundation in Houston, Texas. [Pr 255], and then for a seminar organized by Baxter Healthcare in San Diego, where I had four presentations including a keynote address substituting for Dr. Nolph, who was not able to participate [Pr 256–Pr 259]. Jim Hasbargen, MD, Chief of Nephrology at the Fitzsimons Army Medical Center in Aurora, Colorado, again invited me to present an overview of peritoneal dialysis [Pr 260]. In April we had another meeting at Baxter's headquarters in Deerfield, Illinois, where I had two presentations related to my studies on the exit site [Pr 261] and the Swan Neck catheter [Pr 262]. At the end of that month I attended the 37th Annual Meeting of the American Society for Artificial Internal Organs in Chicago, Illinois, where I delivered three lectures [Pr 263–Pr 265]. In early May I was invited to give a presentation at the Miami Chapter of the American Nephrology Nurses Association [Pr 268]. Later in May, Jim Hauert, Marketing Manager at Baxter Healthcare, organized a peritoneal dialysis seminar for American and Japanese nephrologists in Tucson, Arizona, where I gave a presentation [Pr 269] and participated in the panel discussion [Pr 270].

A similar seminar was organized by Jim Hauert in Lahaina, Maui, Hawaii, in June. The seminar was mostly for Japanese nephrologists, and I provided my slides in advance to have them translated into Japanese and showed by interpreters. I had three presentations there [Pr 271–Pr 273]. Halina was with me in Maui, and we stayed two extra days to enjoy the area. The beaches are wonderful and the waves were ideal for bodysurfing. However, the waves were bigger than those I was used to at the Baltic Sea, and one of them threw me against the sandy bottom — but fortunately only resulting in mild bruising. On Friday, June 21, we went with Dr. Nolph and his wife, Georgia, to Hana. Lahaina is on the west coast and Hana is on the eastern tip of the island. Dr. Nolph rented a car and drove us on the twisty Hana Highway. To use a common expression, it is not the destination that matters, it is the journey itself. The 70-mile highway to Hana features 600 hairpin turns and 54 one-lane bridges with shimmering waterfalls, fragrant flowers and breathtaking cliffs along the way. At the end of our trip I bought the obligatory "I Survived the Road to Hana" T-shirt from the famous Hasegawa General Store, and I felt I really deserved it. As a driver on this twisty road, Dr. Nolph deserved it more, of course.

In July and August I stayed in Columbia, busy with patient care, writing papers and patents, and preparing presentations. One of Halina's friends, Danuta Hoszowska, visited us in August and I took her in our Delta 88 Oldsmobile to Lambert Airport in Saint Louis for her return trip to Poland. In Warrenton, Missouri, the road was under construction and the traffic was slowing down. As I gently applied the brakes, a speeding car slammed into the back of us. The impact was so powerful that I thought we had been hit by a projectile from a cannon. (The Gulf War was in progress at the time, so that was probably the reason for the strange association.) Our car caught fire, and we were not able to remove all our baggage from the trunk before the flames engulfed the vehicle. Ultimately, the car burned out completely before the fire could be extinguished. Halina and I, seated in the front, only had bruises, but Danuta, who was in the rear, had a small infraction in her right hip. It would be the only accident I experienced while driving in the U.S. — and it happened when I was driving very slowly. I say this only because I have gotten a lot of speeding tickets in my life, but my overeager gas pedal has never caused any accidents. Because of our spinal trauma, we were ordered to undergo some chiropractic treatment. Strangely, despite paying for our chiropractic treatment only once, we were reimbursed by our university insurance, by the insurance of the driver who caused the accident, and by our own insurance company. I asked Doug Milner, our insurance agent, why this had happened. He told me that it was the rule, but if I questioned the rule, I might be denied the extra reimbursement. Obviously, I did not see any reason to do that; rules are rules.

In the latter half of the year I traveled to other continents. First was Southeast Asia, but without Halina on this occasion. The trip began with a visit to Seoul, South Korea, for a CAPD doctor seminar organized by Baxter Healthcare in cooperation with Myung-Jae Kim, MD, President of the Korean Society of Nephrology and a professor in the Division of Nephrology of the College of Medicine's Department of Internal Medicine at Kyung Hee University Medical Center.

I remember Denver to Seoul being an incredibly long flight — 16 hours. I also remember my luggage getting lost and having to buy a tie before my presentation, a story that Dr. Ram Gokal would later recount at the American Kidney Fund Torchbearer Award Dinner. All my presentations in Seoul were on September 24 [Pr 274–Pr 277]. The very next day Dr. Gokal and I flew to Hong Kong, which was still a British protectorate. We stayed in the very nice Shangri-La Hotel overlooking the famous Victoria Harbor to the south, but my first presentation was in a seminar organized by Baxter in JW Marriott Hotel on Hong Kong Island [Pr 278], from where we could see the harbor from the other side. The day after, I conducted a workshop with Dr. Gokal in the Shangri-La Hotel on indications of various peritoneal dialysis methods [Pr 279], and I had two more lectures on peritoneal catheters [Pr 280] and the adequacy of peritoneal dialysis [Pr 281]. During the discussion we discovered that the basic form of dialysis in Hong Kong was peritoneal dialysis, as over 80 percent of patients were on this form of therapy. Our stay in Hong Kong was rather short and I could not spend much time sightseeing.

The next day I flew alone to Singapore on the very pleasant Singapore Airlines to Changi International Airport. (I believe Dr. Gokal went to South Africa.) Singapore (Malay *Singapura*, meaning "Lion City"), located off the southern tip of the Malay Peninsula, 85 miles (137 km) north of the equator, is both a city and a country, as the entire island constitutes a single municipality. I did not spend too much time there, but I did note that they had very strict traffic rules. For instance, nobody dared cross the street on a red light for pedestrians. I was told that such strict rules were applied to other transgressions, such as littering, and the fines were never lenient. In any event, I delivered my four presentations on a single day [Pr 282–Pr 285] for the 3rd Scientific Meeting of the Singapore Society of Nephrology — without landing in any trouble with the law.

Two weeks after returning from Singapore I was invited to give a presentation at a conference organized by MEDED (Medical Education) in Aventura, Florida [Pr 286]. Within a week I went to Quito, Ecuador, at the invitation of the Second Congress of the Latin Society of the Peritoneal Dialysis. During my three days there I gave four presentations [Pr 287–Pr 290]. I was not very busy, so I went to visit some places of interest in Quito. The most interesting and unique was La Mitad del Mundo (The Middle of the World), a park lined with statues of members of the famous expedition led by French explorer Charles Marie de La Condamine. The dominant structure in the middle of the park is a 30-meter high monument topped by a bronze globe. There is a red line along one path leading to the monument: if you put one leg on one side and the other leg on the other, you can stand on the Northern and Southern Hemispheres at the same time.

Two days after returning from Ecuador, I went to Vitznau, Switzerland, for the 3rd Baxter Peritoneal Dialysis Symposium, delivering two presentations at the Park Hotel where I was staying [Pr 291, Pr 292]. Halina accompanied me and had some time to take a boat cruise on Lucerne Lake. I had to return to Columbia, but she took the opportunity to go to Poland. In early November I participated in a seminar organized by Baxter Healthcare in Naples, Florida, where I gave a presentation [Pr 293] and contributed to a panel discussion [Pr 294]. A few days later I flew to Venice, Italy, for a peritoneal dialysis workshop to give two presentations [Pr 295, Pr 296]. During my flight home I had tremendous problems with bradyarrhythmia, and immediately after returning I asked cardiologist Dr. Greg Flaker to evaluate me. He did not find anything wrong, except for multiple unifocal premature ventricular complexes (PVCs) and told me that "your heart is telling you something; you have to slow down." I was a little disturbed and decided to take his advice seriously, as I recalled my episode with asystole in 1969 when I was working without rest over a long period. I decided to travel less the following year and to avoid too many rapid changes of time zones. That year I had only two more presentations, but both were in San Antonio, Texas [Pr 297, Pr 298].

1992

I gave only 38 presentations in 1992. For six other presentations I was a coauthor, but they were delivered by the first authors. In the first half of the year I did not travel abroad at all. For our annual conference on peritoneal dialysis in Seattle, I gave three presentations [Pr 299, Pr 300, Pr 302] and participated in the "Quiz the Experts" session [Pr 301]. I had a few day trips organized in the U.S.: I went to Houston,

Texas [Pr 303, Pr 304], attended a local meeting in Columbia, Missouri. [Pr 305], and participated in two meetings organized by the National Kidney Foundation, in Washington [Pr 306] and in Chicago [Pr 307]. In May I was invited to give two presentations during the 38th Annual Meeting of the American Society for Artificial Internal Organs [Pr 308, Pr 309].

My first trip abroad that year was at the end of the first half of the year. In November 1991 I had been invited by Dr. Miguel Nadal, Coordinator of the Sociedad Argentina de Nephrologia, to participate as a guest lecturer in the 8th Argentine Congress of Nephrology in Mar del Plata in June 1992. I arrived in Buenos Aires on June 5 and had half a day to tour the city. I visited the historical city center and also went to La Boca and saw the famous soccer stadium La Bombonera (The Chocolate Box), home ground of Boca Juniors, one of Argentina's most well-known clubs. The next day I attended the congress in Mar del Plata [Pr 310, Pr 311], returning to Columbia the following day. At the end of June I participated in a symposium organized by the National Kidney Foundation of Virginia and delivered two presentations [Pr 312, Pr 313]. My next trip was in Manzanillo, Mexico, for a peritoneal dialysis workshop organized by Baxter Healthcare. It was a two-day meeting where I had only three presentations [Pr 314–Pr 316], so I had time to go on a snorkeling trip in Manzanillo Bay. The next quick trip was for a meeting organized by the Hazel Taylor Chapter of the American Nephrology Nurses' Association in Birmingham, Alabama, where I delivered two presentations on one day [Pr 317, Pr 318].

In September I had two invitations for meetings in Colombia, one from Dr. Roberto D'Achtardo, Sociedad Colombiana de Nefrologia, for the 25th Anniversary Symposium of the Colombian Society of Nephrology in Paipa, and another from Dr. Cesar Pru, to participate as a guest speaker in the 3rd Panamerican and the 1st Venezuelan Congress of Dialysis and Transplantation. My trip to Colombia was not without problems. The idea was to fly to Bogota through Miami, Florida. Halina was not with me, as she had planned to go to Poland. Without her — or anyone else — keeping an eye on me I managed to miss the plane, as I was deeply engrossed in reading and did not hear the boarding announcement. I had to change my flight through

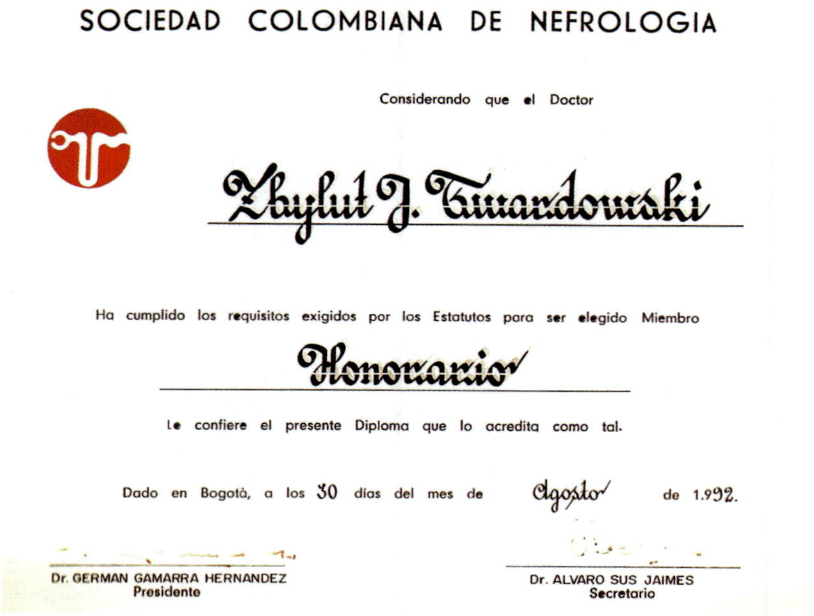
SOCIEDAD COLOMBIANA DE NEFROLOGIA

Considerando que el Doctor

Zbylut J. Twardowski

Ha cumplido los requisitos exigidos por los Estatutos para ser elegido Miembro

Honorario

Le confiere el presente Diploma que lo acredita como tal.

Dado en Bogotà, a los 30 días del mes de Agosto de 1.992.

Dr. GERMAN GAMARRA HERNANDEZ
Presidente

Dr. ALVARO SUS JAIMES
Secretario

Figure 128. Honorary Member Diploma of the Colombian Society of Nephrology.

Caracas, Venezuela, to Bogota, arriving the next morning. The drive to Paipa from Bogota takes about four hours. A nurse gave me a ride and managed the drive in three hours on twisty roads. Regrettably, I do not recall the name of the nurse, but I remember her being an excellent driver. I had three presentations that afternoon [Pr 319–Pr 321]. The Board of Directors of the Sociedad Colombiana de Nefrologia had me designated an Honorary Member of the Society, and society president German Gamarra Hernandez, MD, presented me with a diploma (Fig. 128). I left Paipa in the morning, arriving in Bogota in good time for Viasa Flight 911 to Caracas at 1 pm on September 5, 1992. The next day I had three presentations at the Venezuelan congress [Pr 322–Pr 324] and returned to Columbia on September 7.

The University of Ulm, Germany, was the venue for my next engagement. I was invited by Prof. Dr. H. E. Franz, Medizinische Klinik und Poliklinik, University of Ulm, who had organized a symposium on peritoneal dialysis. I arrived at Frankfurt am Main airport in the morning of September 22 and took train No. 597 at 2:07 pm to

Ulm. I delivered seven presentations the next day, four related to peritoneal dialysis kinetics [Pr 325–Pr 328] and three related to peritoneal access [Pr 329–Pr 331]. My main interest was of course in the dialysis facilities, which were very well equipped. Halina joined me from Poland. Ulm lies at the point where the rivers Blau and Iller join the Danube. It is primarily known for being the birthplace of Albert Einstein, and for a church with the tallest steeple in the world, the Gothic Ulmer Münster (Ulm Minster), which was obviously on our itinerary. We also toured Bavaria and went to Zwiefalten to visit a friend of Halina's, Dr. Zbigniew Oczkowski, with whom she worked in the Psychiatry Department of the Hospital for Miners in Bytom. In Zwiefalten we visited the beautiful Cathedral of Our Beloved Lady.

From Ulm we went directly to Greece for the 7th Congress of the International Society for Peritoneal Dialysis. We spent a night in a very lousy hotel in Piraeus and then took a boat to Thessaloniki. On the way, we visited the famous Santorini Island and rode a mule to the top of the island and back. We eventually arrived in Thessaloniki on October 1. I had one poster presentation [Pr 333], two lectures [Pr 336, Pr 338] and one discussion on the controversy regarding nasal carriage and exit site infections [Pr 337]. Other presentations, where I was a coauthor, were presented by the first authors in the poster forum [Pr 332] and in the slide forums [Pr 334, Pr 335]. We took advantage of our stay in Thessaloniki and visited the Aristotle University, the Archeological Museum and the Tomb of Philip II in Vergina. Legend has it that Philip II was assassinated on the order of his son, Alexander the Great, or his wife Olympia. I was struck by the small size of the tomb, which would seem to indicate the small stature of the king. After the meeting we went to Athens, where we stayed with Charalambos Stathakis, MD, who had worked in our Columbia laboratory in 1983. He acted as our guide and showed us places of interest, including the Acropolis (with its monumental entrance, the Propylaia), the Temple of Athena Nike and the Parthenon. We went to Agora, and if I remember correctly, I stood at the spot where St. Paul gave his talk to the Athenians — St. Paul's meeting place. We returned to Columbia shortly after the meeting. My last presentation of the year was at the 25th Annual Meeting of the American Society of Nephrology in Baltimore, Maryland, in November [Pr 340]. My coauthored presentations were given by Dr. Nolph, the first author [Pr 341, Pr 342]. All in all, in 1992 I changed time zone only once, and the other foreign trips were in South, Central and North America; I had no problems with heart arrhythmia that year.

1993

My travels in 1993 were somewhat limited, amounting to just 30 presentations. As I was working with Rod Kenley on the home hemodialysis machine, I was less involved in peritoneal dialysis research. As a matter of fact, my view was that peritoneal dialysis would not make a great deal of progress, so I had switched to hemodialysis research, including blood access, which I described in previous sections. I eventually stopped providing consulting services to Baxter on March 26. My initial presentations were at our annual conference on peritoneal dialysis in San Diego, California. In conjunction with this conference I received the American Kidney Disease Torchbearer Award, as already mentioned. During the conference I had one presentation [Pr 343], participated in the "Quiz the Expert" session [Pr 344], presented my case in the peritoneal dialysis case forum [Pr 348], and participated in the poster forum [Pr 345–Pr 347]. Over the next few months I took quick trips inside the U.S. to Houston, Texas [Pr 349], Toms River, New Jersey [Pr 350], Salt Lake City, Utah [Pr 351], and Natick, Massachusetts [Pr 353]. As the 39th Annual Meeting of the American Society for Artificial Internal Organs was very close to the Massachusetts presentation, I did not go, and instead Dr. Nolph presented our study on CAPD with a high-flux membrane [Pr 352]. This last one was one of the first presentations on the higher mortality in patients with high peritoneal transport characteristics on the peritoneal equilibration test.

Later in May I traveled to Montevideo, Uruguay, for the 2nd Uruguayan Congress of Nephrology at the invitation of Dra. Teresita Llopart, President of the Congress, and Dra. Emma Schwedt, Organizer of the Peritoneal Dialysis Course, to participate as a guest lecturer in the pre-congress course on peritoneal dialysis. I arrived in Montevideo on Varig Flight 910 from Buenos Aires at 1:50 am on May 11, so I had some time to look around the city the following day as I had presentations the day after that [Pr 354, Pr 355], departing Montevideo at 3:50 pm on Varig Flight 911 back to Buenos Aires. Most striking was the realization that Montevideo, whose name apparently came from the utterance of a sailor (*Montevideo*: I see a hill), is located only about 140 feet (43 meters) above sea level on the north side of the La Plata estuary. I visited the Plaza Independencia (Independence Square), with its various important buildings like the Solis Theatre and the offices of the President of Uruguay. I also saw the Estadio Centenario, a famous soccer stadium where Uruguay had gained numerous victories, including 4:2 over Argentina in the final of the inaugural World Cup in 1930. It is listed by FIFA as one of football's classic stadiums, along with the likes of Maracanã in Rio de Janeiro or Wembley Stadium in the U.K. In early June I went to Phoenix, Arizona, for a seminar organized by Baxter Healthcare where I delivered two lectures [Pr 356, Pr 357].

In mid-June the 12th International Congress of Nephrology met in Jerusalem, and for the first time, the initial results of the presternal catheter were presented. Mrs. Lisa Zellerman, President of Accurate Surgical Instruments (Fig. 129), also showed the catheter for the first time. I only had presentations on one day, Monday, June 14

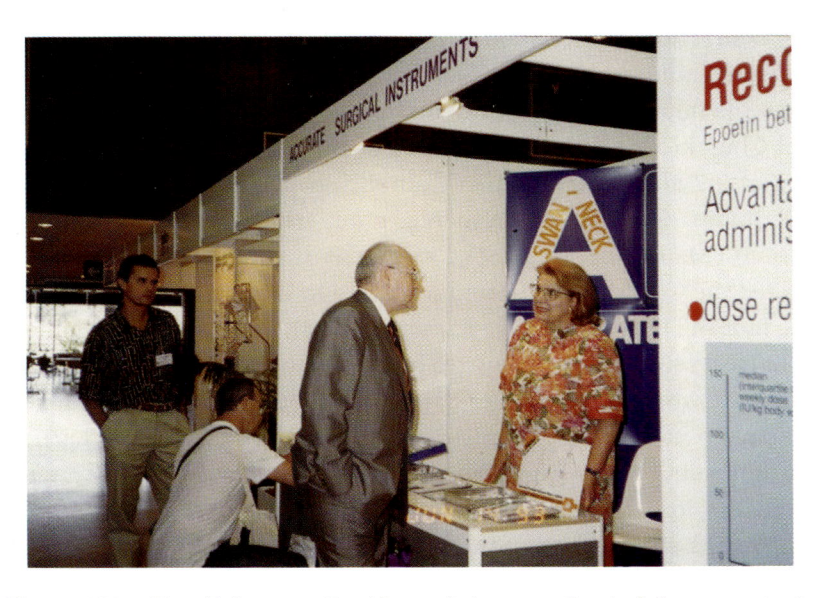

Figure 129. Lisa Zellerman, President of Accurate Surgical Instruments, in Jerusalem, Israel.

[Pr 358–Pr 360]. Halina came with us, and we decided to stay till the end of week to visit a few places in Israel. We took a guided tour with an extremely knowledgeable lady, who knew the Old and New Testaments inside out. On the Tuesday, we saw King David's Tomb and the Room of the Last Supper on Mount Zion. Later we visited the Roman Cardo, the Herodian Quarter and the Western Wall. We walked along the Via Dolorosa to the Church of the Holy Sepulcher, where we spent some time praying. We were stunned to see so many souvenir merchants along the street that Jesus is said to have walked, carrying his cross. Later we proceeded to Mount Scopus and the Mount of Olives, where we were treated to a magnificent panoramic view of the Old City. On Wednesday we visited Yad Vashem, a Holocaust museum with many memorials to those who helped Jews during World War II. It was interesting to note that there were more individuals considered "Righteous Among the Nations" from Poland (6,266 as of January 1, 2011) than any other nationality. This is especially significant since helping Jews in Poland during the war was punishable by death, as I mentioned when describing my father's ordeal as a wartime prisoner (Fig. 3). We then went to Bethlehem, stopped at Rachel's Tomb and visited the Church of the Nativity.

On Thursday we went to Tiberias, saw the impressive Roman aqueduct and visited one Kibbutz there, and then we drove to Capernaum, where we saw the ruins of the synagogue and the octagonal Church of St. Peter. We stopped at the hill near Capernaum, the site of a 20th-century Roman Catholic chapel called the Church of Beatitudes. One person from our group read the Sermon on the Mount (Matthew 5:3–12). The same day we went to Nazareth and visited the Church of the Annunciation. On Friday we drove through the Judean Desert to the Dead Sea, the lowest point on Earth at almost 1,400 feet (420 meters) below sea level. We stopped at Qumran to visit the place where the Dead Sea Scrolls were found. We also decided to take a dip in the Dead Sea. The water is very salty (about 300 g/L of various salts, mostly $MgCl_2$ and $NaCl$) as the delivery of fresh water from the Jordan River occurs at the same rate as evaporation. Of course, the salt concentration changes slightly from year to year. With such a composition, the specific gravity is markedly higher than the specific gravity of the human body, so it is theoretically impossible to drown in the Dead Sea. However, one lady went into the water face down, so her legs came up and she could not recover her position. had to help her to turn around. Some ladies nearby had to help her to turn around. The same day we drove along the shores of the Dead Sea to Masada, which was besieged in 72 AD by the Roman governor of Judaea Lucius Flavius Silva. After failed attempts to breach the wall, they built a circumvallation wall and then a rampart against the western face of the plateau, using thousands of tons of stones and beaten earth. We ascended to the site via cable car and toured the ancient fortress where the Zealots made their last stand against the Romans before committing mass suicide in 73 AD. We contemplated with admiration the Roman military engineering that so frequently brought victory for the Roman legions. On Saturday we observed a day of rest, and on Sunday we went to a Catholic Church in Haifa, where we attended a Mass in Polish.

After our return from Israel I participated in a grand round in our Department of Medicine [Pr 361], and I then traveled to Mexico to deliver several talks at the Conference of Nephrologists of Bajío Province in Leon organized by Baxter Healthcare [Pr 362–Pr 365]. Before going to Mexico I was warned about frequent gastrointestinal infections and advised to take prophylactic doxycycline, which I did. John Moran, MD, who was working for Baxter at the time, also participated in the meeting. When we were in the airport in Guadalajara, he suddenly felt extremely weak and almost fainted. Feeling better after taking some fluids, he told me that he had not heeded the warnings to take some prophylactic antibiotics before leaving. Fortunately, I had some spare tablets he could take.

In September I had only one presentation related to daily home hemodialysis [Pr 366]. The next meeting, which was in Maui, Hawaii, was organized by Reiko Kojima from Baxter's Dialysis Division in Tokyo, and targeted at Japanese nephrologists. I delivered two presentations there [Pr 367, Pr 368]. The year's remaining presentations were in the U.S. The first was at the Consensus Conference on Morbidity and Mortality of Dialysis at the National Institutes of Health [Pr 369]. The day after, in Bethesda, the Scientific Board Meeting of Aksys was convened, and I delivered a presentation on conditions for the revival of home hemodialysis [Pr 370]. I attended a meeting of the Central

Society for Clinical Research on the following day, but our presentation on the reproducibility of the peritoneal equilibration test was delivered without my presence [Pr 371]. My last meeting in 1993 was at Quinton Instruments, where I presented the preliminary clinical results of the vein shape catheter based on our design [Pr 372].

1994

I had just 13 presentations in 1994. Fewer were devoted to peritoneal dialysis and I delivered only nine of them personally. Just three were given outside of the U.S. The first five presentations were at our annual conference on peritoneal dialysis in Orlando, Florida, two of which I gave personally [Pr 372, Pr 373], and three others by the first authors in a poster forum [Pr 375, Pr 376] and a slide forum [Pr 377]. My next presentation was at the 3rd Annual Spring Clinical Nephrology Meetings, Nurse and Technician Program in Chicago, Illionois. [Pr 378]. The first presentation abroad was in Italy. Dr. Nolph and I were invited by Prof. Giuseppe La Greca to participate in the 5th International Course on Peritoneal Dialysis organized by St. Bortolo Hospital in Vicenza, Italy. Halina and I flew with Dr. Georgia Nolph, Dr. Karl Nolph and their son, Chris, to Milan and stayed one night in the Hotel Palace on May 20. On following day we took a train to Santa Margherita Ligure, located on the Italian Riviera, and checked in to Grand Hotel Miramare. The day after, the Nolphs suggested that we walk[11] to Portofino, which was about 3 miles (5 km). Portofino is a picturesque, half-moon shaped seaside village with pastel houses lining the shore of the harbor. A castle sits atop the hill overlooking the village. We hiked through the Parco Naturale di Monte di Portofino (The Natural Park of the Portofino Promontory), taking in breath taking views over Portofino. The following day, May 23, we took a train through Milan to Vicenza and checked into the Viest Hotel on Via Pelosa. The meeting was held

---

11. I remember having tremendous problems with walking, as I had pain in my soles due to flat feet. It had not usually bothered me that much before, but this was my longest walk in a long time. After returning from the trip to Columbia, I acquired insoles from the Featherspring International Corporation in Seattle, Washington, which were made in Germany from Swedish stainless steel. The foot supports relieved the pain significantly, but I had to remove them at airport security checks — even before the incident with the "shoe bomber." These insoles serve me to this day.

in the convention hall of the Banco Ambrosiano Veneto. I delivered a one presentation on exit site care in peritoneal dialysis patients [Pr 379]. In Vicenza we visited several places of interest designed by famous architect Andrea Palladio, including Villa Capra detta "la Rotonda," Basilica Palladiana, Teatro Olimpico and others like Villa Trissino, where Palladio worked as a mason. It is worth mentioning that the main building of the University of Virginia was named "The Rotunda" by Thomas Jefferson in honor of Andrea Palladio. We returned by train to Milan on May 27, again staying at the Hotel Palace for two days. The next day we visited numerous places of interest in Milan, including Piazza de Duomo and the Milan Cathedral. We also went to the monastery of Santa Maria delle Grazie to see Leonardo da Vinci's *The Last Supper*. At the time the mural was undergoing restoration under the direction of Pinin Brambilla Barcilon, and unfortunately, it was not clearly visible. We visited the Museo Nazionale della Scienza e della Tecina "Leonardo da Vinci," with its numerous models, texts, images and exhibits reconstructed from da Vinci's drawings. I also saw an excellent reproduction of *The Last Supper* there. In the evening we decided to visit La Scala. Tickets were obviously not available, but we managed to get tickets from a scalper for Elektra, the single-act opera by Richard Strauss. The scalper helpfully warned us that it was in German, and I retorted that it was of no consequence, as we spoke no Italian either. Besides, the plot of *Electra*, Clytemnestra and Agamemnon were well known to us from the tragedies of Sophocles and Euripides. All in all we thoroughly enjoyed the evening. The next day we returned to Columbia.

I had no presentations that summer. The only invitation I received was from Dr. Andrew M. Weisser, Program Director of the 34th Annual Scientific Symposium on Kidney Disease of the National Kidney Foundation of Southern California. I delivered this presentation in September [Pr 380], and the next two presentations were grand rounds in Indianapolis, Indiana, both unrelated to peritoneal dialysis [Pr 381, Pr 382]. I later received invitations from Poland to present new advances in access for peritoneal dialysis and hemodialysis. The first presentation was for a symposium celebrating the 65th birthday of Prof. Dr. med. Dr. h.c. mult. Franciszek Kokot, organized by Jan Duława, MD, PhD, Andrzej Więcek, MD, PhD, and Rafał S. Wnuk, MD, from the Silesian School of Medicine [Pr 383]. I took the opportunity to spend 10 days in

Poland with Halina, flying via Rome to Kraków on November 12. Dr. Olgierd Smoleński from Krakowski Szpital Specjalistyczny (Specialty Hospital) in Nowa Huta (a subdivision of Kraków) gave us a ride to Szczyrk, the tourist and sports center situated by the slopes of Klimczok Mountain, and asked me to give the same presentation in Polish at a meeting of the Kraków Chapter of the Polish Society of Nephrology to be held in his hospital, which I agreed to do [Pr 384]. We returned to Columbia on November 23, and my last presentation that year was a grand round in our hospital on polycystic kidney disease [Pr 385].

1995

I had 21 presentations in 1995, but I was a coauthor on seven of them and they were presented by the first authors. My first presentation, at New York Medical College, was on the physiology of the peritoneal membrane [Pr 386]. As I mentioned earlier, our annual conference on peritoneal dialysis included, for the first time, the International Symposium on Daily Home Hemodialysis. I delivered an introductory presentation [Pu 394] and gave four additional presentations [Pr 391–Pr 393, Pr 395]; five more were presented by the first authors [Pr 387–Pr 390, Pr 396]. My next trip was to Houston, Texas, at the invitation of Stephen Z. Fadem, MD, FACP, organizer of the National Kidney Foundation of Southeast Texas Update 1995. I talked about major problems surrounding peritoneal dialysis [Pr 397]. In May, in a session of the 41st Annual Conference of the American Society for Artificial Internal Organs called "Vanguard in Dialysis," I presented my concept of a machine for daily hemodialysis [Pr 398]. In the same session Robert Uldall, MD, presented his concept of a machine. As I mentioned earlier, he died suddenly later that year.

My next three presentations were in New Jersey at the invitation of John Burkart, MD, from the Robert Wood Johnson University Hospital and Nephrological Society of New Jersey [Pr 399–Pr 401]. In June I participated in the 7th Congress of the International Society for Peritoneal Dialysis, in Stockholm, Sweden, where several coauthors and I presented three posters [Pr 402–Pr 404]. During the American Society for Artificial Internal Organs Meeting in Chicago, Albert Valek, MD, PhD, DSc, professor of medicine in the Haemodialysis

Centre Háje at Charles University Medical School, Prague, invited me to give a presentation at the CAPD Club Meeting in Wysowa, Poland, organized in cooperation with Prof. Dr. hab. n. med. W. Grzeszczak from Katedra i Klinika Chorób Wewnętrznych i Zawodowych, Śląskiej Akademi Medycznej w Zabrzu (Department of Internal Medicine and Professional Diseases on the Silesian Medical Academy in Zabrze, Poland). I arrived in Warsaw from Stockholm in the evening of June 21 and traveled to Kraków by train, as the airport in Kraków was closed. The next day I was given a ride to Wysowa, a spa resort located among forested hills, two-and-a-half miles from the Slovakian border. The proximity to Slovakia was the reason for organizing this meeting for Polish and Czechoslovakian nephrologists. I gave one presentation [Pr 405]. For my final presentation of the year, I was invited by Jean Ezra, MME, as a featured speaker on daily home hemodialysis for the 7th Annual Network #12 Network Coordinating Council Meeting in Kansas City, Missouri [Pr 406].

1996

In 1996 I delivered 16 presentations, mostly in the U.S. and Europe. The first, at a grand round in our hospital, was on nephrotic syndrome [Pr 407]. For our annual conference on peritoneal dialysis and the 2nd International Symposium on Daily Home Hemodialysis in Seattle, I gave four presentations [Pr 408–Pr 411]. Prof. Dr. H. E. Franz again invited me to give a presentation in Ulm on quality assurance in peritoneal dialysis [Pr 412]. Halina came with us to Ulm, where we spent two days, and then we went to Kraków for three days before flying to Washington, where I had a presentation on same site puncturing of the vascular access in the "Vanguard in Dialysis" session at the 42nd Annual Conference of the American Society for Artificial Internal Organs [Pr 413]. That summer I had no presentations, so I took some time off in June to travel with Halina and my brother Lesław in the Midwestern U.S., a trip I will describe later.

The following three presentations were in the U.S. [Pr 414–Pr 416], while my next international trip with Halina was in Portorož, Slovenia. Dr. Peter Ivanovich, a physician of Slovenian origin who worked at Northwestern University in Chicago, had suggested to the organizers of the 1st Slovene Nephrological Congress that they invite me to speak. Staša Kaplan-Pavlovčič, MD, PhD, Associate Professor at the Department of Nephrology, University Medical Center in Ljubljana, Slovenija, invited me to give a lecture at the congress [Pr 417] and at a workshop for the First Postgraduate Course in Nephrology associated with the congress [Pr 418]. It turned out to be a rather complicated trip. We originally planned to fly to Trieste and rent a car to drive to Portorož, which is about 30 miles (50 km) away. Unfortunately, renting a car in Trieste to drive to what was then considered Eastern Europe was not allowed. We arrived in Trieste on Lufthansa Flight 6847 (operated by Air Dolomiti) at 12:25 pm on October 25, and the organizers had to send a private car to Trieste to take us to Portorož. After the congress, we stayed in the Star Hotel Savoia Excelsior in Trieste on October 27, leaving on Alitalia Flight 1362 to Rome at 6.55 the next morning — without seeing much of Trieste.

The following month we were invited for a meeting in Madrid organized by Dr. Rafael Selgas from La Paz University Hospital in Madrid, in cooperation with Baxter S.A. Valencia. I gave two presentations related to peritoneal dialysis [Pr 419, Pr 420], the former being on our exit site evaluation and care. Some presentations from the hospital indicated that they had used our classification method. While in Spain we took the opportunity to visit some places of interest. In Madrid we visited the Museo del Prado (which houses various paintings by El Greco), the Almudena Cathedral, and the Museo Nacional Cantro del Arte Reina Sofia. We also went to Segovia, a wonderful mix of Roman, Medieval, Renaissance and Modern Spain all rolled into one. Dotted around this UNESCO World Heritage city are three very important sites: a Roman aqueduct, a Gothic cathedral and the Alcázar, not to mention Segovia's multitude of churches and palaces. Built by the Romans between the late 1st and 2nd centuries AD, the aqueduct is an amazing structure designed to bring water from the Frio River, situated in La Acebeda, near the Royal Palace of La Granja. The Romans used no other material apart from stone to hold the structure together, and those stones were as solid in 1996 as they were the day they were first lifted into place. Incredibly, the aqueduct was still functioning when we visited Segovia — and is probably still functioning now. We also visited the Alcázar, a fort founded in 1085 and once a royal residence of Carlos I. It was demolished and restored many times, most recently during the Civil War. Franco had it rebuilt into a military museum. In Toledo we saw the famous cathedral, considered one of the high points of Gothic art. The construction of this monumental building, with a basilica floor plan and five naves, began in 1226, although it was not finished until the 15th century.

I also sent my video for a competition at Videomed '96, and it was accepted for presentation [Pr 421, Vi 5]. From Madrid we traveled by train to Badajoz. Although there appeared to be little interest in the other video presentations, it was gratifying to see the audience swell when it was time to present my video. I was very happy that so many people wanted to see my video, but the reality was a little different. Just before my presentation there was another video showing the wounds acquired during *corrida de toros* (bullfighting) and their treatment. Some of the images were indeed amazing, like blood gushing from a femoral artery punctured by a bull's horn. By the time my video was ready to be shown, the crowd had disappeared and only a few people remained in the audience. In Spain, when it comes to a competition between a video on bullfighting and one on peritoneal catheter implantation and care, there was no contest.

Dr. Umberto Buoncristiani had organized another meeting shortly after. He had invited me to be a member of the Scientific Committee for the Symposium on the Dialysis Schedule in Hemodialysis and Peritoneal Dialysis and to present my take on the influence of different APD[12] schedules on solutes and water removal [Pr 422]. We flew from Madrid via Rome to Perugia on November 24; the return journey would be via Rome to Columbia on November 27. In the evening of November 25 we were invited for dinner at Perugia's renowned La Taverna restaurant on Via Streghe. My presentation had taken place that day, so we had some free time on November 26. Dr. Buoncristiani's wife, Renata, showed us around Perugia. In the morning we saw Fontanna Maggiore and the medieval aqueduct, and then we went by bus to visit Assisi's famous Papal Basilica of St. Francis. We were fortunate to witness the full beauty of the Basilica, as it was seriously damaged in two major earthquakes a year later.

---

12. APD: automated peritoneal dialysis.

1997

I gave 13 presentations in 1997, mostly in the U.S., but I also traveled to Europe and Australia. Our annual conference on peritoneal dialysis with the 3rd International Symposium on Daily Home Hemodialysis was in Denver, Colorado. I had four presentations there [Pr 423, Pr 424, Pr 426], including a presentation of our video made with George Harper [Pr 425, Vi 7]. Przemysław Hirszel, MD, then a professor of medicine in the Nephrology Division of the Uniformed Services University of the Health Sciences, also participated. We had not seen Przemek for many years, so we decided to spend a few days skiing in Keystone, Colorado. In addition to Halina and me, Dr. John Van Stone and Leonor Ponferrada, head nurse at Dialysis Clinic Inc., decided to come. Stephen Z. Fadem, MD, FACP, again invited me to give a presentation at the National Kidney Foundation of Southeast Texas Update 1997 in Houston, Texas [Pr 427]. At the invitation of Rod Kenley I gave a pep talk to bolster the enthusiasm of Aksys employees [Pr 428].

In the middle of 1996, Prof. Dr. H. E. Franz from Ulm, Germany, asked me to organize a half-day symposium on daily home hemodialysis in Cologne, Germany, on Saturday, April 12, 1997. The meeting was meant to increase interest in home hemodialysis in Germany. He guaranteed reimbursement of all expenses to all invited speakers. I invited Umberto Buoncristiani from Perugia and Rod Kenley. I decided to speak about the theoretical background of daily hemodialysis, and I asked Rod Kenley to talk about our machine, and Umberto Buoncristiani to present his long-term clinical results. Each of our talks was to be an hour long with German translation. Many German nephrologists involved in hemodialysis attended the symposium. For the first time I personally met Prof. Dr. med. Gerhard Krönung, chief surgeon at the county hospital in Ottweiler, Germany, whom I mentioned previously when describing the constant site (buttonhole) method of needle insertion. After our presentations, including my own [Pr 429], we had a free discussion about the buttonhole method. Dr. Zbigniew Fałda, already working in Germany at the time, also attended the symposium, so I met him for the first time since our meeting in Warsaw many years earlier. After the symposium I decided to stay for a day in Cologne and among other places visit Cologne Cathedral, officially called Hohe Domkirche St. Peter und Maria. It was a really impressive building: for several years after its completion in 1880 its spires were the tallest man-made structures in the world. During the bombing of Cologne in World War II, the cathedral was damaged, but its spires did not collapse. Zbigniew and I decided to climb the towers. I do not remember how many steps there were, but the climb was no mean feat. I was a little younger than Zbigniew, so I got there quicker than he did. In May during a grand round in our Columbia hospital, I delivered a talk very similar to the one in Cologne [Pr 430].

At the end of May was the 14th International Congress of Nephrology in Sydney, Australia. Our first class tickets were covered by Lisa Zellerman of Accurate Surgical Instruments. She decided not to exhibit her products, but I presented the Swan Neck presternal catheter results and distributed a booklet on its implantation technique. Halina and I decided to take advantage of the long trip and visit a few sights in New Zealand and Australia. We first went to Auckland, New Zealand, and took a guided tour to Rotorua, at the heart of the North Island, where the forces of Nature are on full display. As well as witnessing the impressive geysers, we met a national icon — the flightless kiwi bird — and were introduced to Maori culture. After lunch we visited a sheep farm to observe the mastery of the sheep shearers.

We also went to the Waitomo Glowworm Caves, where thousands of tiny *Arachnocampa luminosa*, glowworms found only in New Zealand, can be seen radiating an unmistakable luminescent light. The *Arachnocampa* species go through a life cycle of eggs hatching to larvae then pupating to become adult flies. They spend most of their lives as larvae. The larval stage lasts about 6 to 12 months, depending on how much food is available. The larva emerges from the egg only about 3 to 5 mm long, and through its life grows to about 3 cm. The larva spins a nest out of silk on the ceiling of the cave and then hangs down as many as 70 threads of silk (called snares) from around the nest, each up to 30 or 40 cm long and holding droplets of mucus, which catches fodder. The larvae can only live in a place out of the wind, to stop their lines being tangled hence caves are their natural environment.

We spent that night in Auckland and flew to Christchurch, the largest city on the Southern Island, the following day. We spent two days there, visiting the Anglican cathedral and a botanical garden. Thereafter, we went to Queenstown and then took a tour to Milford Sound on a sightseeing day cruise, soaking up the unique wildlife, tumbling waterfalls and the towering beauty and majesty of Mitre Peak. Returning to Queenstown, we wanted to take a helicopter to Mount Cook (Aoraki), but such flights are frequently canceled because of bad weather — and ours was indeed unable to go ahead.

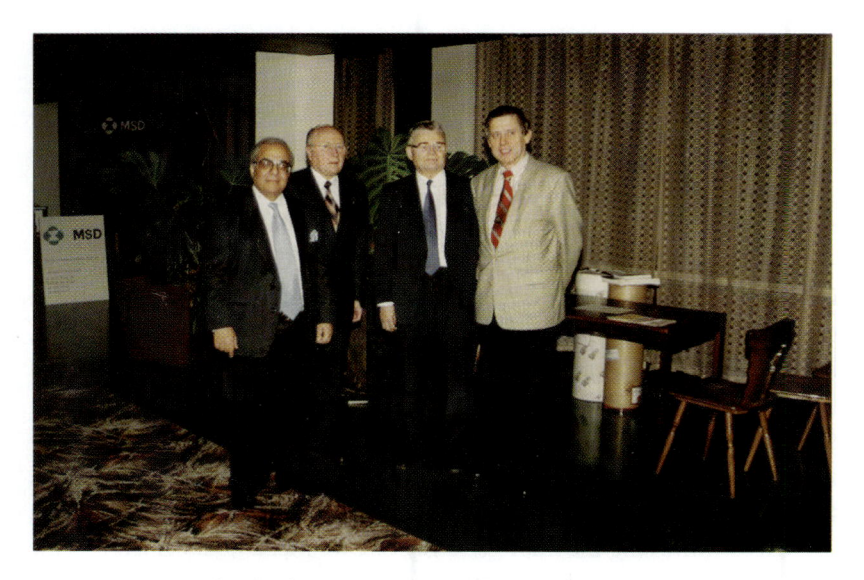

Figure 130. Prof. Shaul Massry, the author, Prof. Franciszek Kokot and Prof. Eberhard Ritz.

From New Zealand we flew to Melbourne, Australia, where Jadwiga Szczepanik, one Halina's cousins, was living. We spent two days there. The main attraction was Melbourne Zoo, which has all the classic Australian animals, especially koalas, kangaroos and wombats. Some say that the koala's life is perfect: 22 hours of sleep, two hours of feeding, and otherwise doing nothing. Koalas eat virtually nothing but eucalypt leaves, and perhaps it is their eucalyptus-only diet that makes them so sleepy. It is a curious thing that some people live their life similar to that of a koala — except that their food is different. In any event, our travels in Australasia came to a conclusion in Sydney. We made the obligatory visit to the Opera House, and I gave my two presentations [Pr 431, Pr 432].

For the Nephrology Summer School in Kraków, organized by Professor Eberhard Ritz, from Heidelberg, Germany, and Prof. Franciszek Kokot, I was invited to present my take on the vascular access for hemodialysis [Pr 433]. Prof. Shaul Massry[13] was also invited to the meeting

---

13. Director of the Division of Nephrology, University of Southern California, Los Angeles, Prof. Massry holds 10 honorary doctorates from universities in Bologna, Marseille, Prague, Pescu, Košice and Szeged, and medical schools in Poznań, Lublin, Gdansk and Katowice. A friend of Poland and Polish people, he has coauthored several of his works with Polish scholars, and many Polish professors have joined the nephrology division at his university as visiting professors. He has also visited Poland several times, giving lectures at numerous meetings.

(Fig. 130). We had a discussion about why the results with hemodialysis are worse in the U.S. than in other parts of the world. In my opinion part of the reason is linked to patient selection, but it also has to do with the generally accepted schedule of short dialysis in the U.S. To attain sufficient dialysis efficiency, high blood flows and sometimes two stack dialyzers have been used. This not only caused problems with achieving a true dry body weight, because of rapid ultrafiltration, but was also very demanding for blood access (high blood flows, large needles). Fistulas sufficient for 200 mL/min or 300 mL/min blood flows were not good enough for 500 mL/min or 600 mL/min blood flows. Such fistulas were replaced by arteriovenous graft access or central venous catheters. In recent years I frequently repeated these reasons for high hemodialysis mortality in the U.S. in papers and presentations, but so far the practice of hemodialysis in the U.S. has not changed. The reasons are ultimately a matter of financing and organization.

In the fall, the 30th Annual Meeting and Scientific Exposition of the American Society of Nephrology was held in San Antonio, Texas. My first presentation was related to the society's Belding H. Scribner Award bestowed upon Dr. Karl D. Nolph [Pr 434]. In my presentation I cited President Eisenhower's categorization of leaders: those who push and those who pull. Followers behave usually like a thread: if a thread is pushed, it wrinkles and goes nowhere; if a thread is pulled, it goes where it is pulled. In my estimation Dr. Nolph was a puller, not a pusher, and richly deserved the award. My next two presentations were in poster forums at the same meeting [Pr 435, Pr 436].

1998

I gave just five presentations in the U.S in 1998. The first, on the symptomatology of acute lead intoxication, was for our hospital's medical grand round [Pr 437]. That year Nashville, Tennessee, was the venue for our annual conference on peritoneal dialysis and the 4th International Symposium on Home Hemodialysis. For the first time we started awarding those who had contributed to the development of hemodialysis. Our first awardee was Vittorio Bonomini, from Bologna, Italy, for his contribution to the development of frequent hemodialysis [Pr 438, Pu 272]. I had three further presentations there [Pr 439–Pr 441].

1999

In 1999 I personally delivered only five presentations, three of which were for our annual conference and the 5th International Symposium on Home Hemodialysis in Charlotte, North Carolina. The first presentation was a tribute to Prof. Paul E. Teschan, our conference's second awardee, for his contribution to the development of frequent hemodialysis [Pr 442, Pu 286]. The next two were related to the problems caused by high dialyzer blood flow [Pr 443] and the influence of frequency and duration of dialysis sessions on patients [Pr 444]. In June I gave two presentations as part of the vascular access training agenda at Kendall headquarters in Mansfield, Massachusetts [Pr 445, Pr 446].

I retired on September 1 and took on a part-time job as chairman of the hemodialysis part of our Annual Dialysis Conference. Dr. Nolph also retired that same year, and Dr. Ramesh Khanna became the director of the division. Dr. Nolph retained a part-time position as the overall chairman of the dialysis conference. I no longer had any follow-up with patients, so I could spend part of my time in Columbia (usually October to April) and part of it in Kraków (usually May to September). Fortunately, various tasks related to the organization of the conference could now be done via the Internet. My tolerance for jet lag had diminished with age, so I decided to give presentations in the Eastern Hemisphere while staying in Poland and the Western Hemisphere when in the U.S. In the latter half of the year I coauthored three presentations that were delivered by the first authors [Pr 447–Pr 449].

2000

I delivered 10 presentations in 2000, but only seven personally. The first was a presentation via the Internet on quotidian dialysis [Pr 450], while the remainder was presented during our annual conference and the 6th International Symposium on Home Hemodialysis, which were in the Moscone Convention Center in San Francisco, California, in February [Pr 451–Pr 456]. After the meeting we decided to visit some places in California, Nevada and Arizona. We rented a car and drove to Yosemite National Park, one of the first wilderness parks in the U.S., best known for its waterfalls. We then visited our son, Przemek, and his wife, Kasia, in Pasadena. After that, we headed to Las Vegas — I remember driving through really heavy torrential rain — and watched a performance by the dance company the Rockettes. I also lost US$20 playing in the casino (that was my rule: stop playing after losing 20 bucks). From Las Vegas we visited Hoover Dam, a really impressive construction. I was surprised to learn that Lake Mead contains enough water to generate power, which is generated in step with, and only with, the release of water in response to downstream water demands. Our next stop was Williams, Arizona, where we took a train to the Grand Canyon, only to find less than ideal weather spoiling the view. From Williams we drove through Sedona to Phoenix and were treated to the colorful rock formations along the way. We left our rented car in Phoenix and took a flight back to Columbia.

My next three presentations, in October that year, were given as posters for coauthored studies. I was in Toronto, Ontario, to participate in discussions on our findings and present the posters during the 33rd Annual Meeting and the 2000 Renal Week of the American Society of Nephrology [Pr 457–Pr 459]. On October 14 we had an executive meeting of the founding members of the International Society for Hemodialysis. In the evening we went to the Prince of Wales Theatre, in the Entertainment District, to see the musical *The Lion King*. The following day we took a tour to the Niagara Peninsula to visit Magnotta Winery Estates. We learned about the production of ice wine and sparkling ice wine, a dessert wine produced from grapes that have been frozen while still on the vine. Later we took a *Maid of the Mist* boat tour to see the Niagara Falls from the Canadian side. The next day, on Monday, we took a tour of Toronto organized by Olde Towne Tours. Among the many attractions, what I most vividly remember were numerous huge, life-sized fiberglass moose sculptures.

2001

I had even fewer presentations in 2001. Our conference changed its name from "Annual Conference on Peritoneal Dialysis" to "Annual Dialysis Conference." For our 21st Annual Dialysis Conference and the 7th International Symposium on Hemodialysis, I delivered just two presentations. The first was related to the Lifetime Achievement Award for Dr. Bernard Charra, who had used long hemodialysis in his patients to achieve the best results ever shown, with excellent blood pressure control and the longest survival rate in the world [Pr 460, Pu 329]. My second presentation was a welcome address on new developments in hemodialysis [Pr 461]. In addition to this, I had one presentation in Kansas City, Missouri. [Pr 462] and one in Kraków, Poland [Pr 463].

2002

In 2002 the 22nd Annual Dialysis Conference was held in Tampa, Florida. My first presentation honored the lifetime achievements of Belding H. Scribner, the father of chronic hemodialysis [Pr 464, Pu 337]. A further two were related to my studies on the tailoring of hemodialysis catheters to patient anthropometrics [Pr 465], and my approach to dialysis adequacy [Pr 466]. I also gave a presentation on daily home hemodialysis during a meeting on "Renal Care in the 21st Century" in St. Louis, Missouri [Pr 467], as well as a presentation in Kraków on my adventures with dialysis therapy [Pr 469]. A coauthored poster presentation for the European Renal Association/European Dialysis and Transplant Association was given by the first author [Pr 468].

2003

In 2003 the International Society for Hemodialysis organized the first International Short Daily Hemodialysis (SDHD) Symposium, one day before our Annual Dialysis Conference. I gave a presentation showing that frequent hemodialysis is not detrimental to blood access [Pr 470]. In the main conference I delivered a keynote address on the fallacies of short dialysis with high dialyzer blood flow [Pr 471] as well as a laudation for Albert Leslie Babb, the father of the proportioning dialysate delivery system for hemodialysis [Pr 472, Pu 344]. I also coauthored four poster presentations that were given by the first authors [Pr 473–Pr 476]. I was also invited by the American Nephrology Nurses' Association to give a lecture on the fallacies of high-speed hemodialysis [Pr 477]. Our last coauthored poster presentation that year was given by Dr. Carl Kjellstrand at the American Society of Nephrology Renal Week in San Diego, California [Pr 478].

2004

In February 2004 the International Society for Hemodialysis again organized a symposium one day before the Annual Dialysis Conference in San Antonio, Texas. I had one presentation at the symposium [Pr 479], and during the main conference I presented a laudation for Dr. Claudio Ronco [Pr 480, Pu 354] and gave two more talks on dialyzer reuse [Pr 481] and global clinical assessment as the best criterion of dialysis adequacy [Pr 484]. In the slide forum, Dr. Kjellstrand presented the results of our two studies related to factors influencing cardiovascular instability in daily hemodialysis [Pr 482] and advantages of hot water reuse of dialyzers over single use or chemical reuse of dialyzers [Pr 483]. He also presented two posters on similar topics in Lisbon, Portugal [Pr 485] and Toronto, Ontario [Pr 486], and in the slide forum during the 50th Anniversary Conference of the American Society for Artificial Internal Organs [Pr 487]. I gave two more presentations on the fallacies of short, high efficiency hemodialysis, in Kraków [Pr 488] and in Chicago [Pr 489].

2005

In 2005 I gave three presentations during our Annual Dialysis Conference [Pr 490–Pr 492] and three in Columbia, Missouri [Pr 493–Pr 495].

2006

In 2006, in accordance with my new post-retirement schedule, I gave three presentations in the U.S. during my stay in Columbia, and four in Europe whilst staying in Kraków. My first presentation on the perfect dialysis access was delivered during our Annual Dialysis Conference in San Francisco, California. I described various accesses for hemodialysis and peritoneal dialysis, stressing the value of accesses based on my studies, such as the Swan Neck peritoneal catheter, the palindrome catheter and the buttonhole method of fistula cannulation [Pr 496]. I was asked to deliver a similar talk [Pr 497] in Columbia, as not everybody from our division was able to attend the San Francisco meeting. Dr. Nolph and I were invited to Vicenza, Italy, for the 15th International Vicenza Course on

Peritoneal Dialysis, which fit my summer schedule as the course was from May 30 to June 1.

Halina and I decided to take advantage of our trip to Italy and visit some interesting places there as well as in Austria. On May 28, we drove in our Opel Astra from Kraków through Slovakia and Austria to Vicenza. Our first stop was in Eisenstadt, Austria, where we stayed in the Hotel Burgenland on Franz Schubert Platz. There is a Holy Trinity column in the square; in the territories that historically belonged to the Austro-Hungarian Empire, it is quite exceptional to find an old town square without such a column. Eisenstadt was a city where many famous musicians lived and performed. Franz Joseph Haydn, for instance, lived there for 14 years. He was the Kappellmeister, the director of music, for Prince Paul Anton and later Prince Nikolaus "the Magnificent." We visited the Haydn Museum, situated close to Haydn's house, and the magnificent Haydnsaal in the Schloss Esterházy (Esterházy Palace), the only remaining residence of that famous Hungarian family, which was known as a great patron of the musical arts. Eisenstadt's musical past is reflected not only in the name of the square (Schubert) but also in numerous streets named after musicians from the 18th century (Haydn) and the 19th century (Franz Liszt).

On the way from Eisenstadt to Villach in Austria we encountered torrential rain, but fortunately the weather was better once we approached Italy. As there was no border control, we could only tell we had left Austria and arrived in Italy when the signposts changed from German to Italian. My Garmin GPS system unfortunately performed mediocrely. It had helped us in Eisenstadt — an old city with no new road works — but failed in Vicenza, where there was some recent road construction. In any event, when we finally entered the old part of Vicenza, the system directed us nicely to our hotel. We arrived at Hotel Boscolo de la Ville in Viale Verona in the afternoon of May 29, the course taking place in the Congress Center Ente Fiera the next day (Fig. 131). I delivered my first presentation in the afternoon [Pr 498]. The next day I had to deliver a talk for Dr. Nolph, who had developed a laryngeal infection and lost his voice, but I was able to use a PowerPoint presentation he had prepared [Pr 499]. In the evening a faculty dinner was organized in Basilica Palladiana. On the last day of the course I gave a talk on the history of peritoneal access [Pr 500]. In this presentation, for the first time,

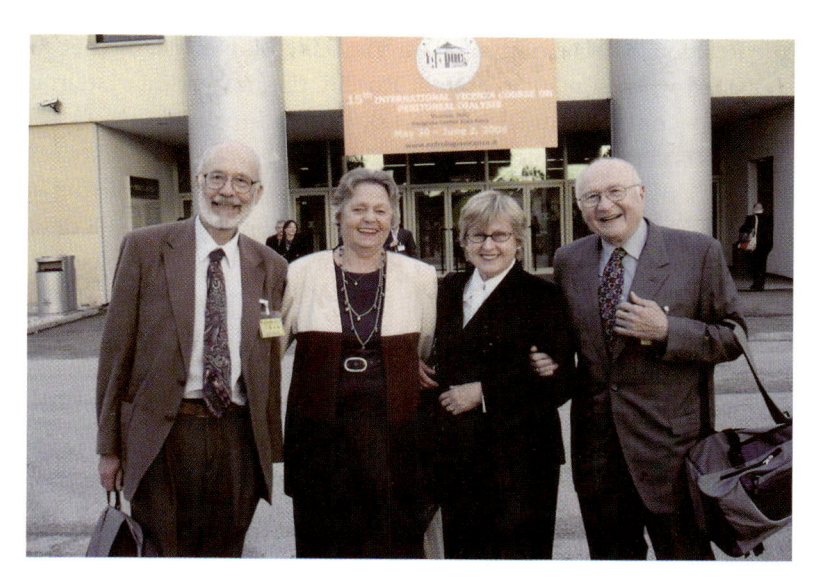

Figure 131. Karl, Georgia, Halina and the author in front of the Congress Center Ente Fiera, Vicenza, Italy.

I compared biological and technological evolution, a comparison that was taken from Stanisław Lem's amazing book, *Summa technologiae* ("Sum of Technology").[14] A new species comes into being imperceptibly, its structure taken from existing forms; new technological solutions also develop from existing forms. The new species gradually changes its form and develops new features adapting to a new environment, which gives rise to new varieties; the new technology also gradually evolves, finding new solutions and performing better for a given intended use. A species (or technology) not adapted to the environment (or requirements) is eliminated and is preserved in fossils (or museums of technology). These similarities are also true in the development of peritoneal access. Later that evening we had a gala dinner in Villa Imperiali Lampertico.

The day after the course we went on a tour through the country. The priority was Florence, as we had never been there before. Using the GPS system with a relatively new map of Italy, I immediately realized that the most recent changes, especially new road construction, are not reflected on even the newest map. We had a hotel reservation

---

14. Lem S. (1984) *Dwie ewolucje, podobienstwa* (Two evolutions, similarities). In: *Summa Technologiae,* 4th ed. Wydawnictwo Lubelskie, Lublin, pp. 14–19.

at the Residence Palazzo Risacoli on Via Delle Mantellate, but because of the road works on Viale Fratelli Roselli, the navigation system got completely confused and I had to ask people for directions. Asking directions is very frustrating for a man. (One of my favorite jokes asks: Why did Moses take 40 years to travel from Egypt to the Promised Land?)[15] The experience confirmed my suspicion that my GPS device was accurate in places unchanged for years but was not so useful in places with new roads and changing traffic directions. Such changes are particularly frequent in cities, so I made a rule of stopping at a gas station just before entering a new city, filling up and buying a recent city map. Hopefully this rule can be relaxed in the near future when navigation systems come with recent maps.

Our hotel was in a very convenient spot within walking distance of places we wanted to see. We first went to the Cattedrale Di Santa Maria Del Fiore on the Piazza del Duomo. I wanted to go to the cupola, one of the most famous domes in the world, built by Filippo Brunelleschi, a renowned architect who created special lifting devices and lewissons for hoisting heavy objects. He also designed a lantern to crown the dome. The project was finished in 1461 by his friend Michelozzo 15 years after Brunelleschi's death. A bronze ball was designed and hoisted on top of the lantern by Andrea del Verrocchio in 1469. It is believed that the young Leonardo da Vinci participated in the design of the ball and made several sketches of the machines used for hoisting the ball. Regrettably, my desire to get to the dome was thwarted by the simple fact that the cupola was under repair at the time.

The next day we visited several museums. We first went to Via Cavour to see *Le Macchine di Leonardo da Vinci*, an exhibition of 50 model machines based on da Vinci's sketches. The collection of inventions, which were displayed in four separate rooms, was unbelievable. It is impossible to describe them all, but at least a few are worth mentioning. There were ball bearings, an anemometer (to measure wind speed), an inclinometer (to determine the elevation of a flying machine in relation to Earth), odometers, hoisters, cogwheels, gear shifts, a machine for cutting files, machines that transform continuous motion

---

15. Answer (because he was a real man after all): He was too stubborn to stop and ask for directions.

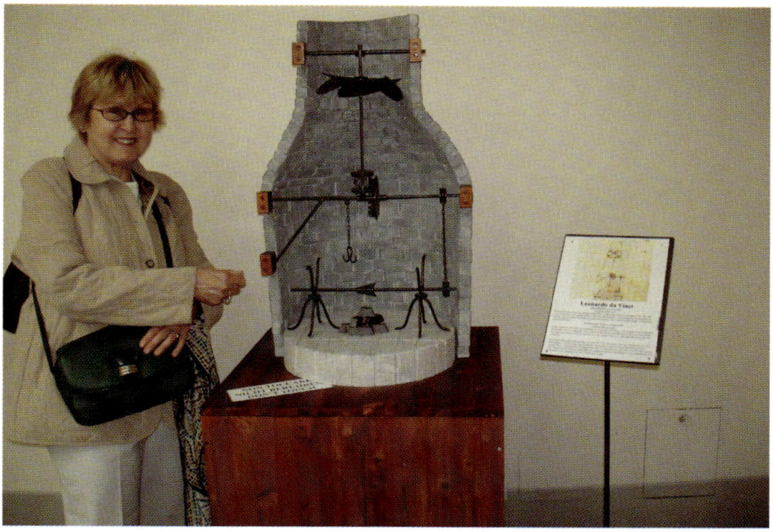

Figure 132. Automated roasting spit (Leonardo da Vinci).

into alternating motion or vice versa (cars work on this principle), tanks, machine guns, submarines, and more. There was even an automated roasting spit (Fig. 132), which impressed Halina. The machine used hot air as a source of energy: the rising air spun a propeller, which engaged a pole with a pulley at the end, which in turn rotated the spit. The more intense the fire, the faster the rotation of the spit. I was also taken with his glider, his arched bridge and a miniature model of the horse that Da Vinci made for Lodovico Sforza, Duke of Milan (Fig. 133). This clay sculpture, which was finished in 1495 and displayed in Milan, was to be cast in bronze, but this was never carried out, as the model was destroyed by an invading French army in 1498. We then went to the Palazzo Medici Riccardi on Via Cavour, where an impressive museum has now been established. The palace was bought by the Medici family in 14th century and embellished by Cosimo the Elder in the mid-15th century and by Lorenzo the Magnificent at the end of that century. In the courtyard, or the courtyard of columns, which lies in the center of the oldest part of the palace, is a statue by Baccio Bandinelli of Orpheus charming Cerberus with his music. The statue was commissioned by Giovanni, Lorenzo's second son, who later became Pope Leo X. In the garden is a sculpture of Hercules, while in

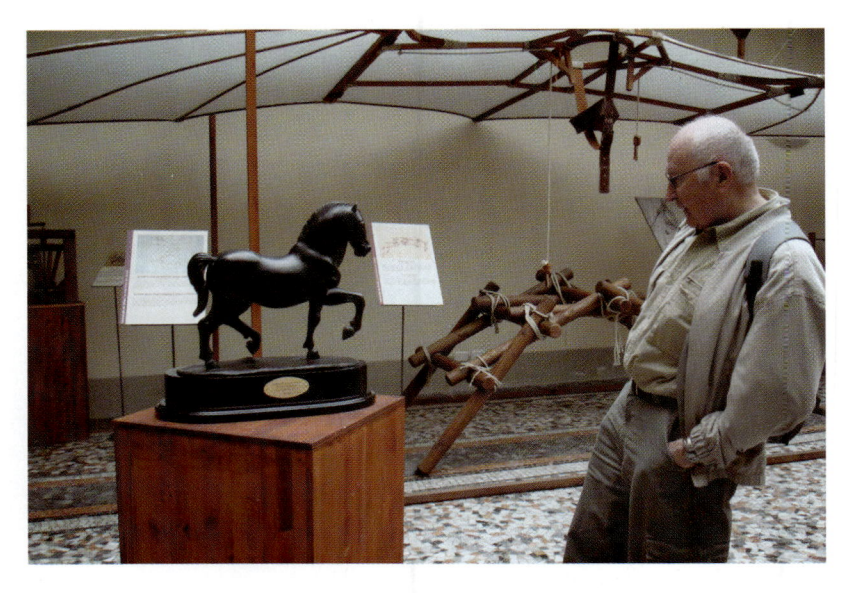

Figure 133. Glider, arched bridge and model of a horse (Leonardo da Vinci).

the basement is the Museum of Ancient Marbles, mostly Greek, created by Riccardo Riccardi (1558–1612), a successful banker and erudite humanist. We also visited the Magi Chapel, the Reception Rooms and Luca Giordano's Gallery, where there are paintings and sculptures representing the "cardinal virtues" and the "capital sins." One had the inscription "*Semper rectus*" (always right), and Halina told me that I probably thought that this inscription was about me, as I was always of the opinion that I was right (which is not true, of course). Halina liked the third one, "*Vitio poena vitium*," as she will always say that fault begets fault, error begets error, malice begets malice, and anger begets anger.

The next stop was the Galleria dell'Accademia (Academy Gallery) on the Via Ricasoli, which was very nearby, but we had to wait in line for two hours before we could get in. One good thing about being old is that in Italy one may enter most museums free of charge. Of course, the museum staff checked our passports very carefully to make sure that we really were old, because looking at us they apparently thought we were youngsters (really?). In any event, we finally made it to the gallery where most of Michelangelo's original sculptures are located. Unfortunately, picture taking, even without flash, was forbidden — though booklets with pictures of the sculptures were available in the souvenir shop. The most impressive sculpture, not surprisingly, was that of David. And it was a huge sculpture: 17 feet (5.17 meters). I was told that Michelangelo made the statue in such a way that the lower part of the body was proportionally smaller than the upper part. In this way looking at the sculpture from below makes the statue appear in perfect proportion. It was a long wait in line, but it was well worth it. We also went to Piazza della Signoria and looked at the copy of the David sculpture in front of Palazzo Vecchio (The Old Palace), where the original sculpture was located in 1504 until it was moved to the Academy Gallery in 1873 to protect it from potential damage. The replica was made by Arrighetti and placed in the original's position in the Piazza della Signoria in 1910.

From Florence we took the A1 (E35 and E45) to Cassino in the Lazio region and checked into Hotel La Pace on Via Abruzzi. Most of the cars drove much faster than the speed limit of 130 kph (81 mph), and many, including me, over 160 kph (100 mph). Halina asked me to slow down, as her cardiac arrhythmia was making her feel unwell. I slowed down to 70 or 80 mph, which made her feel better, but even after we arrived at Cassino multiple premature contractions were present. They seemed more like ventricular than atrial, as I felt compensatory pauses in her pulse. I suspected that in addition to stress, the change in diet with less potassium could have been the cause. A few hours after eating bananas, strawberries and other fruit, her arrhythmia markedly improved.

The only real reason we came to Cassino was to visit Monte Cassino, where one can find the Cemetery of Polish Soldiers commemorating their role in liberating the Abbey from German occupation in 1944 (Fig. 134). At the foot of the cemetery, where 1,051 Polish soldiers are interred, is written an epigram, *Przechodniu powiedz Polsce żeśmy polegli w jej służbie* (Passerby, tell Poland that we fell here faithfully in her service). This spot was important for the German effort to slow down the advancement of Allied forces toward Rome. The monastery had an excellent view of the surrounding hills and valleys, and thus was a natural site for German artillery observers. There were four battles for the site starting in January 1944, with Polish troops ultimately taking the abbey on May 18. We also visited an impressive monastery founded by St. Benedict in 529 AD. The monastery was

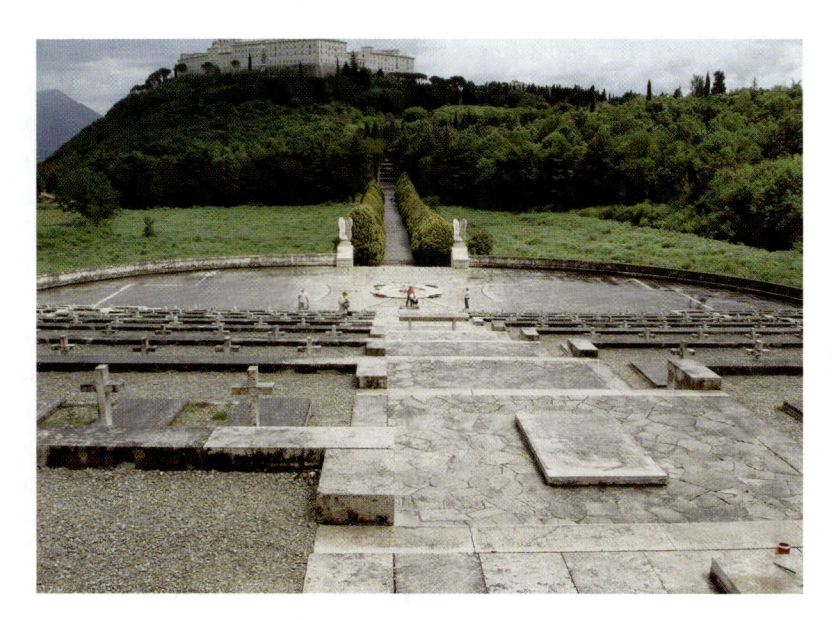

Figure 134. Polish war cemetery in Monte Cassino, Italy.

destroyed by Longobards in 577, then by the Saracens in 833, by an earthquake in 1349, and in a series of heavy Allied air raids on February 15, 1944. The abbey was rebuilt after the war, with financing provided by the Italian state. Pope Paul VI reconsecrated it in 1964.

The next day we drove to Pompeii, located on the Bay of Naples, about 70 miles (110 km) from Cassino (about 150 miles, or 240 km, to the southeast of Rome). The Autostrada Del Sole highway had recently been extended from Rome toward Napoli, so it was not picked up by our GPS system. On the screen it appeared as if we were driving through an open field. Pompeii is in a region called Campania (or Campagna, which means "countryside" in Italian), on a plateau of Vesuvian lava. Most people know about the eruption of Vesuvius in 79 AD, but fewer people know that in 5960 BC and 3580 BC, there were two eruptions that rate among the largest known in Europe. We arrived at the Scavi di Pompeii just before noon on Monday, June 5, to visit the excavations of the old city destroyed by the eruption on August 24, AD 79, according to one version of the text of Pliny's letter. It would be a strange coincidence that it happened the day after Vulcanalia, the festival of the Roman god of fire. There are disputes about the exact date of the eruption, as some archeological excavations indicate that it happened two months later, which is supported by another version of Pliny's letter giving the date of the eruption as November 23. Pliny the Younger lost his uncle, Pliny the Elder, with whom he had a close relationship. His uncle died while attempting to rescue stranded victims. As admiral of the fleet, he had ordered the ships of the Imperial Navy stationed at Misenum to cross the bay to assist evacuation attempts. After thick layers of ash covered the town, it was abandoned and eventually its name and location were forgotten.

The first time any part of the city was unearthed was in 1599, when the digging of an underground channel to divert the river Sarno ran into ancient walls covered with paintings and inscriptions. However, the many lascivious paintings were not considered to be in good taste in the fiercely moralistic and classicist climate of the time and were covered again until they were rediscovered as a result of deliberate excavations in 1748 and later in the following centuries. Later discoveries of household items also had a sexual theme. The ubiquity of such imagery and items indicates that the sexual mores of the ancient Roman culture were extremely liberal. For instance, many bathhouses essentially served as brothels. I was told that the Latin word *fornicatio* (fornication) was coined in Pompeii.[16] The area is huge, so we visited only selected places, including the Forum, the Temple of Apollo, and the Amphitheater. We did not go to the Villa Dei Mysteri (Villa of the Mysteries), which is quite far from the other places; this is where most of the sexually explicit paintings can be seen. The name comes after decorations portraying a "megalography" representing the ancient rituals of the Dionysian mysteries. Among many houses, we saw the House of Venus in the Shell (Fig. 135) and the House of the Faun, where we were greeted with the Latin *have* (meaning "welcome") (Fig. 136). (The Latin word *have* has nothing to do with English "have," so people should not assume that they can take whatever they want.) In the center of the *impluvium*[17] is a bronze statue of the "faun" (Fig. 137). In the afternoon we returned to Cassino.

---

16. The Latin word *fornix*, from which "fornication" is derived, meant "a vault, an arch." The term also referred to a vaulted cellar or similar place where prostitutes plied their trade. This sense of *fornix* in Late Latin yielded the verb *fornicari*, "to commit fornication," from which is derived *fornicatio*.

17. *Impluvium* is a low basin in the center of the household atrium, into which rainwater flowed down from the roof opening (*compluvium*).

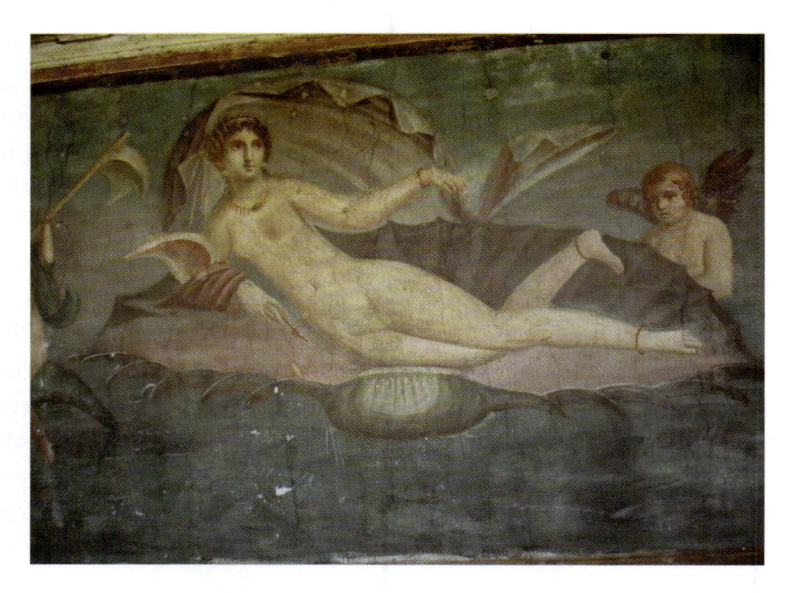

Figure 135. House of Venus in the Shell, Pompeii, Italy.

On Tuesday, June 6, we drove to Rimini. I decided to take a shortcut through the SS509 to the A25 and then on highways along the Adriatic Sea to Rimini. Unfortunately, the entrance to the SS509 from Cassino was under construction, but my GPS system managed to navigate us through various village roads to the SS509. This was evidently because these roads were old enough to be recognized by the system, confirming my experience that such systems are best on old, unchanged roads. In Rimini we stayed in the Mercure La Grandisca hotel on Via Fiume, close to the Adriatic Sea. In the afternoon we went to a beach and I was able to catch some good bodysurfing waves. Later we strolled around town and noted with surprise that one street was named after a Pole, Ludwik Lejzer Zamenhof, the creator of Esperanto (Fig. 138).[18] The next day we

---

18. Ludwik Lazarus Zamenhof was born on December 15, 1859, in the town of Białystok (in Poland, then part of the Russian Empire). The town's population was made up of three major ethnic groups: Poles, Byelorussians and a large group of Yiddish-speaking Jews. Zamenhof was saddened and frustrated by the many quarrels between these groups. He theorized that the main reason for the hate and prejudice lay in mutual misunderstanding caused by the lack of one common language that would play the role of a neutral communication tool between people of different ethnic and linguistic backgrounds. His native languages were Russian, Yiddish and Polish, but he also spoke many other languages. In 1887, he published a book, *Lingvo internacia: Antaŭparolo kaj plena lernolibro* (International language: Foreword and complete textbook), under the pseudonym "Doktoro Esperanto" (Doctor Hopeful), from which the name of the language derives. Zamenhof studied medicine and practiced ophthalmology.

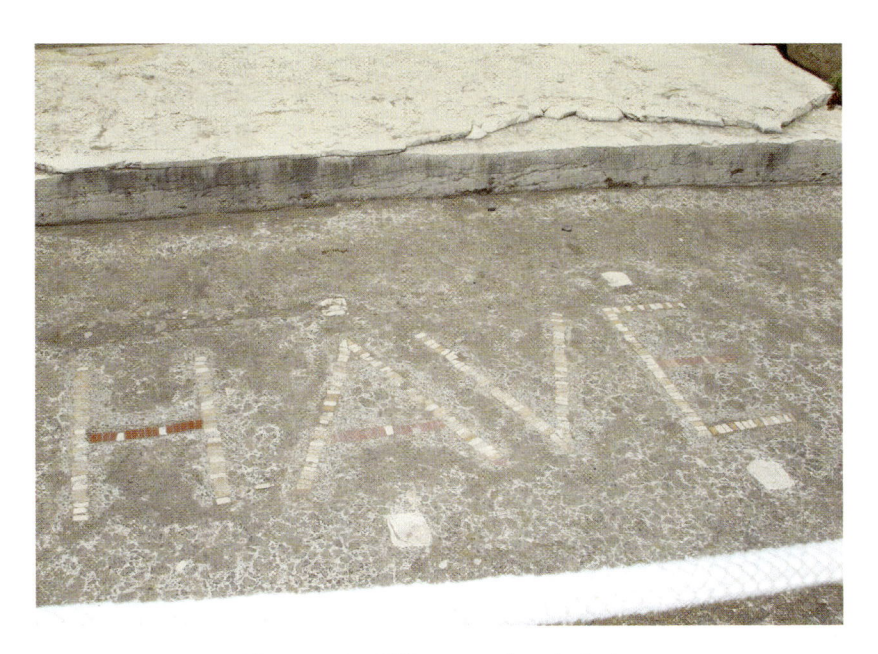

Figure 136. Welcome, or *have* in Latin.

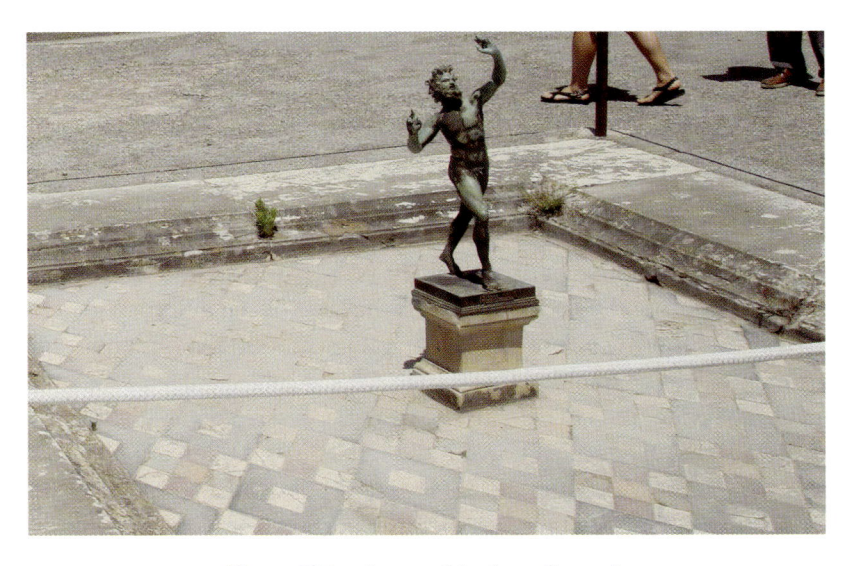

Figure 137. Statue of the faun, Pompeii.

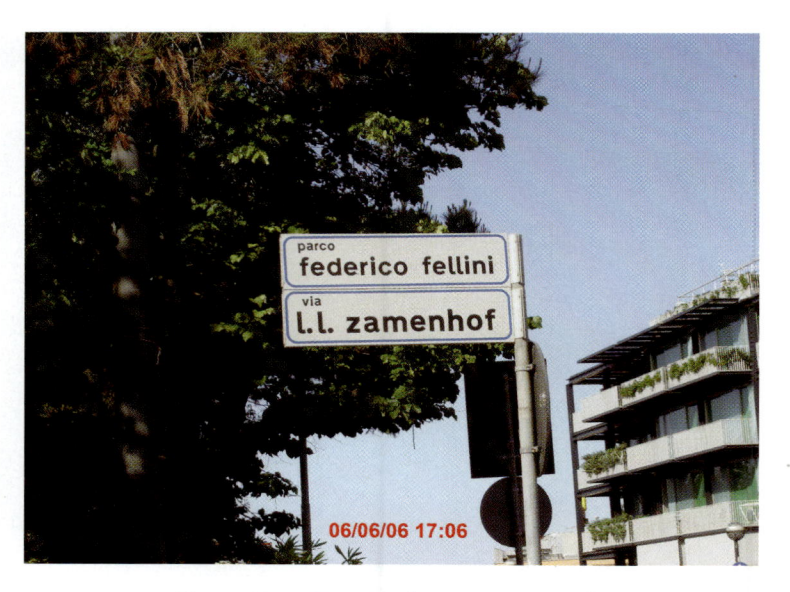

Figure 138. Zamenhof Street, Rimini, Italy.

went to Ravenna, which is about 33 miles (53 km) from Rimini. As the Rubicon River flows from the Apennine Mountains to the Adriatic Sea with an estuary between Ravenna and Rimini, we crossed the Rubicon (Latin: *Rubico*; Italian: *Rubicone*) in both directions, although we did not notice this fact, as there were no signs for the river. Only later did we discover that what was called the Rubicon River is now Fiumicino, which crosses the town of Savignano sul Rubicone. It is amazing that throughout the centuries such an important river, separating the province of Cisalpine Gaul from Italy proper, was almost completely forgotten. During the first century BC, the law obliged a Roman general to disband his army before crossing the Rubicon otherwise both he and his men would be found guilty of high treason and sacrilege, and automatically condemned to death. When Julius Caesar, after assembling his army in Ravenna, decided to cross the Rubicon and uttered the famous phrase "*alea iacta est*" (the die has been cast) on January 19, 49 BC, the civil war with Pompey the Great became inevitable and ended with the defeat of Pompey on the plain of Pharsalus in Thessaly.

Ravenna, situated at the Adriatic Sea, was already an important town in the first century BC, when it was chosen by Emperor

Octavian Augustus as the port for his East Mediterranean fleet. The enormous Porto di Classe was built to provide shelter for what was the strongest fleet in the empire. A huge statue of Octavian Augustus is located in Classe (Fig. 139), close to the Basilica St. Apollinare. In the photo, behind the statue, the bell tower of the basilica with mullioned windows is visible. St. Apollinare came from Antioch in the Roman Province of Syria and was made the first bishop of Ravenna by St. Peter himself. He was persecuted and martyred in AD 79. The basilica bearing his name was built in AD 549. Ravenna became a very important city and by AD 402 was the capital of the Western Roman Empire. Surprisingly, neither Ravenna nor Classe is close to the Adriatic Sea these days. Porto di Classe has been silted throughout the centuries and is now located

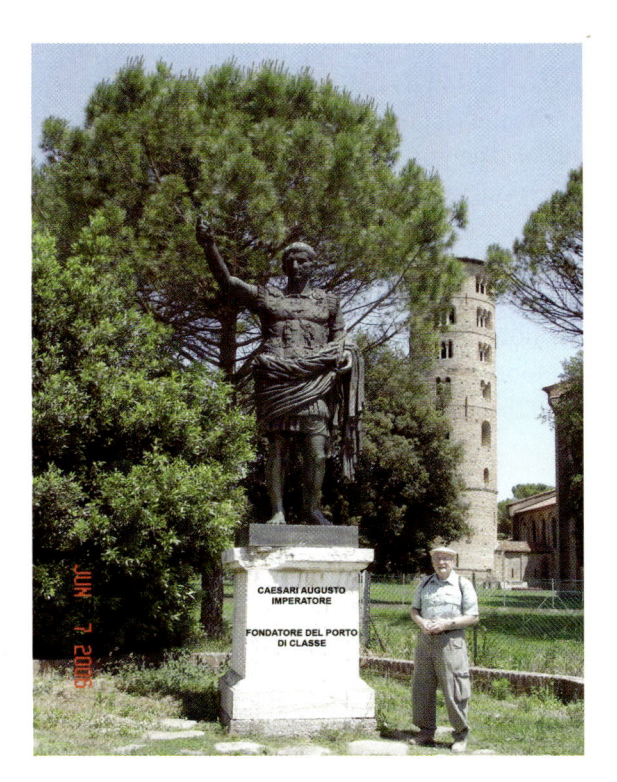

Figure 139. Statue of Octavian Augustus, Classe, near Ravenna, Italy. Behind the statue is the bell tower with mullioned windows.

about 3 miles (5 km) from the sea. We enjoyed visiting many churches and other places in Ravenna and returned to Rimini in the afternoon. On Thursday, June 8, we drove to Villach in Austria, once again surprised that there was no border control and only realizing that we had left Italy when the signposts switched back to German. In Villach we stayed in the Romantik Post Hotel on Hauptplatz. We took Paracelsus Strasse to the car park behind the hotel, and I found the name a little surprising since Paracelsus was associated, in my mind, with Switzerland. I learned that Paracelsus' father, Wilhelm Bombast von Hohenheim, lived and practiced medicine in Villach. His son, having left to study medicine in Basel at the age of 16, lived in many places and is buried in Salzburg, but never returned to Villach. It was a very nice little town with a Marian and Holy Trinity Column (Fig. 140), typical of Austrian towns.

We returned to Kraków the following day, and I gave a presentation at the Progress in Nephrology Symposium jointly organized by Prof. Wladyslaw Sulowicz, the chairman of the Department of Nephrology of the Jagiellonian University Foundation for the Development of Dialytic Treatment in Kraków, the International Society for Hemodialysis, and the Polish Society of Nephrology. I talked about the buttonhole method of needle insertion [Pr 501], my first presentation in Poland on the method. After returning to the U.S. I gave a presentation for our division on the problem of sodium balance, hypertension and the so-called "lag phenomenon," a delay in the decrease in blood pressure after a balance of sodium has been achieved [Pr 502].

2007

In 2007 I gave only five presentations: three in the U.S. and two in Istanbul, Turkey. For the first presentation, I was invited by Nathan W. Levin, MD, the founder of the Renal Research Institute, which is a joint venture of Fresenius Medical Care North America and the Beth Israel Medical Center, New York City. Dr. Levin organizes an annual meeting called Advances in CKD, presenting lectures and moderating debates related to dialysis treatment of chronic kidney disease. He wanted me to debate with Frank Gotch, MD, on the value of urea clearance and blood pressure control in the

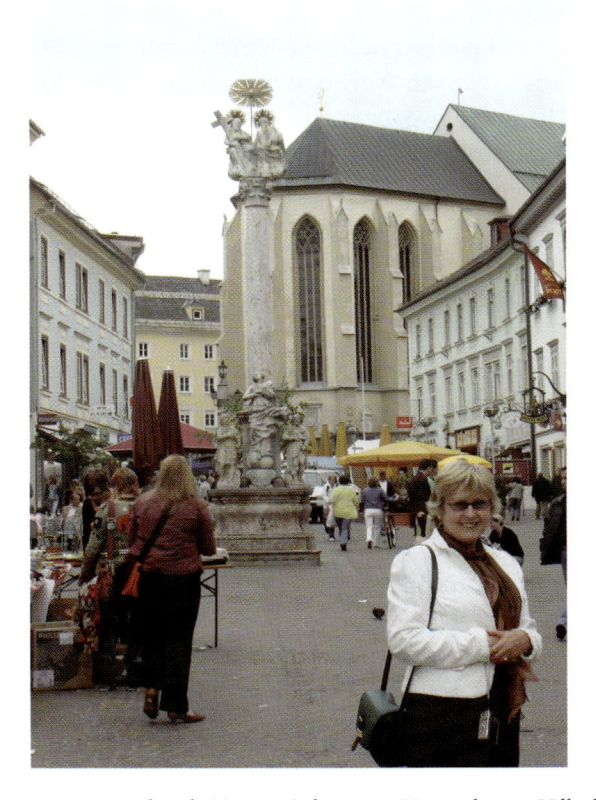

Figure 140. Marian and Holy Trinity Column on Hauptplatz in Villach, Austria.

assessment of dialysis adequacy. In my presentation I insisted that treatment time and ultrafiltration rate are more important in dialysis prescription than small molecule clearance [Pr 503]. Although my opponent in the debate, one of the creators of the Kt/V[19] concept, could not agree completely with me, he admitted that administering dialysis over longer periods of time is important for better control of fluid status and blood pressure. The proceedings

---

19. Kt/V is a unitless index where K is the urea clearance, t is the time of dialysis, and V is the urea distribution volume, which approximately equals total body water. The original idea of the Kt/V concept was that shorter time of dialysis may be compensated by higher urea clearance to maintain the index at its desired value (originally more than 0.95, now about 1.3). Mathematically, it is obviously true, but clearances of other molecules, as well as removal of sodium and water, do not correlate with urea clearance. In hemodialysis, Kt/V may be calculated from predialysis (C_0) and postdialysis (C) urea concentrations {$\ln(C_0/C)$} without even knowing K, t and V.

from the meeting, which contained my presentation, were published in a special edition of *Blood Purification* [Pu 371]. The paper was later translated into German and published in 2008 [Pr 371a, Pr 371b]. The next two presentations were given at our Annual Dialysis Conference. I talked about the features of the ideal hemodialysis catheter [Pr 504] as well as the relationship between sodium balance and blood pressure control in hemodialysis patients [Pr 505].

I had also been invited by Ali Başçi, MD, Professor of Medicine at the Ege University School of Medicine, Department of Internal Medicine, Division of Nephrology in Izmir, Turkey, to give two presentations at the Medical Accreditation Meeting on May 13 organized by Ege University and Fresenius Medical Care. Dr. Başçi was aware of my publications related to the importance of blood pressure control by strict volume control in hemodialysis patients undergoing longer and/or more frequent hemodialyses. The organizers offered to cover all expenses for Halina and myself, including a sightseeing tour of Istanbul. We were asked to come to Istanbul a few days before the meeting. The best means of travel for us was to go from Columbia to St. Louis, then to Chicago, and finally through Warsaw. Unfortunately, Halina developed severe back pain, so she decided to go from Warsaw to Kraków, leaving me to go to Istanbul by myself. I arrived at Atatürk International Airport by LOT Polish Airlines, on LO 135, at 4:30 pm, Tuesday, May 8, and checked into Mega Residence Hotel, located in a new part of the city.

Istanbul is an old city with really fascinating and convoluted history. It was founded in 667 BC by Doric Greeks from Megara and named Byzantium after their king, Byzas. The Roman emperor Constantine the Great made the city the eastern capital of the Roman Empire and conferred the name *Nova Roma*. However, most people called it Constantinople, and it was this name that was used officially by the emperor Theodosius II at the beginning of the fifth century AD. From around the 10th century, when asked, "Where are you going?" local people used the expression $\varepsilon\iota\varsigma\ \tau\alpha\nu$ $\Pi\delta\lambda\iota\nu$ (*is tan polin*, meaning "to the city"). After the Turkish conquest of Constantinople in 1453, the name Istanbul, a corruption of *is tan polin*, began to be used, but Constantinople was only officially renamed Istanbul on March 28, 1930. Istanbul straddles the European part of Turkey, Rumelia, and the Asian part of Turkey, Anatolia. By long tradition, the waters in Istanbul are called "the three seas" — after the Golden Horn, the Bosporus and the Sea of Marmara. The Golden Horn is a deep, drowned valley about 4.5 miles (7 km) in length. Early inhabitants thought it was shaped like a deer horn, but modern Turks call it the Haliç ("Canal"). The narrow Golden Horn separates the old city of Stamboul to the south from the "new" city of Beyoğlu to the north. The broader Bosporus divides European Istanbul from the city's districts on the Asian shore: Üsküdar (ancient Chrysopolis) and Kadıköy (ancient Chalcedon). Two bridges connect the European and Asian parts of Istanbul: the Fatih Sultan Mehmet Bridge and the Bosporus (Bogaziçi) Bridge. The old city and Beyoğlu are connected with two bridges over the Golden Horn: the Atatürk Bridge and the Galata Bridge.

Dr. Başçi arranged a tour of Istanbul with the Creative Company on Wednesday, Thursday and Friday. On Wednesday morning, a van with a driver and freelance guide (Fig. 141) named Esra Cantürk picked us up from our hotel. We began our itinerary with the Hippodrome, the typical starting point of any old city tour. Built by the Romans in about 200 AD, the Hippodrome was originally used for chariot racing and other public events, and the stadium surrounding the track once held over 100,000 people. The Hippodrome was the center of life in Byzantine Constantinople for over 1,000 years, and later of Ottoman life in Istanbul for over 400 years. From the Hippodrome we went to the Sultan Ahmed Mosque, popularly known as the Blue Mosque, which has six minarets containing 16 balconies. The popular moniker comes from the blue tiles covering some interior walls and columns. Construction of the mosque by architect Sedefkar Mehmed Agha began in 1609 and it was completed seven years later. My guide told me that Sultan Ahmed wanted to have five golden minarets and was disappointed when he returned from the Hajj pilgrimage in Saudi Arabia and saw *six* minarets — none of which were golden. Ahga explained that he had misunderstood the order, as in Turkish *altin* (golden) sounds like *alti* (six). But the main

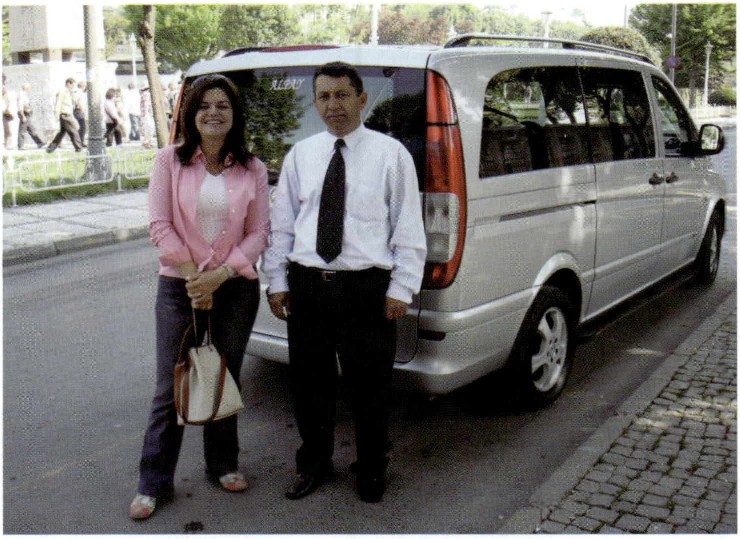

Figure 141. Guide and driver from Creative Co., Istanbul, Turkey.

issue was that the Sacred Mosque in Mecca also had six minarets, so the sultan sent money for a seventh minaret in Mecca and an affront was expiated. In any event, the Sultan Ahmed Mosque is really impressive.

Not far from Sultan Ahmed Square is Hagia Sophia (Greek for "Holy Wisdom"), another building with a long and convoluted history — as can be said of many buildings in Istanbul. Known as the Great Church (*Magna Ecclesia* in Latin), the first church was built by the order of Constantine the Great at the same location a pagan temple had once stood. It was Constantius II who inaugurated the Hagia Sophia on February 15, 360 AD. The church was largely burned down during riots in 404. Theodosius II ordered a second church to be built, inaugurating it on October 10, 415, but this church was completely destroyed during the tumult of the Nika Revolt[20] from January 13 to 14, 532. Only a short time after its destruction, Justinian the Great suppressed the riots, and

---

20. The Nika Revolt, or Nika Riots, started during a chariot race between supporters of different teams — the Blues, the Greens, the Reds and the Whites — but the real reason was the attempt to dethrone Emperor Justinian I, a supporter of the Blues. The name "Nika" comes from the Greek *Nίκα* (meaning "Win!" or "Conquer!"), which was chanted by the rioters. Justinian wanted to resign and flee, but his wife Theodora dissuaded him from surrendering and encouraged him to fight. He restored order with a heavy hand, massacring 30,000 rioters.

decided to rebuild the church. He commissioned two men, Anthemius of Tralles and Isidore the Elder of Miletus, to build a third church at the same location that was greater than its predecessors. Anthemius and Isidore were not real architects, but masters of the science of the mechanics. Anthemius was a mathematician and physicist, and Isidore was a professor of geometry and mechanics. Neither had any building experience before completing the Hagia Sophia, but they created one of the most significant monuments on Earth. The construction started only a short while after the end of the Nika Revolt, and the third church was inaugurated by the emperor on December 27, 537. It was the largest cathedral in the world for a thousand years. Despite several earthquakes, the church survived with only minimal reconstructions. On May 29, 1453, the Sultan of the Ottoman Empire, Mehmed II,[21] conquered Constantinople after a 54-day siege. He ordered the church be transformed into a mosque. Minarets were added; mosaics were not destroyed but covered with plaster. In 1934, the founder of the Turkish Republic, Mustafa Kemal Atatürk, ordered the building to be converted into a museum. The plaster covering the mosaics was pulled down, and floor carpets were removed, revealing the original marble décor. The museum opened on February 1, 1935. There are still some Arabic inscriptions in the church, but the mosaics are almost completely restored (Fig. 142).

The next item on our itinerary was the Topkapi Palace, which was built on the order of Mehmed II in 1470. It was originally named the New Palace, but because of huge cannons placed at the entrance, the people called it *Topkapi* (Turkish for "Cannon Gate"), and the name stuck. The palace complex is located on a promontory overlooking the Golden Horn and the Sea of Marmara with the Bosporus in plain sight from many points of the palace. It was a primary residence of Ottoman Sultans for about 400 years. After the end of the Ottoman Empire in 1921, the Topkapi Palace was transformed by government decree into a museum of the imperial era on April 3, 1924. The site is hilly and one of the highest points close to the sea. The palace is really huge, with four courtyards and numerous buildings, so it took me the whole afternoon to do it justice; seeing everything would likely have taken several days. I was intrigued by the chamber of the chief physician

---

21. In modern Turkish, Fatih Sultan Mehmet.

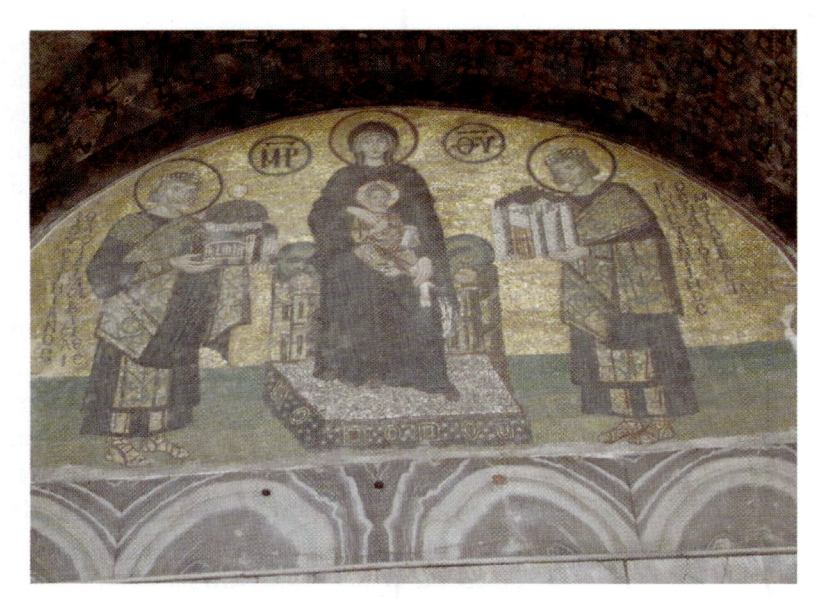

Figure 142. Tenth-century Mosaic in Hagia Sophia, Istanbul: Virgin Mary with a child, Emperor Justinian with model of Hagia Sophia (left) and Constantine the Great with model of Constantinople (right).

and the drugstore already operating in the 15th century. I visited the Imperial Treasury in the Second Courtyard, where one can see the Spoonmaker's[22] Diamond, an 86-carat (17 g) diamond, one of the prides of Topkapi. I later went to see the Basilica Cistern, which I knew from the famous 1963 Bond movie, *From Russia with Love*. In the film, it is referred to as being constructed by the Emperor Constantine, with no reference to Justinian, who really built the cistern. In the film the intricate details of the cistern were visible, but I was disappointed to find it very dark and was unable to take a photo of any value. It presumably takes a good deal of skill and effort to take the kind of pictures that one sees on postcards and tourist brochures.

---

22. The name comes from the following story of debatable veracity. A very poor man found an attractive stone on a rubbish heap of Egri Kapi in Istanbul and bartered it to a spoonmaker for three wooden spoons. The spoonmaker sold the stone to a jeweler for 10 silver coins. When the story about the stone came to the attention of Sultan Mehmed IV, he ordered the stone be brought to the palace — and promptly took possession of it. Whether he paid for it or not remains a mystery.

The next morning I was taken for a ferry cruise on the Bosporus, the channel connecting the Black Sea (Kara Deniz) to the Mediterranean (Ak Deniz) by way of the Sea of Marmara (Marmara Deniz) and the straits of the Dardanelles. During the cruise I learned that there is a constant flow of water through the Bosporus between the Black Sea and the Sea of Marmara. Connected with the Mediterranean Sea, the Marmara Sea is saltier than the Black Sea. While the evaporation in the Mediterranean Sea is faster than the inflow of river water, the inflow of river water to the Black Sea is faster than the evaporation. The temperatures are also different, higher in the Marmara Sea than in the Black Sea. The water of the Marmara Sea flows on the bottom of the Bosporus, because it is heavier despite being warmer; the water from the Black Sea flows on the surface, as it is less salty and lighter. It is customary to divide the Bosporus into two parts: the Southern Bosporus (from the Golden Horn and city center to the Bosporus Bridge) and the Northern Bosporus (from the Bosporus Bridge to the Black Sea). There are many places of interest that can be seen from the boat, including the Galata Tower seen from the Southern Bosporus; the Rumeli Fortress, close to the Fatih Sultan Mehmet Bridge; and in the Northern Bosporus, numerous impressive seaside mansions worth millions of dollars each.

In the afternoon I visited the Beyoğlu district, starting with the Adam Mickiewicz Museum on Tatli Badem Street. Adam Mickiewicz (1798–1855) was a great Polish poet, patriot and political activist. In the summer of 1855 he came to Istanbul to help form a Polish legion to fight Russia in the Crimean War. Following a trip to a military camp, Mickiewicz fell ill. He died on November 26 that same year — probably of cholera or possibly (as some suspect) of acute arsenic poisoning. On the 100th anniversary of his death, a museum was opened in the house where he died. The museum is small but the life and works of Mickiewicz are very well presented. Later we went to Galata Tower, located just to the north of the Golden Horn. A high, cone-capped cylinder, it dominates the skyline and affords a panoramic vista of Old Istanbul and its environs. I took several pictures from the tower. I discovered that it was the place where the first trial flight of the 17th century was attempted. During the reign of Murad IV (1612–1640) legendary aviator Hezârfen Ahmet Çelebi apparently flew using artificial wings from Galata Tower over the Bosporus to the slopes of Üsküdar on the Anatolian side, nearly five kilometers away. We also visited Istanbul's famous Spice Bazaar (also called Egyptian Bazaar), constructed between 1597 and 1664. I bought some very expensive Iranian saffron, which was the best in the world, or so I was told.

The next day we went to Polonezköy (literally "Polish village" in Turkish), located about 25 miles (40 km) from the center of Istanbul (about one hour by car). The village was founded on March 19, 1842, by Prince Adam Czartoryski, chairman of the National Uprising government and leader of a political emigration party, known under the name of Hôtel Lambert. The village was initially called Adamköy or Adampol and was inhabited by 12 Poles, military emigrants after the collapse of the November Uprising (1830–1831) in Poland against Russian occupation.[23] It is worth remembering that the Ottoman Empire, in spite of previous wars with Poland, never formally recognized the Polish partitions and the deprivation of Poland's sovereignty.[24] Today's inhabitants are descendants of the early settlers and combatants for the independence of Poland; a group of soldiers from the Polish division of Ottoman Cossacks settled there at the end of the Crimean War in 1856, as well as participants in the insurrection of January 1863 and other insurrections in the 19th century. The village was established on the outskirts of Istanbul, and it is now part of the city. Mustafa Kemal Atatürk visited the village in 1937, and newly elected president Lech Wałęsa visited after Poland regained independence from Soviet domination. Originally, the inhabitants of the village were farmers, but it eventually became a popular spot for tourists and vacationers. People like spending their weekends at Polonezköy's country clubs and hotels as well as trying the local food in its famous restaurants and picnic areas. I visited the various places of interest,

---

23. After the partitioning of Poland in 1795, the country ceased to exist as an independent political entity. Poles never accepted the situation, and uprisings against the occupiers were conducted during the 19th century. Without help from the outside, however, all of them were defeated.

24. I was told that at the annual reception of ambassadors in the Topkapi Palace, when the Polish ambassador was called by the sultan, a master of ceremonies would always say, "The ambassador from Lechistan has not arrived yet." Fevzi Ersoy, Professor of Medicine at Akdeniz University in Antalia, with whom I talked in Istanbul, told me that he had heard the same story. Poland was called Lechistan in the Ottoman Turkish language.

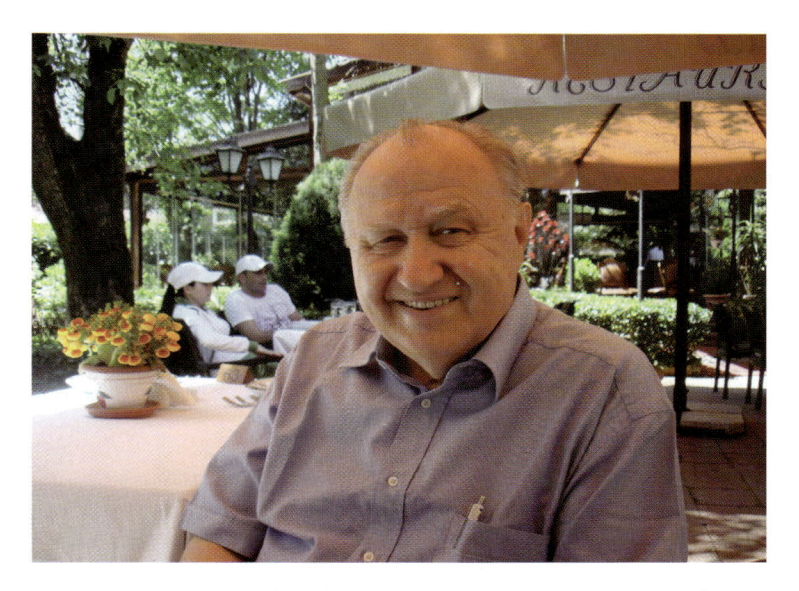

Figure 143. Leonardo Dohoda in his restaurant, Polonezköy, Turkey.

including the cemetery, the Church of Our Lady of Częstochowa, and the house in which Atatürk stayed during his visit. I also spent some time in discussion with Mr. Leonardo Dohoda, a descendant of one of the original settlers and owner of a restaurant and guesthouse (Fig. 143). His Polish was perfect, but not all inhabitants speak good Polish; some only speak Turkish.

In the afternoon Profs. Ali Başçi and Ercan Ok (Fig. 144) invited me for dinner at the Bosporus Restaurant. During the dinner I was surprised when Prof. Ok asked me to move to Izmir and work in their department. For many years they had benefited from having Dr. Evert Doorhout Mees work at Ege University after retiring in 1990 from Utrecht University in the Netherlands. Dr. Mees was about to conclude his time there, and they thought that I could offer some help of a similar nature. I was intrigued by the idea, but I wanted to learn more about the conditions in Izmir. I contacted Dr. Mees, who described very enticing conditions for work in Izmir, including the possibility of doing research much more easily than in Europe, and the presence of an excellent team under the leadership of Prof. Ok. He praised Izmir as "the most Western city" in Turkey, with amazing

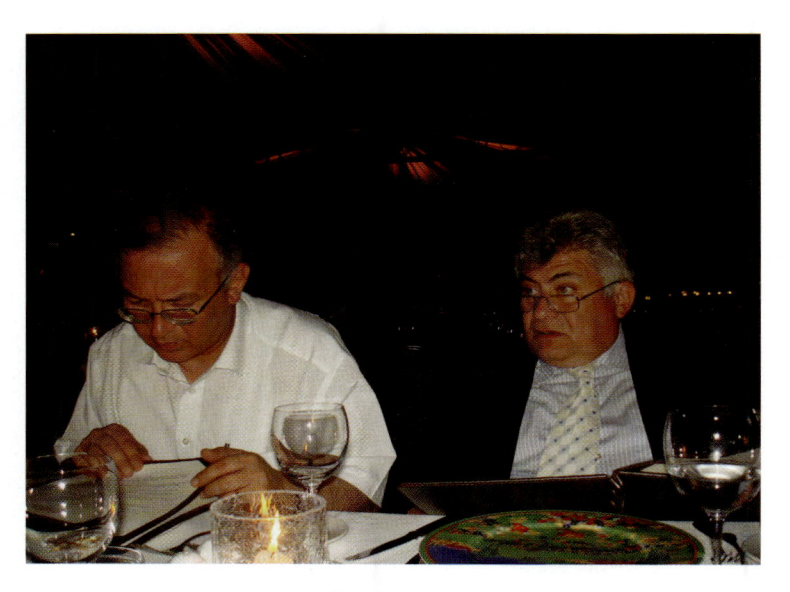

Figure 144.   Professors Ercan Ok and Ali Başçi.

hospitality and respect for his religion. But there were several potential problems with my coming to work in Izmir. First of all, I still worked part-time co-organizing our Annual Dialysis Conference, so I needed to be in the U.S. for at least a few months. Secondly, Halina wanted to be in Poland for several months and did not relish the prospect of living in a third country. Taking all the factors into account, I decided not to accept the proposal, but I eventually spent a few weeks in Izmir during the summer to help with several projects.

The next day I was transferred to Klassis Hotel on the European side of Istanbul. In the evening we had dinner with many eminent Turkish nephrologists and managers from Fresenius Medical Care in Turkey. I had an opportunity to talk with Fevzi Ersoy, our former fellow at the Division of Nephrology in Columbia, who later became Professor of Medicine and Nephrology, and Director of Akdeniz University Hospital at the Akdeniz University School of Medicine in Antalia (Fig. 145). On Sunday, May 13, I gave two talks at the Medical Accreditation Meeting. The first was on the importance of blood pressure control in hemodialysis patients by controlling volume with gentle ultrafiltration [Pr 506]. The second was on the difference

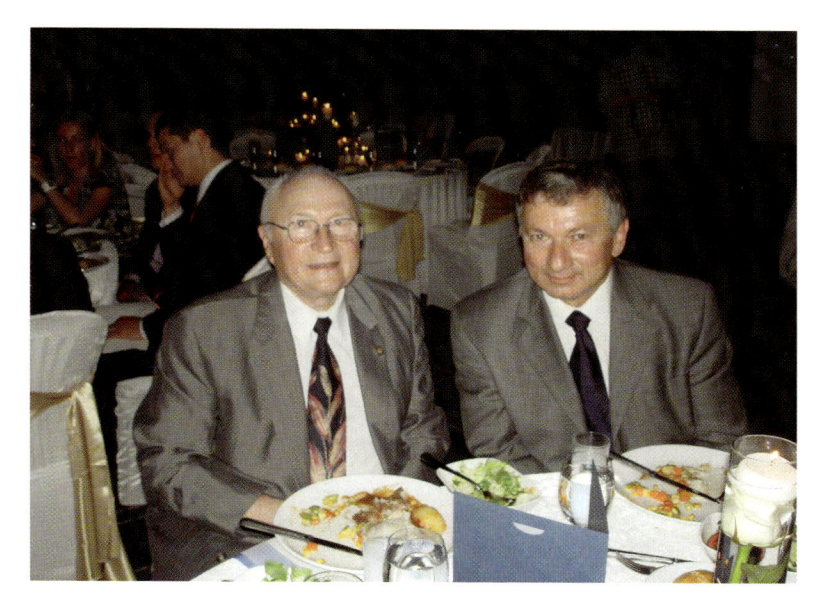

Figure 145. Fevzi Ersoy and the author at a dinner in Klassis Hotel, Istanbul.

between optimal and adequate dialysis and how best to achieve them [Pr 507]. I expressed the opinion that the term *adequate* should be abandoned, as it indicates "barely satisfactory or sufficient," in favor of *optimal*, which indicates "the best possible."

2008

In 2008 I had only one presentation at our Annual Dialysis Conference. I presented various inferential data indicating that high dialyzer blood flow is detrimental for blood access survival [Pr 508].

2009

I had only six presentations in 2009. Four were in the U.S., one was in Poland and one was in Turkey. Our Annual Dialysis Conference was in Houston, Texas, and for the first time Barb was not at the conference. She was able to prepare most of the nursing session, but a few weeks before the conference she passed away. Dr. Nolph paid tribute

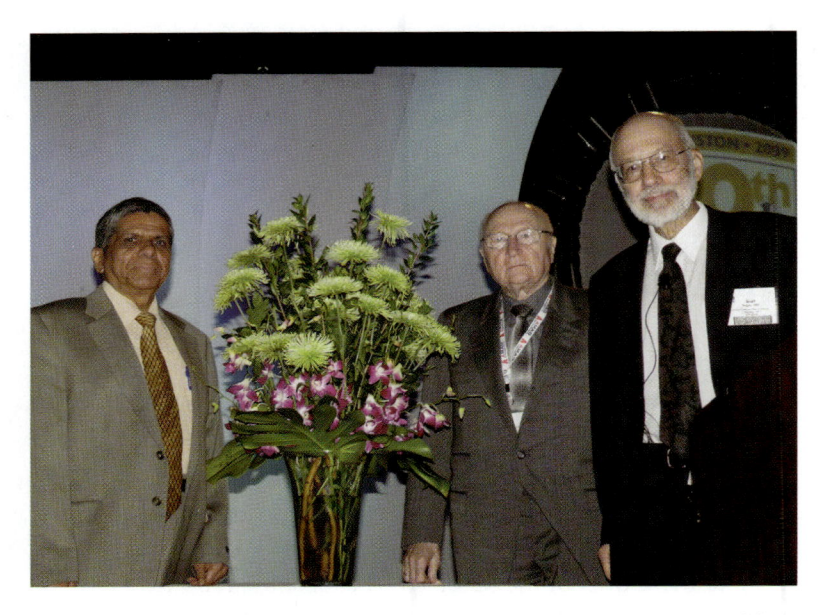

Figure 146. Podium at a conference in Houston: Dr. Khanna, a collection of flowers for "Barb," the author and Dr. Nolph.

to her with a minute of silence, and a collection of flowers was in her place on the podium (Fig. 146). My first presentation was on urea transport in dialysis. On the basis of multiple studies, I argued that urea is not toxic in concentrations encountered in dialysis patients; that its intercompartmental transport through the aquaporins AQ3, AQ6 and AQ7 is faster than any real uremic toxin including phosphorus, guanidines, beta-2 microglobulin, sodium, and water; and that the blood concentrations of urea do not reflect concentrations of uremic toxins in dialysis patients [Pr 509]. My next presentation was on the evolution of peritoneal dialysis catheters with emphasis, naturally, on my Swan Neck abdominal and presternal catheters. I predicted that there was still some room for further improvement in catheter design [Pr 510]. In my third presentation I criticized the current belief that only randomized controlled trials were needed to prove that some device or treatment method was superior to others. In contrast to the study of pharmaceuticals, when studying treatment methods, randomized controlled trials are not better than observational studies, mostly due to the fact that patients are asked to perform procedures and there are tremendous numbers of exclusions, both of which make these studies unreliable. The genesis of this presentation was the fact that the clearly superior method of dialysis performed every day or night instead of three times weekly was not approved for higher reimbursement and a randomized controlled trial was ordered instead by the National Institutes of Health in 2001. Although nine years had elapsed, the trial had not been completed [Pr 511]. The last presentation was a commentary on the role of the peritoneal equilibration test in the selection of appropriate peritoneal dialysis modality and technique [Pr 512]. After the meeting we took advantage of being in Houston and visited NASA's Lyndon Johnson Space Center. We went with Roberta Satalowich, who delivered a presentation at the conference and whose husband, Florian, had worked in the space center in the past. The visitor's center presents the history of space exploration in a truly impressive way. Some of the exhibits are really huge, like the model of the Saturn V rocket shown in Fig. 147.

My next presentation was at the 18th Scientific-Teaching Conference of the Polish Society of Nephrology in Warsaw. Delivered in Polish, it focused on the future of hemodialysis [Pr 513]. I predicted

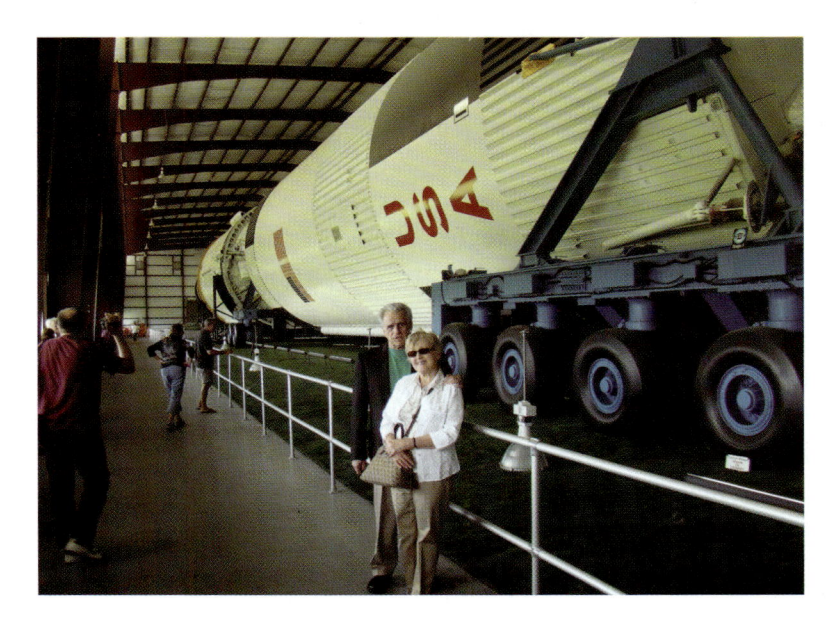

Figure 147.   Halina and Florian with the model of the Saturn V rocket.

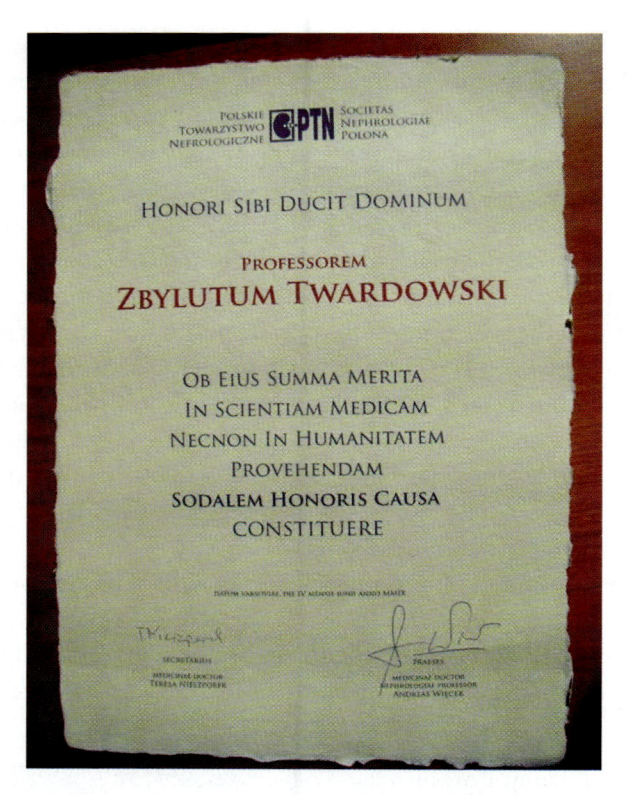

Figure 148. Certificate of Honorary Membership of the Polish Society of Nephrology.

that the improvement in hemodialysis results would not be as a consequence of technological progress alone, but rather by more frequent and longer dialysis sessions, and by the rejection of Kt/V as an index of dialysis quality. During the conference, the Polish Society of Nephrology (Societas Nephrologiae Polona) bestowed on me Honorary Membership (*Provehendam Sodalem Honoris Causa Constituere*) for highest merit in medical science and humanities (*Ob Eius Summa Merita, In Scientiam Medicam Necnon In humanitatem*) (Fig. 148).

In August I went to Ege University in Turkey for a week to review drafts and projects related to hemodialysis prepared by Prof. Ercan Ok and his team, and I then gave a presentation. I also suggested performing a study ultimately putting an end to the Kt/V index as the measure of dialysis quality, a study that I was unable to undertake in

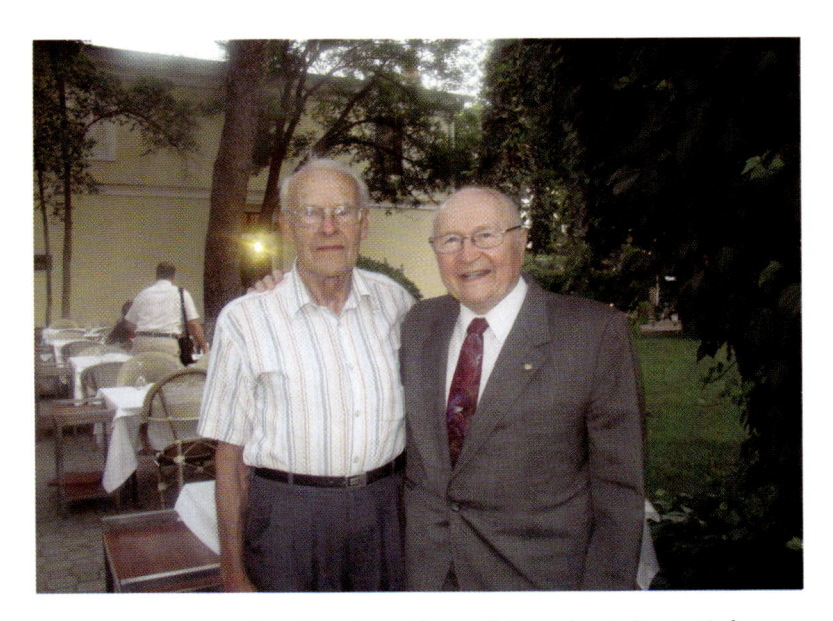

Figure 149. Dr. Evert Doorhout Mees and the author in Izmir, Turkey.

the U.S. I suggested doing a randomized controlled trial in two groups treated three times weekly with the same Kt/V of about 1.3 per session. In one group I proposed a dialysis time of 190 min and a blood flow of > 400 mL/min and in another group a blood flow of 200 mL/min and a dialysis duration > 360 min to achieve the same Kt/V. The exact blood flow and dialysis duration were to be adjusted taking into account V (urea distribution volume related to body mass) in individual patients. My strong belief, then as now, is that such a study would show much better results with longer dialysis and slower blood flow. I flew from John Paul II Airport in Balice, Kraków, through Munich, arriving at Adnan Menderes Airport in Izmir on Lufthansa Flight 3370 at 3:40 pm on August 17. I was taken by a nephrology fellow, Fatih Kircelli, to Ege Palace Hotel. The next day another fellow, Mümtaz Yilmaz, took me to the university. I met Dr. Evert Doorhout Mees personally for the first time (Fig. 149). His work at Ege University has been honored by naming the dialysis center after him. Each day of my visit Mümtaz gave me a ride to the university and I reviewed manuscripts related to dialysis written by various fellows, including Ender Hür, Fatih Kircelli and Hamad Dheir.

In a meeting on August 20 I presented the bases of my strong conviction that Kt/V should not be used as a measure of dialysis adequacy [Pr 514], but after discussing the proposal with Prof. Ok and various faculty members and fellows, it was clear that a study to put an end to Kt/V would not be possible at Ege University. The most important reason was that Turkish Government regulations fixed the dialysis time at four hours. It was a disappointing outcome for me, but I had to yield to it. I suspect the concept of the Kt/V index is so deeply entrenched and accepted by those who pay for dialysis that it will be extremely difficult to challenge it — a problem I will return to again later.

In addition to my work at the university, I was taken out for dinner every night by Prof. Ok, Dr. Mehmet Özkahya and Dr. Ali Başçi. On Saturday and Sunday some fellows would take me to visit various places of interest. I was most interested in Smyrna, the original name of the city, which later became Izmir in Turkish. Smyrna was probably founded by Tantalus[25] to the northeast of the present-day city in 1430 BC. I was interested in Smyrna in particular because in 146 AD Cornelius Galen began the study of medicine, and in about his 20th year he left Pergamum for Smyrna, in order to place himself under the instruction of the anatomist and physician Pelops, and of the peripatetic philosopher Albinus. Galen, a prolific writer, was the personal physician to the emperor Marcus Aurelius and his son Commodus. In his book on the functions of body parts, he clearly stated that urine is secreted from the blood by the kidneys and passes through ureters to the bladder, from which it is intermittently discharged. This was one of the first notes on the role of kidneys in making urine. Unfortunately, the Smyrna of ancient times no longer exists. Only after the WWII, in 1948, were important excavations carried out by the British Archaeological Institute of Athens and, after 1960, by the Turkish Historical Association. However, very little was excavated (Fig. 150). At 10:45 am on August 24 I flew back to Kraków from Izmir through Munich on Lufthansa Flight 3336. All in all I really enjoyed my stay in

---

25. According to Greek mythology Tantalus was a cruel king who was condemned to Hades for his crimes, to stand in water that receded when he tried to drink, and to have fruit hang above him that moved away when he reached for it. From his name we have received the word *tantalize*, meaning to excite or tease someone with the promise of something unobtainable.

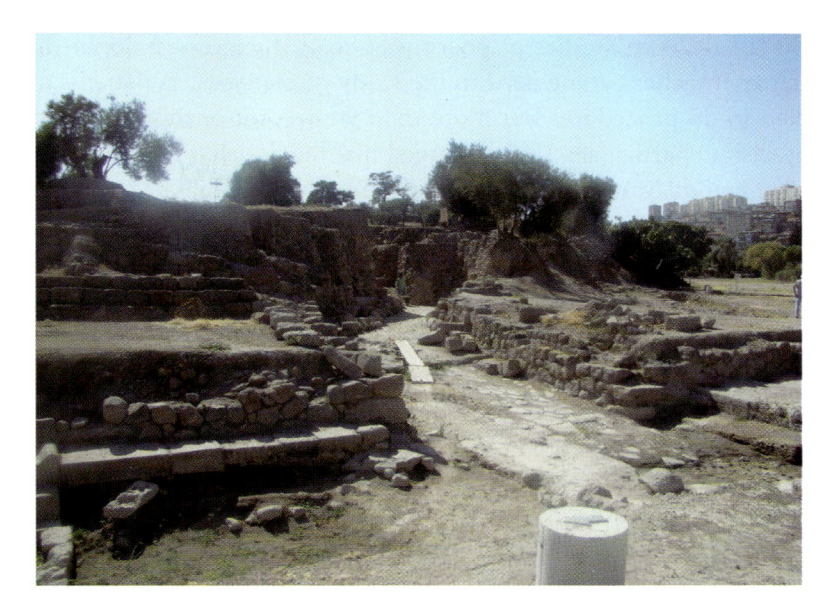

Figure 150. Ruins of Smyrna, Turkey.

Izmir, and I promised to return for a short time in the future if I would be of some help.

2010

In 2010 I delivered only nine presentations, four in the U.S. and five in Europe. In our Annual Dialysis Conference I delivered a presentation where I harshly criticized randomized controlled trials (RCTs) as inappropriate for determining whether a daily or three times weekly dialysis schedule is superior [Pr 515]. My studies performed in Bytom 40 years earlier had found, in consecutive observations (before and after design; A → B) in the same small group of patients, that more frequent dialysis is better than less frequent dialysis. There have been hundreds of similar observations and nobody has been able to show me anything to the contrary. Moreover, such conclusions are logical because kidneys work continuously and more frequent dialysis therefore better resembles the functions of the kidney and alleviates fluctuations of body fluids and chemistries. While recognizing the value of RCTs in studies of pharmaceuticals, I expressed doubt that such approaches can be used in the study of methods, as patients are asked to do procedures but more than 90 percent of those asked do not wish to participate. I even charged that the decision to undertake a daily hemodialysis study resembles the Tuskegee Syphilis Experiment[26] with one difference, namely that the control group receives at least some treatment.

Another presentation was in the session commemorating the 50th anniversary of the first chronic hemodialysis treatment, which was undertaken in Seattle on March 9, 1960. The session was divided into two parts. In the first part, survivors or family members of the group who contributed to the achievement spoke about their memories of that time. In the second part, several speakers from all over the world presented their recollections and the impact of the developments in Seattle on their work. I presented my memories from Kraków and Bytom [Pr 516]. My presentation on the statistics in dialysis research was very well received, and I was asked to present the material with slight modifications during our local conference at the division [Pr 517] and as a grand round at our Department of Medicine [Pr 518]. The title for the talk comes from one part of the presentation during which I presented examples called — by Joseph Berkson from the Division of Biometry and Medical Statistics at Mayo Clinic — the Traumatic Interocular Test.[27] One of these examples was the first use of chronic dialysis in the treatment of a patient. The patient, Clyde Shields, treated under the direction of Belding Scribner, survived over 10 years, whereas all patients with advanced chronic renal failure without dialysis survived only a few weeks.[28]

In September 2009 I received an e-mail from Dr. Marek Rawa, a former surgeon at the Hospital for Miners in Bytom and with whom

---

26. A clinical study conducted between 1932 and 1972 in Tuskegee, Alabama, by the U.S. Public Health Service. When the study began in 1932, standard medical treatments for syphilis were toxic, dangerous and of questionable effectiveness. By 1947 penicillin had become the standard treatment, yet the study continued for 40 years even after it was obvious that nontoxic penicillin was effective. Most of the subjects were poor and black, and were never given any treatment.

27. If the difference is impressive, the distinction hits you between the eyes and you do not need fancy "P" values or other statistical tools to say, "Yes that's a real difference."

28. "Successful treatment of Clyde Shields represents one of the few instances in medicine where a single success was all that was required to validate a new therapy" — p. 513 in Scribner BH. (1990) A personalized history of chronic hemodialysis. *Am J Kidney Dis* **16**: 511–519.

I created some arteriovenous fistulas in the early 1970s. He later immigrated to Morocco and became a leader in the creation of arteriovenous fistulas in that country. In his e-mail he informed me about his leading the introduction of the buttonhole method of needle insertion in Morocco and his presentation on the topic during the congress of the Société Francaise des Abords Vasculaires (SFAV) in Ajacco, Corsica, France. He was looking at my early publication on the topic and asked me to participate as an honorary guest of the 2010 Congress of SFAV in Tours, France. I tentatively agreed, as the congress was supposed to be in June, during my stay in Kraków, so it would be in line with my rule to travel within the same time zone. In October I received an official invitation from Dr. Pierre Bourquelot, President of SFAV, and I accepted. I eventually agreed to give a presentation on the history of the buttonhole method in the plenary session and conduct a workshop with three other presentations related to blood access. Halina decided to go with me and we planned to take advantage of the congress location and visit the castles of the Loire Valley and later do some sightseeing in Paris. I also wanted to visit Tours because of its history: the Battle of Tours was a decisive battle to preserve Christianity in Europe.[29] I was a little surprised to find that not too many people in Tours seemed to know about this important battle. Our arrival in Kraków was somewhat delayed owing to the volcanic ash thrown up in the atmosphere by the eruption of the Icelandic volcano Eyjafjallajökull. We had planned to arrive on April 20, but only got there on April 28. In any event, it was well before the congress in Tours from June 14 to 16. We departed from Kraków at 7:55 am on LO 343 and arrived in Paris De Gaulle Terminal 1 at 10:10 am on June 13. There were no flights to Tours, so we took a train departing from Terminal 2 at 1:37 pm and arriving at Saint Pierre Des Corps Station in about two hours, and later arriving by taxi at the Holiday Inn in Tours at about 4 pm.

---

29. The Battle of Tours (October 10, 732), also called the Battle of Poitiers, was fought in an area between the cities of Poitiers and Tours. The location of the battle was close to the border between the Frankish realm and then-independent Aquitaine. It pitted Frankish and Burgundian forces under Austrasian Mayor of the Palace, Charles Martel (The Hammer), against an army of the Umayyad Caliphate led by 'Abdul Rahman Al Ghafiqi, Governor-General of al-Andalus. The Franks were victorious, 'Abdul Rahman Al Ghafiqi was killed, and Charles subsequently extended his authority in the south.

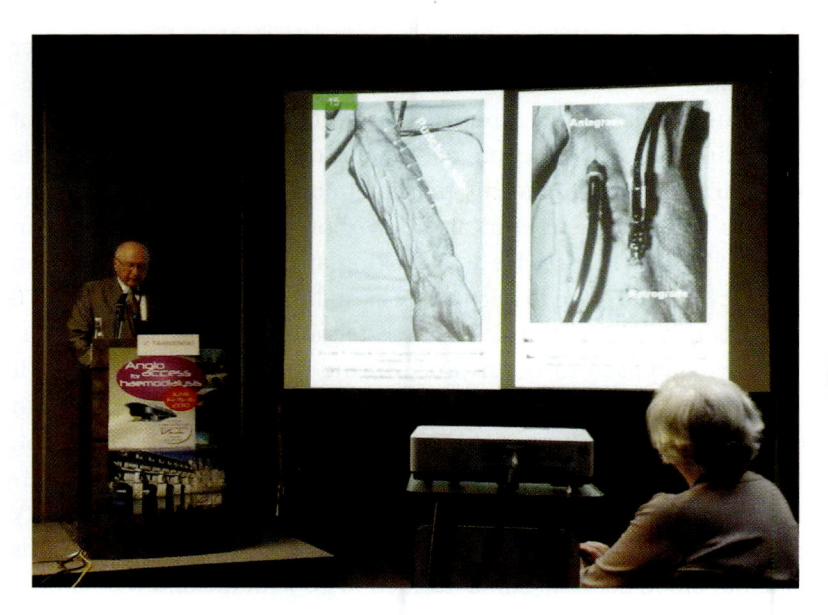

Figure 151. Presenting the history of the buttonhole technique (Plenary Session 3) in Tours, France.

The congress, which took place at the Vinci Centre International de Congrès, began the following day. The first day was mostly devoted to the importance of creating arteriovenous fistulas in the forearm. Most sessions were in English, but there were sessions in French, Italian, Spanish and Portuguese. My first presentation was on the history of the buttonhole technique [Pr 519] (Fig. 151), covering essentially what I have described in previous chapters of this book. In the afternoon I held a workshop with Dr. Marek Rawa. He talked about his experience with the buttonhole technique in Morocco (Fig. 152); I presented the worldwide experience and use of this technique [Pr 520], intravenous catheter design and problems [Pr 521], and the detrimental effect of high dialyzer blood flow on blood access [Pr 522]. In my second presentation I talked about the history of intravenous catheter development and my studies leading to the design of Palindrome catheter and its advantages. The last presentation on the possible detrimental influence of high dialyzer blood flow on blood access was based on many observational studies showing that the best results with blood access have been achieved in Japan,

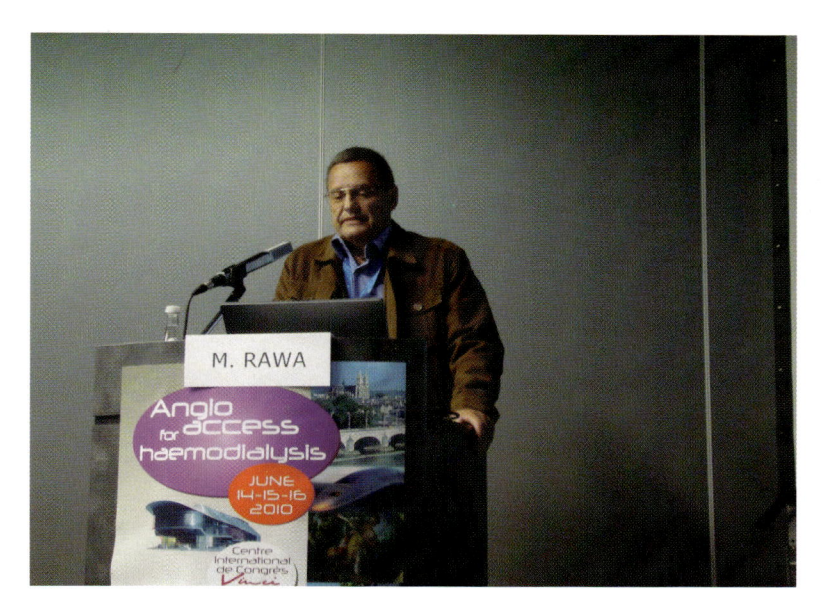

Figure 152. Dr. Rawa's presentation in Tours, on the buttonhole method in Morocco.

where dialyzer blood flow is about 200 mL/min, slightly worse in Europe, with dialyzer blood flow of 300 mL/min, and the worst in the U.S., where dialyzer blood flow is 400 mL/min or more. One criticism of the comparison between different continents is that there are different populations. I received strong support on this notion from the Dialysis Outcome and Practice Patterns Study (DOPPS) presented by Dr. Rajiv Saran during his State of the Art Lecture at our Annual Dialysis Conference in Seattle. Indeed, I had suggested to the organizing committee that they invite him to make this presentation and ask him to analyze the data with this notion in mind. He found that regardless of the particular country, centers using lower dialyzer blood flow achieved better access results.

My presentations were well received. I was subsequently invited by Dr. Jan Tordoir to give a presentation at the European Vascular Access Course in Maastricht from March 2–4, 2011. Another invitation was from Drs. Jean-Pierre Becquemin, Pierre Bourquelot and Jean Marzelle with respect to a presentation at a session on Controversies and Updates in Vascular Surgery in Paris from January

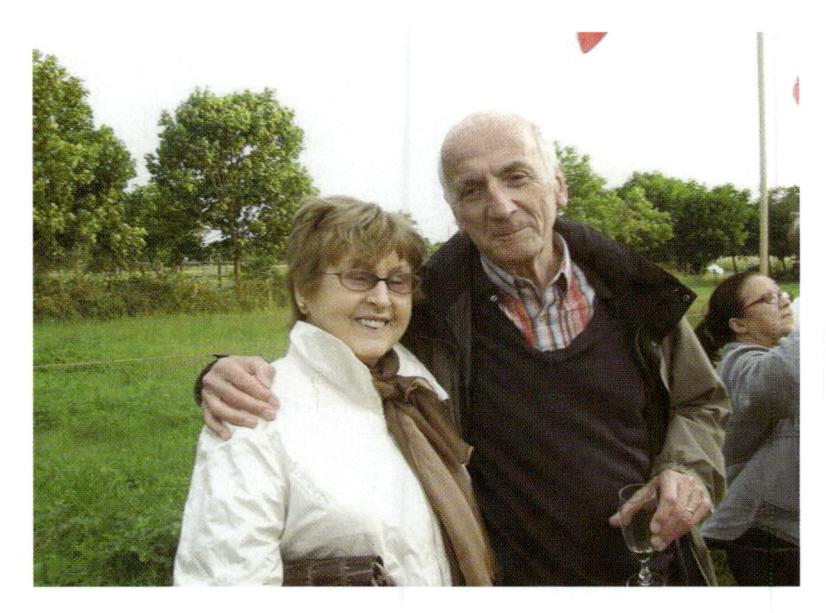

Figure 153. Halina and Dr. Bourquelot.

27–29, 2011. Unfortunately, the dates were at the time when I would be in the U.S. close to our Annual Dialysis Conference in Phoenix in the middle of February, so I had to decline. On Monday and Tuesday evenings, Dr. Luc Turmel, an interventional radiologist, organized a "speakers' dinner" at his beautiful estate not far from Tours. The atmosphere was friendly (Fig. 153) and jovial (Fig. 154) with music, dancing (Fig. 155) and excellent food.

After the Wednesday afternoon meeting, we took a minibus to visit two châteaux, Villandry and Azay-Le-Rideau. Villandry is famous for its garden (Fig. 156); Azay-Le-Rideau was built on an island on the Indre River from 1515 to 1527, and its foundations rise straight out of the water (Fig. 157). On Thursday we took another tour to visit Chenonceaux, Amboise, Langeais and Ussé. The Château de Chenonceaux was not particularly impressive, but it was the only castle with a visitor's guide in Polish. We were more taken with Ussé, which served as Charles Perrault's inspiration when writing the classic fairytale *Sleeping Beauty*, and the Langeais, where the stylish marriage

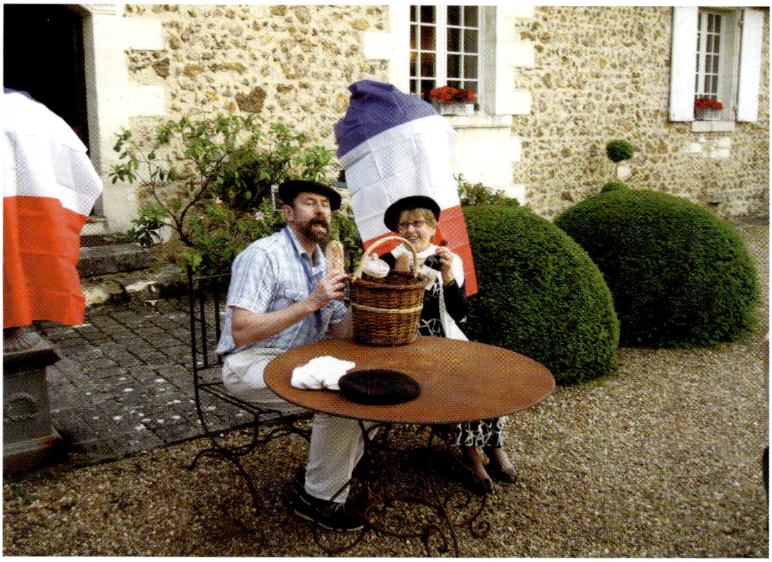

Figure 154. Luc Turmel dressed as d'Artagnan with Halina.

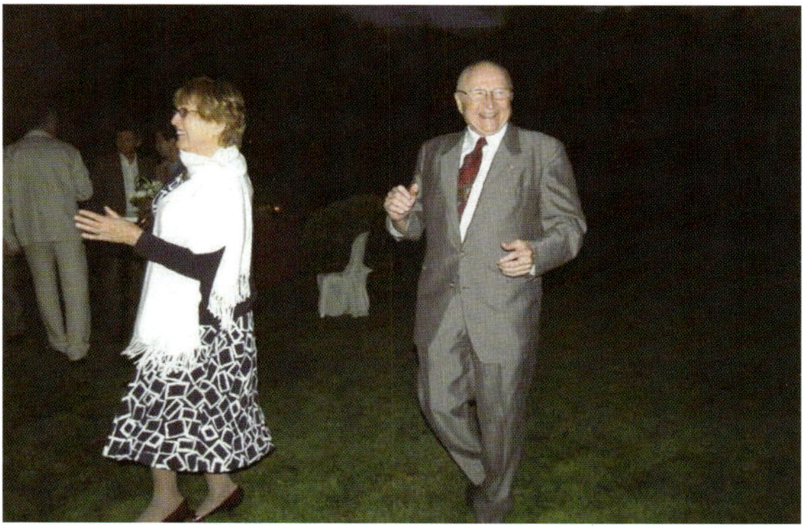

Figure 155. Halina and the author dancing at the Speakers' Dinner.

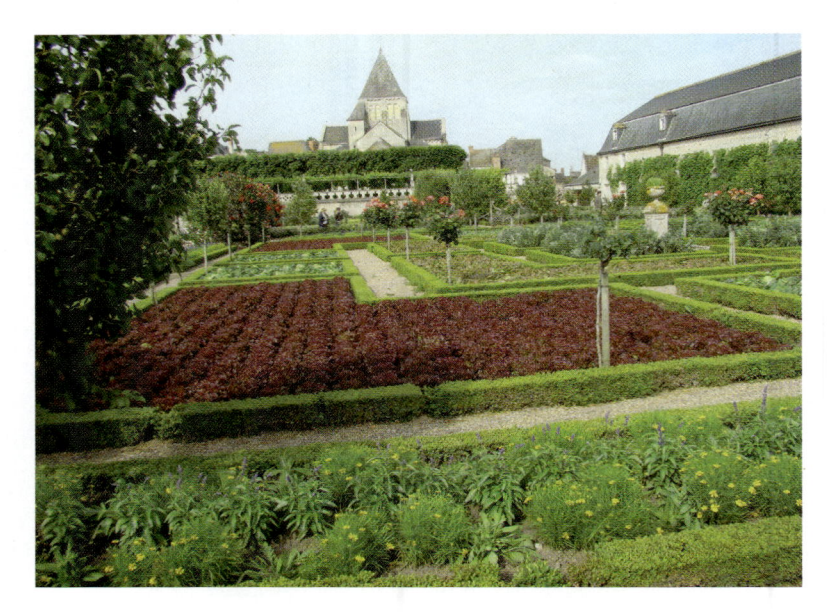

Figure 156. The Gardens of the Château de Villandry.

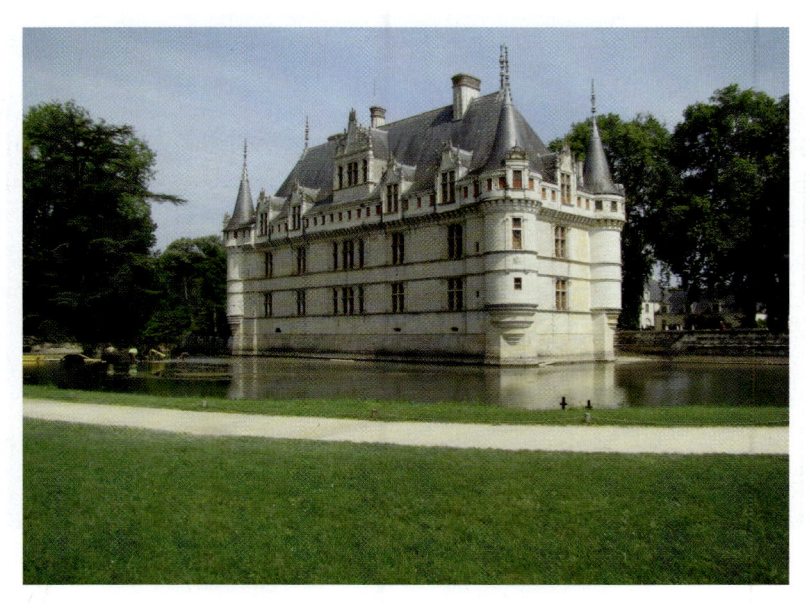

Figure 157. Château d'Azay-le-Rideau.

ceremony between Charles VIII and Anne of Brittany on December 6, 1491, was elaborately reconstituted. I was intrigued by the contrasting nose shapes of the couple: the aquiline of Charles VIII and retroussé of Anne. I was very interested in Château d'Amboise, where Leonardo da Vinci spent the last three years of his life as a guest of King Francis I. Da Vinci came in December 1515 and lived and worked in the nearby Clos Lucé, which was connected to the château by an underground passage. Da Vinci worked primarily on inventions and engineering projects, discussing philosophy with the king, who paid him visits using the secret passage. Da Vinci died on May 2, 1519, and was buried in the Chapel of Saint-Hubert, adjoining the château. We had a choice of visiting either the castle or the da Vinci museum in Clos Lucé; everyone on the tour, ourselves included, elected to see the second. Most rooms had been restored to their original 15th-century simplicity: a small chapel, a studio and hall where Francis I and Leonardo discoursed, a kitchen, and the bedroom where da Vinci died. The most interesting exhibits were replicas of his inventions produced from his drawings by IBM engineers. The large-scale models included a breech-loading cannon, an armored tank, a portable suspension bridge, a barometer, and a three-speed gear, as well as several flying machines and even an air conditioner. I have to say that I was more impressed with the exhibits in the da Vinci museum in Florence, which I had seen three years earlier, and considered them to be of higher quality. We were told that Leonardo brought with him, and left for the king, two portraits: the *Mona Lisa and the Virgin of the Rocks*, both now in the Louvre in Paris. In any event, to a great degree I had fulfilled a dream that I had since graduation and after reading about da Vinci's life in books, as I had witnessed first-hand his amazing accomplishments in Milan, Florence and Amboise.

On Friday, June 18, we took a train from Tours to Paris Montparnasse Station and then checked into Hotel Lotti on 7 Rue de Castiglione. The next day we took a two-hour tour called "Paris at a Glance." We had an excellent driver-cum-guide who spoke several languages including excellent English and occasional Russian; it was just us and a Russian couple in the minibus. The tour took us quickly past the Champs-Élysées, the Arc de Triomphe, Place de la Concorde, Les Invalides, the Trocadéro and the Opéra. We spent a little more

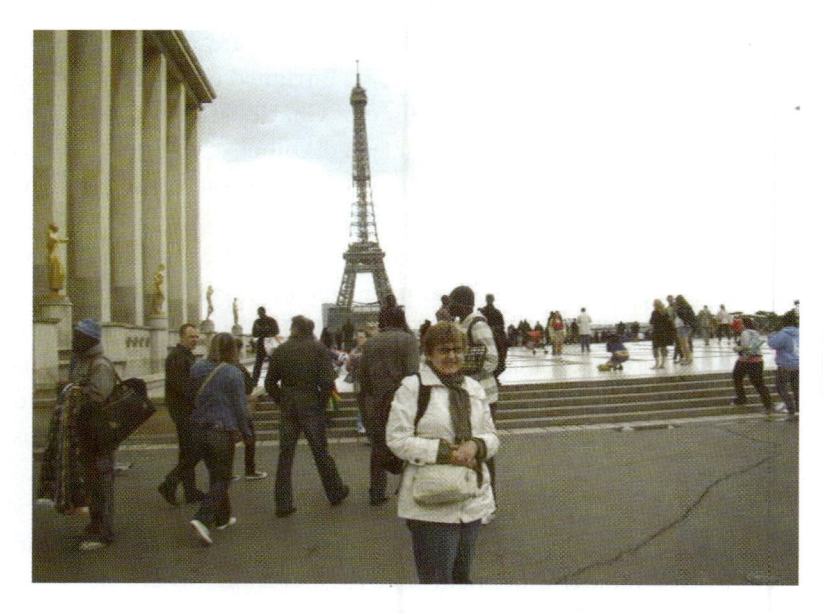

Figure 158. Halina at the Eiffel Tower, Paris.

time at the Eiffel Tower (Fig. 158), and we were taken through Place Vendôme to see the column originally erected by Napoleon I between 1806 and 1810. The present statue from 1874 depicts Napoleon as a Roman emperor (Fig. 159), as did the original statue installed on the column, but it was replaced by various other statues in between. As our guide told us, Frédéric Chopin was one of Place Vendôme's famous residents; he passed away in the house at No. 12 in 1849. As our hotel was close by, the next day I went to look for a sign commemorating the event but found none. I asked several passersby, but nobody knew about it. I thought that our guide was perhaps mistaken, but on our next tour, "Historical Paris," another guide said the same thing. In the evening we went to the Moulin Rouge cabaret (Fig. 160) and were entertained by its famous dancers, acrobats, magicians and clowns.

On Sunday we went to the Church of Saint Roch on Rue Saint-Honoré. There was a wonderful Mass marking the end of the school year, after which schoolchildren gave a performance (Fig. 161). In the afternoon we walked through the streets of Paris. I was very impressed

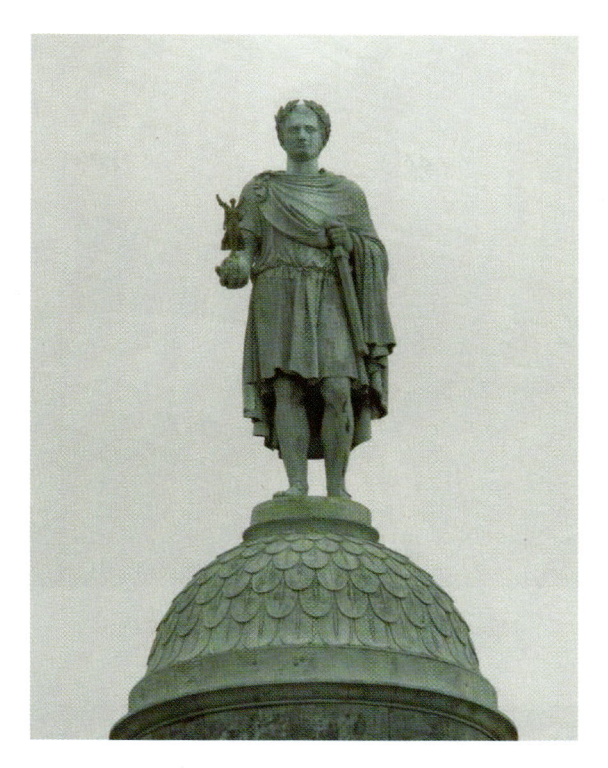

Figure 159. Column of Napoleon dressed as a Roman emperor at Place Vendôme, Paris.

with the beautiful condition of buildings erected in the previous centuries. I took photos of many of them. The Palais Garnier (Fig. 162), which houses the Paris Opera, is a beautiful example of 19th-century architecture, while Forum des Halles (Fig. 163, taken from where Rue Saint-Honoré meets Rue des Halles) is typical of the controversial buildings that were erected in the 20th century. The next day we took the Grand Louvre Museum Walking Tour, beginning at the visitor's center just below the famous glass pyramid. We managed to see the three famous ladies of the Louvre: the *Mona Lisa*, the *Winged Victory of Samothrace* (or *Nike of Samothrace*), and the *Venus de Milo*. We saw more of da Vinci's paintings: the *Virgin of the Rocks,* the *Virgin and Child with St. Anne,* and *St. John the Baptist.* As anyone knows who has tried tackling it, the Louvre is a huge museum. We only saw a fraction of the exhibits, but what we saw was really impressive.

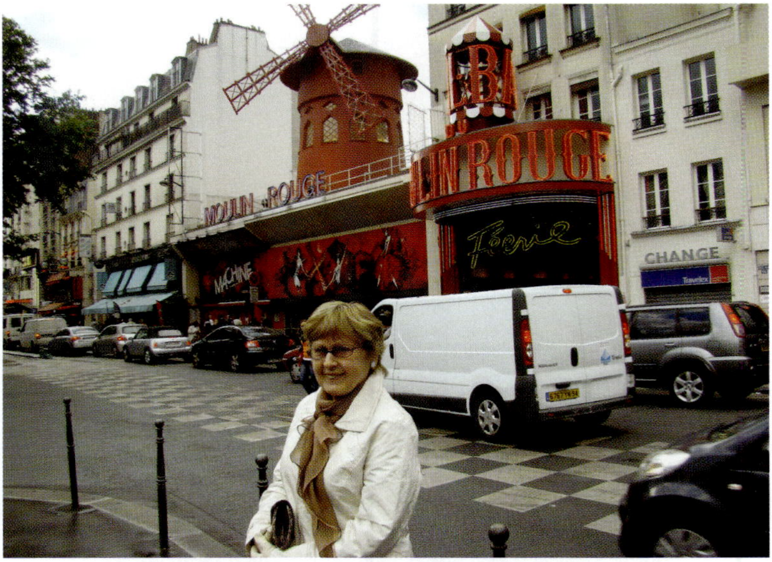

Figure 160. Halina at Moulin Rouge, Paris.

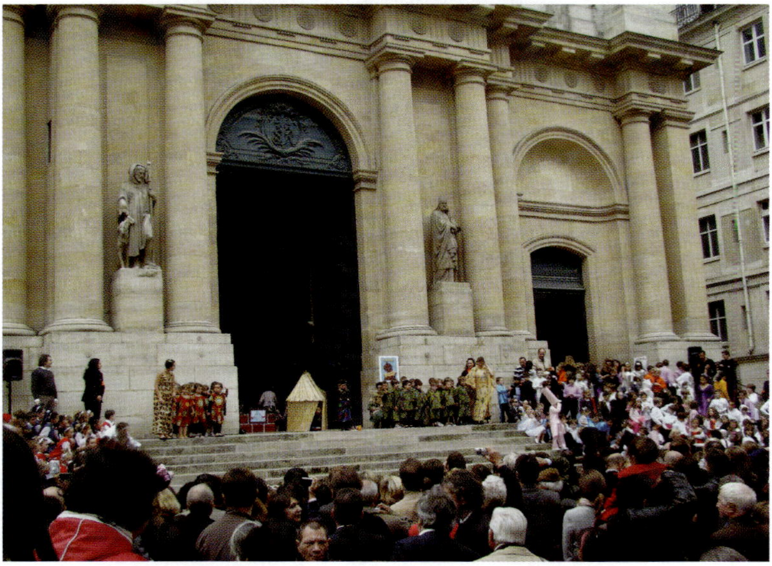

Figure 161. Schoolchildren perform at to the Church of Saint Roch, Paris.

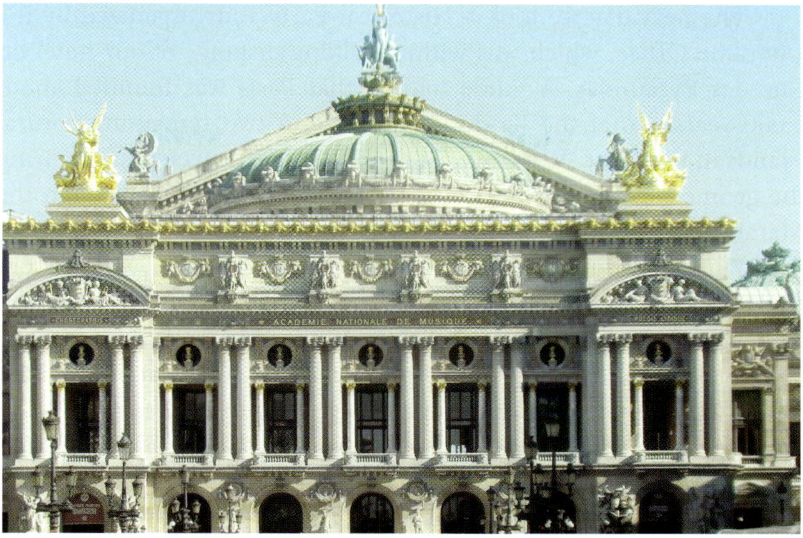

Figure 162. Palais Garnier, which houses the Paris Opera.

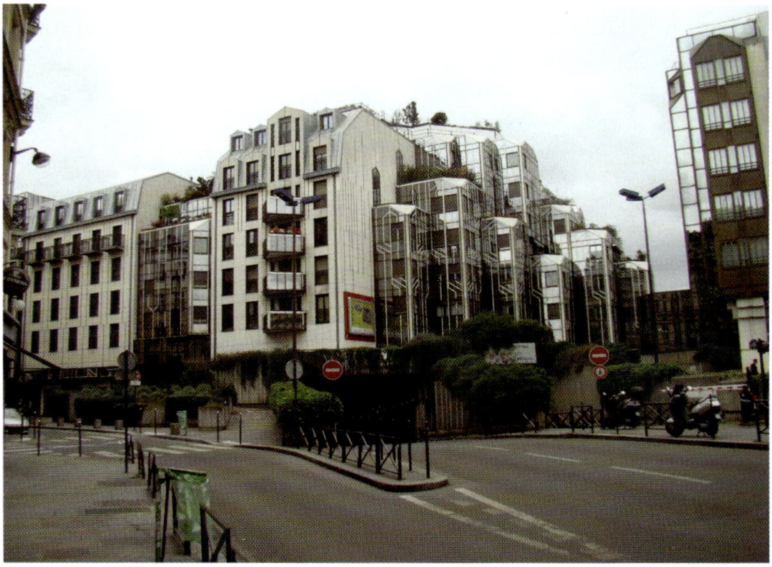

Figure 163. Forum des Halles, Paris.

The next day we took a Historical Paris Tour organized by the Cityrama Office, which was within walking distance of our hotel on Rue des Pyramides. A guide told us that Paris was founded about 2,000 years ago at the Île de la Cité, one of two remaining natural islands in the Seine. We drove through the oldest parts, first admiring the geometric design of Place Vendôme. We then went through the Marais district and its "hotels," private townhouses of the nobility of the 17th and 18th centuries, crossed the Latin Quarter, with its old university (the Sorbonne), along the Luxembourg Gardens, and into Saint-Germain-des-Prés, with its famous cafés and Romanesque church. Afterwards, we went to the Île de la Cité and went on a guided tour of the interior of Notre Dame, where I photographed a model of the cathedral. Notre Dame de Paris stands on the site of a Christian basilica, which was in turn built where a Roman-era temple once stood. It really is in the heart of Paris. There were visitor's guides in various languages, including Polish, but it was "out of stock," unfortunately. Later we took a Batobus for a cruise on the Seine, and I got a shot of Notre Dame from the boat (Fig. 164).

On Wednesday we decided to visit Montmartre. We took a taxi from our hotel to Place Saint-Pierre, and our driver suggested we take

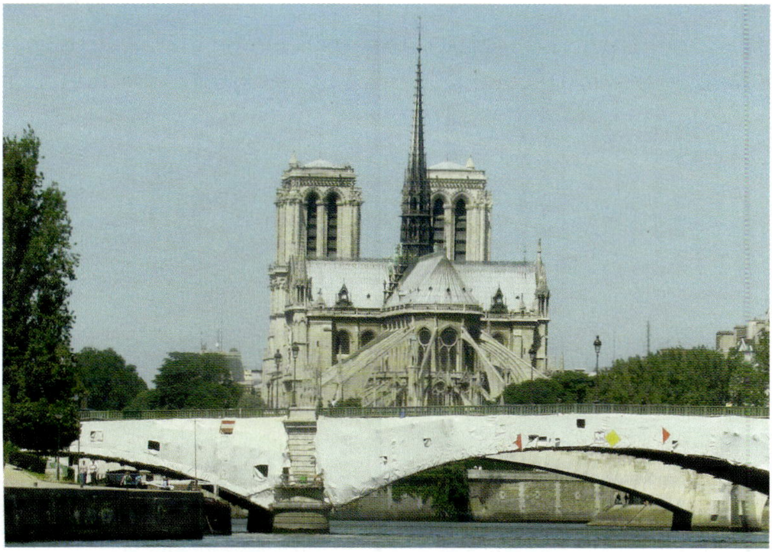

Figure 164.   Notre Dame, as photographed from a Batobus, Paris.

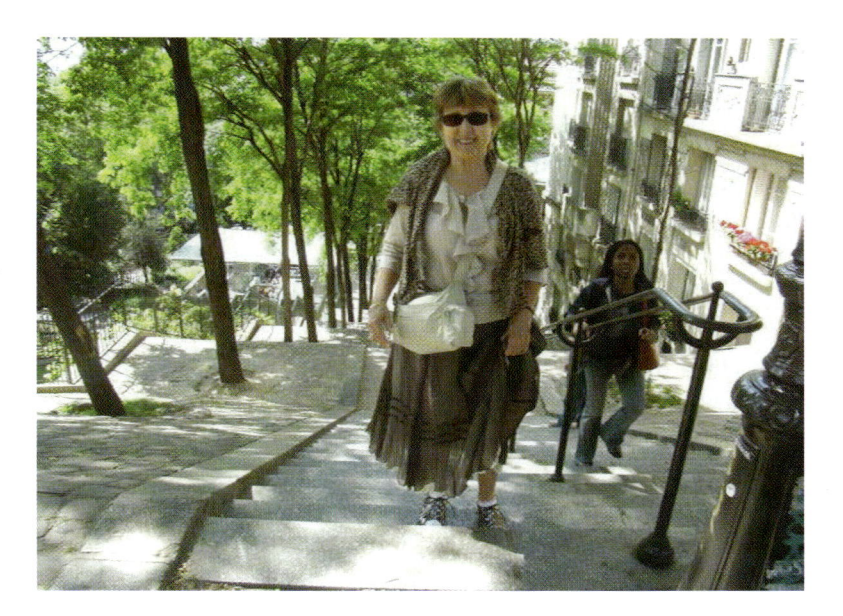

Figure 165. Halina climbs stairs on Rue Foyatier, Paris.

the Montmartre funicular to the top of the hill. Unfortunately, there was a long line, so we decided to climb the stairs alongside on Rue Foyatier (Fig. 165) — which only a few other people had elected to take — up to Rue Azaïs. At the top of Montmartre hill is the majestic Sacré-Cœur Basilica (Fig. 166). The basilica took more than 40 years to build, with construction beginning in 1875 and consecration only in 1919. After enjoying the views of the city, we visited Galerie Montmartre on artists' square before returning to Rue Azaïs and taking a streetcar to the Pigalle Métro station (Fig. 167). We wanted to go to Place Pigalle because of the well-known episode *"Hasło"* (Password) of Polish TV serial *"Stawka większa niż życie"* (Playing for High Stakes). Very successful in its native Poland, this black and white TV series was about the adventures of a James Bond-like Polish secret agent, Hans Kloss (real name: Stanisław Kolicki; code name: J-23), played by Stanisław Mikulski, who acts as a double agent in the German intelligence organisation *Abwehr* in occupied Poland during WWII. In this particular episode Hans was supposed to meet another secret agent in Paris and receive important information. The agent was supposed to say the password "*W Paryżu najlepsze kasztany są na Placu Pigalle*" ("In Paris the best chestnuts are sold on Pigalle Square") and Hans'

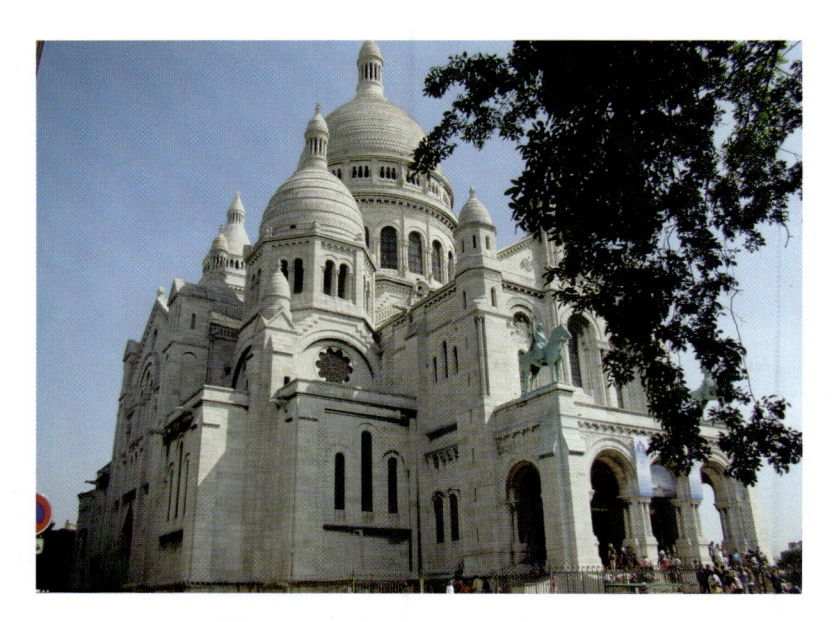

Figure 166. Sacré-Cœur Basilica, Paris.

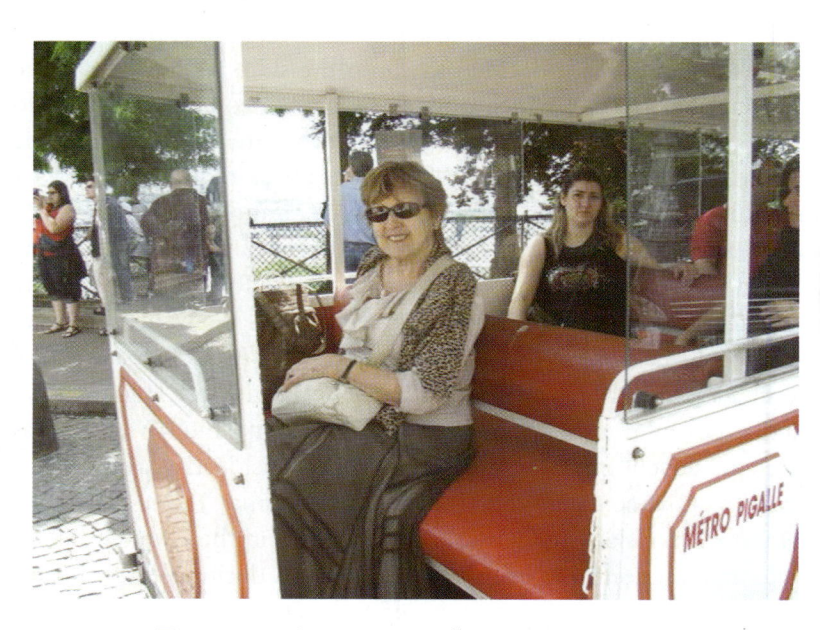

Figure 167. Streetcar to Pigalle Métro station, Paris.

response was supposed to be *"Zuzanna lubi je tylko jesienią — Przysyła ci świeżą partię"* ("Zuzanna likes them only in the fall — She is sending you a fresh batch"). This exchange is familiar to every Pole who watched the series in the late Sixties and early Seventies (almost everybody) and later in reruns and on DVD. (I still have all 18 episodes on DVD.) Our whirlwind tour of Paris came to an end the following day, and we flew back to Kraków on LOT Flight 344.

My final presentation for 2010 was at a meeting in Kraków, IX Krakowskie Dni Dalizoterapii (The Ninth Cracovian Days of Dialyzotherapy). The organizer, Prof. Olgierd Smoleński, asked me to present the history and current status of the buttonhole method of needle insertion, a topic I had talked about in Kraków in 2006, but in English. This time it was to be in Polish; it was actually my first talk in Poland, in Polish, on the method that had been invented in Poland 38 years earlier [Pr 523].

2011

In 2011 I gave just four presentations, all for the Hemodialysis Symposium alongside our Annual Dialysis Conference in Phoenix, Arizona, from February 19 to 22. I was asked to discuss exit site classification and its role in appropriate exit site care [Pr 524], and in two further presentations I summarized the influence of dialysis time on blood pressure control [Pr 525] and the impact of required dialyzer blood flow on blood access results [Pr 526] in five centers on four continents. It was apparent that longer dialysis and slower dialyzer blood flow are beneficial for patients. My last talk was a substitution for Dr. Carl Kjellstrand, who could not make it to Phoenix. The presentation offered multiple reasons why Kt/V_{urea} should not be used as a measure of dialysis adequacy, the most important being that K_{urea} (clearance of urea) and t (time of dialysis) influence dialysis performance in different ways and changes in t cannot be compensated with K. Standardized Kt/V_{urea} (std Kt/V_{urea}) is calculated from predialysis (C_0) and postdialysis (C) concentrations of urea, so-called urea reduction ratio (URR = C/C_0), even without knowing the value of clearance, time of dialysis, and volume (V) of urea distribution [Kt/V_{urea} = $\ln(C_{0\ urea}/C_{urea})$]. It has been always surprising to me that something

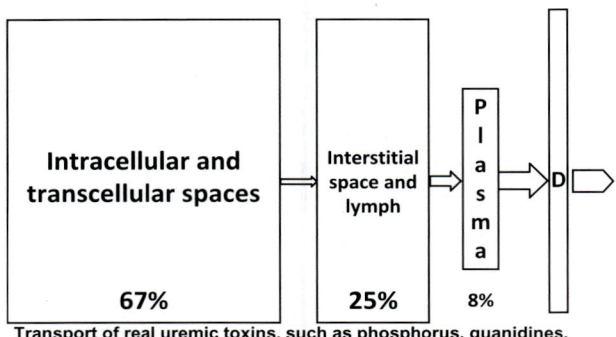

Intracellular and transcellular spaces ⇒	Interstitial space and lymph ⇒	P l a s m a	⇒ D ⇒
67%	25%	8%	

Transport of real uremic toxins, such as phosphorus, guanidines, and beta-2 microglobulin is similar to that of sodium and water

Figure 168. Fluid spaces, sodium and water transfer in hemodialysis patients.

mathematically correct has been widely accepted despite the fact that physiologically it does not make any sense [Pr 527].

The major problem with this index is that the transfer of urea between fluid spaces or compartments is much faster than of any real uremic toxin. Figure 168 illustrates three fluid spaces and their changes during short hemodialysis. The three spaces are in equilibrium before a hemodialysis session. The situation is completely different during short, efficient hemodialysis. The widths of the arrows between the spaces illustrate the speed of sodium and water transfer during dialysis: rapid from plasma to dialysate, slower from interstitial space to plasma, and very slow from intracellular to interstitial space. In one of my papers for dialysis patients, I compared this arrangement to the multiple swimming pools in a large natatorium [Pu 369]. Let us imagine that the natatorium is composed of three pools: large, middle-sized and small. The large pool represents the intracellular water (the water found in each of the body's cells and so-called transcellular space), the middle pool represents the interstitial water and lymph (the water found in organs and tissues between cells), and the small pool represents plasma. Now, let us imagine that these three pools are connected by narrow pipes. The movement of water between the pools is controlled by gravity: the greater the difference in the amount of water contained in the pools, the more the water will flow from one pool into the other. In other words, the water will flow from a pool that is filled up to one that is not. Finally, let us imagine that the water from the small pool (plasma) is being removed very rapidly. Because of the narrowness of the pipes, the water from the middle pool (interstitial space) cannot refill the

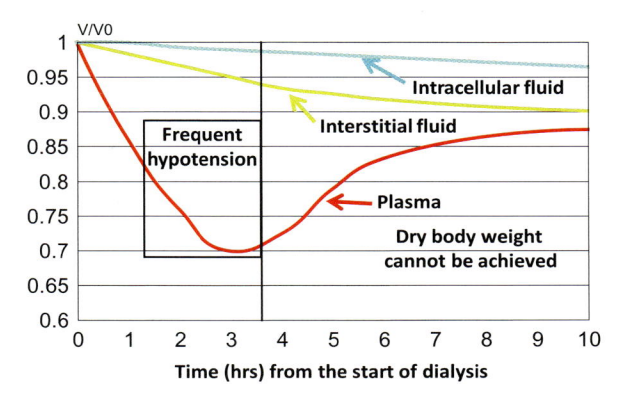

Figure 169. Volume changes during short hemodialysis.

water in the small pool (plasma) quickly enough, so the volume of water in plasma rapidly decreases until it falls below a critical level, resulting in hypotension. The pipe between the large pool and the middle pool is even narrower, so the refilling of the middle pool is even slower.

The consequence of this rapid removal of water from the plasma during short hemodialysis is illustrated in Fig. 169. In this diagram V/V_0 represents the ratio of volume at particular time to volume at the start of dialysis. Plasma volume decreases rapidly and is slowly replaced from the interstitial fluid, which is even more slowly replaced from the intracellular fluid. Hypotensive episodes are frequent, with 20–30 percent plasma volume loss, so the real dry body weight (the correct amount of volume in the interstitial fluid compartment) cannot be achieved. Volume changes during long dialysis with slow ultrafiltration are shown in Fig. 170. Plasma volume decreases slowly and is replaced from the interstitial fluid, which is in turn replaced from the intracellular fluid. There are no hypotensive episodes and dry body weight can be achieved. It is important to realize that the transport of urea, which is not toxic in concentrations encountered in dialysis patients, is much faster than the transport of real uremic toxins, such as phosphorus, guanidines, beta-2 microglobulin and other charged and higher molecular weight solutes. The transport of these molecules is similar to that of sodium and water. In my presentation [Pr 527] I predicted that Kt/V_{urea} will be rejected as a measure of dialysis quality and that the time of dialysis will be increased in a few years' time.

In early April I was invited by Dr. Jan Tordoir to participate as a member of the PhD committee for Mrs. Magda van Loon, who was to

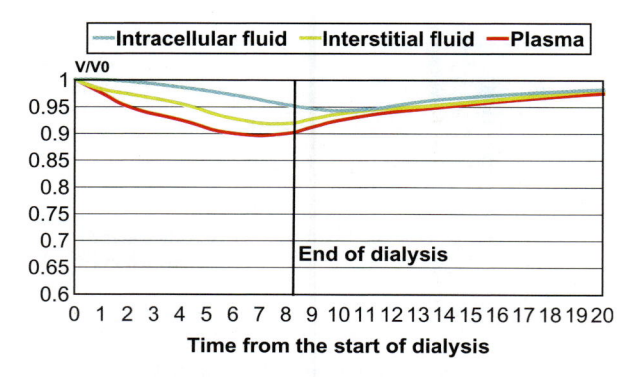

Figure 170. Fluid compartment volume changes during long dialysis.

defend her thesis entitled "Cannulation techniques and complications of hemodialysis vascular access" on Thursday, May 26, in Maastricht. Mrs. van Loon, a nurse in the Department of Surgery, University Hospital Maastricht, is one of the pioneers of the buttonhole technique in the Netherlands, and it was for this reason that Dr. Tordoir, co-supervisor of her PhD thesis, asked me to become a committee member. I flew with Halina from Kraków to Brussels and then by taxi to the Kruisheren hotel on Kruisherengang in Maastricht on May 25. Our taxi driver, a Belgian, passed the hotel a few times as it looked like a church. After we checked in, we discovered that the hotel had been converted in 2005 from a Kruisheren cloister, which was built by order of the Crutched Friars in the 16th century. At the end of 18th century the Crutched Friars were driven away when the French occupied the city, and the monastery was used to house French soldiers. For the next two centuries the buildings served as shops and for other purposes, until 2005 when the cloister and church were converted into the hotel. Maastricht is considered by many to be the oldest city in the Netherlands. It was built over the walls of a Roman settlement, *Traiectum ad Mosam*, at the crossroads of several international trading routes. By the early Middle Ages, Maastricht had become a city. The name *Traiectum* is preserved in the "– tricht" of Maastricht — the town on the river Maas (or Meuse).

The PhD ceremony took place the following day in Minderbroeders chapel at Maastricht University, with Mrs. van Loon successfully defending her thesis (Fig. 171), and in the afternoon we were invited for a very enjoyable celebration dinner. We returned to Kraków the next day.

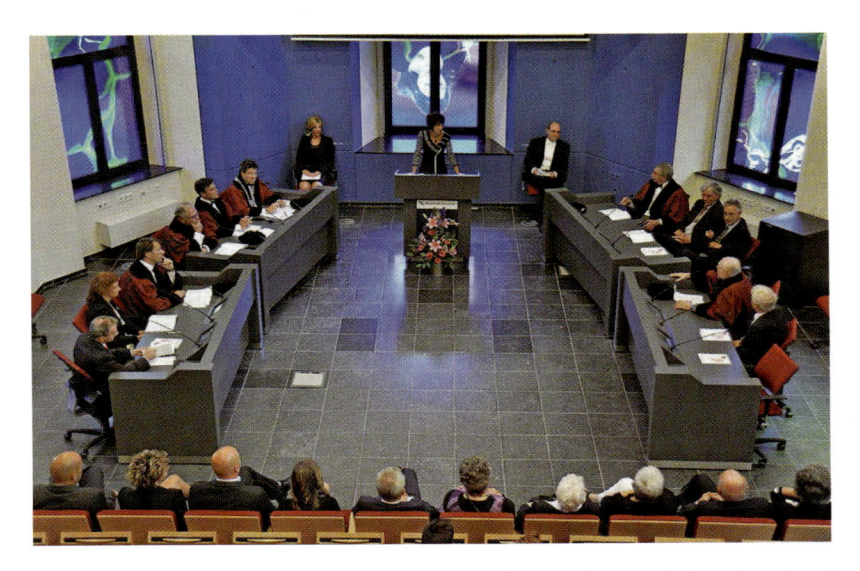

Figure 171. Magda van Loon defends her PhD thesis in the Minderbroeders chapel at Maastricht University, Netherlands.

In 2012 I gave four presentations. Two of them were made during our Hemodialysis Symposium of the Annual Dialysis Conference in San from Antonio, Texas, February 25–28. In the first presentation, I provided inferential data that prescribed high dialyzer blood flow increases access related complications and shortens its survival [Pr 529]. The second was on the history of buttonhole technique [Pr 529].

In May Prof. Władysław Sułowicz, with the cooperation of the Polish Society of Nephrology, organized a Conference on the 50th Anniversary of the First Hemodialysis in Krakow and an educational course on dialysis therapy and kidney transplantation, supported by the European Renal Association-European Dialysis and Transplant Association (ERA-EDTA). In this conference, I gave a presentation on my memories from the first hemodialysis in Kraków, which I described in detail in the Chapter 2 [Pr 530], and participated in the session on "Meet the Experts [Pr 531]".

At the opening of this conference I was honored by the Rector of the Jagiellonian University with a medal "Plus Ratio Quam Vis" and diploma (Fig. 172), which reads: "Nos, Rector Universitatis Jagiellonicae Cracoviensis, Pro Magnis Merits in Nostram Universitatem, Virum illustrissimum, Zbylutum Twardowski, Nummo Plus Ratio Quam Vis Ornavimus. Carolus Misiol, Universitatis Jagielonicae Cracoviensis,

Pro Magnis Merits in Nostram Universitatem, Virum Illustrissium, Zbylutum Twardowski, Nummo Plus Ratio Quam Vis Ornavimus. Carolus Misiol, Universitqatis Jagielonicae Cracoviensis Hoc Tempore Rector Magnificus. Dabamus Cracoviae Die Decima Mensis Mai Anno Bis Millesimo Duodecimo (We, the rector of the Jagiellonian University of Cracow, for extraordinary merit in our university, decorate the illustrious man Zbylut Twardowski with the medal "reason is greater than force." Karol Musioł, at this time, the most excellent rector of the Jagiellonian University is of Cracow). We have given this in Cracow on the 10th day of the month of May in the year 2012.

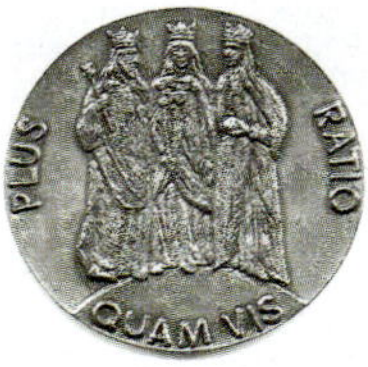

Averse

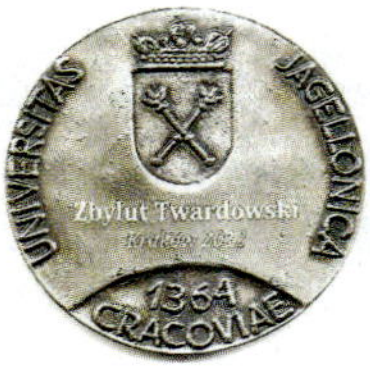

Reverse

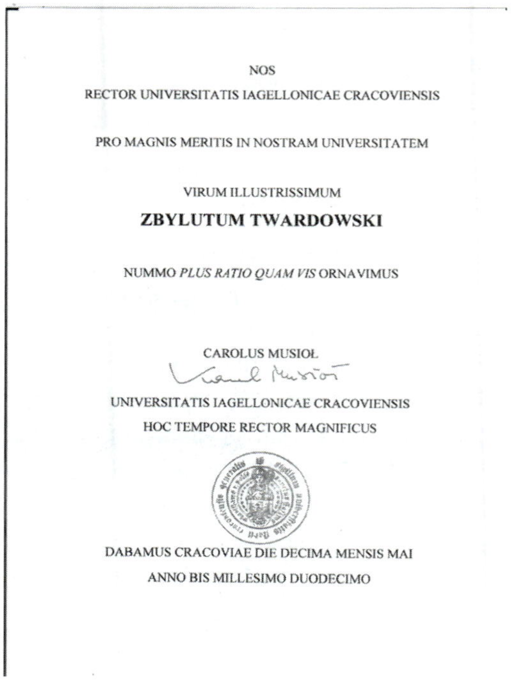

NOS
RECTOR UNIVERSITATIS IAGELLONICAE CRACOVIENSIS

PRO MAGNIS MERITIS IN NOSTRAM UNIVERSITATEM

VIRUM ILLUSTRISSIMUM
ZBYLUTUM TWARDOWSKI

NUMMO *PLUS RATIO QUAM VIS* ORNAVIMUS

CAROLUS MUSIOŁ

UNIVERSITATIS IAGELLONICAE CRACOVIENSIS
HOC TEMPORE RECTOR MAGNIFICUS

DABAMUS CRACOVIAE DIE DECIMA MENSIS MAI
ANNO BIS MILLESIMO DUODECIMO

Figure 172. Medal and Diploma of the Jagiellonian University. On averse: King Casimir the Great, King Władysław II Jagiełło (Ladislaus II Jagiello), St. Hedwig, Queen of Poland, and motto of the Jagiellonian University: "Reason is greater than force." On reverse: University coat of arms — crossed Rector Scepters, my name, place and date.

Translation of Diploma: We, the rector of the Jagiellonian University of Cracow, for extraordinary merit in our university, decorate the illustrious man Zbylut Twardowski with the medal *"reason is greater than force."* Karol Musioł. At this time, the most excellent rector of the Jagiellonian University of Cracow. We have given this in Cracow on the 10th day of the month of May in the year 2012.

Chapter 13

Vacations and Travel Unrelated to Business

As I mentioned I had so many business trips that I did not take too much vacation time during my employment in Columbia. They were short, usually a week, sometimes 10 or 14 days. It was different when I worked in Poland, where vacations were usually longer, up to four weeks. The situation has changed again after my retirement.

1989 — Kuźnica

My first vacation was at the seaside in Kuźnica on the Hel Peninsula in Poland, in July 1989. It was just after the first "semi-free" elections in Poland on June 4.[1] At that time, services were extremely cheap in Poland as the dollar was extremely strong relative to the Polish zloty. I remember that for a two-week stay in a private home in Kuźnica we paid only the equivalent of US$50. It was the last year the Polish zloty was so weak. With the development of the Polish economy after the collapse of communism in Poland, the currency started to gain strength. I was never able to get such a bargain again.

1992 — Keystone

In January 1992 we decided to spend a few days skiing with Leonor Ponferrada, John C. Van Stone and their friends, and we rented a house in Keystone, Colorado. Everyone was a non-smoker, except for me. By then I had been a pack-a-day smoker for more than 40 years. It was not a problem when I was in Poland as most people were smokers, but the situation was different in the U.S., particularly at the hospital and the Dialysis Clinic, where the majority did not smoke. It had begun to get a little uncomfortable for me, as many colleagues complained about the smell of the smoke. The situation became even more awkward when Halina came in 1985, as she had quit smoking while in Poland and did not like the smell either.

---

1. In many countries the fall of the Berlin Wall on November 10, 1989, is considered the end of communism in Eastern Europe. However, the demise of communism actually began in Poland with the Solidarity movement and the establishment of the free Polish Sejm (Parliament) after the free elections of June 4, 1989, five months before the fall of the Berlin Wall. The emergence of a free Poland separated the Soviet Union from East Germany.

I decided to quit as well. I had smoked for so many years that it was very unlikely I could quit abruptly, as I was probably addicted. So I decided to go slowly by restricting places I could smoke, like home, the office and in cars. By imposing such restrictions I gradually came down to 15, 12 and then 10 cigarettes per day, and going to Keystone with a group of non-smokers encouraged me to quit completely. It turned out to be easier than I had originally thought. I gave up and never considered returning to the habit. In fact, I changed the diagnosis: I came to the conclusion that I was not addicted but merely habituated and probably could have quit earlier — speculation, of course, which cannot be proven. The only consequence of quitting was some weight gain, which is a well-known phenomenon, although not completely explained. One explanation is that while smoking cigarettes a person is not inclined to munch, so he or she consumes fewer calories. A more scientific explanation was given by Angela Hofstetter and her colleagues in a study published in the *New England Journal of Medicine* in 1986.[2] The study was performed on eight cigarette smokers who spent two 24-hour periods in a metabolic chamber, once not smoking and once smoking 24 cigarettes. The energy expenditure was approximately 200 kcal higher during the smoking period, concomitantly with increases in diurnal excretions of norepinephrine and epinephrine, most likely stimulated by nicotine, and cotinine. They calculated that people who stop smoking 24 cigarettes per day may be expected to gain 10 kg of body weight within a year if diet and exercise patterns remain unchanged. I was already gaining weight when I was cutting down, but after quitting I started to gain more weight and eventually reached 99 kg (218 lbs) after Christmas 1994.

1993–1994 — Branson

I do not remember going anywhere on vacation in 1993, but I had some business travel, as already described. In summer 1994 we invited Halina's sisters, Joanna and Barbara, and her nieces, Barbara's daughters Justyna and Karolina, for a two-week stay in Columbia. During their stay we visited the State Capitol in Jefferson City, the Lake of the

---

2. Hofstetter A, Schutz Y, Jéquier E, Wahren J. (1986) Increased 24-hour energy expenditure in cigarette smokers. *N Engl J Med* **314**(2): 79–82.

Ozarks, Silver Dollar City, and Branson. These were short trips over the weekends. In Branson we attended the Yakov Smirnoff Show and the Shoji Tabuchi Show. Yakov Smirnoff, a Russian comedian who immigrated to the U.S., was particularly entertaining.[3] On the way back we went to the Animal Paradise Family Fun Park, where exotic animals from around the world roam free, and you can observe from the safety of your car. We saw zebras, buffaloes and other wild animals, though I do not remember seeing any predators there. The name "Animal Paradise" comes from the fact that the situation is the opposite of what happens in a normal zoo, where animals are in cages and people are free to roam.

1995 — Canada and Alaska tour and cruise

In 1995 I had only one presentation in the second half of the year, so we decided to join Georgia and Karl Nolph on a tour and cruise of Canada and Alaska organized by Boone County National Bank in Columbia. We took a flight to Calgary, Alberta, on September 5, and then joined a bus tour. From Calgary we went to the Banff National Park and stayed a night in one of the hotels. For nephrologists Banff is very significant place, as one of the early classifications of the renal pathology in lupus erythematosus was established at the so-called "Banff Conference." The next day we went to see Lake Louise, which is an incredibly beautiful emerald color due to the light reflecting off the "rock flour."[4] The next day we drove to the city of Kelowna at Okanagan Lake in British Columbia. There is a legend that a giant serpent-like creature named Ogopogo lives in the lake. The legend predates Nessie, the Scottish Loch Ness Monster, by more than 80 years. We heard different stories about Ogopogo — including one claiming that the creature is a brother or cousin of Nessie — but we

---

3. I remembered Smirnoff from an interview on TV, when I first came to Columbia in 1976. An interviewer asked him whether he spoke English before coming to the U.S. He answered that he did not speak a word. The interviewer had continued, "So how did you learn to speak such excellent English?" Yakov answered, "I listened to the TV. The problem was that after three months I realized that it was a Spanish channel."

4. The glaciers at the head of the valley that are the source of Lake Louise's water grind up the limestone into a fine glacial silt known as "rock flour." This finds its way into the lake and gives it its characteristic color.

were not lucky enough to see it. We spent only a night and a day in Kelowna before heading to Vancouver on Saturday, September 9. On Sunday we visited Queen Elizabeth Park to see its numerous species of plants, trees and shrubs. I remember being impressed by the beautiful topiary of various animals and other structures.

On Monday we boarded a Holland America Statendam ship for a cruise to Alaska. Purchased from the Russian Empire on March 30, 1867, for US$7.2 million (2 cents per acre), Alaska has an interesting connection to the Polish people. According to several sources, the first administrator of Alaska, the largest state in the U.S. by area, was Włodzimierz Krzyżanowski, the first cousin of Frédéric Chopin (Polish: Fryderyk Szopen or Chopin).[5] The posting was a reward for his performance as the personal representative of Secretary William H. Seward during the negotiations for the purchase of Alaska. Krzyżanowski was a Polish immigrant, military leader and a brigade commander in the Union Army during the American Civil War. President Lincoln promoted him to the rank of brevet brigadier general on March 2, 1865, for his accomplishments during the war. On March 30, 1867, the Russian flag was lowered and the American flag was raised. The land went through several administrative changes before becoming an organized territory on May 11, 1912, and the 49th state of the U.S. on January 3, 1959. Sitka, the previous capital of Russian Alaska, remained the capital until 1912, when it was moved to Juneau, which was founded by gold prospectors from Sitka, Joe Juneau and Richard Harris, in 1880.

Our first stop was Ketchikan, a city with the world's largest collection of standing totem poles. It is also known for having the highest annual rainfall in the U.S., so much so that rain is called "liquid sunshine" by the locals and the average rainfall is measured in feet, not inches. It was sunny weather when we arrived, though, and our guide told us that she could not show us typical Ketchikan weather. To be honest we were not disappointed. Our next stop was Sitka. We visited the Alaska Raptor Center, where we could see bald eagles under care and rehabilitation in the hospital. Some of them could not be completely rehabilitated and released, so they were kept as "Raptors-in-Residence."

---

5. Chopin's mother, Justyna Krzyżanowska, was the sister of Włodzimierz Krzyżanowski's father.

Juneau was our next stop, and from there we took a helicopter excursion to the Mendenhall Glacier. We were astonished to learn from our guide that the glacier started to recede from its greatest size as early as 1750, many years before so-called man-made global warming first began sometime in the 20th century. As usual the food on board was excellent, and we also had the opportunity to visit an ice cream parlor and indulge in a chocolate extravaganza. But all this good food had some unpleasant consequences for me. Before the cruise I lowered my weight to 94 kg (207 lbs), but afterwards it went up to 97 kg (214 lbs). I also checked my fasting glucose and it had gone up to 140 mg/dL. I was concerned about developing diabetes and decided I had to reduce my calorie intake and do more physical activities (swimming, walking, cycling and lifting weights). This regimen has worked slowly but surely, and at the time of writing, in September 2011, my weight is 82 kg (181 lbs) and my fasting blood glucose is below 90 mg/dL.

1996 — Trip with my brother, Lesław, through the American Midwest

As I mentioned previously, in the summer 1996 I had no presentations, so I took 15 days off to travel with Halina and my brother Lesław in the Midwestern U.S. in June. He arrived in St. Louis on TWA255 at 18:22 on Saturday, June 1, and I picked him up in our Pontiac Bonneville. On Sunday we went for Mass in our parish, the Sacred Heart Church, and in the afternoon we went to Jefferson City to visit the Capitol building. The next day I showed him our hospital and Dialysis Clinic at 3300 LeMone Industrial Blvd. On Tuesday we started our tour through Kansas City and then followed large portions of the Lewis and Clark Trail.[6] Our first stop was in Omaha, Nebraska, where we visited the Lewis and Clark National Historic Trail on

---

6. After the Louisiana Purchase, President Thomas Jefferson commissioned the Corps of Discovery as a scientific and military expedition to explore the newly acquired land. Jefferson selected U.S. Army Captain Meriwether Lewis and his aide and personal friend, to lead the Corps of Discovery. Lewis selected William Clark as his partner. The expedition started in May 1804 and ended in St. Louis in September 1806. The expedition covered approximately 3,700 miles, beginning near Wood River, Illinois, and passed through portions of Missouri, Kansas, Iowa, Nebraska, South Dakota, North Dakota, Montana, Idaho, Oregon and Washington.

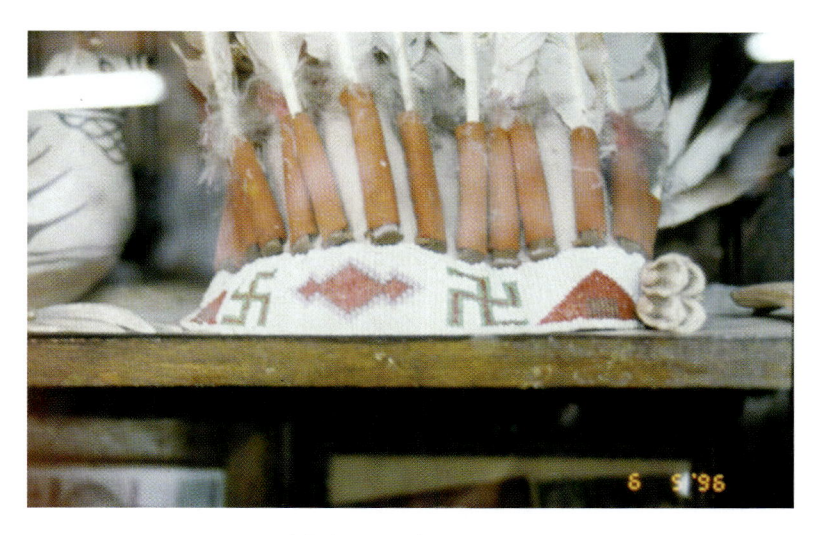

Figure 173.   A left-facing Indian swastika on a headdress.

Woolworth Avenue. We stayed one night on the other side of the Missouri River at Days Inn in Council Bluffs. The next day we drove along the trail through Sioux City, Iowa, then continued on Interstate 29 (I-29) through Sioux Falls, South Dakota, and then on I-90 to Best Western Lee's Motor Inn in Chamberlain, South Dakota. On the way we stopped at the Old West Museum. In the Indian Artifact section, I spotted a headdress with a swastika symbol (Fig. 173). I was quite astonished, as I had always thought that it was a symbol of the Nazi Party in Germany. How could it have been a symbol used by American Indians?[7]

On Thursday we drove through Rapid City, South Dakota, to Ramada Limited at 608 E 2nd Street in Gillette, Wyoming. On the way we returned to Keystone to see Mount Rushmore National Memorial, located in the Black Hills region of South Dakota. Mount Rushmore features 60-foot (18-meter) sculptures of the heads of

---

7. Only later did I learn that this symbol was known in antiquity in Iran, China, India, Japan and southern Europe. In the Middle Ages, in the Slavic countries as well as western and northern Europe, it was well known, though not commonly used, and had many different names: *Hakenkreuz* in Germanic princedoms, fylfot in England, *crux gammata* in Latin countries, and tetraskelion or gammadion in Greece. Both clockwise (from the center) angled and counter-clockwise angled swastikas have been used. American Indians used this symbol in the 19th century or maybe even earlier.

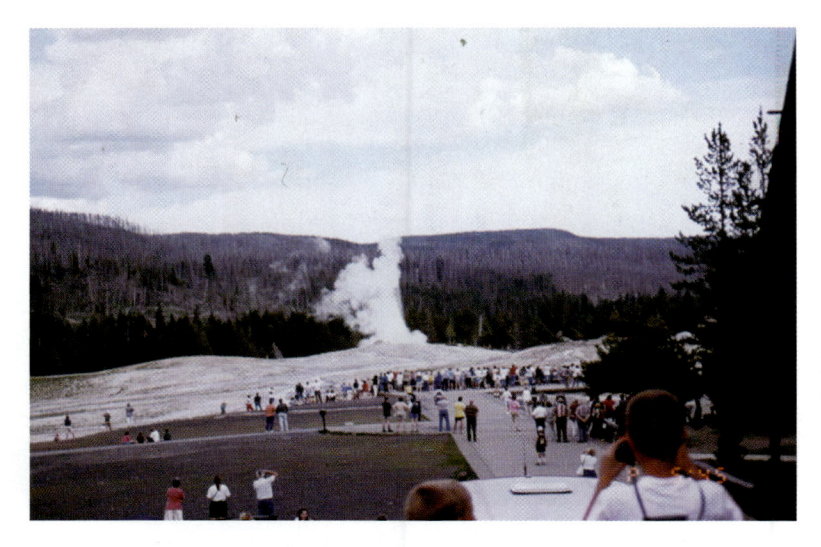

Figure 174. The Old Faithful Geyser in Yellowstone blows its top.

former U.S. Presidents George Washington, Thomas Jefferson, Theodore Roosevelt and Abraham Lincoln. The sculptures were completed between 1934 and 1939. We then visited a site in the Black Hills where Korczak Ziółkowski started his attempt to create the largest sculpture in the world of famous Indian Chief, Crazy Horse. At the time of our visit Ziółkowski's sons were continuing his work following their father's death in 1982. At that time the work was very far from completion.

From Gillette we went to Yellowstone National Park and stayed for two days and three nights in Grand Village Motel. The park, established in 1872, is centered over the Yellowstone Caldera,[8] the largest supervolcano on the continent. There are numerous geysers in the park, the most famous being Old Faithful, so called because of its tendency to erupt rather regularly, as it did when we visited (Fig. 174). Hundreds of species of mammals, birds, fish and reptiles inhabit the park, and the vast forests and grasslands also include unique species of plants. We managed to see grizzly bears, wolves and free-ranging herds of bison and elk, observed from a distance,

---

8. The caldera is considered an active volcano. It has erupted violently several times over the last two million years.

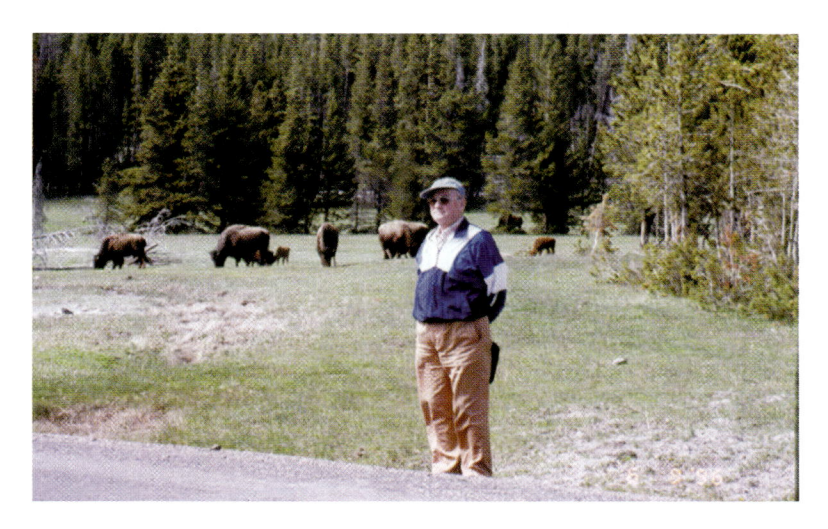

Figure 175. My brother, Lesław, and grazing buffaloes.

of course (Fig. 175). On Sunday we went to Jackson Hole, driving through the valley in Grand Teton National Park. The valley is surrounded by high mountains and crowned by three peaks named the Pilot Knobs by beaver trappers from Missouri, or Les Trois Tetons[9] by French trappers. It is believed that the Missouri trappers dubbed the valley Jackson,[10] and they frequently referred to a valley surrounded by high mountains as a "hole." Thus Jackson's Hole, or later Jackson Hole, was born.

On Monday we went to Billings, Montana, where we stayed for one night in the Dude Rancher Lodge at 415 N 29th Street. The following day we drove to Bismarck on I-94. At the time there was no speed limit in Montana, so I wanted to test the maximum speed of my Pontiac Bonneville. I could not get over 110 mph (177 kph). In Bismarck we stayed two nights in the Comfort Inn at 1030 E. Interstate Ave. and spent a few days with the family of our older son, Radek. On Wednesday morning we visited the Capitol. On display in the Capitol are portraits of famous North Dakotans, one of which was of Phil

---

9. So called because they resembled female breasts to the French!

10. David Edward Jackson served in the War of 1812 under the command of his cousin, Colonel Andrew Jackson (later the seventh President of the U.S.), and in 1826 became co-owner of the beaver trapping company Smith, Jackson and Sublette.

Jackson, who started his athletic career in Williston, North Dakota,[11] and later became known as the winner of the most championships in NBA history as a player and as a head coach. I was a fan of Phil Jackson from the time he was coaching the Chicago Bulls, but I was not aware of his association with North Dakota until we visited the Capitol in Bismarck. In the afternoon we went to the Fort Abraham Lincoln State Park in Mandan, which is across the Missouri River from Bismarck. In the park is the house of General George Armstrong Custer, whose adoration by North Dakotans is not quite clear to me. He was admitted to West Point in 1858, where he graduated last in his class and he was defeated and killed at the Battle of the Little Bighorn in 1876, fighting against a coalition of Native American tribes under the command of Crazy Horse and White Bull. On Thursday we drove to Minneapolis, Minnesota, and stayed at Econo Lodge on 2500 University Ave. SE. The next day we visited the Capitol in St. Paul and the largest mall in the world at the time, the Mall of America, in Bloomington. On Saturday, June 15, we drove to Chicago and stayed one day with our younger son, Przemysław, and his wife, Kasia, at 4061 Sheridan Road. The following day, we drove Lesław to his wife's sister, who lives in Chicago, and on Monday we drove back to Columbia. Our trip was over 3,240 miles (5200 km) in total.

1997–1999 — Retirement and apartment in Kraków

I did not take any vacations in 1997 and 1998, since I had various travel-related presentations, as already described. Halina and I also started to prepare for longer stays in Poland after my retirement. We agreed that after my retirement we would spend at least three months in Poland, and we decided upon a retirement date of June 1999, when I would be 65. There were some other incentives to retire at that time. Obviously, I could not have dialysis patients under my care with me not being in Columbia for prolonged periods. Besides, practicing medicine in a hospital setting was becoming rather unpalatable. Even when I was attending in the hospital, I was not the only one who decided how long a patient should stay. There was a committee that

---

11. The high school in Williston now has a sports complex named after him.

reviewed notes and if, in their opinion, they believed it to be the case, they would notify me that the patient should be discharged. If I felt that the patient should stay longer, I had to give further justification as to why the patient should stay. I found this irritating, as it was my opinion that only the attending physician could determine whether a patient was stable enough to be discharged. For me, writing additional explanations for a committee was a waste of time. This practice, as well as disruptions to attending rounds, is even more disagreeable these days.[12] Also, by retiring I could do some extra work, like editing *Hemodialysis International*, writing papers and participating in the organization of our Annual Conference. The Internet became an important method of communication. My e-mail address stayed the same regardless of where I was, so I could work from Poland as well. Finally, my salary was rather low, and royalties became my main source of income. I am supposed to be paid these royalties well into my 90s — or, more likely, for my beneficiaries.

Taking all these factors into account, we decided to buy an apartment in Kraków. As Poland's economy had opened up only a decade earlier, the building of apartments had just begun. At the end of April 1996, while in Kraków, Halina's sister, Basia, found an advertisement for a new building with about 20 apartments and garages in the basement close to Wawel Castle. We started to inquire whether the building contractor was reliable enough to risk a down payment, but our inquiries were negative and we decided to wait for another opportunity. In August 1997, while we were in Kraków for a presentation at the Nephrology Summer School, Basia told us about a similar advertisement for a building, close to the other one, being constructed by the same contractor. We again heard some negative opinions about the building developer, Mr. Wandyga, but the first building that we had decided against was progressing well and all the apartments had already been sold. I decided to take a risk. In the new building all the apartments except one were available, and we decided to buy one on the fifth floor with a garage in the basement.

Most of our payments had been settled by June 1998 when we visited Kraków. All the apartments had been sold at that point. When

---

12. The current problems were recently described in: Sarosi GE. (2010) On being a doctor: Attending rounds. *Ann Intern Med* **153**: 482.

we went to see the building, we found that the roof had been completed, but our apartment was not yet ready. As the weather was very hot, I asked whether it would be possible to install air conditioning. At the time not many people in Poland thought about air conditioning. I was told that it was possible, as our apartment was unfinished and the job could be relatively easily done, with condensers and compressors located on the balconies and cooling and dehumidifying units in the rooms. The moisture from the dehumidifiers was taken via piping under the floors to the bathrooms. It turned out to be an excellent purchase because summers sometimes get very hot in Kraków. The apartment, with all its appliances and furniture, was ready in the summer of 1999, just after I retired.

2000 — Great Britain and Ireland

We went on our first long tour of Europe in 2000, when I was already retired and we were living in Kraków during the summer months. Our grandchildren, Anna (Ania) and Adam, wanted to go with us for our tour of Great Britain and Ireland, which was organized by Trafalgar Tours (Fig. 176). Ania was 14 years old and Adam almost 10. On July 20, we picked them up from Puławy, where they were visiting their other grandfather, and drove to Kraków. The next day we flew from Balice Airport to London Gatwick on British Airways Flight No. BA4473. We were met at the airport by the Trafalgar representative and transferred to the Forum Hotel on Cromwell Road. The following day we had a morning sightseeing tour of London, taking in the Changing of the Guard at Buckingham Palace, the Houses of Parliament, Big Ben, and Trafalgar Square, with its statue of Lord Nelson on a huge Corinthian column. The statue commemorated his many victories in battles including over the French fleet at Trafalgar. On Sunday, July 23, we joined a bus tour, with an excellent driver called Noel Hitchman, and our tour guide, Rona Fitzpatrick, whose knowledge of the history of Great Britain and Ireland was amazing. We first visited Hampton Court, which was originally built for Cardinal Wolsey but later passed to King Henry VIII when Wolsey fell from favor. The impressive gardens were laid out in Dutch style for William III (reign: 1689–1702). Our next stop was Stonehenge, a monumental circular setting of large standing stones surrounded by a circular earthwork,

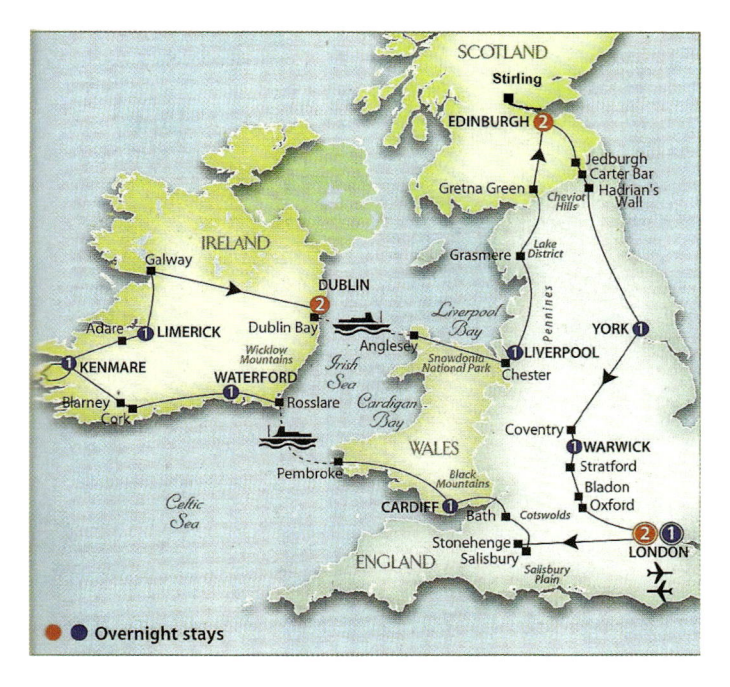

Figure 176. Our tour Great Britain and Ireland.

built in prehistoric times (anywhere from about 3000 BC to 2000 BC) and located about 8 miles (13 km) north of Salisbury, Wiltshire (Fig. 177). The purpose of the structure is uncertain.

From Stonehenge we visited Salisbury Cathedral, built in only 38 years from 1220 to 1258. The seat of an Anglican bishop, the cathedral has one of the four surviving original copies of the Magna Carta and contains the world's oldest working clock from 1380. Made without the use of a single screw, the clock has an iron frame that is held together by arbor pivots, rivets and wedge bolts. It also has no face, since all clocks of that time rang out the hours on a bell.[13] We next went to the city of Bath. The hot mineral springs (120°F or 49°C) at the site attracted the Romans, who founded Bath as *Aquae Sulis*,

---

13. It has to be mentioned that the word "clock" bears the mark of its initial way of indicating time. The Middle English *cloc* came from the Middle Dutch word for bell and is a related to the German *Glocke*, which means bell [Daniel J. Boorstin. (1985) *The Discoverers*. Vintage Books, A Division of Random House, New York, p. 37]. It appears to me that the word is onomatopoeic.

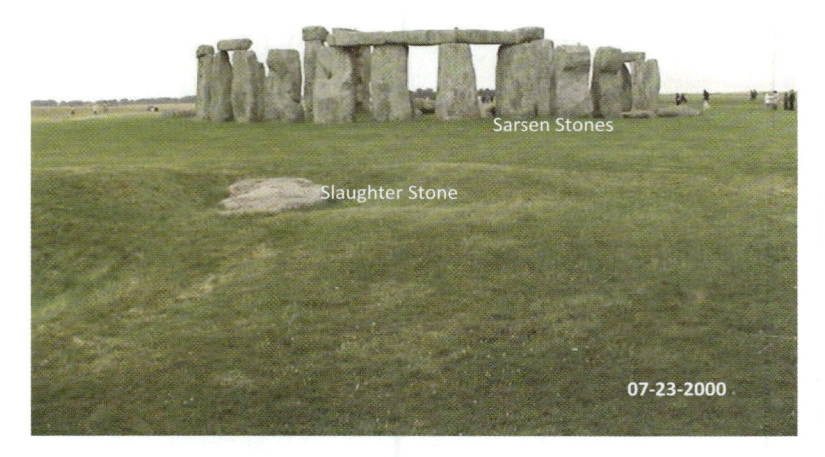

Figure 177. Stonehenge, as viewed from the Heelstone through the Slaughter Stone to the circle of sarsen stones.

dedicated to the deity Sul (Minerva). The Saxons built an abbey on the site at which Edgar, first king of all England, was crowned (AD 973). The Normans subsequently rebuilt the church between 1088 and 1122. Much later it became popular as a spa during the Georgian era, which led to a major expansion that left the exemplary Georgian Architecture crafted from Bath Stone. A unique structure is the Royal Crescent, a residential road of 30 houses laid out in a crescent. We visited the majority of sites of interest, including the Abbey, the Crescent, the Flower Garden and the Great Bath. From Bath we rode to the Quality Hotel on Merthyr Road, Tongwynlais, in Cardiff (Welsh: *Caerdydd*). I discovered that in Wales the names of streets and towns are written in English and in Welsh — and that the Welsh versions are not easy to pronounce.

Cardiff is the capital of Wales. The Romans built a small fort (c. AD 75) there, where their Gloucester-Carmarthen road crossed the Taff River, and strengthened it in the face of seaborne attacks from Ireland. The town began its continuous existence with the arrival of the Normans in the 11th century. By 1150 a stone keep was erected on

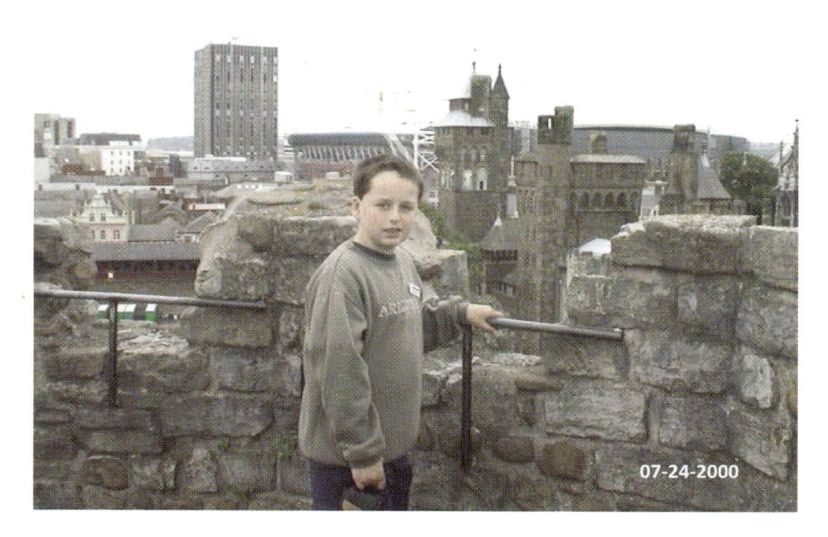

Figure 178. Adam on the top of the Keep in Cardiff Castle.

the mound, one of the finest surviving examples of its kind in the country. In the morning we visited Cardiff Castle, going through the Great Hall and the Roof Garden, and to the top of the Keep (Fig. 178). We then headed across South Wales via Carmarthen, the birthplace of Merlin the Wizard,[14] to Pembroke, where we boarded our ferry to Rosslare in Ireland. From Rosslare we rode again by coach to the Majestic Hotel in Tramore, Waterford County (Irish: *Port Láirge*).

The next morning we visited the Waterford Crystal Showroom, which exhibits famous crystal products manufactured from 1729. We were told that Waterford glass, particularly the early variety, is characterized by thick walls, deeply incised geometric cutting, and brilliant polish. The smoky, bluish gray color of early Waterford glass was considered uncomplimentary, so clear crystal was produced after 1830. It is the darkened glass, however, that is most prized by modern collectors. The next stop was in Blarney Castle (Irish: *An Bhlarna*) (Fig. 179). The greatest attraction over there is the Blarney Stone

---

14. An enchanter and wise man in Arthurian legend and romance of the Middle Ages.

Vacations and Travel Unrelated to Business

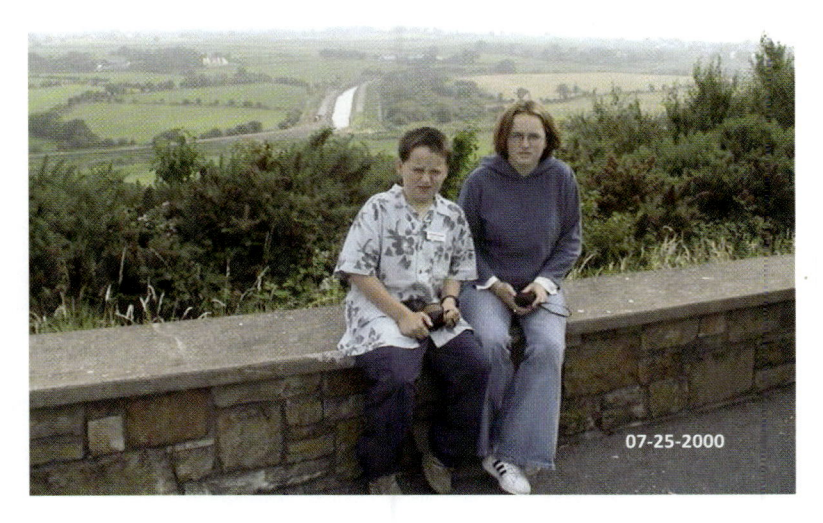

Figure 179. Adam and Ania in Blarney Castle.

(Irish: *Cloch na Blarnan*), reputed to provide the "gift of the gab" (confer eloquence) to those who kiss it, a feat that can only be achieved by ascending to the castle's peak, leaning over backwards on the parapet's edge and hanging one's head downward. An accident once occurred when someone was trying to kiss the stone, but it has now been fortified with an iron bar. And if that is not enough, there is also a Keeper of the Stone to physically restrain and support the kisser. I kissed the stone, but I did not think that it helped me, probably because I was already 66. Adam and Ania also kissed the stone, and it seems to have been successful, but they were young. Halina did not even need to try kissing the stone, as she was very eloquent anyway. In any event, mystery surrounds the story of the stone. The most commonly accepted story is that, in gratitude for Irish support at the Battle of Bannockburn in 1314 (when the Scottish defeated the English), Robert the Bruce gave a portion of the Scottish Coronation Stone (Stone of Scone or Stone of Destiny) to Cormac McCarthy, King of Munster. Installed at McCarthy's stronghold, Blarney Castle, it became known as the Blarney Stone. A century later, in 1446, King Dermot McCarthy

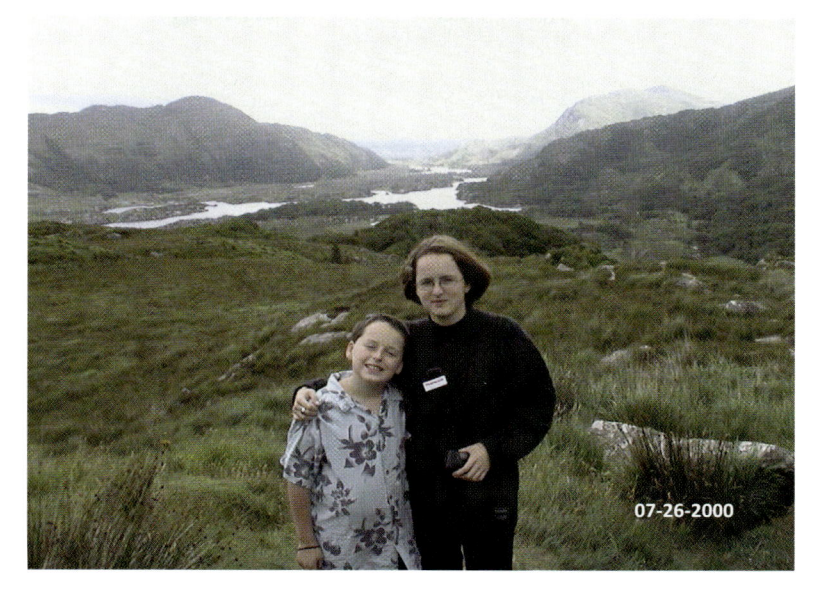

Figure 180. Ania and Adam enjoy a scenic view of the lakes at Killarney National Park in Kerry.

installed the stone in an enlarged castle he constructed.[15] Later that day we drove through Cork and Youghal to Riverside Hotel in Killarney (Irish: *Cill Airne*). In the evening we went to the Irish Pub in Killarney for the Larry Mathews Show.

The next day we were taken on a scenic coastal drive around the Ring of Kerry (or Iveragh Peninsula), and Killarney National Park, founded in 1932 and designated a UNESCO Biosphere Reserve in 1981 (Fig. 180). We were told that Irish vegetation is famous for having 40 shades of green. Some were identifiable in the park, others as we drove through Limerick county (Irish: *Luimneach*). Much of Limerick lies within the Golden Vale, famed for its rich pastures and dairy products. In many areas almost all the land is under grass and hay, for the main wealth lies in the dairy herds. En route Adam and Ania participated in the *Riverdance* at Kathleen's Irish Ceilidh in Bunratty Castle Hotel. We stayed the night at Ryan Hotel on Ennis

---

15. There is also a legend that the stone is not actually the local Scottish one but was probably brought by the Crusaders, and in reality it was the Stone of Jacob taken from Haran and used as a pillow on which Jacob dreamed of his ladder. This story seems far-fetched to me.

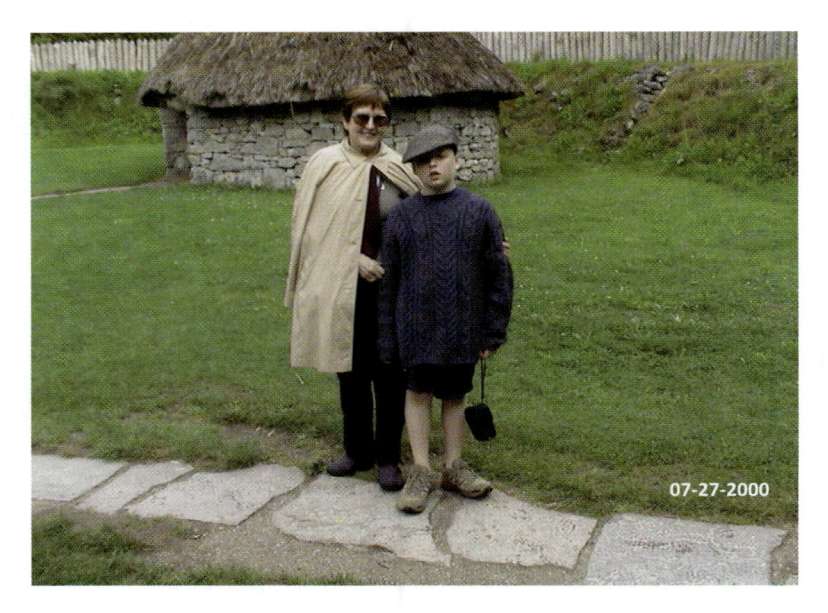

Figure 181. Halina and Adam in the ringfort of Craggaunowen Celtic Village.

Road in Limerick. The county is also associated with the invention of limericks, humorous and sometimes dirty verses.[16]

On Thursday, July 27, we drove across County Clare en route to Galway Bay. On the way we stopped in Craggaunowen Celtic Village, which offers a taste of Celtic life, with a reproduction of a Bronze Age village, set beside the 16th-century Craggaunowen Castle. One of the interesting features of this village was an example of a ringfort, a homestead where families and their servants lived. A ringfort was protected by an earthen bank alongside a trench with a gap for an entrance sealed off by a sturdy wooden gate; a robust wooden wall was put on the top of the bank (Fig. 181). Our next stop was in Bunratty Castle, which is situated at the River Shannon, also in County Clare, and we strolled through the Bunratty Folk Park located within the castle grounds. Before noon we reached Galway Bay and admired the scenic views. Then, driving east across Ireland from the Atlantic Ocean to the nation's

---

16. Limericks consist of five anapaestic lines. Lines 1, 3 and 5 have seven to ten syllables and rhyme with one another. Lines 2 and 4 have five to seven syllables and also rhyme with each other.

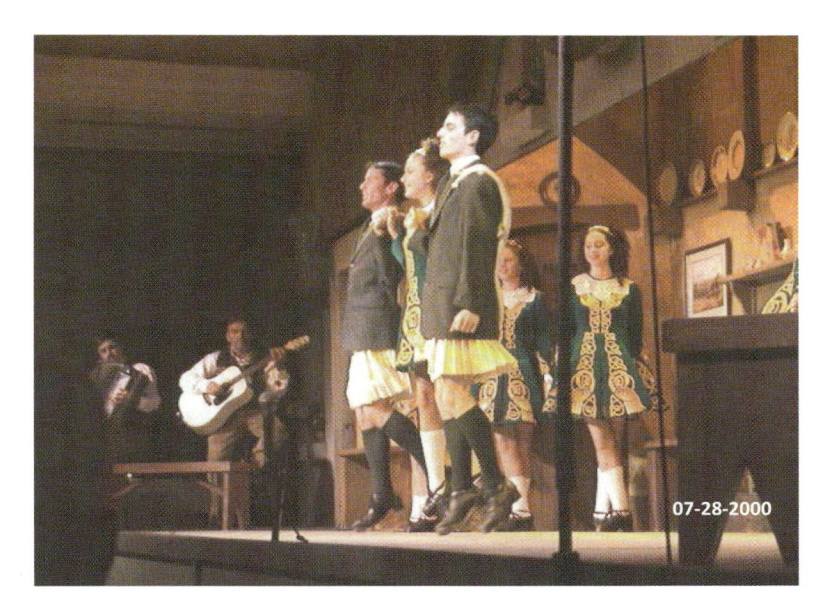

Figure 182. *Riverdance* at the Dublin Dinner and Cabaret.

capital at the Irish Sea, we finally reached Dublin, where we settled into the Gresham Hotel on O'Connell Street.

The next morning was devoted to seeing Dublin's sights, including Trinity College, St. Patrick's Cathedral and Phoenix Park. In the early afternoon we spent some time shopping and then visited the Guinness Brewery, producer of beer and stout, the nation's largest private employer and its largest industrial exporter. I wanted to visit the brewery, as I admired famous statistician William Sealy Gosset, who was hired by Claude Guinness to cheaply monitor the quality of his beer brews.[17] Gosset (known by his pen name *Student*) invented what is called the unpaired and paired t-test. I consider these tests, particularly the paired t-test, the most valuable for analyzing dialysis results. Later that evening we went for the Dublin Dinner and Cabaret featuring *Riverdance* (Fig. 182), which we found hugely entertaining.

---

17. William Sealy Gosset was hired because of Claude Guinness's innovative policy of recruiting the best graduates from Oxford and Cambridge to apply biochemistry and statistics to industrial processes. Gosset published the *t-test* in *Biometrica* in 1908, but was forced to use a pen name by his employer, who regarded the fact that they were using statistics as a trade secret.

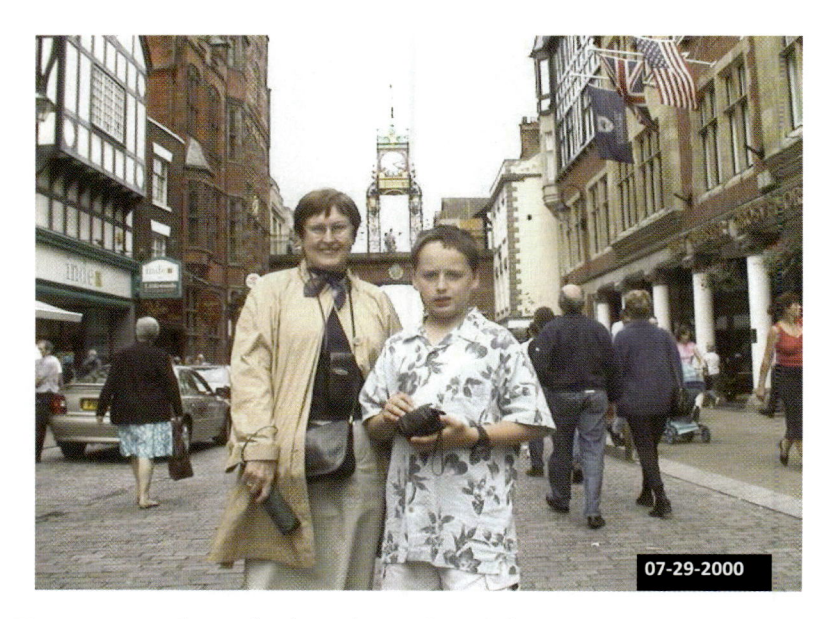

Figure 183. Halina and Adam admire Chester's famous Rows and a clock on the Roman Wall.

On Saturday, July 29, we took a ferry across the Irish Sea to the Welsh island of Anglesey. We then crossed Britannia Bridge to the mainland and continued past Snowdonia National Park to the historic Roman city of Chester, where we stopped to see the Tudor architecture and galleried shops known as the "Rows." The entire 2-mile (3-km) circuit of Chester's ancient walls is intact. The street plan of the central area is Roman in origin, with four main streets radiating at right angles. Perhaps the most distinctive feature of the town is the Rows, a double tier of shops with the lower ones set back and the upper ones projecting over them (Fig. 183). We continued on to Liverpool, where we planned to spend the night at Thistle Liverpool Hotel on Chapel Street. In the evening we went to the Parish Church of Our Lady and St. Nicholas for Mass. At the time *Christ on a Donkey* (Fig. 184), a controversial fiberglass sculpture by Brian Burgess, stood in the churchyard overlooking Chapel Street. I recently learned that the fiberglass figure started to deteriorate and eventually collapsed. There were not many people at the Mass, mostly older people; there

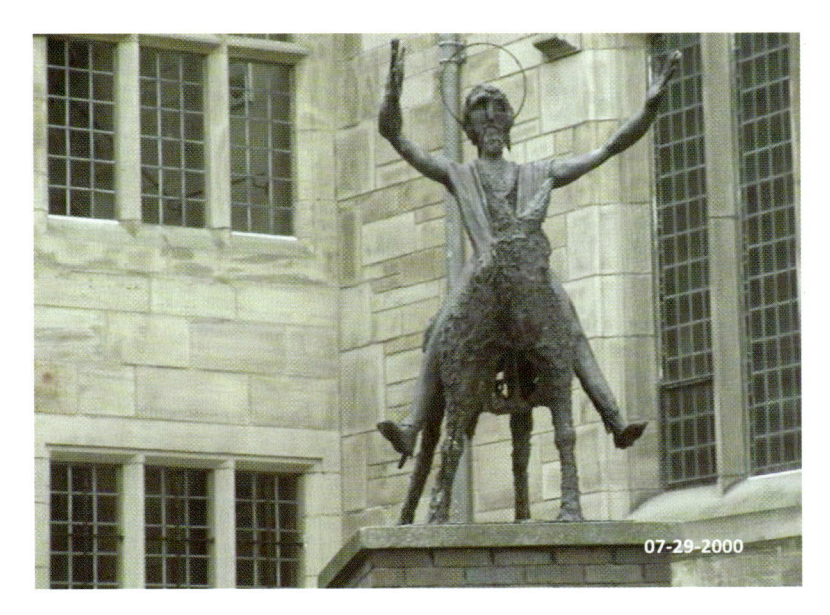

Figure 184 Brian Burgess' *Christ on a Donkey*.

were only two children in the church, aside from Adam and Ania. The pastor announced that two parishes would have to combine, as there were not enough priests or money to keep both. The situation in the Liverpool church resembled that which we observed in Amsterdam in 1988 when we were in the company of just a few Mass attendees and we were the youngest. It was completely different in the U.S. and Poland, where churches are usually full and there are large numbers of youngsters.

On Sunday, July 30, we drove through the beautiful English Lake District to visit Grasmere, and we took a trip on a boat on Grasmere Lake. From there we crossed the Scottish border at Moffat Woolens and visited Gretna Green before heading to the Scottish capital, Edinburgh, where we stayed at the Post House Hotel on Corstorphine Road. That evening we had a wonderful meal at the world famous fish and chip restaurant Harry Ramsden's. The next morning we went to "*Braveheart* country," driving through the Trossachs, home of Scottish folk hero Rob Roy MacGregor and famous Scottish knight William Wallace, and continuing on to Stirling Castle, known for its connections with William Wallace, Robert the Bruce and Mary Queen of

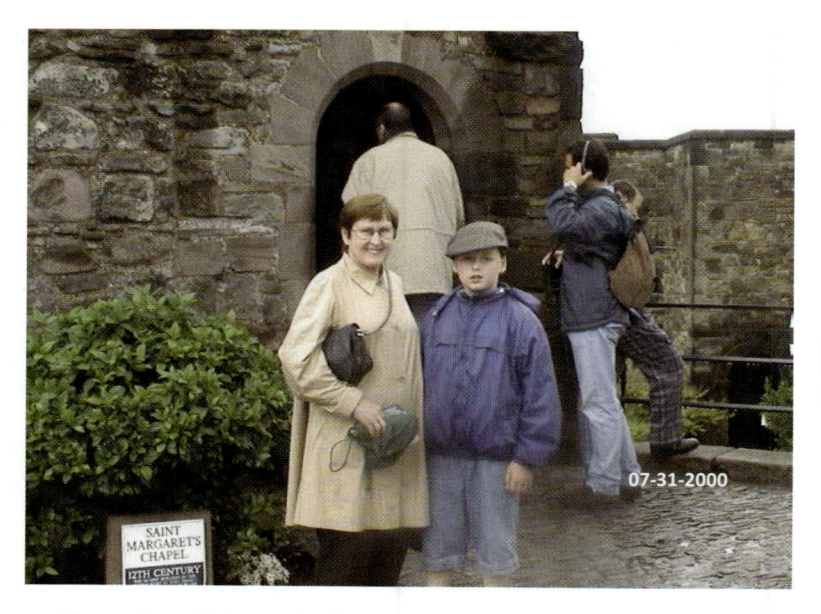

Figure 185. Halina and Adam at the entrance to St. Margaret's Chapel.

Scots. In the afternoon we visited Edinburgh's Princes Street Gardens, laid out between the Old and New towns, and Edinburgh Castle, with St. Margaret's Chapel on the rock's highest point, the oldest building in Scotland (Fig. 185).

We visited numerous places in Edinburgh Castle, including the famous Stone of Destiny, kept securely behind armored glass surrounded by a sophisticated security system. We wanted to see the "other half" of the Blarney Stone. The story we heard here about the stone was a little different. We were told it was originally kept in the village of Scone as a Coronation Stone, taken to England by King Edward I in 1296 and returned to Edinburgh in 1996. The stories about the stone are somewhat conflicting, however. According to the story I had heard in Blarney, the Blarney Stone was part of the Coronation Stone and was given to Cormac McCarthy by Robert the Bruce in 1314, 18 years after the stone was already supposed to be in England.[18] In the evening we invited Halina's relatives from Edinburgh for dinner at Posthouse Hotel Restaurant (Fig. 186).

---

18. We will probably never know the truth about the origins of the stone.

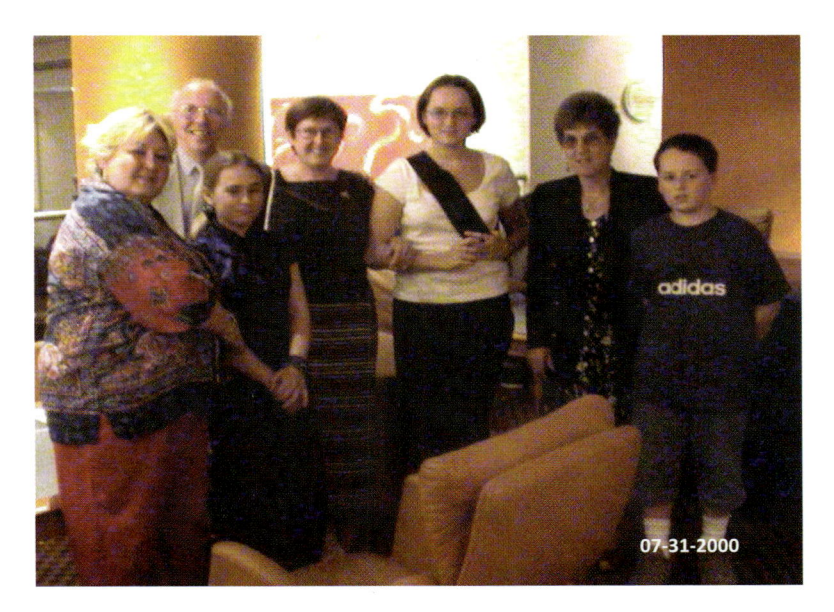

Figure 186. Anna, Patrick, Ann, Halina, Ania, Barbara and Adam before the dinner at the Posthouse Hotel Restaurant in Edinburgh.

On Tuesday, August 1, we drove south through the Scottish Borderlands and stopped to see the ruined Jedburgh Abbey, and then into England, through the rugged landscape of Northumberland National Park for a photo stop at Hadrian's Wall (Fig. 187). Hadrian (r. AD 117–138), the third of the Five Good Emperors (Nerva, Trajan, Hadrian, Antonius Pius and Marcus Aurelius), who traveled extensively during his reign, came to Britain in AD 122 and decided to build a defensive barrier that guarded the northwestern frontier of the province of Britain from barbarian invaders. The wall extended from coast to coast across the width of Britain; it ran for 73 miles (118 km) from Wallsend (*Segedunum*) on the River Tyne in the east to Bowness on the Solway Firth in the west. The wall was made of stones and was about 10 feet (3 meters) wide. At every one-third of a mile there was a tower, and at every mile a fortlet (milecastle) containing a gate through the wall, presumably surmounted by a tower, and one or two barrack-blocks. Building continued through most of Hadrian's reign. The wall was abandoned in favor of the Antonine Wall (constructed about 100 miles, or 160 km, to the north) under Hadrian's successor,

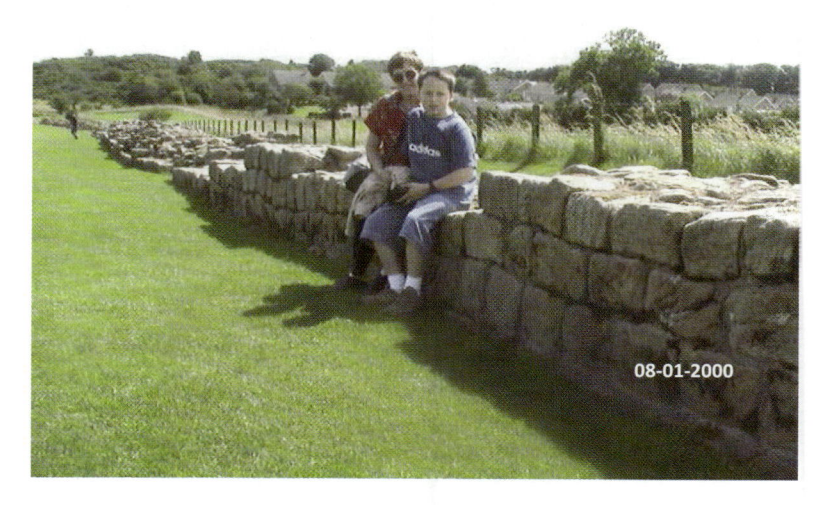

Figure 187. Halina and Adam on the Hadrian's Wall.

Antoninus Pius (r. AD 138–161), but thereafter continued to be used during Marcus Aurelius' reign and later until about the end of Roman Britain in AD 410. There are only fragments of the wall left as a tourist attraction; most of the stones have disappeared, used for road building and other construction.

In the afternoon we drove to York, where we stayed in Swallow Hotel on Tadcaster Road. York lies at the confluence of the Rivers Ouse and Foss, about midway between Edinburgh and London. The Romans occupied the site in AD 71 and built a fortress and wall, traces of which remain. Under the name *Eboracum*, the settlement served as the Romans' northern military headquarters until they withdrew in about 400. Anglo-Saxon rule followed and the Danes conquered York in 867. The city's present name was derived from the Danish Jorvik. We visited Shambles, an old twisty street with overhanging timber-framed buildings, some dating back to the 14th century. It was once known as the Great Flesh Shambles from the Anglo-Saxon *Fleshammels* (literally "flesh shelves"), the word for the shelves that butchers used to display their meat. We could find no butcher shops when we visited. We also toured the city's cathedral,

York Minster. The largest Gothic church in England, it was built between the 13th and 15th centuries.

On August 2 we headed for the Britannica Hotel on Cathedral Square in Coventry. On the way we stopped at Wedgwood Pottery Center, established by Josiah Wedgwood at Burslem, at Etruria, and finally at Barlaston, all in Staffordshire. In the decade of its first production, the 1760s, Wedgwood ware attained a world market, which it continues to hold. The company perfected the cream-colored earthenware called creamware, or Queen's ware, as a consequence of royal patronage. Mass-produced, it was nevertheless of high quality, being light, durable and tasteful both in terms of shape and decoration. We decided not to buy any pottery. In the afternoon we went to Coventry. Probably established in Saxon times, Coventry is known for the 11th-century story of Lady Godiva (*Godgifu*, meaning "gift of God" in Old English) in which she rode naked through the town on a white horse as a protest against high taxes imposed by her husband, Leofric, Earl of Mercia. The people were not supposed to look at the lady. Only one person, a tailor ever afterwards known as Peeping Tom, disobeyed her proclamation in one of the most famous instances of voyeurism; he bored a hole in his shutters and saw Lady Godiva pass and was struck blind. World War II saw the destruction of Coventry, and the air raids of November 1940 and April 1941 wiped out much of the city, including St. Michael's Cathedral, except for its tower and spire. I recall that during the bombing of Cologne in WWII its cathedral was damaged but the spires also did not collapse. Could the bombs have slid down the sides of the spire, damaging the buildings but leaving the spire intact? Or is this far-fetched? It would be difficult to confirm or reject the hypothesis. In any event, the city of Coventry had been rebuilt by the time we visited.

On Thursday, August 3, we headed back to the Forum Hotel in London, but on the way we visited several places. First, we visited Stratford-upon-Avon, the birthplace of William Shakespeare, who was born in a half-timbered house on Henley Street in 1564. In 1597 Shakespeare returned from London to the house known as New Place, where he died in 1616. His grave is in the parish church of the Holy Trinity. After seeing these places for ourselves, we went to Warwick Castle and later saw Sir Winston Churchill's grave in Bladon on our

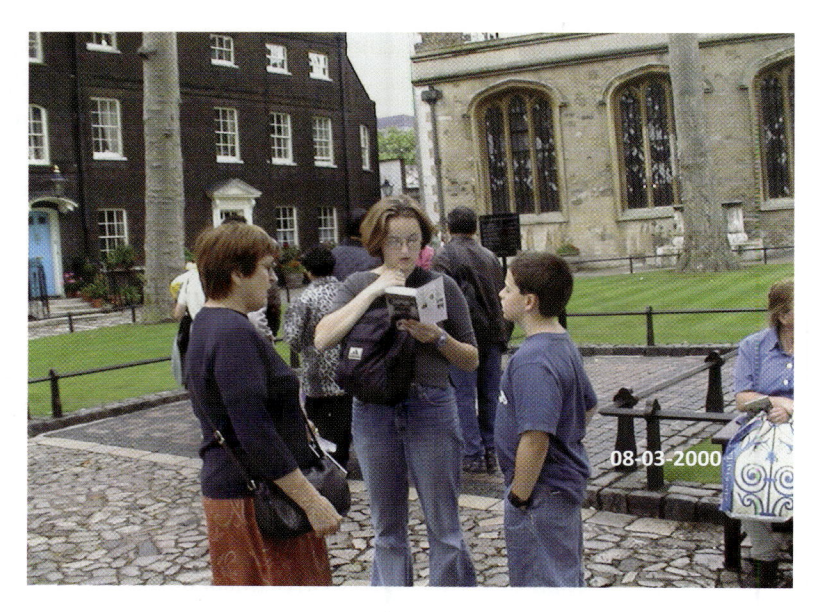

Figure 188. Halina, Ania and Adam at the Scaffold in the Tower of London.

way to Oxford. We visited Oxford University's library and chapel, and then drove through Runnymede and past Windsor before reaching our hotel. In the afternoon we went to the Bloody Tower, otherwise known as the Tower of London, which served as a prison and a place of execution between 1388 and 1747 (Fig. 188). Some prisoners were given the privilege of a private execution on the scaffold inside the Tower Yard. The first was Anne Boleyn, Queen of England from 1533 to 1536, whose crime was her failure to produce a male heir for Henry VIII. Falsely accused of adultery, she was executed on May 19, 1536. Feeling some remorse about her imminent death, Henry hired a skilled French swordsman from Calais, who sliced off her head with one blow.

The final day of the tour was the following day, and our group flew to the United States. We stayed one more day to visit the Madame Tussauds. There were a number of Poles at the wax museum at the time, including Solidarity leader Lech Wałęsa and Pope John Paul II. We also visited the Sherlock Holmes Museum on Baker Street and the British Museum. Seeing the many exhibits took a good deal of time. The Rosetta Stone (Fig. 189), a fragment of an Ancient Egyptian granodiorite stele that was discovered in 1799 by a soldier of the Napoleonic

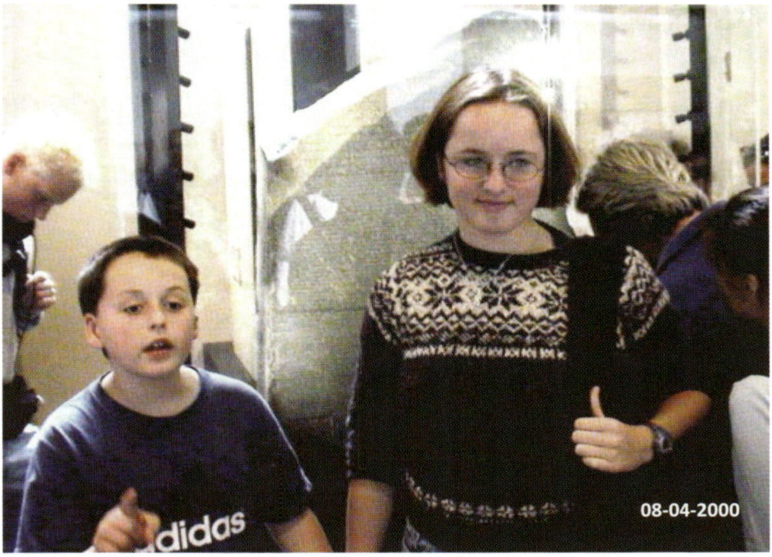

Figure 189. Adam and Ania observe the Rosetta Stone in the British Museum.

Expedition, was one of the highlights. Immediately acknowledged as an important finding, it bears three inscriptions in ancient Egyptian hieroglyphs, Egyptian demotic script and in ancient Greek. When British troops defeated the French in Egypt in 1801, the stone came into British possession during the Capitulation of Alexandria, was transported to London, and has been displayed in the British Museum ever since. Indeed, it is the most-visited object in the museum. Many people have tried to decipher the text on the stone. The most successful were Thomas Young[19] and Jean-François Champollion.[20] On August 5, at 12:20 pm, Ania and Adam departed from London Gatwick to Minneapolis on Northwest Flight No. NWA45, and then continued on to Bismarck. We departed the next day at 10:50 am from London Gatwick on BA4474 to Kraków Balice.

---

19. Thomas Young was a physician and a physicist who established the principle of interference of light and thus resurrected the century-old Huygens' wave theory of light. He was also an Egyptologist.

20. A polyglot who spoke a dozen or so languages, Jean-François Champollion had extraordinary linguistic talent. He ultimately translated the whole hieroglyphic grammar based in part upon the earlier work of Young.

2001 — Jurata, Gdańsk and Malbork; Father John Long in Kraków

In 2001 I was still busy with editing *Hemodialysis International* and organizing our annual conference, so it was July 10 before we arrived in Kraków. While in the U.S. I had arranged the purchase of a car, an Opel Astra, and we bought it immediately after our arrival. It may sound implausible, but just one day before our arrival the value of the Polish zloty dropped from 4.00 zl to US$1 to 4.40 zl to US$1. The price of the car was 78,150 zl, and as we paid in Polish currency, the sudden change in the exchange rate saved us about US$1,777. Intriguingly, a few days later the exchange rate came back to 4.00 zl to the dollar.

Taking our new car, we decided to spend some time on the Hel Peninsula. We booked a room in Hotel Neptun in Jurata from July 21 to July 31. Our medical school friends, Teresa and Staszek Januś, were in Jurata at the same time. I remember the weather being good and for a few days the waves were good enough for bodysurfing. We played volleyball with Staszek and his grandson Wojtek. It reminded us of the lovely time we had had several decades earlier in Chałupy, another spot on the Hel Peninsula where we had vacationed with our sons. On July 31 we went to the Hotel Hanza in Gdańsk and stayed there for three days.[21] We visited several places of interest, including the Long Market with Neptune's Fountain (Fig. 190). We also went to see St. Mary's Church, the largest brick church in the world with its famous 15th-century astronomical clock.

On August 1 we drove to Malbork Castle,[22] which is about 40 miles (64 km) from Gdańsk. A classic example of a medieval fortress, it is the

---

21. Founded in the 10th century, Gdańsk is one of the oldest Polish cities. It was under control of the Teutonic Knights from 1308 and joined the Hanseatic League in 1358. After the defeat of the Teutonic Knights at the battle of Grunwald (Tannenberg) in 1410, the city came under the control of the Polish Kingdom and of the Polish-Lithuanian Commonwealth. The city was later under Prussian rule and also enjoyed the status of "free city" between the First and Second World Wars. During WWII it was part of Nazi Germany and became a Polish city once again after 1945. Gdańsk is also the cradle of the Solidarity movement, which liberated Poland and other Eastern European countries from Communist rule.

22. Malbork (German: Marienburg) was founded by the Teutonic Knights on the bank of the river Nogat in 1274. Its fate was very convoluted, as were most places in the region. The castle belonged to Poland from the 15th century until the First Partition of Poland in 1772. Under continuous construction for nearly 230 years, the castle complex is actually three castles nested in one another. Severly destroyed during WWII, it now belongs to Poland and is continuously being restored.

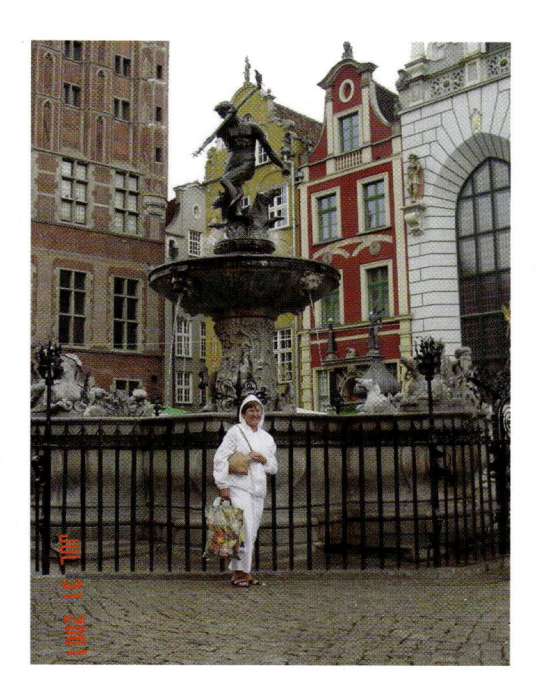

Figure 190. Halina at Neptune's Fountain; the town hall is to the left.

world's largest brick castle and one of the most impressive of its kind in Europe (Fig. 191). For the first time we saw the very impressive medieval latrines that were built by Teutonic Knights in their castles. Located in a special toilet tower (*dansker*), complete with private toilet stalls, the latrines emptied into the castle moat. Cabbage leaves, placed above the wooden toilet seat, served as medieval toilet paper.

We invited Father John Long, our pastor from the Sacred Heart Church in Columbia, for a 10-day visit to Kraków. He arrived on August 16 and checked into Hotel Copernicus on Kanonicza Street. Something that is quite common, I suspect, is that people who live in a particularly interesting city, as Halina and I do, often do not take the opportunity to visit places of interest. So on the occasion of Father John's visit, we decided to do some sightseeing with him to become better acquainted with Kraków and its surroundings. We visited various churches, including St. Mary's Basilica (Polish: Kościół Mariacki) with its famous wooden altarpiece carved by Veit Stoss (Wit Stwosz), and St. Adalbert's Church (Kościół Św. Wojciecha), built in the 10th

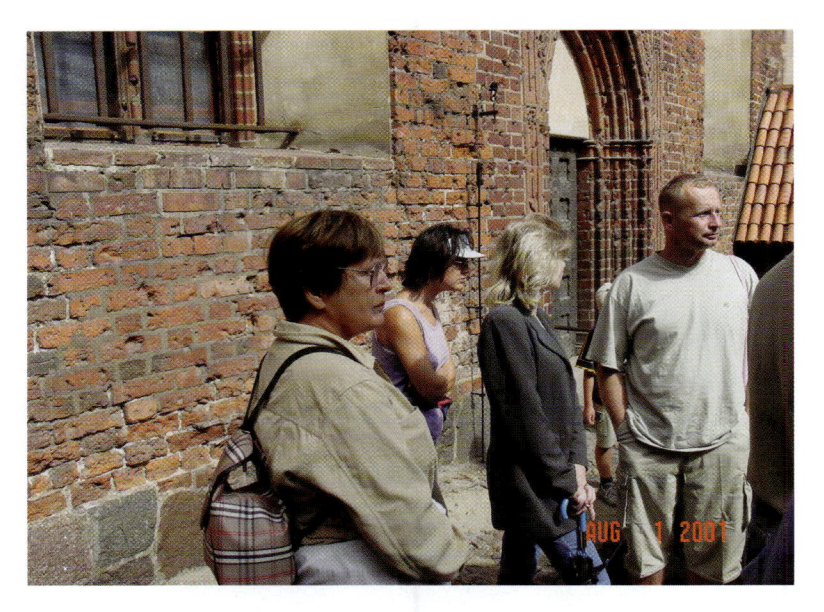

Figure 191. Halina visits the enormous Malbork Castle.

century. We also went to Wawel Castle, the Wieliczka salt mine and to Wadowice, the birthplace of Karol Wojtyła, who became Pope John Paul II. The house where Karol Wojtyła lived is now a museum (Fig. 192). We got back to Columbia on October 2, leaving enough time for me to review all 299 abstracts (sent in by fax at that time) before the abstract meeting on October 11.

2002 — Jurata, Slovakia and New York

Arriving in Kraków on June 24 that year, we again went to Jurata for a two-week break. Again, we stayed in Hotel Neptun from July 16 to July 30 and had quite good weather with waves suitable for bodysurfing (Fig. 193). Teresa and Staszek Janusiowie and their grandchildren were also in Jurata. We only had American passports at that time and were supposed to be in Poland for a maximum of 90 days; otherwise we needed permission to extend our stay. We had booked our return tickets for September 24, so the permitted time would have been exceeded by two days. However, if we came out of the country, even for few hours, we come back in to Poland and renew the 90-day period. The closest

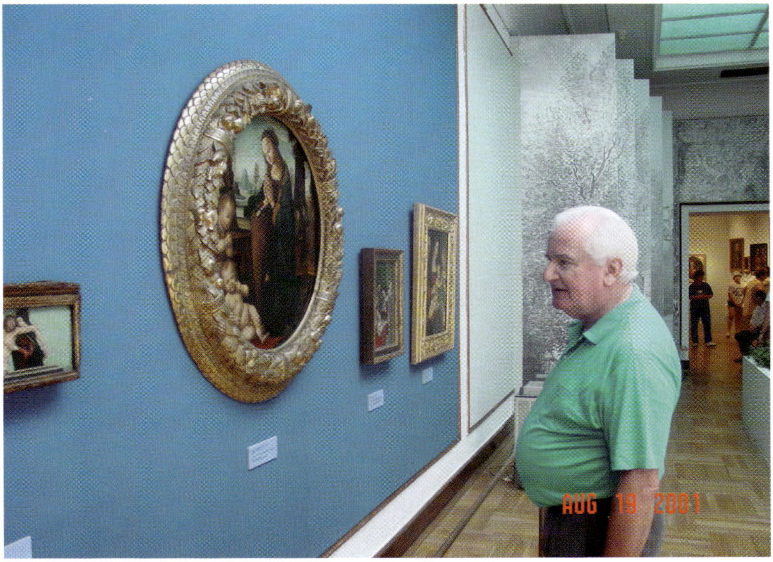

Figure 192. Father John Long in the museum in Wadowice where Karol Wojtyła once lived.

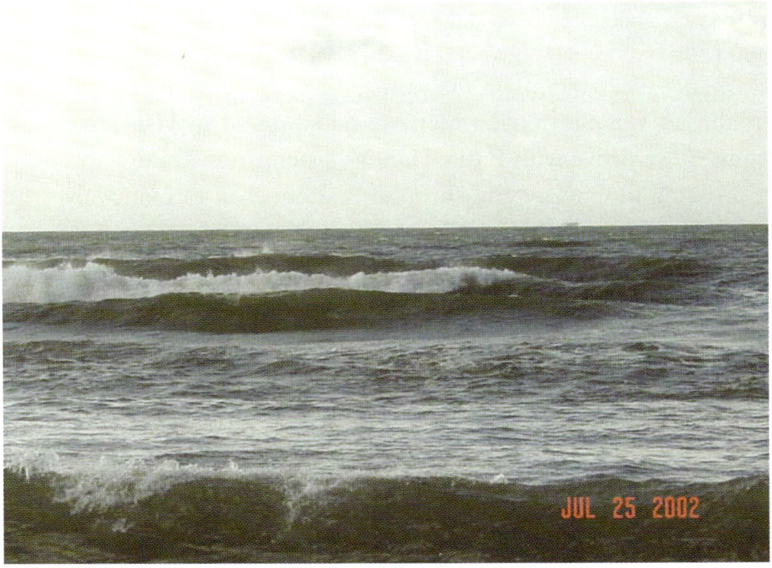

Figure 193. Time for the bodysurfers to hit the waves.

Vacations and Travel Unrelated to Business | 421

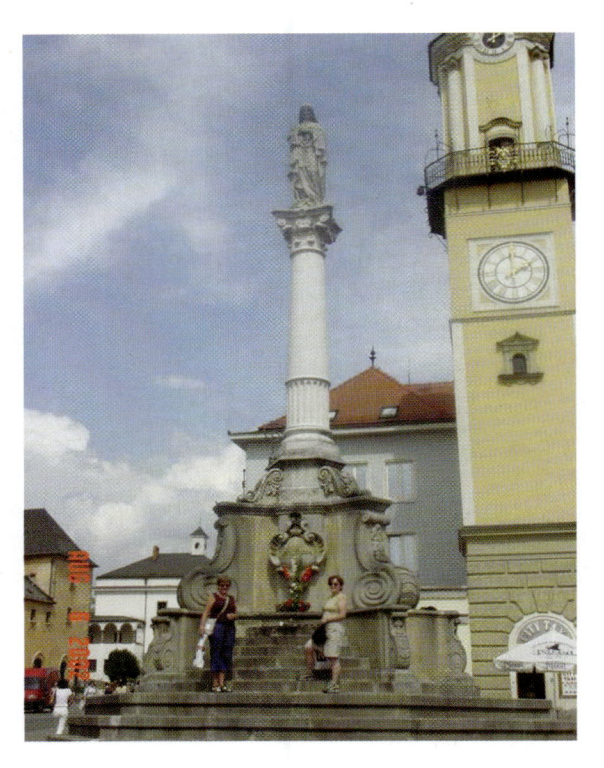

Figure 194. Halina and Basia at the "plague column" with the nearby leaning clock tower.

trip abroad was Slovakia, which we had wanted to visit anyway. On August 5, we drove with Basia, Halina's sister, from Kraków to the border crossing in Chyżne and through Ružomberok to Donovaly, where we stayed in the Sport Hotel Donovaly for three days.

On the Tuesday, we drove to Banská Bystrica, a very pretty, small town, founded in the 9th century. Most of the historical monuments are concentrated near its central, picturesque SNP Square (Námestie SNP). The square is dominated by its leaning clock tower, whose top leans some 16 inches (40 cm) off the perpendicular. The "plague column" (*morový stĺp*) was erected in the square in the 18th century in gratitude to the Virgin Mary for ending a deadly plague[23] (Fig. 194).

---

23. Interestingly, before the visit of the Soviet leader Nikita Khrushchev in 1964, the column was temporarily removed because a religious symbol was considered to be an inappropriate background for the Communist leader's address. Fortunately, the column was not damaged in the process.

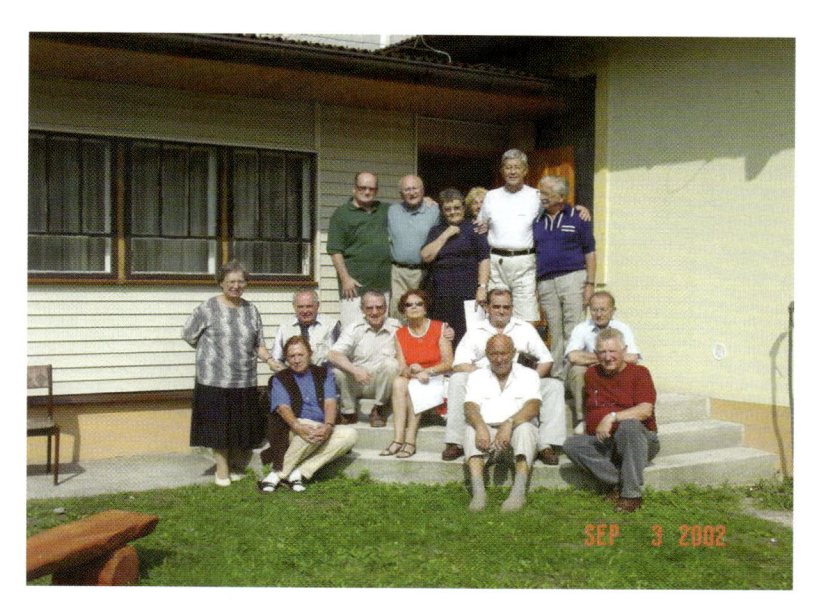

Figure 195. Fifteen graduates from the class of 1952.

We returned to Kraków on Wednesday, obtaining fresh stamps indicating our arrival in Poland on August 7.

That particular year it was the 50th anniversary of my class graduation from high school, and a committee had been created to organize celebrations from September 1 through 3. The head of the committee, Mieczysław Kalisz (nicknamed Mahdi), had arranged the event to take place in Buczkowice near Szczyrk, about 60 miles (100 km) from Kraków. Forty students graduated from our class, but only 26 were still alive. Many were abroad and could not come, so ultimately only 15 participated (Fig. 195), with seven coming with their spouses. It was a wonderful party, with many recollections from our student years and our lives after graduation. Returning from Buczkowice the following day, I attended the meeting in Kraków and gave a presentation [Pr 469]. We returned to Columbia on September 24, and I immediately started reviewing the 316 abstracts submitted for the coming meeting in Seattle.

In May, before our departure to Poland, we had booked a tour with Boone County Bank Classic to New York for November 17 to 22, staying at the Marriott Marquis Hotel on Times Square. We managed

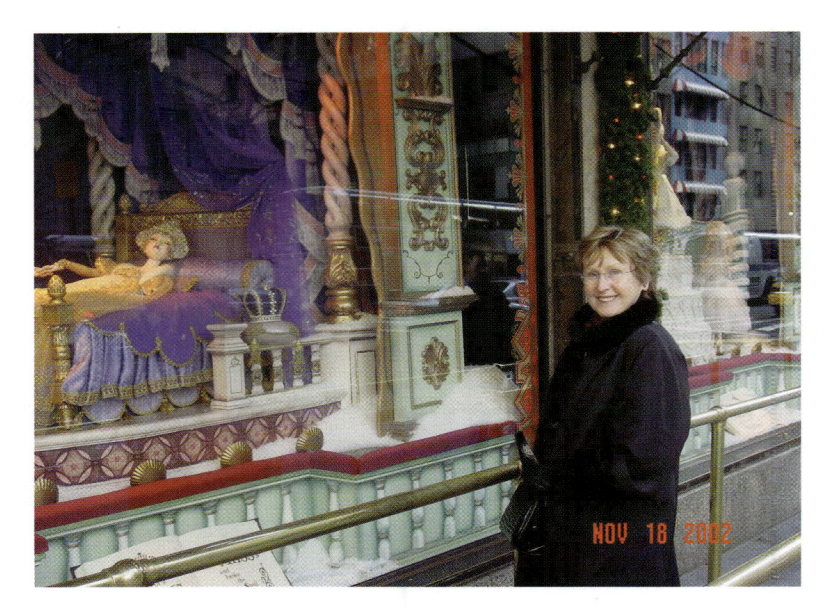

Figure 196. Halina at Sleeping Beauty on Fifth Ave.

to get good tickets (Grand Tier seats B25, B27) for a performance of *Aida* at the New York Metropolitan Opera. The day after our arrival, on Monday, we went on a long walk through the city, visiting St. Patrick's Cathedral, Times Square and Fifth Avenue (Fig. 196), and had to have a good rest in a Starbucks café afterwards. We went to the opera that evening. One thing that really impressed me was the personalized screen displaying the subtitles (built into back of the seat in front). I usually do not understand the words in songs, even in Polish or English and obviously not at all in Italian and other languages, so the subtitles really helped us follow the plot. It was the first time I had seen such a system, but I later found out that other opera companies have similar systems in place nowadays.[24] On Tuesday morning I went to a stand-up show by comedian Jackie Mason, who made a lot of jokes about the relations between the Jews and Gentiles. He reminded me of our visit to Starbucks when, referring to the coffee chain, he

---

24. If La Scala in Milan had used this system for *Electra* when we were there in 1994, it would not necessarily have helped us unless the subtitles had been in Polish or English, since we understood neither German nor Italian.

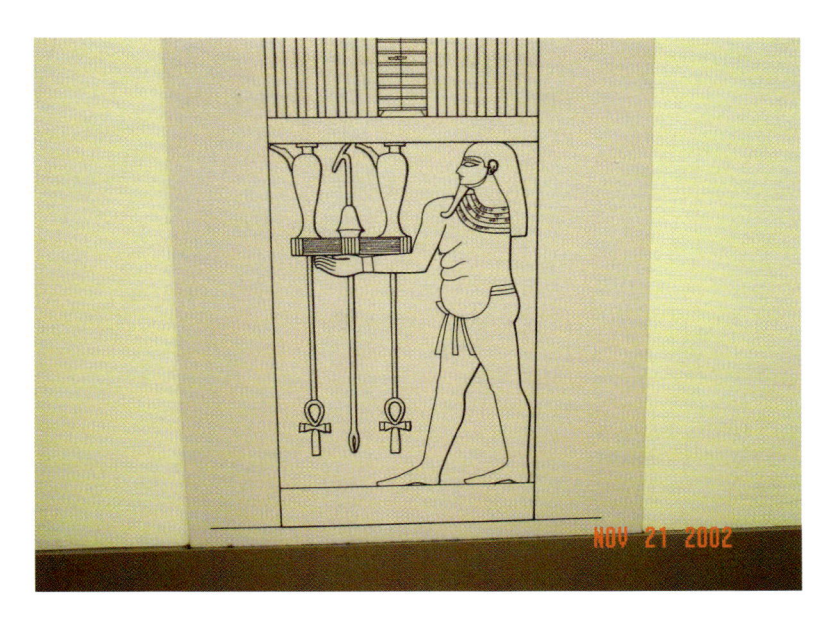

Figure 197   A picture of an Egyptian in the Metropolitan Museum of Art.

said: "The less you get, the more it costs. By the time they give you nothing, it's worth four times as much." In the evening we caught the Broadway Musical *Mamma Mia*, while on Wednesday we went for the Rockettes Radio City Christmas Show. The day after, we visited the Metropolitan Museum of Art. I was struck by a picture of an obese Egyptian (Fig. 197), as in my mind all ancient peoples from Egypt and Europe were lean.

2003 — Scandinavia, St. Petersburg and Estonia

I was still editing *Hemodialysis International* in 2003, so I could not be out of Columbia for more than about three months. We arrived in Kraków on July 3, having already arranged a tour with Trafalgar Tours through Scandinavia, Finland, St. Petersburg and Estonia (Fig. 198). We needed visas to Russia, which we arranged through AAA. On July 17 we arrived in Copenhagen and were transferred to the Radisson Falconer/Scandinavia Hotel. We met up with Barbara Van Meter and her husband Marshall, who were already at the hotel. Barbara is Halina's cousin, the daughter of Wira and Adolf, who I

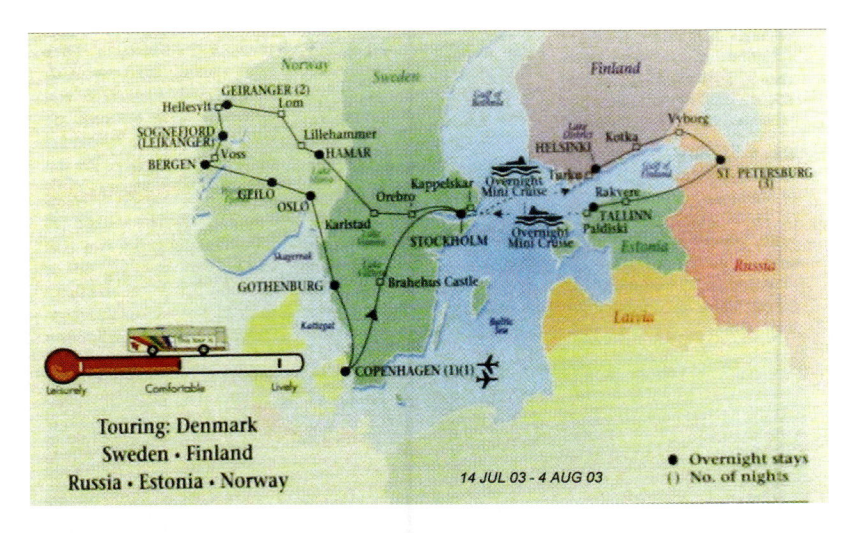

Figure 198. Our tour of Scandinavia, Finland, St. Petersburg and Estonia.

already mentioned when I described our first trip to Edinburgh in 1969. We had planned the trip with them well in advance. In the afternoon we visited the Town Hall Square, and then went to Tivoli Gardens and had a traditional Danish dinner there. On July 18 we traveled from Copenhagen to Helsingør and then by ferry across Øresund to Helsingborg in Sweden (Fig. 199). On the way we passed Kronborg Castle, the Elsinore Castle of Shakespeare's *Hamlet*. From Helsingborg we went by bus to the Birger Jarl Hotel, where we were staying in Stockholm, stopping for lunch close to Huskvarna at Vättern Lake.

Sweden's capital and largest city, Stockholm is located at the junction of Mälaren (Lake Mälar) and Saltsjön (Salt Bay), an arm of the Baltic Sea, opposite the Gulf of Finland. The city consists of a mainland portion in addition to numerous islands. By virtue of its location, it is regarded as one of the most beautiful capital cities in the world. Stockholm was first mentioned as a town in 1252 and was largely built by the Swedish statesman Birger Jarl.[25] It came to be officially regarded as the Swedish capital in 1436. After conflicts between the Danes and

---

25. Birger Jarl is revered by Swedes, and many hotels and places are named after him. We stayed in the Birger Jarl Hotel.

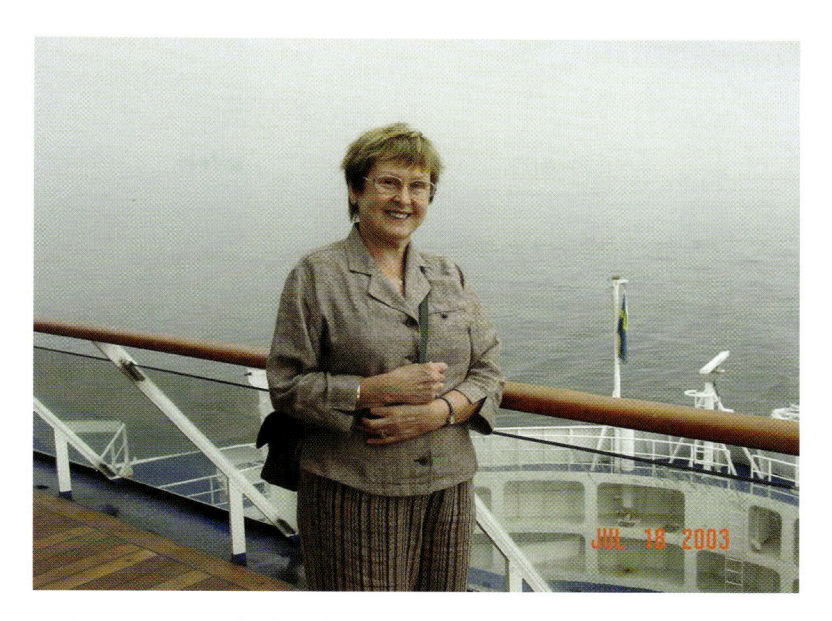

Figure 199. On the ferry from Helsingør to Helsingborg across Øresund.

Swedes for many years, Stockholm was liberated from Danish rule by Gustav I[26] in 1523. The original nucleus of the city is the "city between the bridges," Gamla Stan (Old Town), consisting of Stads Island, Helgeands Island and Riddar Island. We wandered through the Old Town in the evening (Fig. 200) and enjoyed the 16th- and 17th-century buildings in the area. The well-preserved city nucleus, with the original network of streets and many of its buildings dating from the Middle Ages, is legally protected from alteration. Stads Island contains the Royal Palace, while the House of Parliament and the National Bank are on Helgeands Island.

---

26. Gustav I (r. 1523–1560), born Gustav Eriksson Vasa, was the first monarch of the House of Vasa, a Swedish (and Polish) royal dynasty. His descendants reigned in Sweden until 1818. One of Gustav's grandsons became King of Poland (r. 1587–1632) as Sigismund III Vasa, and also ruled Sweden between 1592 and 1599. He was succeeded as King of Poland by his sons, Wladyslaw IV Vasa (r. 1632–1648) and John II Casimir Vasa (r. 1648–1668), after which the dynasty ended in Poland. Held in high regard in Sweden, the Vasa dynasty was less revered in Poland. Before visiting the Vasa Museum, I was under the impression that the name "Vasa" came from the Latin *vasa* (vessels), but it is actually from the Swedish word meaning "sheaf of grain," as seen on the Vasa ship emblem.

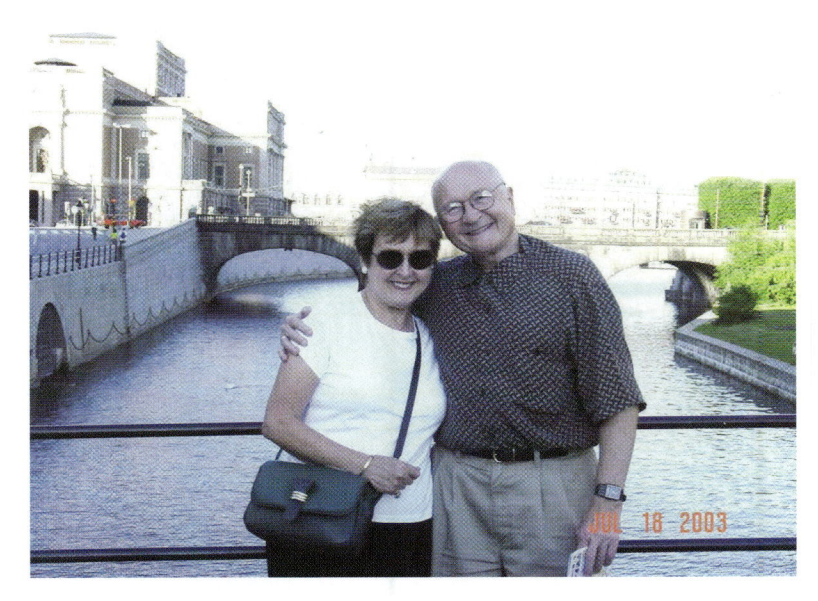

Figure 200. The view from Vasabron (Vasa bridge) over Riksbron (Riks bridge) and the island of Helgeandsholmen.

The next day, Saturday, July 19, we took a Grand Tour of Stockholm, which included visits to the Stadshuset (City Hall), with its beautiful Gyllene Salen (Golden Hall), and the Blue Hall, used for the banquet held after the annual Nobel prize award ceremony, and Kungliga Slottet (Royal Palace), where we observed, among other things, the changing of the guard. Later, we went to the island of Djurgården, a cultural-recreational area that has several museums, including the Skansen and the Vasa Museum, which houses a salvaged Swedish warship built from 1626 to 1628 (Fig. 201). Poorly balanced, the ship foundered and sank after sailing less than a nautical mile (2 km). It was supposed to assist in the battles with Poland when the Swedish navy was defeated at the Battle of Oliwa in 1627. At the time the Thirty Years' War was being waged and Sweden was also involved.

In the evening we boarded a Silja Line ship for a short overnight cruise to Turku in Finland (Swedish: Abo), a bilingual city that has universities for Swedish speakers and Finnish speakers, several specialized institutes of higher education, art galleries, libraries and museums. We only had breakfast and did not visit the city. From there it was a short

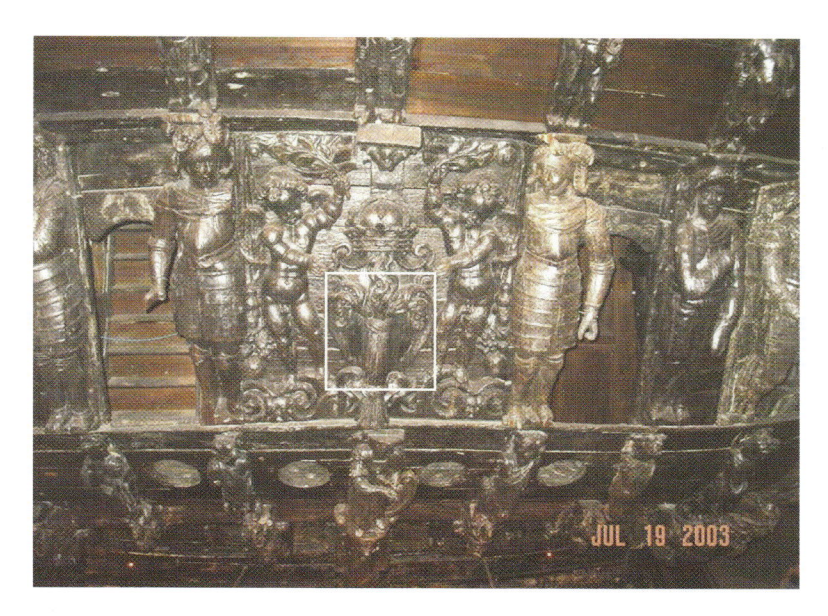

Figure 201. The coat of arms on the Vasa ship comprising the Vasa emblem (a sheaf of grain) supported by cherubs.

drive to Helsinki (Swedish: Helsingfors), the Finnish capital. Founded in 1550 by King Gustav I of Sweden, Helsinki was originally located at the mouth of the Vantaa River. It has a convoluted history, having been under both Swedish and Russian rule. In 1809 Finland was ceded to Russia and in 1812 the Russian Czar Alexander I moved the capital of the grand duchy of Finland from Turku to Helsinki. In December 1917 Finland declared independence from Russia, and a brief but bloody civil war ensued in the capital between Finnish troops and Russian units occupying the city. Conditions soon became more stable, with the Helsinki parliament electing Finland's first president in 1919. In subsequent decades the city developed into an important center of trade, industry and culture, a process interrupted only by WWII. We stopped at the Senate Square and Sibeliuksenpuisto (Sibelius Park), with its monument to the composer Jean Sibelius (1865–1957) created by Eila Hiltunen (Fig. 202), and in the afternoon we visited Hvitträsk Museum in Kirkonummi, located about 20 miles (32 km) to the west. Built between 1901 and 1903 by architects Herman Gesellius, Armas Lindgren and Eliel Saarinen, the museum is a glorious example of

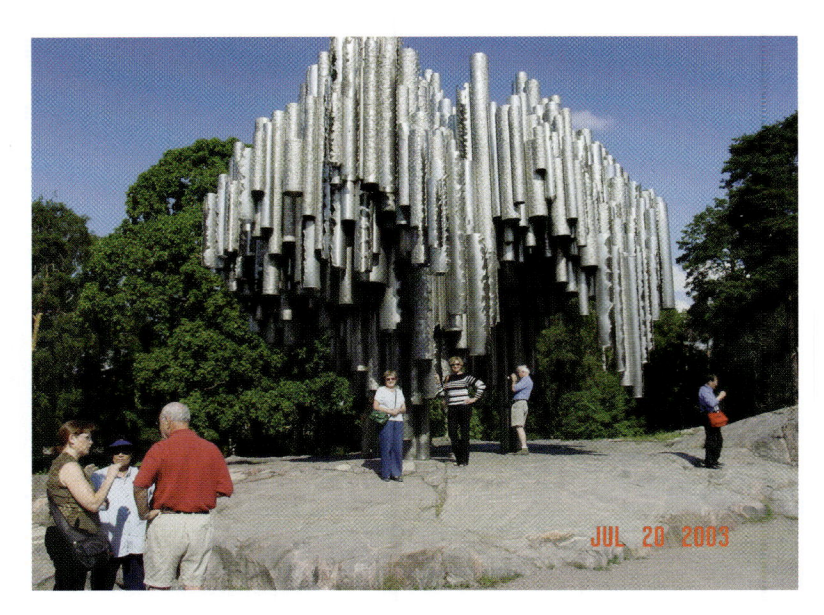

Figure 202. Halina and Barbara in front of the steel pipes of Eila Hiltunen's Sibelius Monument.

Finnish Art Nouveau at its best and a celebration of peasant culture. During the early decades of its existence, the main building served as both an architectural office and as a cultural home. It was visited by such esteemed figures as Jean Sibelius, Finnish painter Akseli Gallen-Kallela and Russian and Soviet author Maxim Gorki.

On Monday, July 21, we headed to St. Petersburg, driving through the province of Karelia (Finnish: Karjala; Russian: Kareliya). On the way we passed the timber center in Kotka before crossing the Russian border and stopping in Vyborg for lunch. We arrived in St. Petersburg in the late afternoon. St. Petersburg has played a vital role in Russian history. Founded as St. Petersburg by Peter the Great in 1703, it was the capital of the Russian Empire for two centuries (1712–1918). It was the scene of the February and October Revolutions in 1917 and was a besieged and fiercely defended city during WWII. Today, the city is an important cultural and industrial center and serves as the nation's largest seaport. In 1924 the name of the city was changed to Leningrad, after Soviet leader Vladimir Lenin, but it reverted to its original name in 1991. It is situated on the delta of the Neva River where it debouches into the Gulf of Finland, about 100 miles (160 km) from the Finnish border.

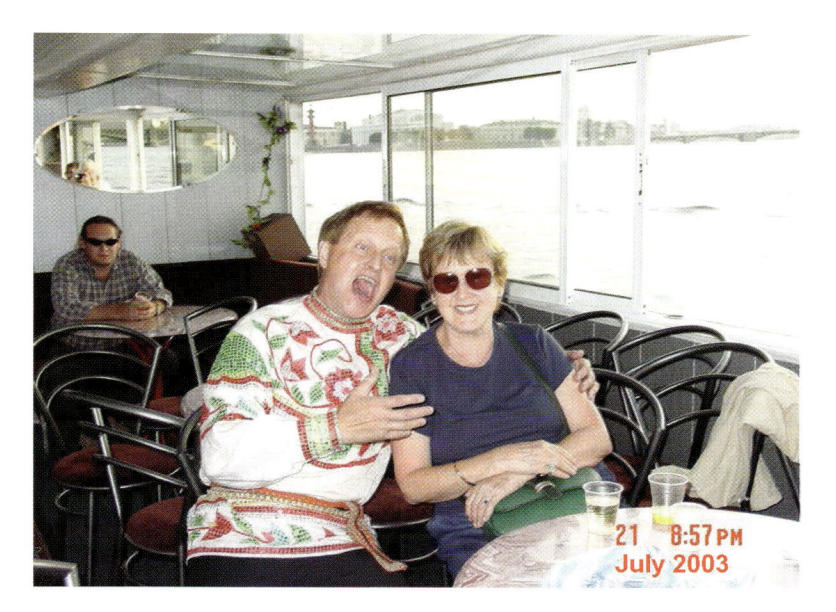

Figure 203. Wladimir Chmielnicki's vocal performance; our guide, Xavier, is in the background.

On July 22 we took a sightseeing bus tour of St. Petersburg. The remarkable richness of its architecture is exemplified in buildings such the Peter and Paul Fortress, the Summer and Winter Palaces, Nevsky Prospect, Smolny Convent, the Vorontsov and Stroganov Palaces, Kazan and St. Isaac's Cathedrals, the Smolny Institute, the new Admiralty, and the Senate. What impressed me most was the sheer number of gold-plated domes on the cathedrals and churches — indicating, of course, that Russia was a very affluent country in the 18th and 19th centuries. We had never seen so many anywhere else and have not since. In the evening we took a canal cruise and saw a number of interesting bridges and houses, including a house containing an apartment owned by one of the greatest Russian-born American dancers, Mikhail Baryshnikov. During the cruise we listened to a vocal performance by one Wladimir Chmielnicki[27] (Fig. 203).

---

27. Our singer was not aware that a man with the same last name, Bogdan Chmielnicki, led an uprising against the Polish-Lithuanian Commonwealth (1648–1654). He was interested in the story and appreciated the information.

On Tuesday morning, July 22, we visited the Church of the Resurrection of Christ, Savior on the Spilt Blood,[28] and then dropped in to the Onegin Art Store on 11 Italianskaya Str., where Halina bought a beautiful Fabergé Egg. Afterwards, we visited the Cathedral of St. Isaac of Dalmatia[29] on St. Isaac's Square. It is amazing that the cathedral was damaged neither during communist rule nor during the siege of Leningrad during WWII. A guide told us that the gold-plated dome was painted gray to avoid attracting attention from enemy aircraft. In the early afternoon we went to the Hermitage ensemble and saw the Winter Palace (the former state residence of the Russian emperors), the Small Hermitage, the Old Hermitage and the New Hermitage. Among many displays we saw two great works (1490–1491) of Leonardo da Vinci in the Leonardo Room on the first floor: *Madonna with a Flower* (*Benois Madonna*) and *Madonna and Child* (*Madonna Litta*). In one room of the New Hermitage there is a clock that stopped at 2:10 am at the beginning of the Bolshevik Revolution on the night of October 25–26 on the Julian calendar (November 7–8 on the Gregorian calendar) (Fig. 204). Later that day we were treated to various dances in a Russian Folklore Evening. There is no question that Russian music and dance are very enjoyable.

The following day we took a tour to Tsarskoe Selo and Peterhof, two suburban estates founded by the Romanov Czars, both surrounded by extensive landscaped gardens with diverse and fascinating decorative architecture. We started by visiting the Catherine Palace, built for Empress Elizabeth by Bartolomeo Rastrelli, the architect of St. Petersburg's Winter Palace. Undoubtedly Tsarskoe Selo's top attraction, the palace is particularly renowned for its extraordinary Amber Room. I was again impressed with the gold-plated[30] domes of the church in the palace. The town of Pushkin, which surrounds the Tsarskoe Selo estates, is St. Petersburg's most charming suburb. It was

---

28. Czar Alexander II was assassinated at this spot on March 1, 1881. His son Alexander III decided to build a church there, hence the name.

29. I was a little surprised that the cathedral is named after St. Isaac of Dalmatia, and not Isaac, son of Abraham and Sarah. I should not have been, however, as Isaac of Dalmatia was the patron saint of Peter the Great, who was born on the saint's feast day.

30. I adore the color and luster of gold. By the same token, I am not fond of copper-plated surfaces, as they are oxidized quickly and become covered with patina, valued by some for its dull greenish color, but not appreciated by me.

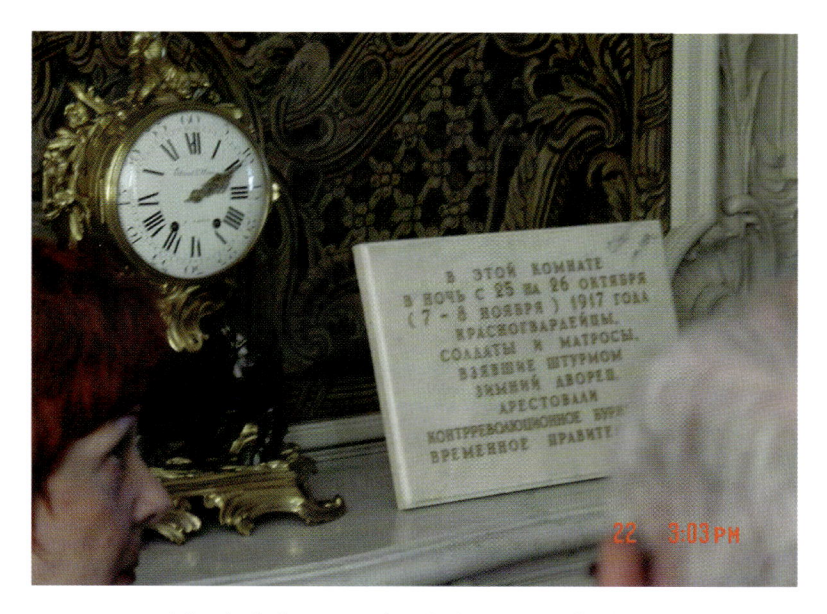

Figure 204. The clock that stopped at the beginning of Bolshevik Revolution.

renamed in Soviet times to honor Russia's great poet, Alexander Sergeyevich Pushkin. Next we went to Pavlovsk, 3 miles (5 km) further down the road from Tsarskoe Selo. Named after the son of Catherine the Great, Pavlovsk is the youngest of the grand Imperial estates around St. Petersburg. At the entrance to the Great Palace is a statue of Czar Pavel (Paul I). The affluence of the paintings and decorations is unbelievable, as the photo of the dining room in Fig. 205 shows. Our next stop was the statue of Kirov[31] in Peterhof, after which we spent several hours in the vast park. Again, the opulence is impressive, with gold-plated statues surrounding the Great Cascade and the Great Samson Sea Canal (Fig. 206).

The next morning, on Thursday, July 24, we went to the Peter and Paul Fortress and visited the Peter and Paul Cathedral, stopping at the tombs of Elizabeth I, Catherine I and Peter I, and the tomb of Czar Nicholas II and his murdered family in St. Catherine's Chapel.

---

31. Sergei Kirov, the head of the Bolshevik Party in Leningrad and a rising star in the Soviet Union, was assassinated on the order of Joseph Stalin, whose *modus operandi* was to eliminate all potential rivals to his absolute rule (*cf.* Footnote 60).

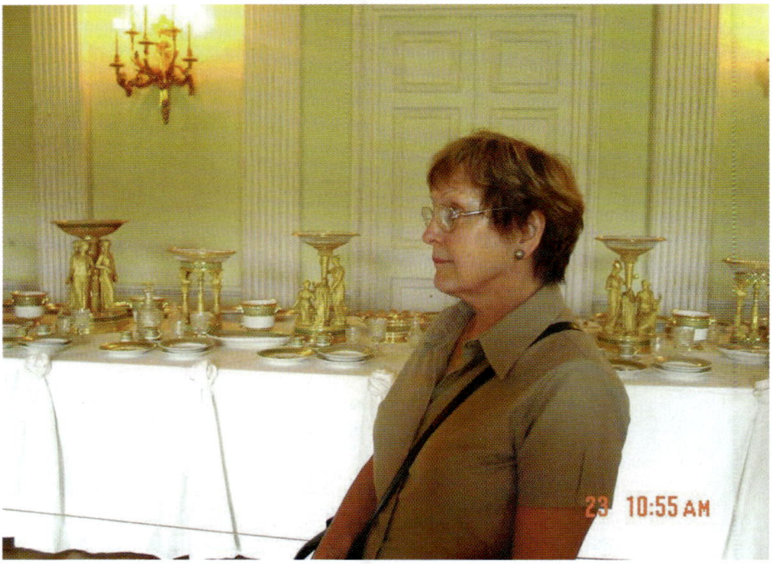

Figure 205. The impressive dining room in Pavlovsk Palace.

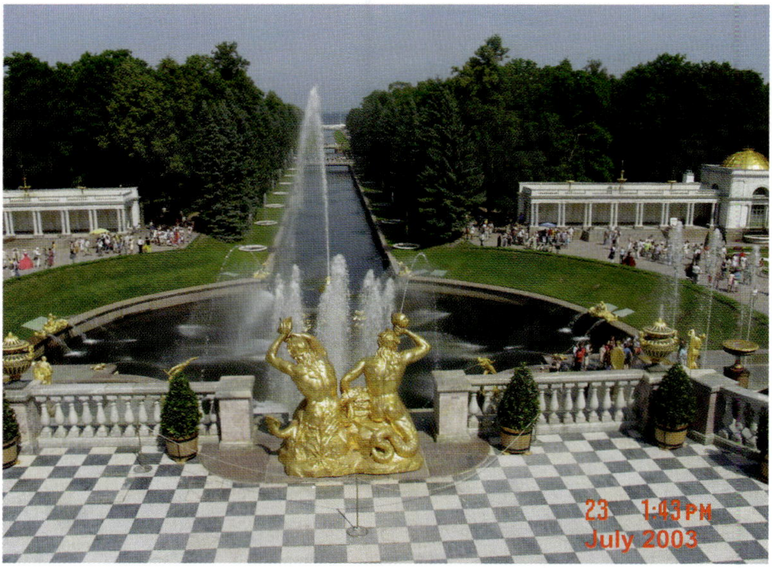

Figure 206. The Great Samson Sea Canal in Peterhof.

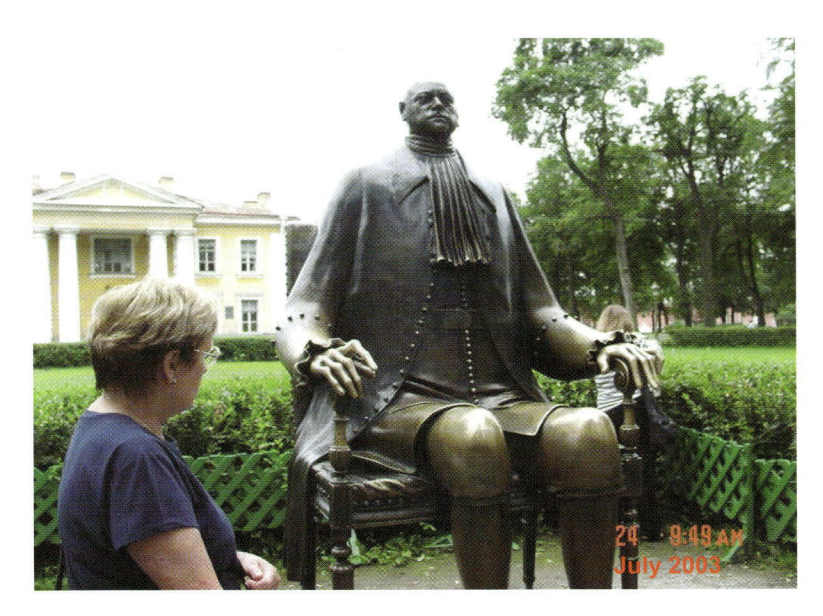

Figure 207. The Monument to Peter the Great by Mikhail Shemiakin, erected in 1991; the head was recreated from the Tsar's own death mask.

In a ceremony in St. Catherine's Chapel that could not have happened during Soviet rule, the remains of Czar Nicholas and his family were laid to rest in 1998 with then-President Boris Yeltsin in attendance. With a choir of monks singing for us as we left the cathedral, we went to see the monument of Peter the Great — and squeezed his right index finger for luck, of course (Fig. 207). We then visited the Yusupov Palace on the Moika Embankment. Among the many attractive exhibits was a wax figure of Grigori Yefimovich Rasputin.[32]

In the afternoon we made our way to Tallinn, the capital of Estonia. Estonians belong to the Finno-Ugric peoples (as do Finns

---

32. In the palace we were told the story of the murder of Rasputin. On December 16, 1916 (Julian calendar), having decided that Rasputin's influence over the Tsarina had made him a threat to the empire, a group of nobles led by Prince Felix Yusupov lured Rasputin to the Yusupov's Moika Palace and tried to poison him with cyanide. The poison apparently did not work, so Yusupov shot Rasputin in the back with a revolver, supposedly left him for dead and went for other conspirators to throw him into the Neva River. The conspirators were surprised to find Rasputin still alive and attempting to strangle Yusupov, so they shot him again. They proceeded to club him and then wrapped him in a carpet and threw him into the icy Neva River. When Rasputin's body was recovered three days later and subjected to an autopsy, it was found that water was in his lungs, and the cause of death was declared to be drowning.

and Hungarians), which probably arrived from the east many centuries ago. In his *Germania*, written in the 1st century AD, Tacitus mentioned a people called the Aesti. Mina, our Estonian guide, told us that some Finno-Ugric people decided to travel further: "The cold-resistant Finns to the north and the heat-resistant Hungarians to the south: only the lazy ones decided to stay where they had arrived." Estonians had an independent nation until the 13th century. The country was then successively conquered by Denmark, Germany, Poland (the southern part, called Livonia, 1580–1629), Sweden, and finally Russia, whose defeat of Sweden in 1721 resulted in the Uusikaupunki Peace Treaty, granting Russia rule over what became modern Estonia. The country was independent from 1918 until 1940, was briefly occupied by the Germans during WWII, and was then annexed by the Soviet Union in 1944 until it regained its independence in 1991. When Estonia became independent in 1918, the name of the capital was changed from Reval to Tallinn. On the morning of July 25, we walked through the Lower Town, dropped by the city hall, and then walked through Pikk Jalg (Long Leg) street to the Toompea (Upper Town), where we visited Toompea Castle, Alexander Nevsky Orthodox Cathedral, and the House of Parliament (Fig. 208). Afterwards, we walked from the Upper to the Lower Town through Luhike Jalg (Short Leg) street. In the afternoon we drove to Paldiski port to board our ship for an overnight cruise to Sweden.

The following morning we arrived at Kappelskär port, north of Stockholm, and drove westwards by bus through the scenic surroundings. We stopped for lunch in Arboga and visited the medieval city of Örebro, seeing its fine castle from the outside. We continued on to Karlstad, the capital of Värmland county, in southwest-central Sweden. The city is located on the island of Tingvalla and on the northern shore of Lake Vänern at the mouth of the Klar River. We stopped there for a while and then drove northwest to Morokulien, where we stopped at the Peace Monument erected in 1914 to commemorate the peace treaty of 1905 between Norway and Sweden (Fig. 209). The "kingdom" of Morokulien, as it is sometimes called, is a 15-acre (6 ha) enclave and border crossing between Sweden (Värmland) and Norway (Hedmark). The name *Morokulien*

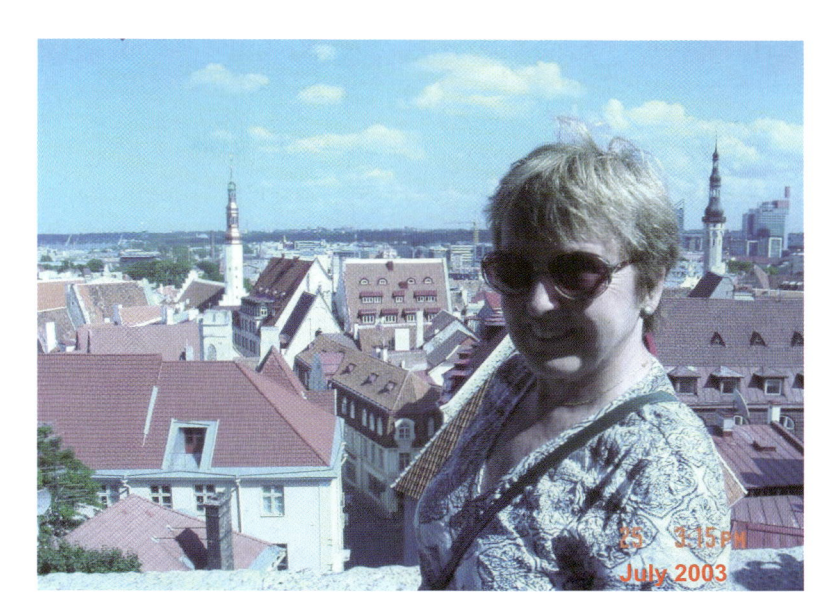

Figure 208. The view over the Lower Town from Toompea, Tallinn.

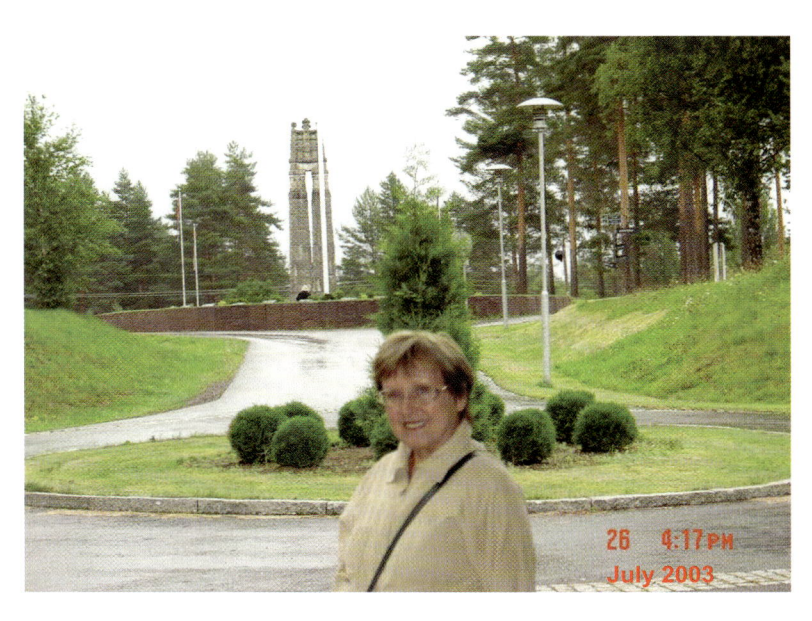

Figure 209. The Peace Monument (Fredsmonument) in the Kingdom of Morokulien enclave on the Swedish-Norwegian border.

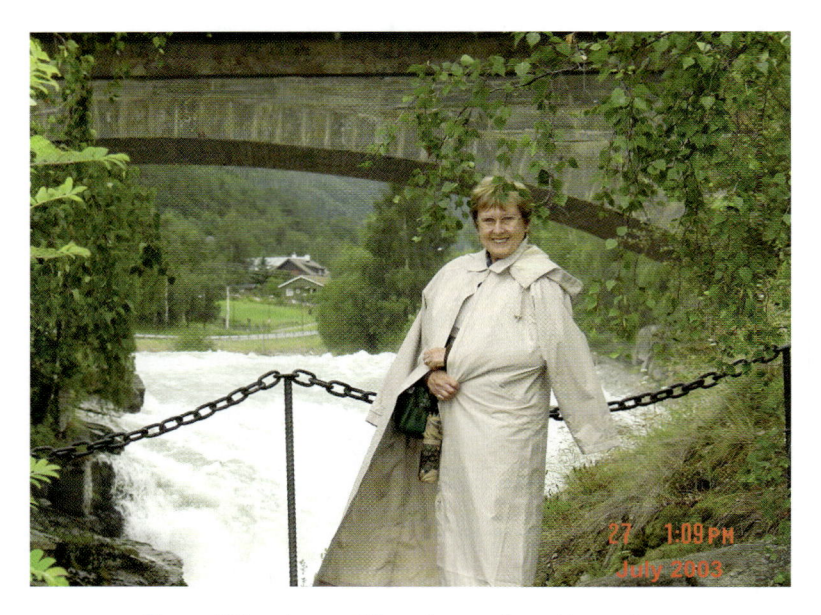

Figure 210. A waterfall on the way from Otta to Lom.

combines the Norwegian word (*moro*) and Swedish word (*kul*) for "fun." We then drove further northwest following the Glomma River and Lake Mjøsa, the largest lake in Norway, to Hamar. We visited Hamar Cathedral (Lutheran), consecrated in 1866, and stayed overnight in the town.

On July 27 we went to Lillehammer, host of the 1994 Winter Olympics, and spent a little time looking at the Olympic Museum and the ski jump. Next we drove through the scenic Gudbrandsdal Valley, passing the mountains of Jotunhaimen (English: The Home of the Giants). On the way, we drove through Otta (Fig. 210) and stopped in Lom to visit a stave church (Norwegian: *stavkirke*), a medieval wooden building whose load-bearing posts (*stav*) have lent their name to the construction technique. The rest of the way to Geiranger was through a beautiful scenic region of mountains, waterfalls and passes. Geiranger is located at the Geiranger Fjord, famous for the Seven Sisters Waterfall (Syv Søstrene), which consists of seven separate streams that have their sources in Geit Mountain. The water flows over a high perpendicular cliff and plunges several hundred feet into Geiranger Fjord below.

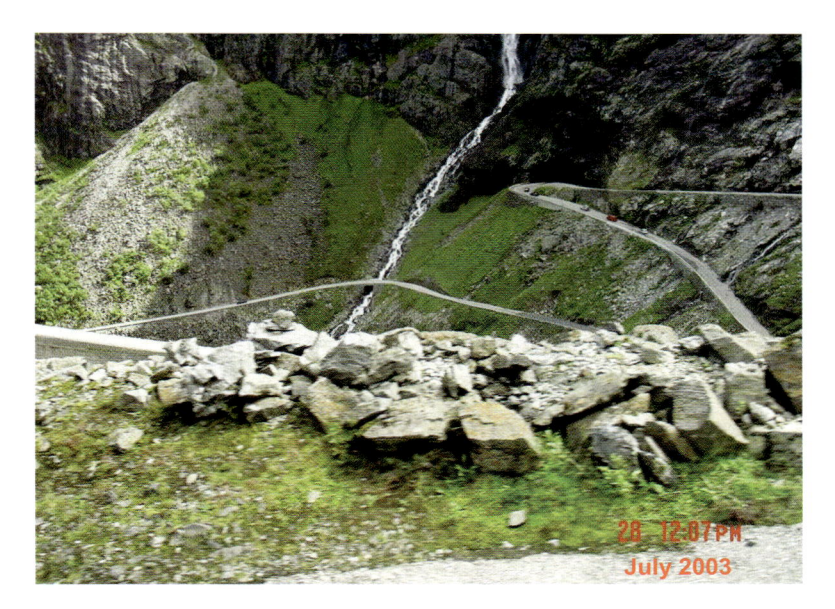

Figure 211. Trollstigen, or Troll Ladder, and Stigfossen waterfall.

The following day we did a full-day Trollstigen excursion. Trollstigen, or Troll Ladder, is a steep mountain road (9 percent incline) with 11 hairpin bends encircled by lofty mountains. Names such as Kongen (the King), Dronningen (the Queen) and Bispen (the Bishop) confirm their majesty. Stigfossen (Stig Waterfall) gushes down the mountainside towards the Isterdalen Valley. In the middle of all this, Trollstigen winds its way up to Stigrøra, 858 meters above sea level (Fig. 211). A number of warning signs (Fig. 212) alert motorists about the dangerous serpentine nature of the road — as well as the possibility that trolls[33] may cross unexpectedly.

On Tuesday, July 29, we took a short ferry cruise along Geirangerfjord to Hellesylt, where we could take a good picture of the Syv Søstrene (Fig. 213). Back on the coach, we drove through the Jostedal Mountains and past Lake Jolstra, stopping to see Bøyabreen (Bøya Glacier) before driving along the shores of Sognefjord to

---

33. In Scandinavian, particularly Norwegian, mythology, trolls are creatures related to elves, dwarves or monsters.

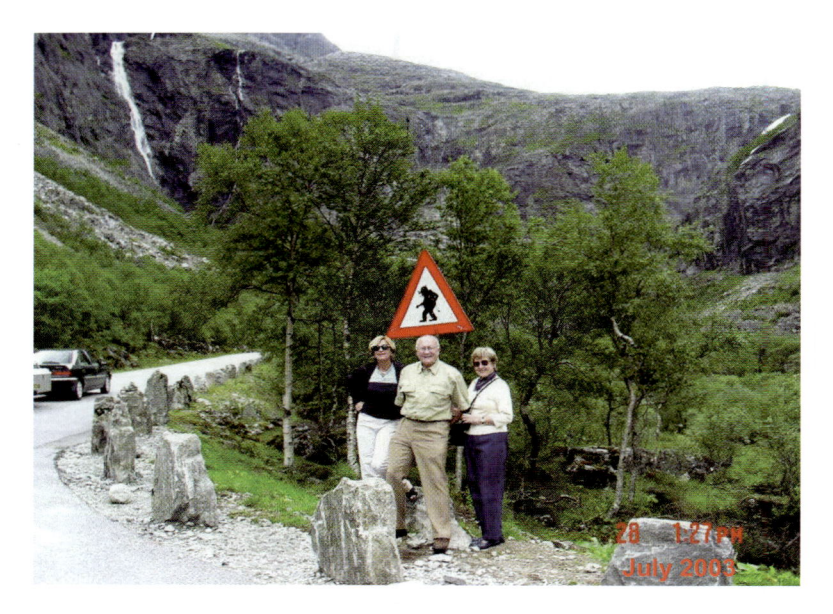

Figure 212. A typically Scandinavian warning sign.

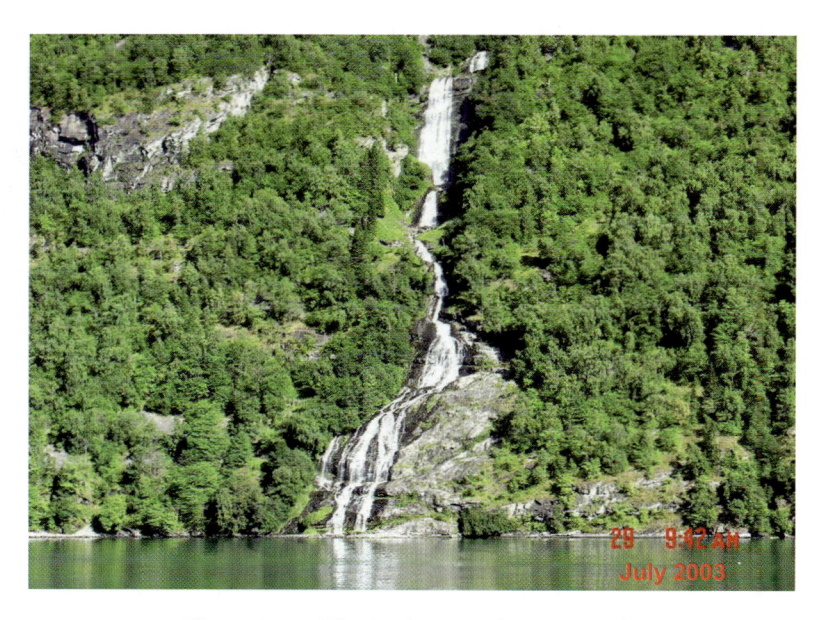

Figure 213. The Syv Søstrene (Seven Sisters).

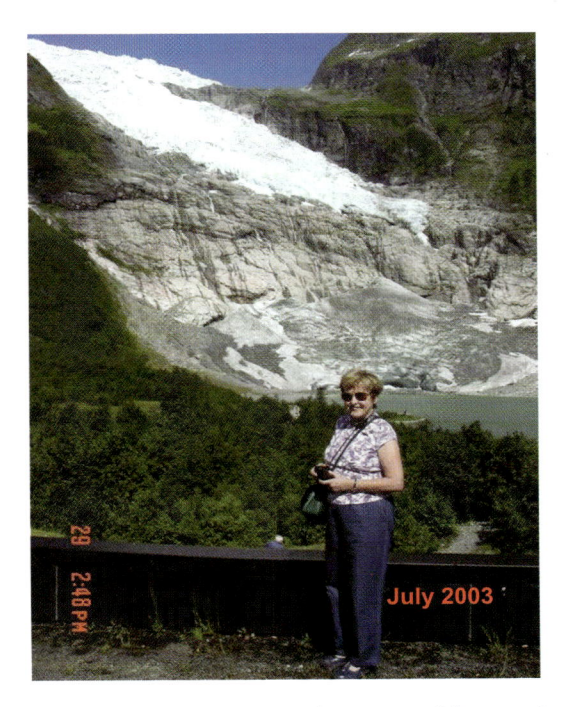

Figure 214. The magnificent Bøyabreen Glacier, part of the giant Jostedalsbreen.

Leikanger. We were told that glaciers in the region were advancing, not receding, and parts of the glaciers were used as podiums during the 1994 Winter Olympics. The spectacular blue Bøyabreen (Fig. 214) is advancing faster than others, and if one is lucky enough — unfortunately, we were not — one may witness glacial calving, as a mass of ice suddenly breaks away and tumbles into the meltwater lagoon beneath the glacial tongue. We arrived at Leikanger at about 5 pm and decided to go for a swim in the Sognefjord. The water was about 72°F (22°C) — no colder than the Baltic Sea — which was surprising as I did not expect such comparatively warm water to be associated with glaciers. The next day began with a ferry trip among the spectacular mountains and waterfalls of the Sognefjord, with attendant seals on the banks. We arrived at Flåm, situated at the innermost part of the Aurlandsfjord, a tributary of the Sognefjord. We took the Flåmsbana (Flåm Railway) to

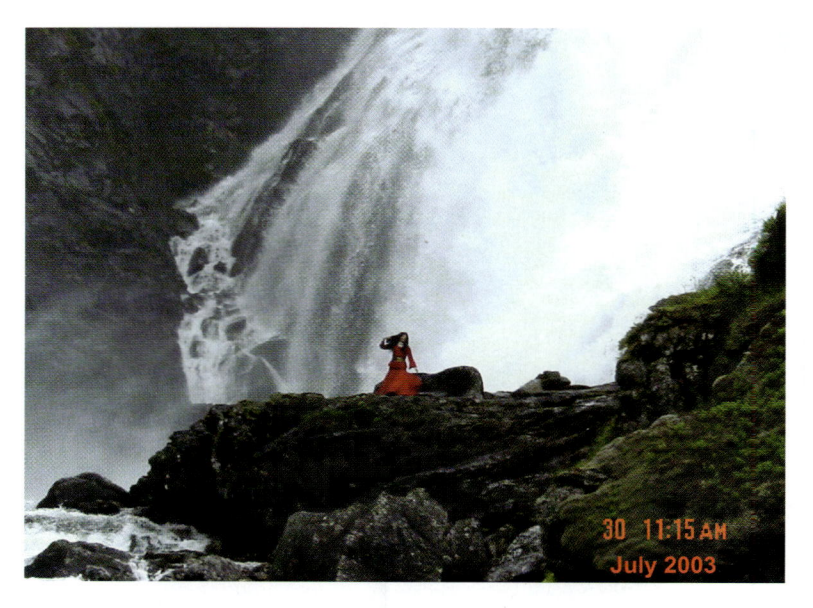

Figure 215.   A mysterious huldra at Kjosfossen.

Myrdal to observe the mystical huldra[34] dancing under the amazing Kjosfossen (Kjos Waterfall) (Fig. 215). From there we made our way to Bergen, walked through the city, and visited the colorful harbor and the Hanseatic Museum at Bryggen, the main street of Bergen.

Bergen, originally called Bjorgvin, was founded in 1070 by King Olaf III. About 1100 a castle was built on the northern edge of the Vagen harbor, and Bergen became commercially and politically important. It was Norway's capital in the 12th and 13th centuries, and in the 14th century it joined the Hanseatic League and became the most important port on the west coast of Norway. Bergen was the birthplace of the composer Edvard Hagerup Grieg (1843–1907), and we decided

---

34. Considered part of the troll family in Scandinavian folklore, the huldra is a mysterious, seductive forest creature. She is fair-haired and alluring, and were it not for her cow's tail, she would look like an ordinary girl, though an exceptionally beautiful one. Occasionally, she tries to hide her tail in order to lure young human men into marrying her. Legend has it that once the young man agrees and they are married in a church, the huldra's tail will fall off. But the true nature of the troll remains in the huldra. If he does not treat her well, she will turn incredibly ugly, and the man will suffer throughout his marriage and regret being tricked by a huldra. So men, watch out! You never know when the next beautiful woman you see is actually a huldra in disguise.

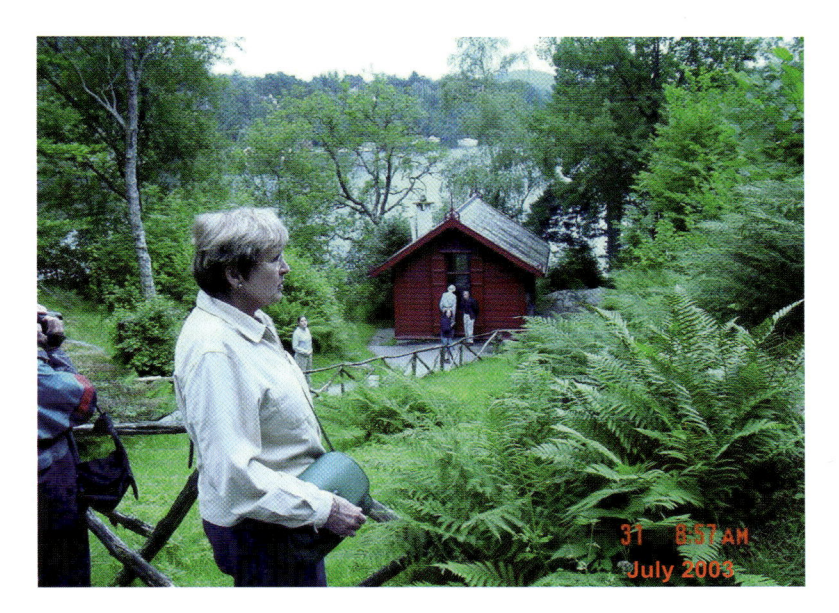

Figure 216. Little garden hut of Norwegian composer, Edvard Grieg, on Troldhaugen.

to visit his summer home, Troldhaugen[35] (Fig. 216), on an optional excursion on July 31. The house has been perfectly conserved with the aim to celebrate the life and works of the great composer. It remains as he left it, with his manuscripts lying about in various rooms. His Steinway grand piano, which he received as a present for his silver wedding anniversary in 1892, can be seen in the comfortable drawing room. They also had a little garden house (Fig. 216) Grieg's and his wife's ashes are entombed in a mountain crypt near the house. Afterwards, we made another excursion to see the surroundings of Bergen. We first went to Mount Fløyen, with its beautiful views of Bergen, souvenir shop and a huge troll statue (Fig. 217). Then we visited two churches, the ecumenical Korskirken (Church of the Cross) and St. Olav's (Lutheran) Cathedral. In the afternoon we drove on to Geilo, enjoying more fabulous views of the surrounding mountains and waterfalls, including the giant Vøringsfossen. On the Hardangervidda mountain plateau, in the middle of nowhere, we encountered a kiosk (Fig. 218). We arrived in Geilo that evening.

---

35. Troldhaugen means "hill of trolls." It has been speculated that Grieg gave it that name because he and his wife Nina were of rather short, troll-like stature.

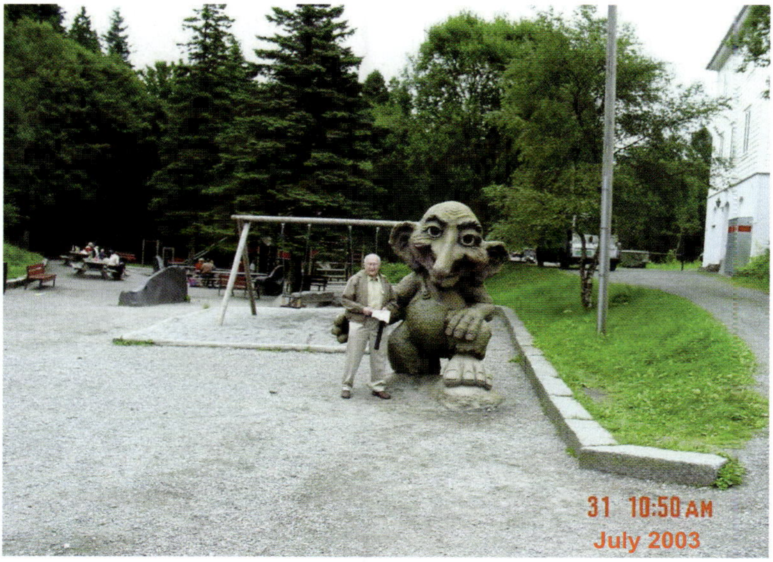

Figure 217. The large troll guarding Mount Fløyen.

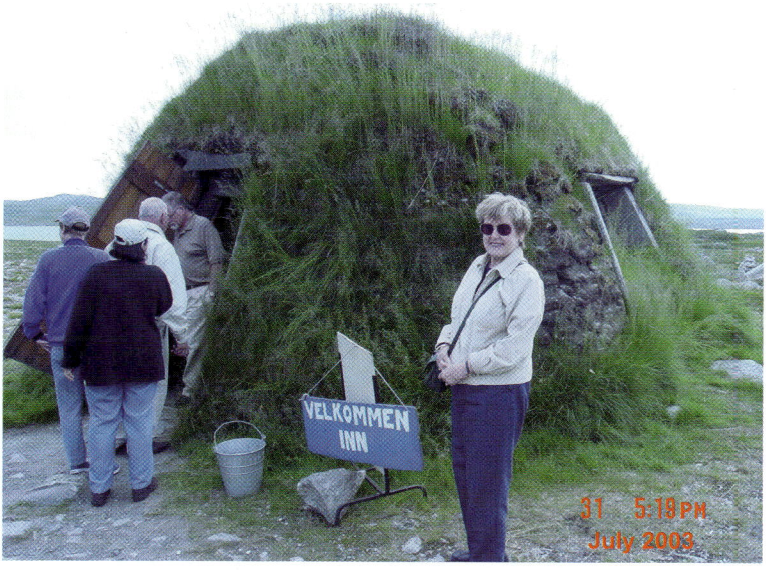

Figure 218. A kiosk in the middle of nowhere on Hardangervidda.

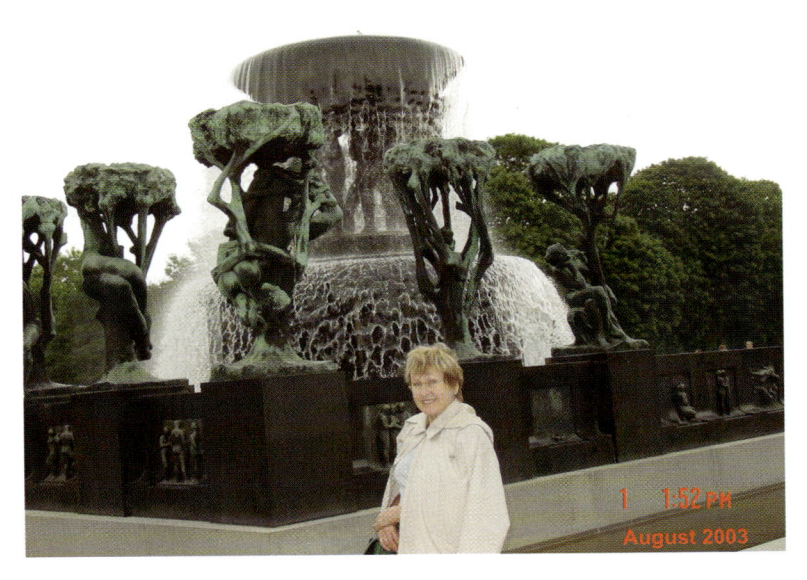

Figure 219.   *The Tree of Life* sculpture at Vigeland Park in Oslo.

On August 1, we drove to Oslo, Norway's capital. Our itinerary included the Oslo Rådhus (City Hall), the statue of King Christian IV of Denmark and Norway (founder of Christiania, later renamed Oslo), and the Vigeland Park, with its huge collection of sculptures, such as the *Tree of Life* (Fig. 219). Later that afternoon we went to see the Vikingskipshuset (The Viking Ship Museum), the Norsk Sjøfartsmuseet (the Norwegian Maritime Museum), and the nearby *Kon-Tiki*, used by Norwegian explorer Thor Heyerdahl, and *Fram*, used in expeditions of the Arctic and Antarctic. As a young man I read a book in Polish called *Fridtjof, co z ciebie wyrośnie?* (Fridtjof, who you will be when you grow up?), a biography of Norwegian explorer and humanitarian Fridtjof Nansen by Alina and Czesław Centkiewicz, so I was keen to see his famous ship (Fig. 220). After that, we strolled through the city and saw Nationaltheatret (National Theater), Stortingsbygningen (the building housing the Storting, Norway's parliament) and the Holmenkollen ski jump.

The next day, after breakfast, we traveled through the farmlands of Oslofjord to Sweden's 350-year-old city of Gothenburg (Göteborg),

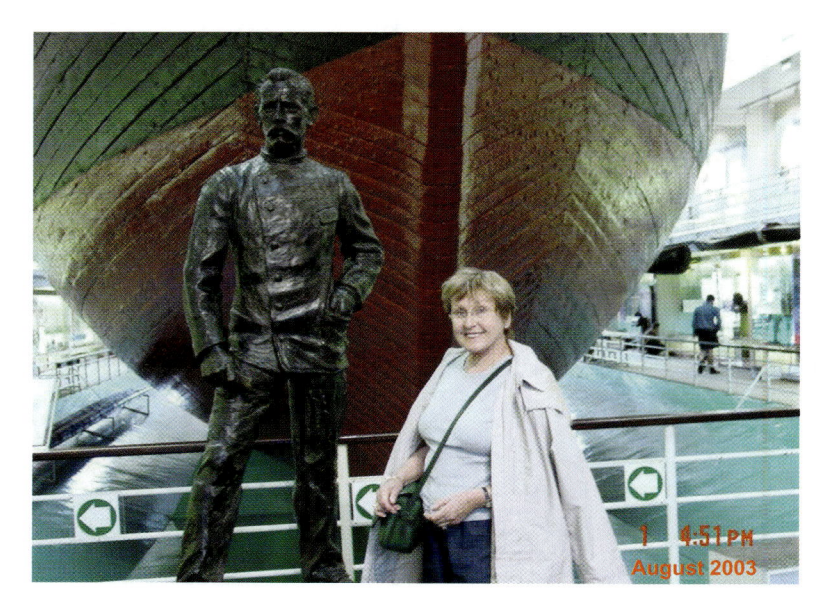

Figure 220. The Fridtjof Nansen statue in front of Fram in Frammuseet on Bygdøy.

arriving late in the afternoon. I had already been to the city in 1989, but we still walked through the Gotaplatsen with its statue of Poseidon (Neptune) in the middle. The following day we took the Helsingborg-Helsingør ferry back to Denmark, going by coach to Copenhagen. We were on Danish soil: our guide reminded us that cyclists have complete right of way on cycle paths, so pedestrians have to take great care not to get in the way. Our afternoon tour took in Edvard Eriksen's famous statue at Langelinie, The Little Mermaid (Fig. 221), and Amalinborg Palace, home of the Danish royals. Later in the afternoon we went to the islet of Slotsholmen in central Copenhagen to see Christiansborg Palace, seat of the Folketing (parliament), the Prime Minister's Office and the Supreme Court. Nearby we saw one of the oldest buildings in Copenhagen, the Old Stock Exchange, which was built by King Christian IV between 1619 and 1640 and housed the Danish stock market until 1974. Our next stop was Frederiksborg Castle in Hillerød, originally built as a royal residence for King Christian IV and now the Museum of National History. In the Mint Tower of the museum we saw the celestial globe from 1657, with the planets moving according to the Sun-centered Copernican system

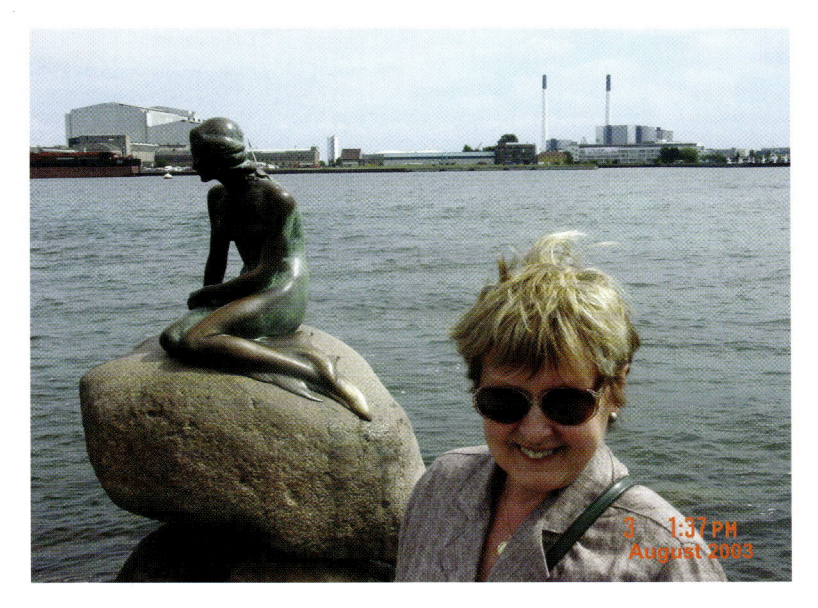

Figure 221. *Den Lille Havfrue* (The Little Mermaid) by Edvard Eriksen at Langelinie in Copenhagen.

(Fig. 222). We also saw another Fountain of Neptune, which was in the courtyard behind the castle's Princess's Wing. We ended our trip to Scandinavia that evening with a farewell dinner in the Bernstorff Restaurant in Tivoli. The next day, August 4, we left Copenhagen at 9:55 am and flew to Poland, with one stop in Warsaw and arriving in Kraków at 3:05 pm.

On September 13 our son Przemek and his wife Kasia spent two weeks with us in Kraków. They also visited Kasia's parents in Rzeszów. We returned to Columbia on October 9, with Jola Ostrowska Jaźwiecka, a school friend of Halina's, traveling with us. We spent some time in Columbia and visited the State Capitol in Jefferson City. On October 16 we went to Branson and stayed at the Honeysuckle Inn, 3598 Shepherd of the Hills Expressway, dropping by the Ozarks on the way. On the morning of October 17 I went to the theater on 3750 West Highway 76 to see Yakov Smirnoff perform. After a thoroughly enjoyable show, I managed to have my picture taken with Yakov (Fig. 223). In the afternoon we all went to the Shoji Tabuchi Show in the Shoji Tabuchi Theater, 3260 Shepherd of the Hills Expressway (Fig. 224). Aside from

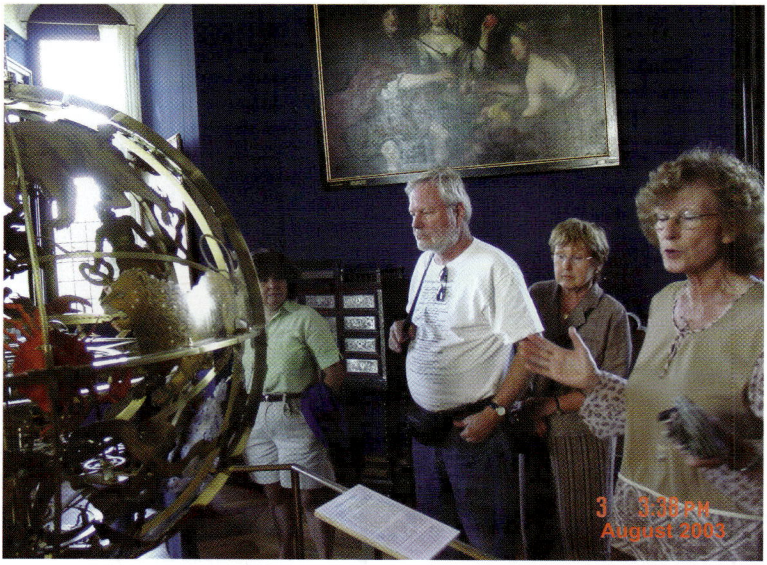

Figure 222. The celestial globe at the Mint Tower, Frederiksborg Castle. The planets move according to the Copernican system.

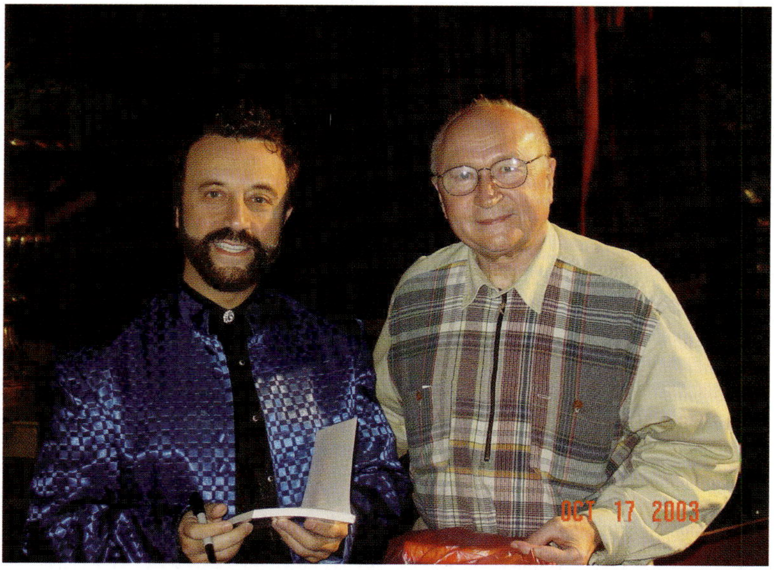

Figure 223. The author with Ukrainian-born American comedian Yakov Smirnoff.

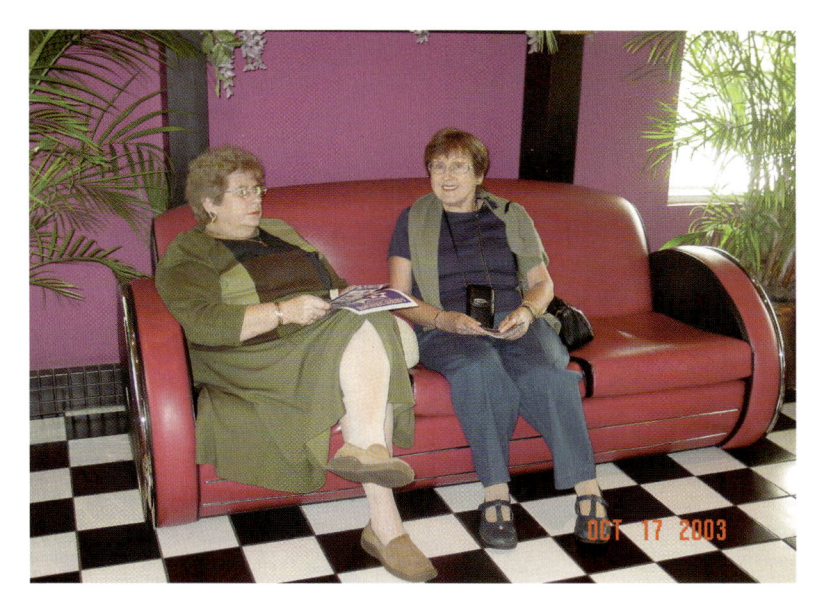

Figure 224. Jola and Halina at the Shoji Tabuchi Theater.

this wonderful performance, the theater is famous for having one of the most comfortable and lavish restrooms in existence. The ladies' powder room is complete with wainscoting and ceiling reproduced from the 1890s Empire period. The gentlemen's lounge is no less impressive, with black lion head sinks imported from Italy, black leather chairs and a marble fireplace. Leaving Branson the next morning, we headed to the Silver Dollar City theme park, where we saw the Harvey Water Clock patented in 1798 (Fig. 225) and a variety of nice farmers' products. Later we went to see the Fantastic Caverns north of Springfield, with its impressive stalactites and stalagmites. Jola returned to Poland on Thursday, October 30.

2004 — Father Edvin Cole's Kraków visit and our Portugal tour

In 2004 we left for Poland on March 31, as it was possible to leave Columbia earlier in the year having resigned from my post as editor of *Hemodialysis International*. We invited Father Edwin Cole, our pastor from the Sacred Heart Church in Columbia and Father John Long's successor, to come to Kraków. Our program was similar to that

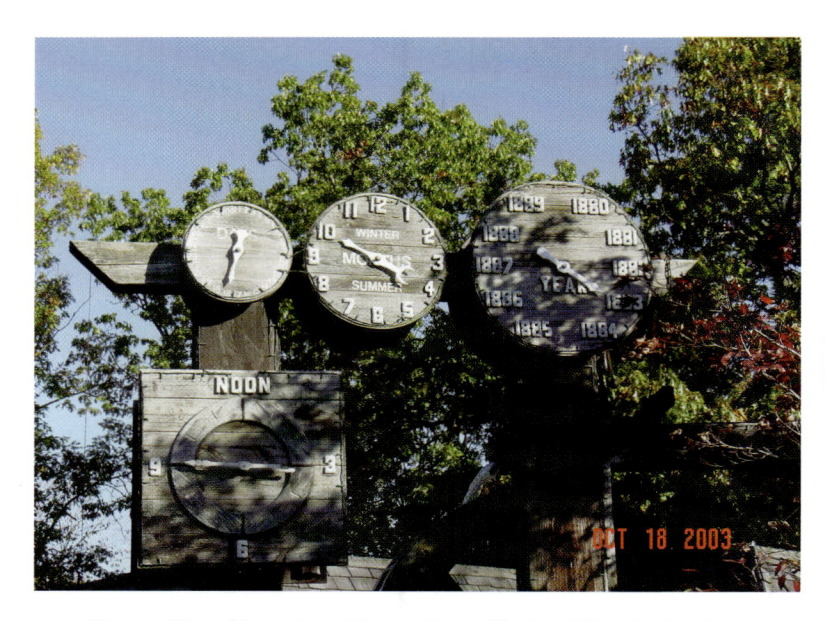

Figure 225. The unique Harvey Water Clock at Silver Dollar City.

involving Father John three years earlier. Father Edwin arrived on June 9 and checked into the Novotel Hotel on Kościuszki Street. This time we also decided to accompany the pastor and see places of interest in Kraków and the vicinity. We visited various churches, including Kościół Św. Anny (St. Anne's Church), Kościół Franciszkanów (the Franciscan Church), 10th-century Kościół Św. Wojciecha (St. Adalbert's Church) and Kościół Mariacki (St. Mary's Basilica), which houses a famous wooden altarpiece carved by Wit Stwosz (Veit Stoss). On June 11 we visited Wawel Castle, and the following day we went to Wadowice, Kalwaria Zebrzydowska and also the Sanctuary of the Divine Mercy in Łagiewniki. On Sunday, June 13, we attended Mass in Kościół Dominikanów (the Dominican Church) and visited the National Museum and the Czartoryski Museum, where da Vinci's *Lady with an Ermine* is on display. The day after, we went to the Wieliczka salt mine, which was built after Bochnia's in the 12th century but was much bigger and established itself in the 13th century as the epicenter of Polish salt production until 1970. In 1978 it was designated a UNESCO World Heritage Site. The discovery of salt there is connected with St. Kinga, third daughter of King Béla IV of Hungary, patroness of Poland and Lithuania. There are several legends related to the discovery, but our guide in the salt mine, Dominika, told us the following version. When St. Kinga was traveling to marry Bolesław V Wstydliwy (Bolesław V the Chaste), the Prince of Kraków, she lost her engagement ring. After her wedding in Kraków, Kinga went for a trip to the nearby town of Wieliczka. She ordered that a well be dug, but the well diggers had to stop work because they encountered hard stone. Kinga told them to raise a chunk of the stone to the surface, and what emerged was a piece of pure salt with her ring trapped inside. After the miraculous incident, Kinga became the patroness of salt miners, and in spite of the marriage, the devout couple took up a vow of chastity. During her reign Kinga involved herself in charitable works such as visiting the poor and helping lepers. When her husband died in 1279, she sold all of her material possessions and gave the money to the poor. Pope Alexander VII beatified Kinga in 1690, and she was made chief patroness of Poland and Lithuania in 1695. On June 16, 1999, she was canonized by Pope John Paul II. The Wieliczka salt mine features a 3.5-km touring route for visitors (less than 1 percent of the length of the mine's passages) that includes historic statues and mythical figures. The oldest sculptures were carved out of rock salt by miners. More recent figures have been fashioned by contemporary artists (Fig. 226).

On June 15 we visited the Kazimierz district, which lies to the south of the Wawel Castle and was once a town in its own right inhabited mostly by Jews. Founded in 1335 by King Kazimierz (Casimir) the Great, the town was a center of prosperity and tolerance, with splendid churches and synagogues. But after the Nazi invasion of Poland in September 1939, the Jewish population was almost completely exterminated. Recently, Kazimierz has undergone a major renaissance, and both its Jewish and Christian heritage is being restored. We visited Kościół Bożego Ciała (Corpus Christi Church) and the Temple Synagogue, and then we went to Kościół na Skałce (Church on the Rock), Poland's holiest place save for Częstochowa. Here, in 1079, Poland's chief patron saint, St. Stanisław, was martyred at the hands of King Bolesław II the Bold. On June 16, we drove to Częstochowa to see Czarna Madonna, or Matka Boska Częstochowska (The Black Madonna of Częstochowa). The Black Madonna is

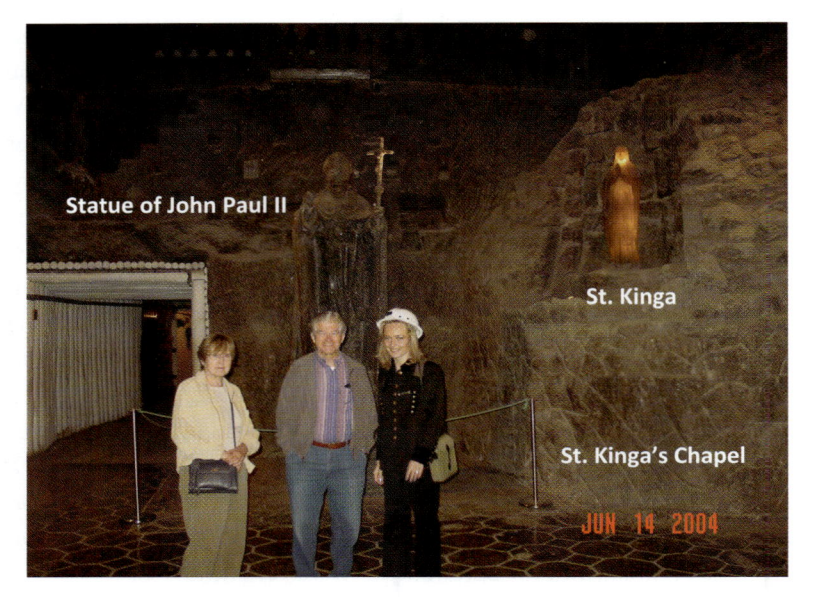

Figure 226. Halina, Father Edwin and our guide, Dominika, in St. Kinga's Chapel.

credited with miraculously saving the monastery of Jasna Góra (Bright Mount) in Częstochowa from a 17th-century Swedish invasion called Potop (Deluge), which actually changed the course of the war. The event led King John II Casimir Vasa to crown the Black Madonna as Queen and Protector of Poland in the Latin Cathedral of Lwów (now Lviv in Ukrainian) on April 1, 1656. We spent the whole day exploring the monastery. Father Edwin returned to Columbia the following day.

Around that time I was reading a fascinating book on prominent "discoverers" by Daniel Joseph Boorstin.[36] I was captivated by one story about Portugal in the 15th and 16th centuries, particularly the achievements of Henry the Navigator. Indeed, I had not learned much at all about that country during high school as our universal history course had not included Portugal. The country's name derives from the Roman name Portus Cale. Cale was the name of an early settlement located at

---

36. Boorstin DJ. (1983) *The Discoverers: A History of Man's Search to Know his World and Himself*. Vintage Books, A Division of Random House, New York.

the mouth of the Douro River, which flows into the Atlantic Ocean. During the Second Punic War, after the defeat of Hasdrubal by Scipio Africanus at Ilipa in 206 BC, the Romans took the Iberian Peninsula from the Carthaginians and in the process conquered Cale, renaming it Portus Cale (Port of Cale). During the Middle Ages the region around Portus Cale became known to the Visigoths as Portucale, and the name evolved into Portugale during the seventh and eighth centuries. By the ninth century, that term was used extensively to refer to the region between the rivers Douro and Minho, the latter flowing at the northern border between Portugal and Spain.

Little is known about the first inhabitants of the Iberian Peninsula. It is known that in the first millennium BC, several waves of Celts invaded Portugal from central Europe and intermarried with the local population, forming numerous ethnic groups, with many tribes. Chief among these tribes were the Calaicians, or Gallaeci, of northern Portugal, the Lusitanians of central Portugal, the Celtici of Alentejo, and the Cynetes, or Conii, of the Algarve. Some small, semi-permanent coastal settlements, like Tavira in the Algarve, were founded by the Phoenicians-Carthaginians in the southernmost part of the country. The first Roman invasion of the Iberian Peninsula occurred in 219 BC. Within 200 years, almost the entire peninsula had been annexed to the Roman Empire. As mentioned above, the Carthaginians were expelled from their coastal colonies during the Second Punic War. Rome installed a colonial regime. During this period, Lusitania grew in prosperity and many of modern-day Portugal's cities and towns were founded. In 27 BC, Lusitania gained the status of a Roman province. Later, a northern province called Lusitania was formed, and it came to be known as Gallaecia, with its capital in Bracara (today's Braga). In the early fifth century, Germanic tribes invaded the peninsula, namely the Suevi, Vandals and Sarmatian Alans. Another wave of Germanic invaders, the Visigoths, conquered all of the Iberian Peninsula and expelled or integrated the Vandals and the Alans. The Visigoths eventually conquered the Suevi kingdom and its capital city Bracara (Braga) in 584–585.

In 622, an Islamic expansion started, but did not reach the Iberian Peninsula until a century later in the spring of 711, when Islamic Moors (Berbers and Arabs) landed near Algeciras, on the Bay of Gibraltar in current Spain, and destroyed the Visigothic kingdom. Many of the ousted Gothic nobles took refuge in the unconquered north Asturian highlands in the northern Iberian Peninsula. From there they aimed to reconquer their lands from the Moors: this war of reconquest is known in Portuguese and Spanish as the Reconquista. This Reconquista was made easier by the typical error of all empires: stretching the borders beyond real capabilities. The Muslim rulers of al-Andalus (Andalusia) decided to extend their territory north, beyond the Pyrenees, in the early eighth century. They were punished by the Franks under the command of Charles Martel at Tours and Poitiers in 732 and had to retreat (see above). In 868 Count Vimara Peres reconquered and governed the region between the rivers Minho and Douro, the county known as Portucale.

In 1095, Portugal separated almost completely from the Kingdom of Galicia.[37] Its territories, consisting largely of mountains, moorland and forest, were bound in the north by the Minho and in the south by the Mondego. At the end of the 11th century, the Burgundian knight Henry became Count of Portugal and defended his independence, merging the County of Portucale and the County of Coimbra. Henry declared independence for Portugal while a civil war raged between León and Castile, but he died without achieving his aims. Real Portugese national origins trace to June 24, 1128, with the Battle of São Mamede, when Portugese forces led by Afonso I defeated forces led by his mother, Teresa of León. Afonso proclaimed himself the first Prince of Portugal and in 1139 the first King of Portugal. By 1143, with the assistance of a representative of the Holy See at the conference of Zamora, Portugal was formally recognized as an independent state, with the prince recognized as Dux Portucalensis. In 1179 Afonso I was declared king by the Pope. The king ruled from Guimarães, the first capital of Portugal. Later, when Portugal was already officially independent, he ruled from Coimbra. From 1249 to 1250 the Algarve

---

[37]. There was also a historical region of Eastern European called Galicia, which is in present-day southern Poland and western Ukraine. The territory was populated in Roman times by people similar to those in the Iberian Peninsula, including various tribes of Celto-Germanic admixture, such as the Celtic Galice (or Gaulics) — hence, most likely, the name. During the great migration coincident with the fall of the Roman Empire, various people invaded the area, including Scythians, Sarmatians, Huns, Avars and, in the seventh to eighth centuries, the Slavs. Central Anatolia, modern-day Turkey, north of Phrygia and Cappadocia, was also populated by Gauls from Thrace and called Galatia.

(*al gharb* in Arabic means "the west"), the southernmost region, was finally recaptured by Portugal from the Muslims. In 1255 the capital shifted to Lisbon. Neighboring Spain would not complete their Reconquista until 1492, almost 150 years later. Portugal's land-based boundaries have been notably stable in history. The border with Spain has remained almost unchanged since the 13th century. The Treaty of Windsor in 1386 created an alliance between Portugal and England that remains in effect to this day. Since early times, fishing and overseas commerce have been the country's main economic activities. Henry the Navigator's interest in exploration, together with some technological developments in navigation, made Portugal's expansion possible and led to great advances in geographic, mathematical and scientific knowledge and technology, more specifically naval technology.

Henry, born in 1394, was the third child of King John I of Portugal, the founder of the Aviz dynasty, and of Philippa of Lancaster, the daughter of John of Gaunt. Henry encouraged his father to conquer Ceuta, a Muslim port on the North African coast across the Gibraltar. Prince Henry, only 19 at the time, was assigned the task of building a fleet in Porto. After two years of preparation the Crusade against Ceuta was launched on July 25, 1415, and this date is considered the beginning of the Portuguese Empire. Ceuta was conquered on August 24, with minimal losses to the Portuguese but tremendous casualties among the Muslims. For the first time Prince Henry could see the enormous wealth lying hidden in Africa that was being delivered by caravans. In addition to the usual booty of gold, silver and jewels, there were exotic stores of pepper, cinnamon, cloves, ginger and other spices. Ceuta became a Christian city, but the caravans stopped arriving and the Portuguese were in possession of a profitless city. Either they had to cooperate with the surrounding tribes or conquer the hinterland. Prince Henry gathered information about the interior lands from where the treasures had come. Most likely then came his plans to expand Portuguese trade. He resigned from joining the court in Lisbon and went to Portugal's most southwesterly point, Cape Saint Vincent. Ancient geographers had given it the name *Promontorium Sacrum* (Sacred Promontory). The Portuguese, translating it into Sagres, made it the name of a nearby village. The prince

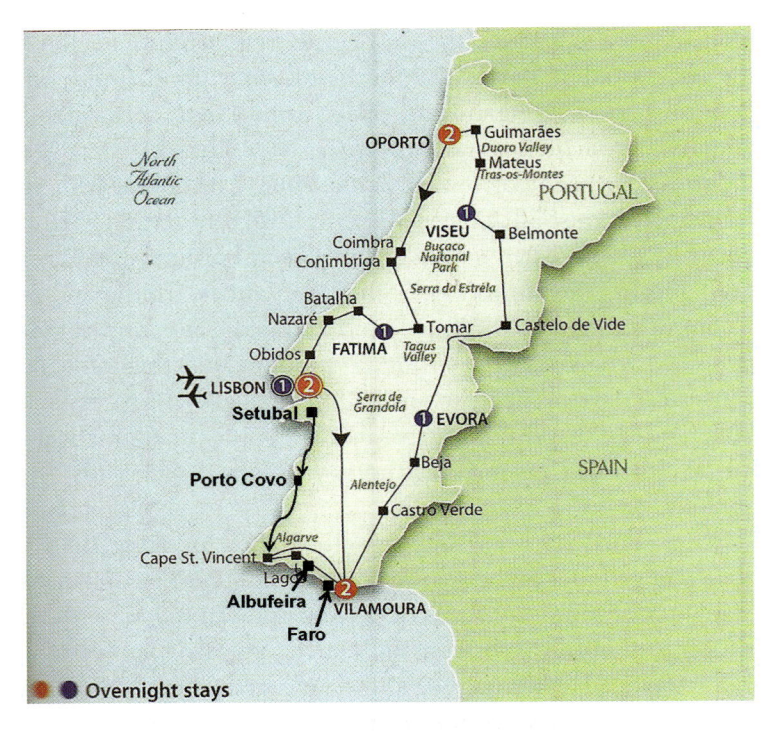

Figure 227. Our Portugal tour.

made his headquarters there for 40 years and became known as Henry the Navigator. From here he initiated, organized and commanded expeditions that would make Portuguese sailors famous.

We decided to take a tour of Portugal with our preferred tour company, Trafalgar Tours, flying out from Kraków on Lufthansa LH3337 to Munich and then LH4540 to Lisbon, and arriving at 1:30 pm on June 23. When we got there, we took a taxi to the Marriott Hotel on Avenida dos Combatentes. The tour (Fig. 227) was not exactly as shown on the map, as we were told that some small deviations were needed for organizational reasons. Traveling south the next day, our first stop was in Setúbal, once a prosperous center of the fish-salting industry, located in the former Roman town of Cetobriga. In the town we visited Igreja de Jesus, a Gothic church with a wonderful high altar. In front of the altar stood triple columns twisted to create spirals carved in Arrábida pink stone from

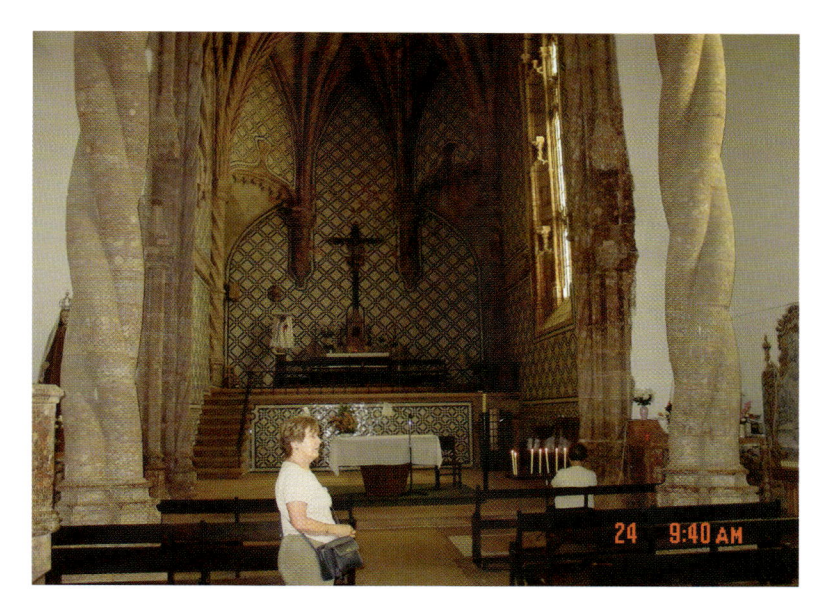

Figure 228. The high altar at Igreja de Jesus Gothic church in Setúbal.

the nearby quarry. The architect Diogo Boitac designed this wonderful example of the Manueline[38] style in 1494 (Fig. 228). We also stopped at a monument honoring Luisa (Rosa) d'Aguiar Todi, one of the great Portuguese opera singers. Our next stop was Porto Covo, a little village on the Atlantic Ocean with many wonderful beaches. We had lunch there and then went further south to the territory where Henry the Navigator had his headquarters in Sagres: Cabo de São Vicente (Cape St. Vincent) (Fig. 229) and Lagos. Located approximately 3.5 miles (5.6 km) from the village of Sagres, Cape St. Vincent is a landmark for ships traveling to or from the Mediterranean. The present lighthouse, one of the most powerful in Europe (its two 1000-watt lamps can be seen as far as 37 miles, or

---

38. The Manueline style is named after King Manuel I (r. 1495–1521), whose reign coincided with its development. The style is also called "Portuguese Late Gothic" and marks the transition from Late Gothic to Renaissance. It was much influenced by the astonishing successes of Portuguese navigators, drawing heavily on the style and decorations of East Indian temples, and was largely financed by proceeds of the lucrative spice trade with Africa and India. As seen in the photo of the high altar in Igreja de Jesus, the beginnings of this style preceded the reign of King Manuel I.

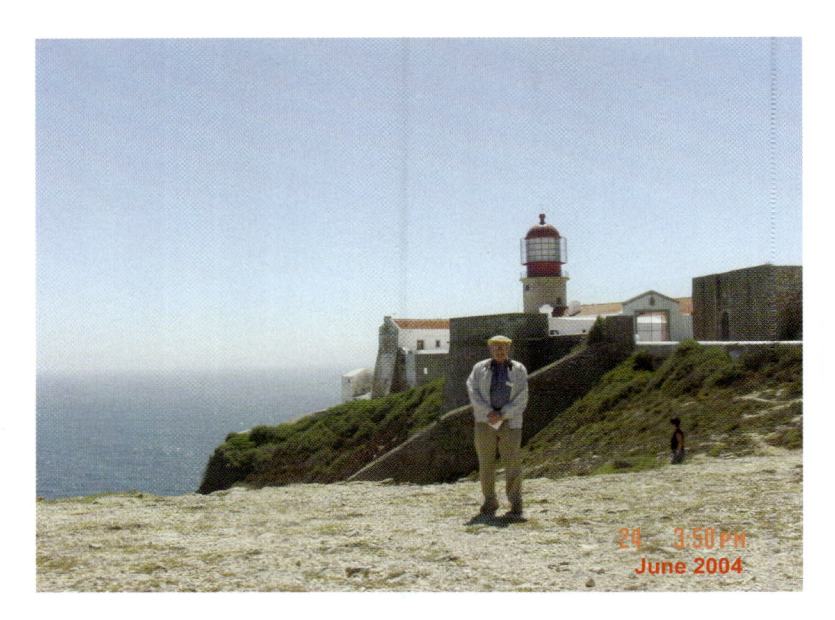

Figure 229. The lighthouse at Cabo de São Vicente.

60 km, away), was built over the ruins of a 16th-century Franciscan convent. All existing buildings, including the Vila do Infante of Henry the Navigator, fell into ruins during the Great Lisbon Earthquake.[39] In the evening we arrived in Albufeira and stayed the night at Hotel Montechoro.

On Friday, June 25, we spent the morning at the beach in Montechoro. In the afternoon we went to visit the Church of St. Lawrence of Almancil. The main nave of the church is covered in blue and white glazed tiles (azulejos) depicting the life and death of the saint (Fig. 230). We discovered that the Romans had condemned St. Lawrence to death by burning, or "grilling." Afterwards, we visited the Sao Lourenço Cultural Center with its beautiful garden, and later in the afternoon we went to see the Sé Cathedral in Faro. The original Moorish name Ossonóba was changed to Faro following King Dom Afonso II defeat of the Moors in 1249. There is a nice view of King Dom Afonso III Square from the belfry of the church (Fig. 231). Note

---

39. The epicenter of the earthquake was in the Atlantic Ocean, 120 miles (200 km) from Cape St. Vincent, closer than to Lisbon, but the name comes from the greatest devastation and casualties in Lisbon than in any other affected place.

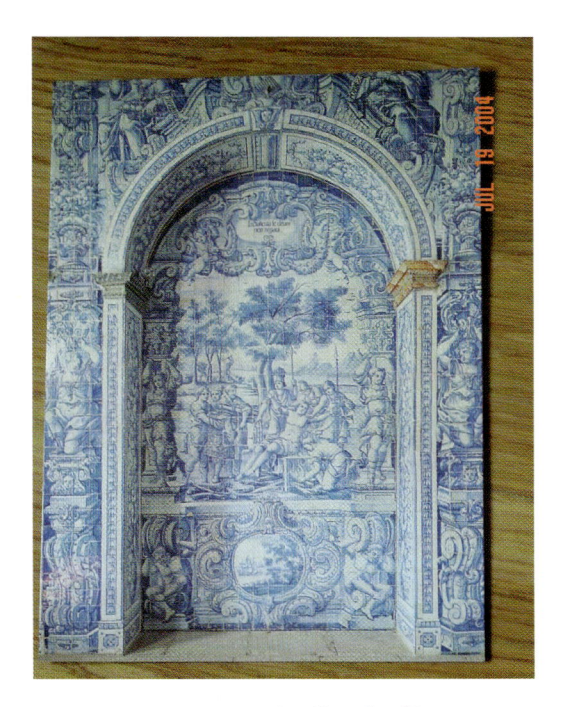

Figure 230. St. Lawrence on a grate in the Church of St. Lawrence in Almancil.

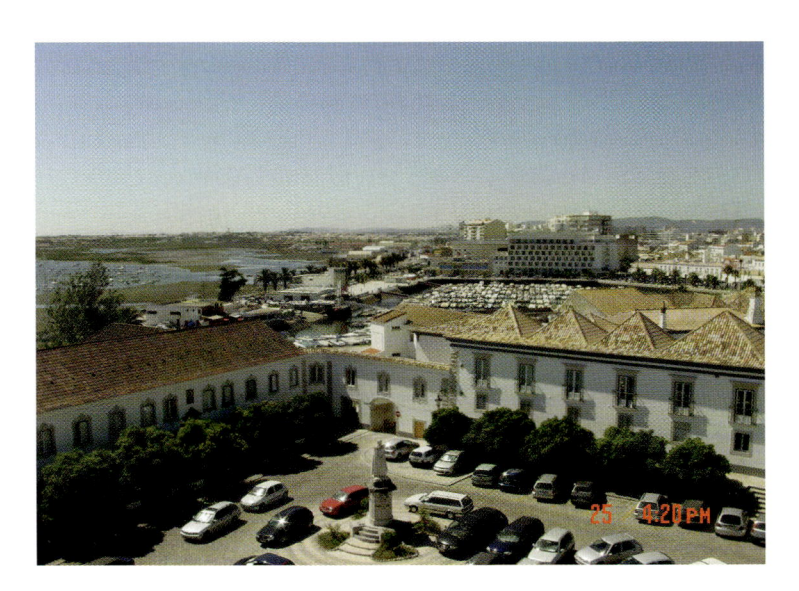

Figure 231. The view from Sé Cathedral's belfry over King Dom Afonso III Square.

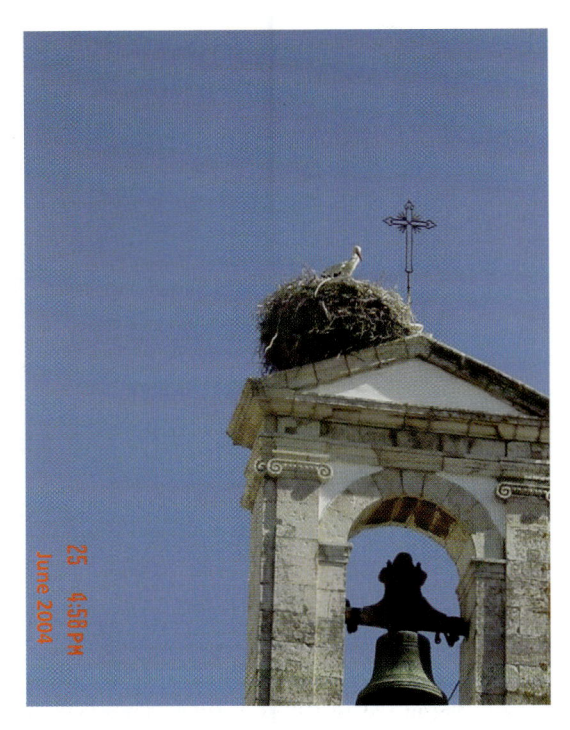

Figure 232. A stork claims the belfry as its own.

the shape of the roofs on the Paço Episcopal, which are unique to Faro. We also spotted a stork in its nest on the belfry of the cathedral (Fig. 232). In the evening we returned to Hotel Montechoro.

The next day we headed to Évora, located in the south-central region of Alentejo. On the way, in Beja, we visited the Royal Monastery of Our Lady of the Conception from the Holy Order of St. Clara under Franciscan Jurisdiction, which was transformed into the Regional Museum in 1927–1928. We visited an exhibition of Mariana Alcoforado (1640–1723), a nun who was seduced by and fell in love with a French officer. Her *Letters of a Portuguese Nun* (French: *Les Lettres Portugaises*) were translated into many languages, including into Polish by Stanisław Przybyszewski in 1920 (Fig. 233). Afterwards, we continued on to Évora, an old city dating back more than two millennia. The city may have been named after ivory workers. The Lusitanians, who made the town their regional capital, called it Ebora. The Romans conquered the

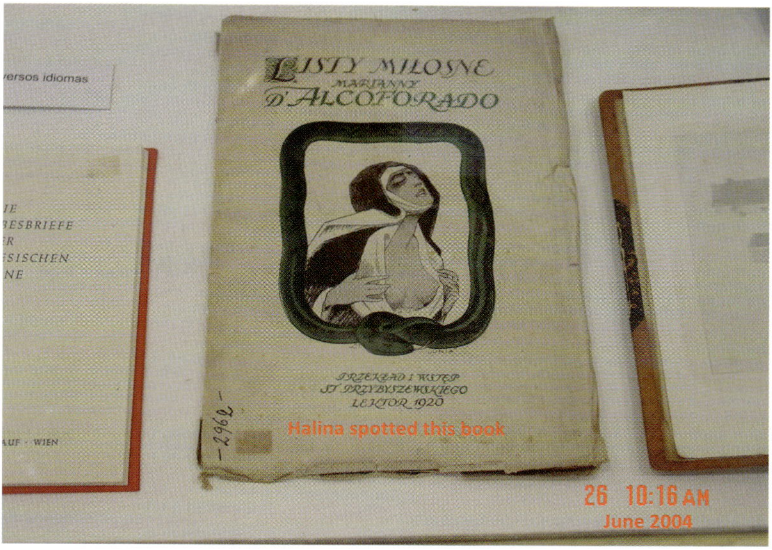

Figure 233. An exhibition of *Les Lettres portugaises* translated into Polish.

town in 57 BC and expanded it into a walled town. Vestiges from this period — city walls and ruins of Roman baths — still remain. Julius Caesar called it *Liberalitas Julia* (Julian generosity). During his travels through Gaul and Lusitania, Pliny the Elder also visited the town, calling it Ebora Cerealis (because of the surrounding wheat fields) in his book *Naturalis Historia*. With Ebora flourishing in the first century, the monumental Corinthian Temple of Diana in the center of the town was erected in honor of Emperor Augustus. The ruins of the temple (Fig. 234) and the very well preserved city walls are just some of the many remnants from Roman times. The Silver Water Aqueduct, built not during Roman times but in 16th century, was also impressive. We visited a cloister and the beautiful Sé Cathedral with its gilded altar, and Igreja Real de Sao Francisco (St. Francisco Church) with its Capela dos Ossos (Chapel of Bones) (Fig. 235). Our overnight stay was at Hotel Albergaria Vitoria, Rua Diana de Liz, in Évora.

On Sunday, June 27, we continued our tour from Évora north to Viseu. On the way we went through the region where cork is collected from *Quercus suber* (cork oak). Our guide, Isabel, told us that the bark of the tree can be harvested every 9 to 12 years, and that the tree can

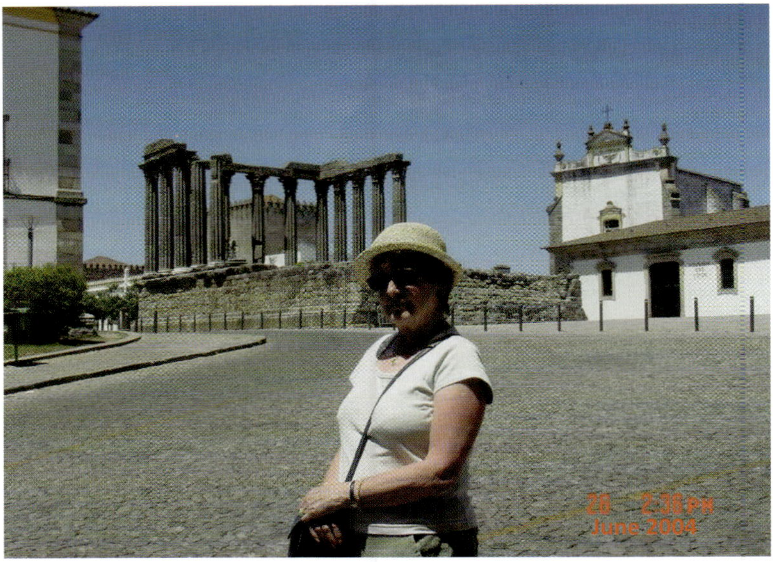

Figure 234. The ruins of a Roman Temple of Diana in Évora, Alentejo.

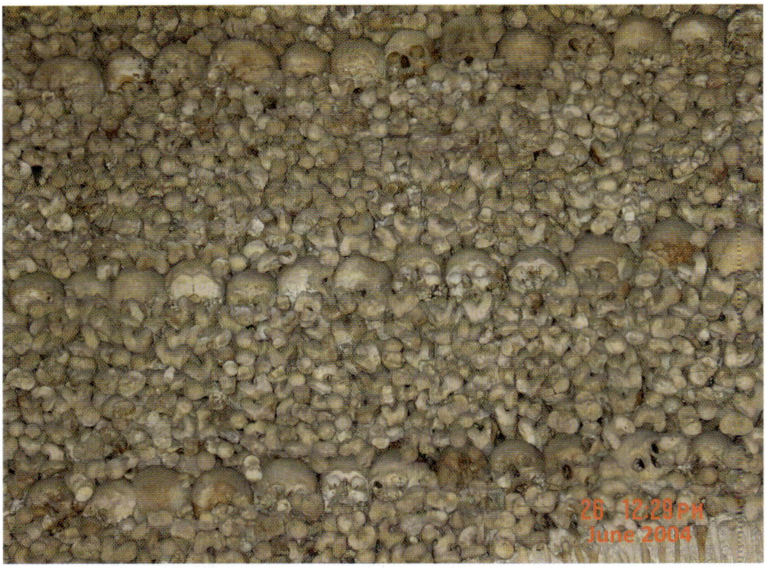

Figure 235. Capela dos Ossos at the Igreja de Sao Francisco in Évora.

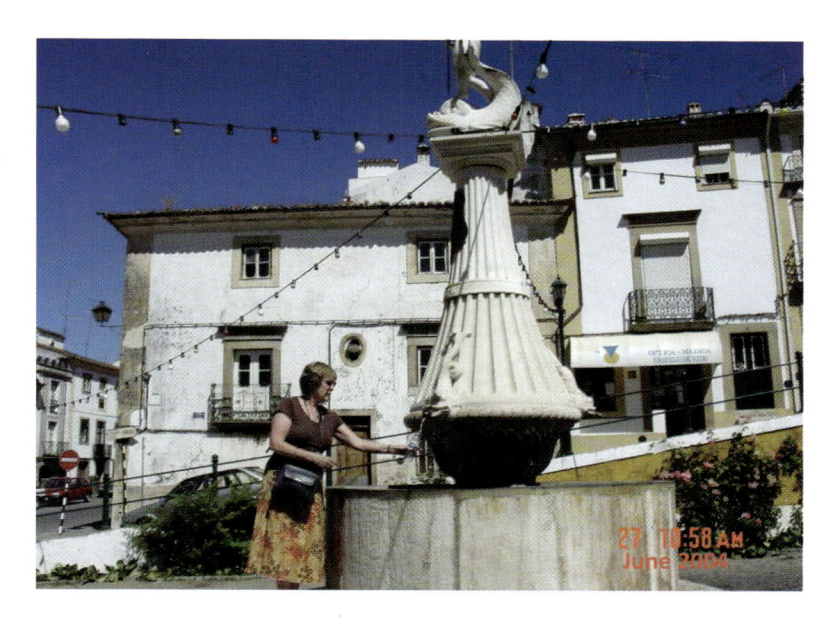

Figure 236. A well with excellent drinking water in Castelo de Vide.

still bloom after recent stripping. We also passed several marble quarries. We then reached Castelo de Vide, famous for its original medieval architecture and Jewish quarter. Climbing up to the castle, we were treated to one of the most magnificent panoramas in the province of Alentejo. We stopped at Sinagoga Sefardita, a medieval synagogue of the Sephardic Jews, and walked through the city, enjoying its many remnants of medieval architecture. We noted several fountains supplied with drinking water from wells (Fig. 236). Next we continued north, passing forests of eucalyptus trees regenerating after a fire in 2003, and stopping at Torre de Centum Cellas in Belmonte, Beira, well-preserved ruins of an unusual three-story Roman building at least 16 centuries old (Fig. 237). The nearby Belmonte Castle, which we did not see, contains the tomb of navigator and explorer Pedro Álvares Cabral, whose most remarkable achievement was the discovery of Brazil. Later that afternoon we arrived at Viseu and visited the Grão Vasco Museum, which occupies the old seminary building beside Viseu Cathedral. The museum is named after one of the most important Portuguese painters of the Renaissance, Vasco Fernandes,

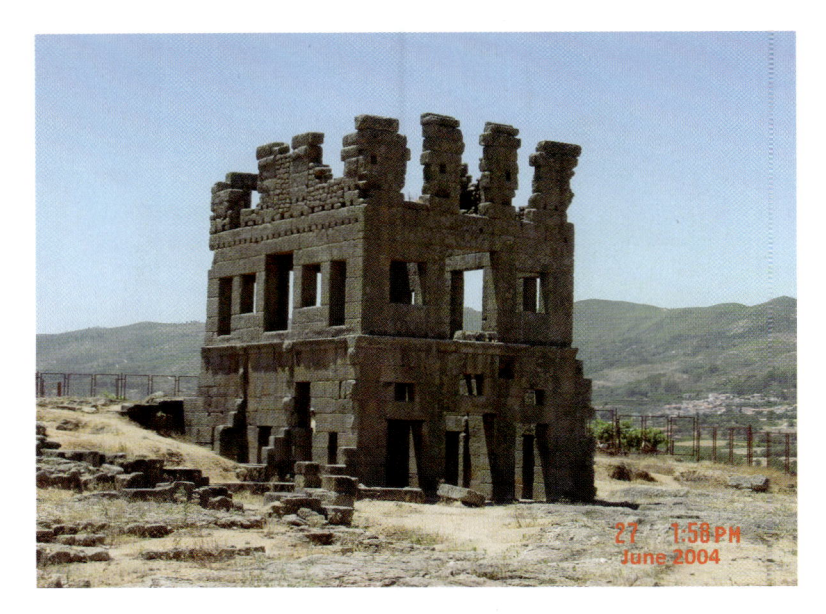

Figure 237. Torre de Centum Cellas, an unusual three-story Roman building in Belmonte.

or Grão Vasco, who had his workshop in Viseu. We overnighted in Melia Confort Grão Vasco on Rua Gaspar Bareiros.

On Monday we first traveled north to Vila Real and then west to Porto through Amarante and Guimarães. On the way we crossed the Douro River and admired the vineyards on the southern mountain slopes near Vila Real. Grapes from the Douro Valley are processed for the production of port, and only the sweet dessert wine from these grapes is considered real port wine. We then visited Palácio de Mateus in Vila Real with its very impressive garden and the most amazing topiaries we had ever seen. One tunnel-like form, made from Mexican cypress trees (*Cupressus lusitanica*),[40] was fashioned to resemble the trunk and neck of a huge animal (Fig. 238). After that, we went to Amarante, where we had lunch and visited Igreja da São Gonçalo de Amarante (Monastery of St. Gonçalo) (Fig. 239). The patron saint of Amarante is revered mostly for his many healing miracles and is also known for the promotion of love and marriage. Every summer on

---

40. The Latin name *lusitanica* (of Lusitania or of Portugal) comes from the fact that this evergreen conifer tree was imported from Mexico to Portugal in the early 17th century.

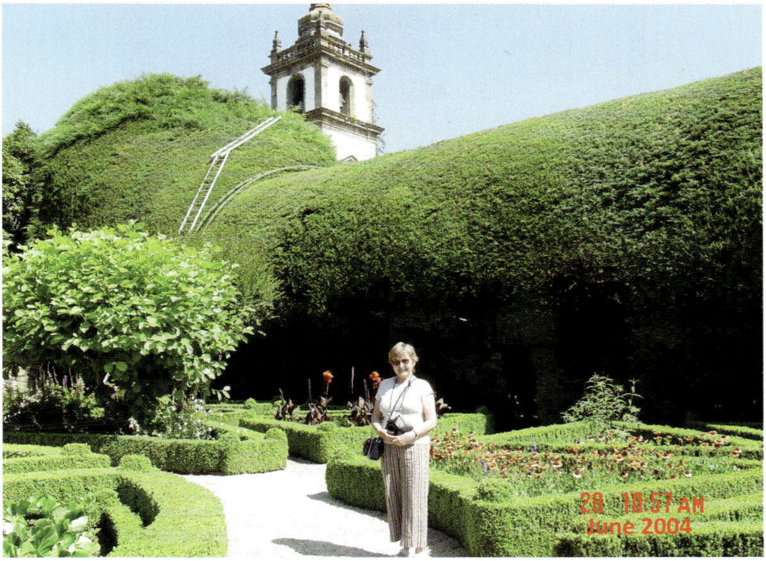

Figure 238. A huge topiary in the garden of Mateus Palace; the ladders belong to gardeners trimming the neck.

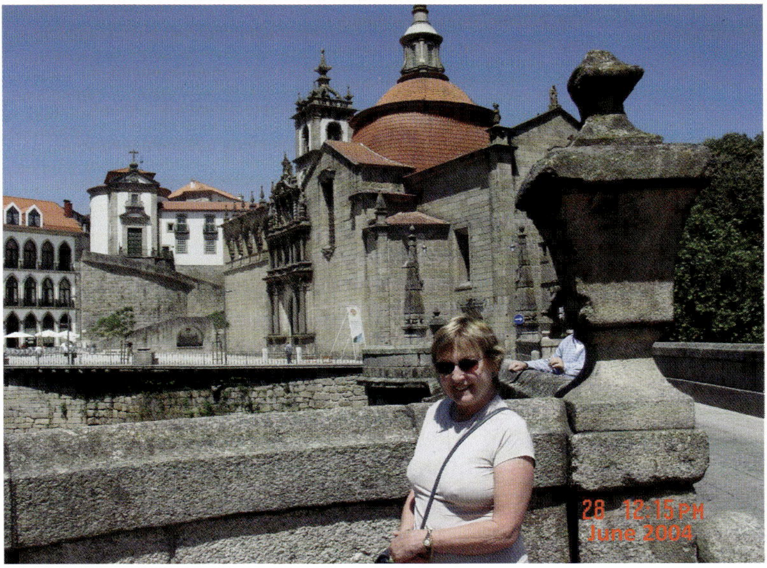

Figure 239. The Monastery of St. Gonçalo in Amarante.

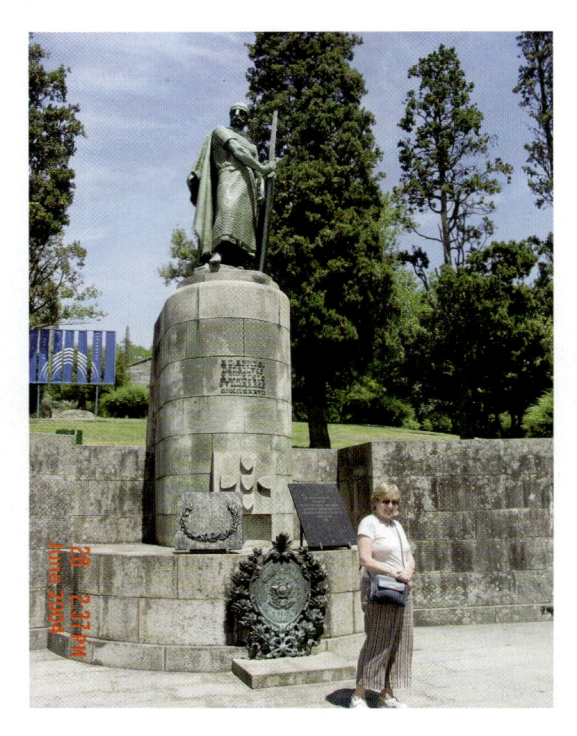

Figure 240. A statue of King Afonso Henrîques, Portugal's first king.

the first Saturday and Sunday of June, there is a festival involving men giving phallic shaped pastries to the womenfolk — a festival we unfortunately missed by three weeks. Our next stop was Guimarães, birthplace of Afonso Henrîques, the first king of Portugal. King Afonso is honored there, as in the whole of Portugal, with a memorial-like statue (Fig. 240) and a baptismal font in St. Michael's Chapel (built by his father, Henry), where he was baptized in 1109 or 1111. In the late afternoon we headed to Vila Nova de Gaia on the A28, crossing a bridge over the Douro River estuary, and reached our hotel for the night, the Mercure Porto Gaia.

We spent Tuesday sightseeing in the area. First we crossed the Douro River north to Porto, Portugal's second largest city. In the morning we visited Igreja de S. Francisco, and Palácio da Bolsa, where the head offices of the Porto Chamber of Commerce and Industry are located. Just before the noon we crossed the Douro River again to Vila Nova de Gaia. We visited the famous Sandeman Cellars, where countless barrels of Porto are stored and aged, and then the Sandeman Museu do Douro, where we were shown a film on the company and its Porto production. The current Chairman of the House of Sandeman, George Sandeman, is the eldest of the seventh generation of the family linked to the port wine and sherry business. The company was founded in London at the end of the 18th century by his ancestor, also named George Sandeman; he then went on to found a winery in Porto. Port wine is fortified by the addition of a neutral grape spirit known as *aguardente* (fiery water), which boosts the alcohol content and stops fermentation, leaving residual sugar in wine. As for all wines, some years are better for growing grapes, and the wine produced from the grapes harvested in those years is considered of higher quality and is used in the bottling of vintage ports. We also learned that the cork stoppers are important in classic wines classified for aging in bottles, as in the case of vintage port. For wines consumed within a few months after bottling, cork stoppers are less important, and other types of closure may be preferred by the makers of such wines. After the movie, we tasted some red and white port wines and bought some vintage bottles (Fig. 241). In the evening we took a cruise on the Douro River after enjoying some lovely views over Porto from Vila Nova de Gaia (Fig. 242) as well as the fine bridges connecting the two cities, Ponte D. Luis I, Ponte da Arrabida, Ponte S. Joao and Ponte D. Maria Pia. This last bridge was constructed by Gustave Eiffel (Fig. 243).

On June 30 we traveled on to the province of Bairrada, driving through the Parque Nacional do Bucaçao (Bucaçao National Park), and then through Coimbra and Conímbriga to Tomar. The forest in the Serra do Bussaco was settled by Benedictine monks in the sixth century. The Discalced Carmelites, an order of barefooted monks, took over in 1628, built a monastery and surrounded the 250-acre (100-ha) forest with a wall. The region is known as a place liberated by British and Portuguese soldiers under the command of the Duke of Wellington during the unsuccessful Napoleonic invasion of Portugal in 1810. The monastery and forest fell into government hands in 1834, when monasteries were abolished throughout Portugal and the Bucaçao National Park was established. Over the centuries, the monks

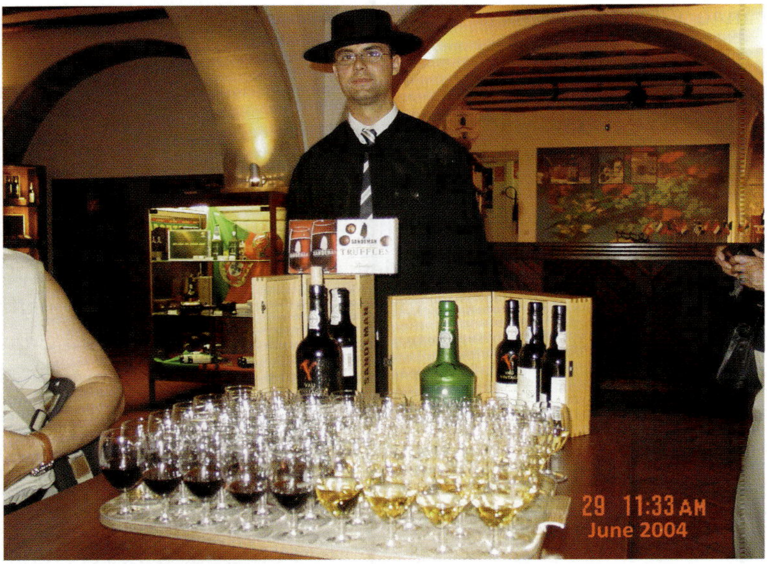

Figure 241. White and red port wines for tasting and vintage port in boxes.

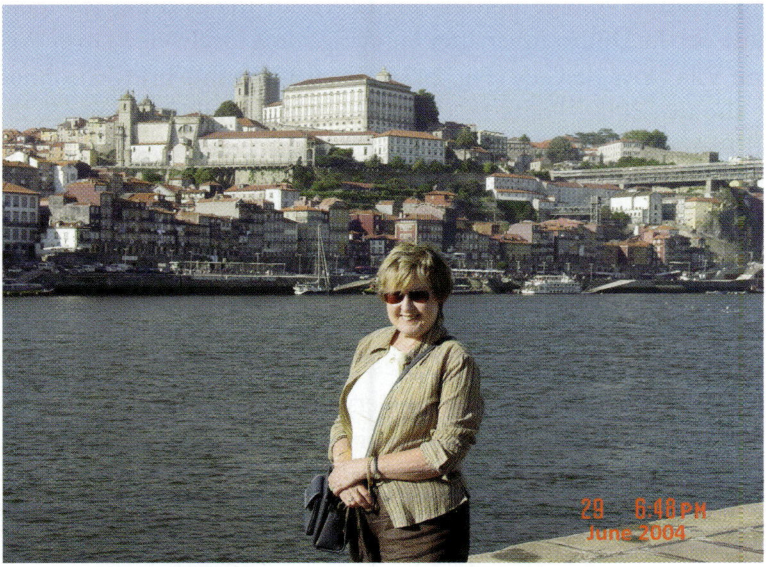

Figure 242. The view from Gaia over Sé Cathedral and Seminary.

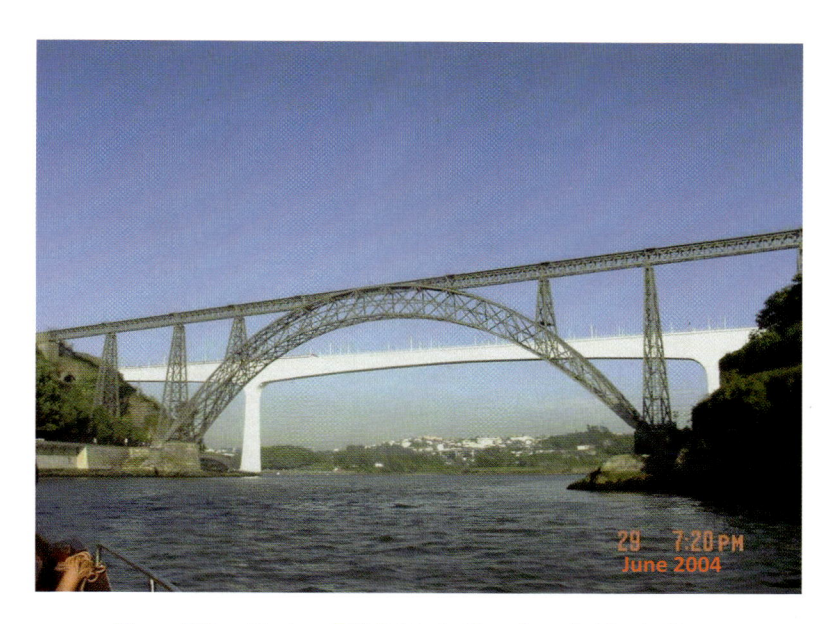

Figure 243. Gustave Eiffel's Maria Pia railway bridge in Porto.

and the government foresters who succeeded them have planted trees and shrubs from all over the world. We spent a short time there and then drove to Coimbra, which was the capital of the country between 1139 and 1256, and a place where six of Portugal's kings were born. The University of Coimbra was founded by King Dinis on August 13, 1290. It was moved to Lisbon and back to Coimbra several times until 1537 when Dom João III (King John III) transferred the university permanently to Coimbra. Entering the university through Porta Férrea (Iron Gate), the first thing we encountered was a statue of King John III. We spent most of our time in the very impressive Biblioteca Joanina and in the chapel. After leaving the university, we spotted a statue of King Dinis. At the time of our visit, Portugal was hosting the UEFA European Football Championship, and the hosts won the match that day (Fig. 244). (Portugal went all the way to the final only to lose 1–0 to underdog Greece in the final on July 4.) Our next stop was Conímbriga, the best-preserved Roman city in Portugal. Some of the ruins are in a remarkably good condition (Fig. 245).

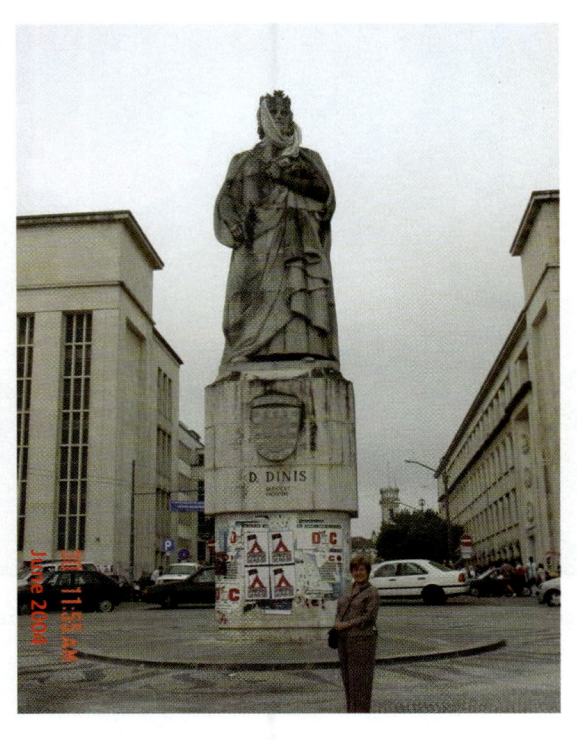

Figure 244. A statue of D. Dinis (1261–1325), who founded the Universidade de Coimbra in 1290. A scarf was wrapped around the king's head after the Portuguese won a UEFA Championship soccer game.

After lunch we went to Tomar's Convent of Christ. Tomar Castle was built as part of a Templar defense system to secure the border of the Christian kingdom against the Moors of Iberia. It was founded by Gualdim Pais, provincial Master of the order of Knights Templar in Tomar, in 1159. In return for the help in defense, the knights received lands and political powers that became their eventual undoing, as their strength and wealth became too much of a threat to the Church. In 1313 Pope Clement V decided to act and suppressed the Order. King Dinis promptly reacted by creating the new Order of Christ, which was given the assets and power of previous Knights Templar. Henry the Navigator was made the Governor of the Order in 1418 and made liberal use of their funds (together with their logo of a white cross) to finance his explorations of the world. The original church in

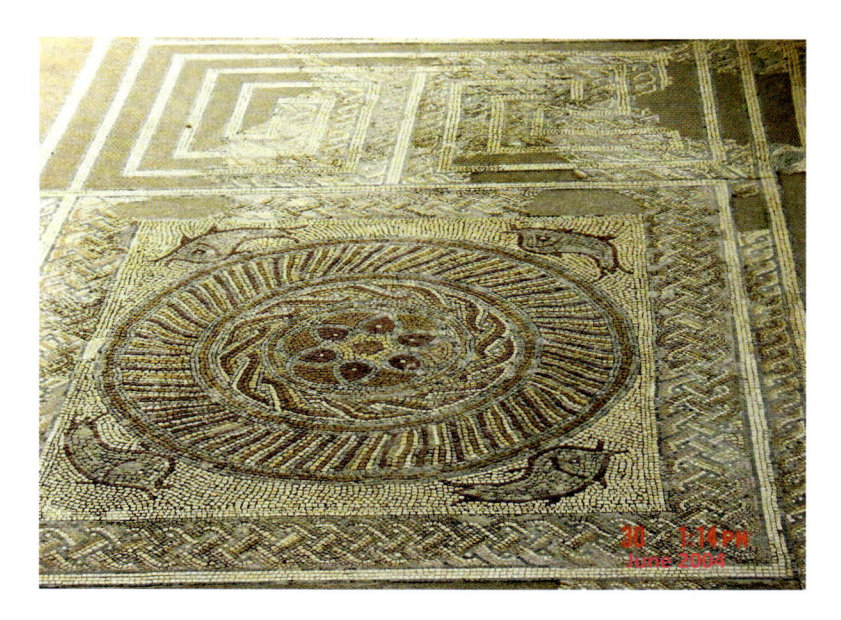

Figure 245.   A floor mosaic at Conímbriga's fifth-century Roman ruins.

Tomar was based on a polygonal ground plan of 16 bays including an octagonal choir with an ambulatory: it is one of the typical "rotondas" of Templar architecture of which all too few examples are still extant in Europe. The Manueline influence was, as elsewhere, decisive and compelling. The convent and the church are now museums. An example of Manueline style can be seen in the photo of the Western Church Façade ornamented with the emblem of the Order of the Garter in Fig. 246. Later that afternoon we settled in to our room at Hotel dos Templários on Largo Cândido dos Reis in Tomar, and from our balcony there was a nice view of the Convento de Cristo. Walking in the city in the evening, on the pavement there were Templar crosses — the logo used by Henry the Navigator — almost everywhere we looked (Fig. 247).

On July 1, we went from Tomar to Lisbon, and on the way we visited Fátima, known for its famous Chapel of Apparitions. According to Catholic belief, three young shepherds, Lúcia dos Santos and her cousins Francisco and Jacinta Marto, saw an apparition of the Virgin Mary on May 13, 1917. The Lady appeared and spoke to the children again in Cova da Iria on the 13th days of June, July, September and

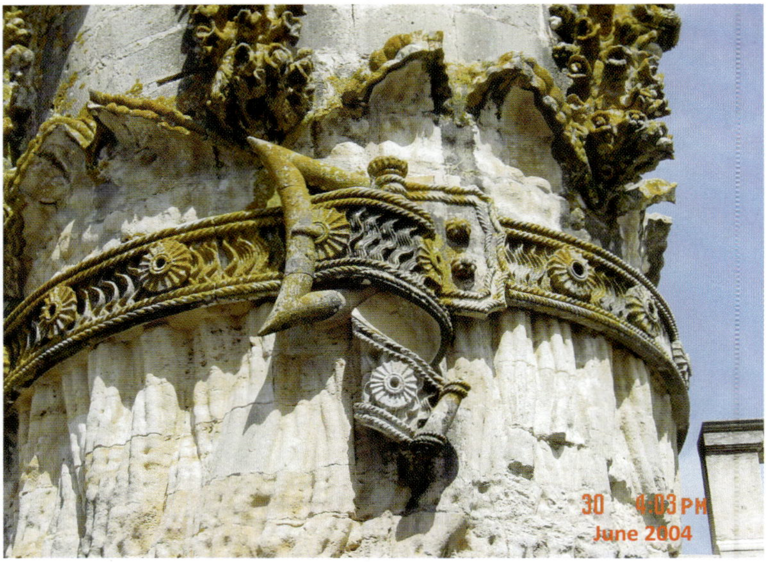

Figure 246. The emblem of the Order of the Garter (established by King Edward III of England in 1348) on the Western Church Façade at the Convento de Christo in Tomar. D. Manuel I was one of the Order's members.

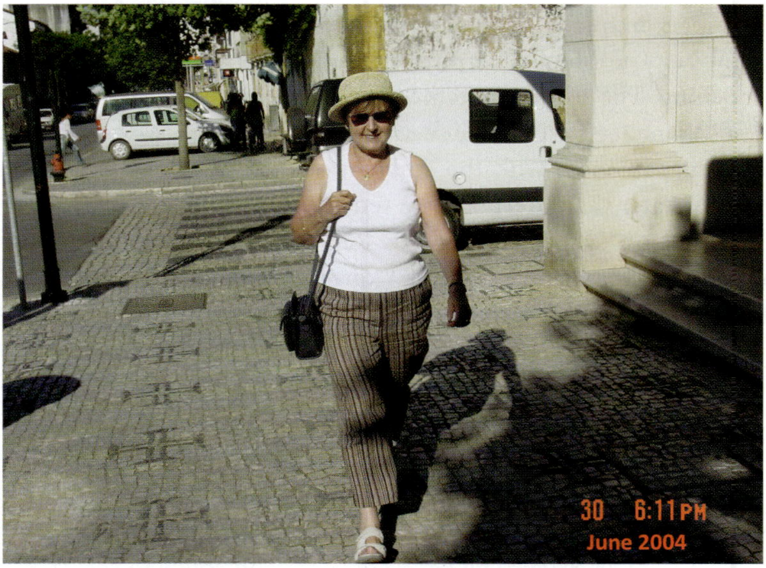

Figure 247. Templar crosses on the pavement.

Around the World with Nephrology

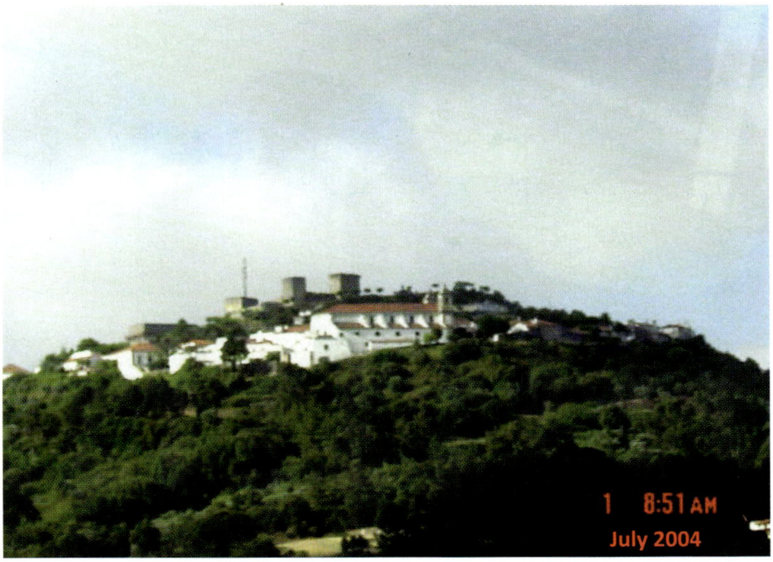

Figure 248. Ourém Castle as seen from our bus on the way from Tomar to Fátima. Shepherds Lúcia, Jacinta and Francisco, who witnessed a series of apparitions of the Virgin Mary, were kept here in August 1917.

October; there was no apparition in August, as the children were kept in Ourém Castle (Fig. 248). Of the three shepherds, Jacinta and Francisco died from pneumonia at a young age, but Lucia lived in Coimbra till her death in 2005 at the age of 97. We went to see the Chapel of Apparitions (Fig. 249) as well as the neighboring basilica. Our trip continued with a visit to Batalha, where the monastery of the Dominicans of Batalha was built to commemorate the victory of the Portuguese over the Castilians at the Battle of Aljubarrota in 1385 (Fig. 250). The Batalha Monastery, built in Late Gothic and Manueline styles, contains a number of important tombs, including that of Prince Henry the Navigator (Fig. 251). Our next stop was the famous coastal fishing village of Nazaré. The locals told us that the village was settled by the Phoenicians in the 12th century BC and that the name of the village was Nazareth up until 500 years ago. En route to Lisbon we stopped at Óbidos, a fortified medieval city once at the seashore, now six miles inland. We also dropped by Our Lady of Piety Oratory and Igreja da Misericórdia as well as observing the work in a porcelain shop.

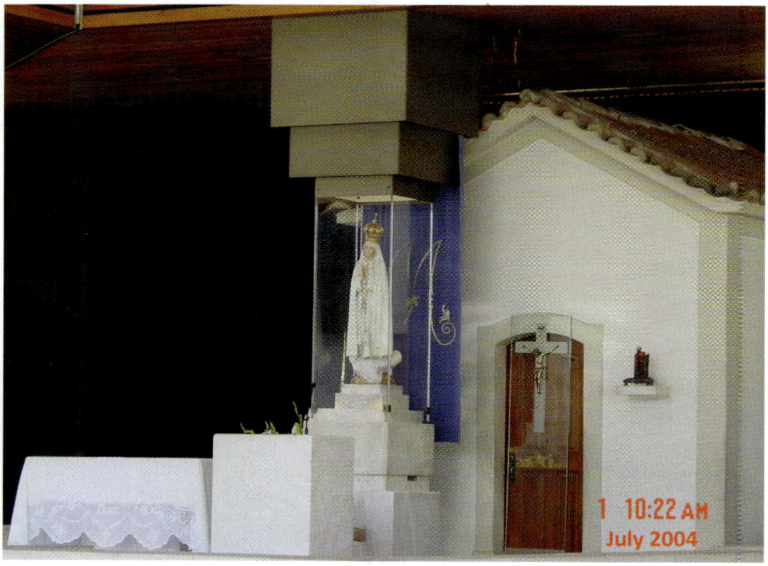

Figure 249. The Statue of Our Lady in the Chapel of Apparitions was built where the apparitions took place above a large oak tree at the Cova da Iria.

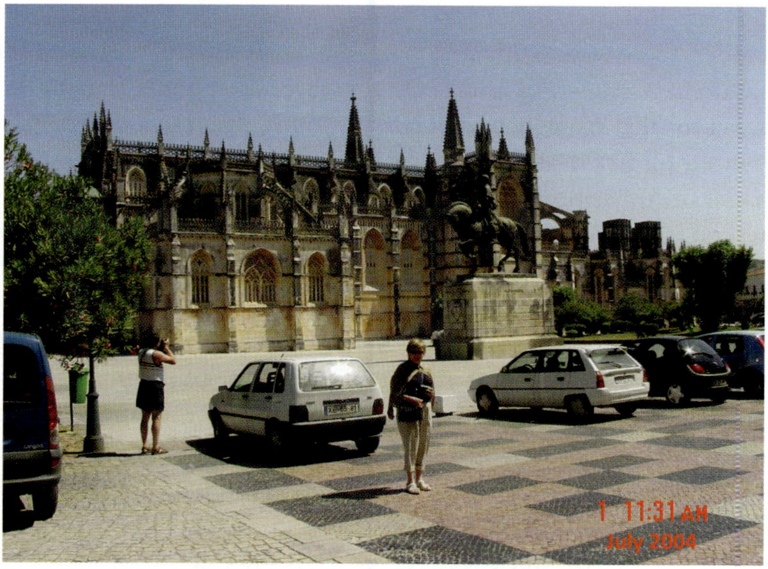

Figure 250. The Batalha Monastery's statue of Dom Nuno Álvares Pereira (1360–1431), commander at Aljubarrota in 1385.

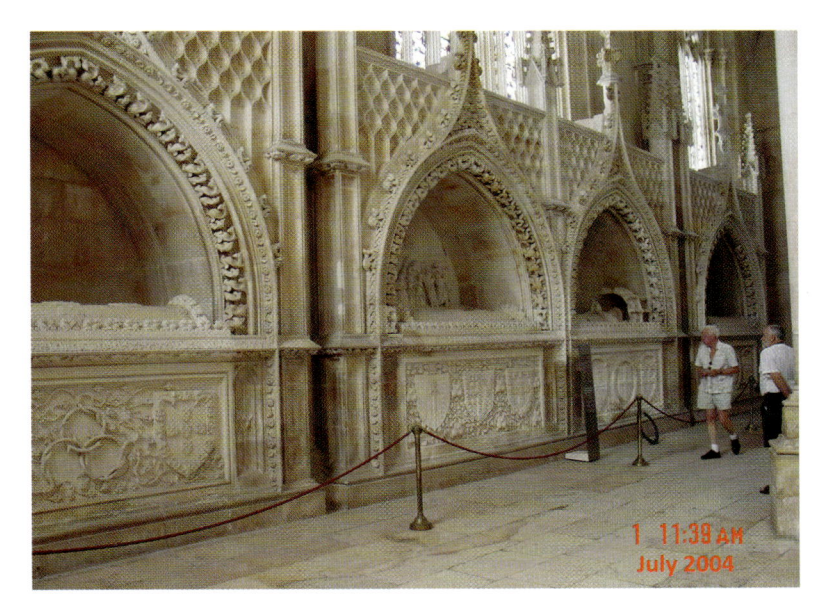

Figure 251. The tombs of the sons of King João I and Queen Philippa of Lancaster. Their third child was Prince Henry the Navigator (1394–1460).

That night we stayed in Lisbon at Metropolitan Hotel on Rua Soeiro Pereira Gomes.

On Saturday morning, July 2, we did a sightseeing tour of Lisbon, paying particular attention to the achievements of the King Manuel I, nicknamed "o Venturoso" (the Fortunate). His reign came about unexpectedly when King John II, after the death of his son, Prince Afonso, named his cousin an heir to the throne in 1493. Thus, he became the king through fortunate circumstances. Manuel would prove to be a worthy successor to his cousin, King John II, supporting the Portuguese exploration of the Atlantic Ocean and the development of Portuguese commerce. During his reign, Vasco da Gama discovered the maritime route to India in 1498, Pedro Álvares Cabral discovered Brazil in 1500, Francisco de Almeida became the first viceroy of India in 1505, and Afonso de Albuquerque secured a monopoly of the maritime routes for Portugal in the Indian Ocean and the Persian Gulf. Manuel I also ordered the construction of several buildings in the Manueline style in many places, including Lisbon.

The next morning we drove east, passing the Torre de Belém, an essential part of the defensive system for the Tagus River estuary. The tower's construction began in 1514 and was completed during the reign of King Manuel I. We then went to Belém, a suburb of Lisbon on the bank of the Tagus, to see Padrão dos Descobrimentos (Monument to the Discoveries), inaugurated in 1960 during celebrations of the 500th anniversary of the death of Henry the Navigator (Fig. 252). Its design resembles the prow of a ship about to sail, with the main statue of Henry the Navigator in front, statues of other explorers and discoverers on the left, and monks and scientists and Henry's mother on the right (Fig. 253). Also in Belém, we visited Praça do Imperio and saw the Monastery of Santa Maria, known locally as the Jerónimos Monastery. The old name of Belém was Rostello, and it was from here that Vasco da Gama set out to discover a sea route to India. A chapel had been built on the spot by Henry the Navigator, and to it King Manuel I and his court went in procession on July 8, 1497. On the same day Vasco da Gama embarked; he

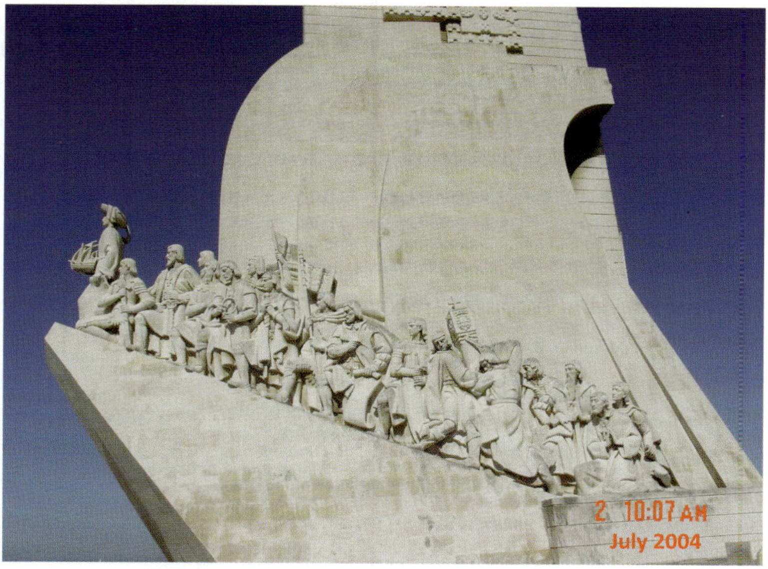

Figure 252. The left-hand side of the Monument to the Discoveries with Henry the Navigator in front. The statues on this side are of important explorers and discoverers.

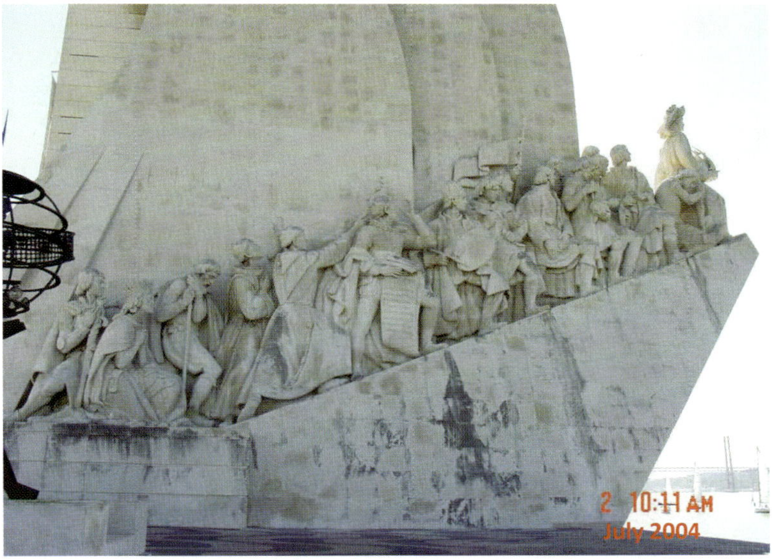

Figure 253. The right-hand side of the Monument of Discoveries depicts monks and scientists. The only woman is Philippa of Lancaster, daughter of John Gaunt and mother of Infante Dom Henrique.

returned in September 1499 having rounded the Cape of Good Hope. To immortalize the event King Manuel I built a monastery near Prince Henry's chapel, changed the name of the locality to Belém (Bethlehem) and gave the new building to the monks of St. Jerome, hence the name Jerónimos (Fig. 254). The style of the architecture is pure Manueline: a mixture of Late Gothic, Renaissance and Moorish. We obviously paid a visit the church, where the remains of Vasco da Gama now rest.

I should mention here that there were discussions between Spain and Portugal at the end of 15th century about the best way to get to India. In 1484, Portugal officially rejected Christopher Columbus' idea of reaching India from the west, as it was seen as unreasonable. Some historians have claimed that the Portuguese had already performed fairly accurate calculations concerning the size of the world and therefore knew that sailing west to reach the Indies would require a far longer journey than navigating to the east. However, this continues to be debated. After Columbus discovered the New World in 1492,

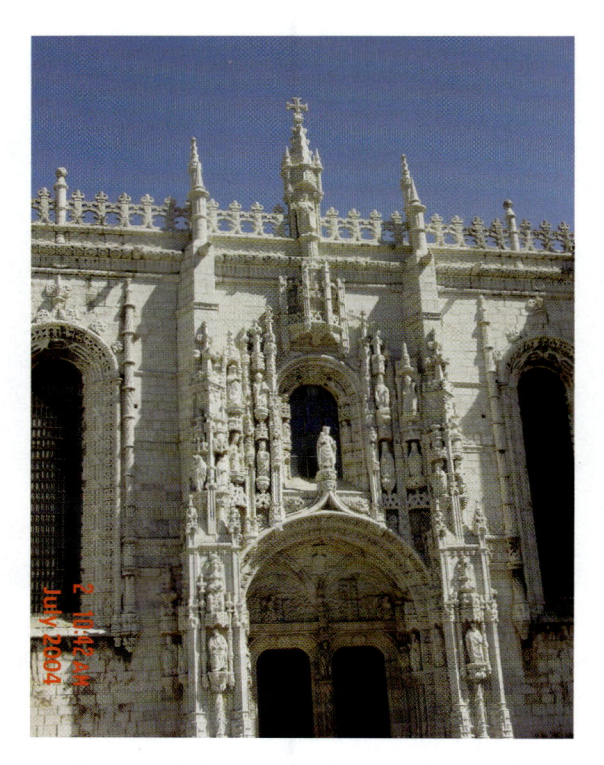

Figure 254. A close-up of the exuberantly decorated portal of the Church of Os Jerónimos.

it was clear that conflict would soon arise over land claims by Spain and Portugal. On May 4, 1493, Pope Alexander VI took action to clear up any confusion that may have arisen over territorial claims. He issued a decree establishing an imaginary line running north and south through the mid-Atlantic, 100 leagues (480 km or 300 miles) from the Cape Verde islands. Spain would have possession of any unclaimed territories to the west of the line and Portugal would have possession of any unclaimed territory to the east of the line. Thus began a long-lasting dispute that eventually resulted in the signing of the Treaty of Tordesillas with Spain in 1494. The treaty divided the (largely undiscovered) world equally between the Spanish and the Portuguese, along a north-south meridian line 370 leagues (1,770 km or 1,100 miles) west of the Cape Verde islands, with all lands to the east belonging to Portugal and all lands to the west to Spain. In this

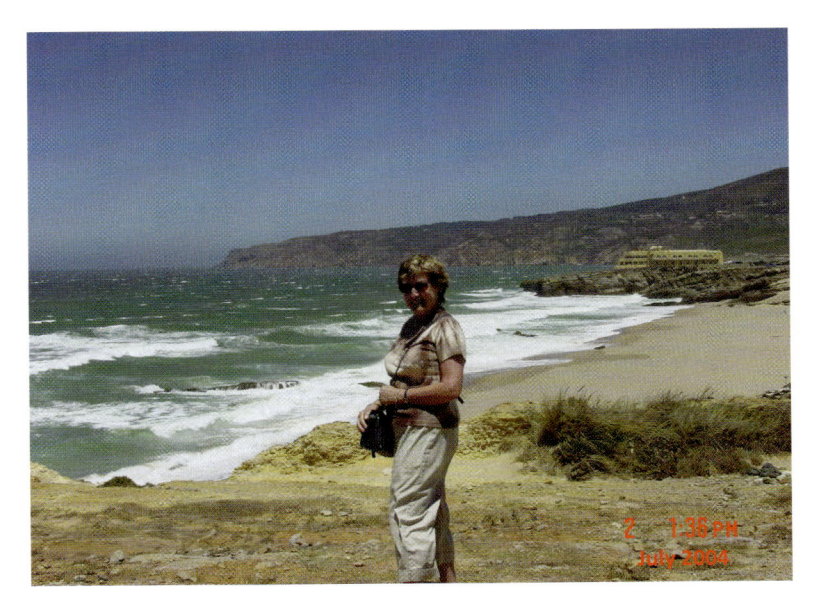

Figure 255. Cabo da Roca, the westernmost point of the European continent (latitude: 38°46'5" North; longitude: 9°29'54" West).

way western South America belonged to Spain and eastern South America (Brazil) belonged to Portugal. In the afternoon we drove to Sintra, a residence of Portuguese monarchs in the 15th century and now a museum. On the way we passed Cabo da Roca, the westernmost point of continental Europe, which the poet Luis de Camões defined as "where the land ends and the sea begins" (Fig. 255). In the evening we returned to the Metropolitan Hotel in Lisbon.

As on previous trips organized by Trafalgar Tours, we were very happy with the service provided by our tour company. The bus and hotels were very comfortable and the bus driver was extremely skilled, typical for Trafalgar. Also, our guide, Isabel, was very knowledgeable and we learned a lot from her. She spoke four languages and was well versed in Portuguese history, architecture, fauna and flora.

As I mentioned, the UEFA Europa League was taking place in Portugal, and we watched several games on TV during our trip. We watched the final between Greece and Portugal on Sunday, July 4, the day after returning to Kraków. We spent two months in Poland and returned to Columbia on September 12. I went for a short meeting in

Vacations and Travel Unrelated to Business   479

Chicago, and then I was busy with abstracts for our Annual Dialysis Conference in Tampa in February 2005.

2005 — New England tour, Adam in Kraków, and our trip to Bismarck for Thanksgiving

In 2005 we decided to go to Poland later because we wanted to tour the northeastern U.S. by car, as we did not know the area too well. We planned to drive at most 4 to 6 hours a day (200–400 miles). Lynne Schwartze from AAA Travel in Columbia made all our hotel reservations and prepared maps for the journey from MapQuest. The whole tour, without the details, is shown on the map in Fig. 256. At the time we had a Cadillac STS (Fig. 257) with in-car navigation system to help us with directions. Having two methods of finding directions was a really good idea, although some newer places and hotels were not located on either. We started from home at 9:07 am on Saturday, May 7. We did the first 222 miles on our first day in about 4 hours and 45 minutes with one stop in Silver Lake Rest Area on the I-70. Our hotel reservation was for the Country Inn & Suites, 1200 North Raney,

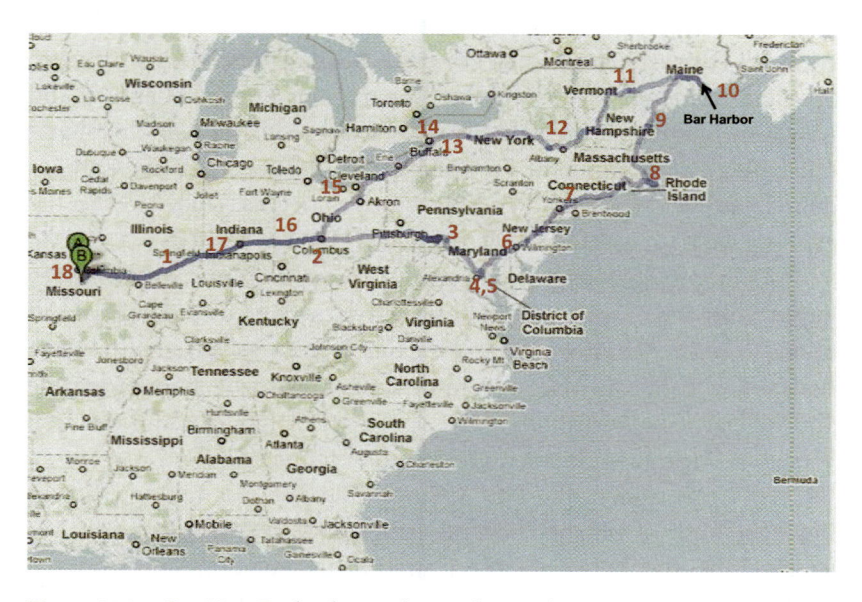

Figure 256. Our New England tour; the numbers indicate the numbers of nights in hotels.

480 Around the World with Nephrology

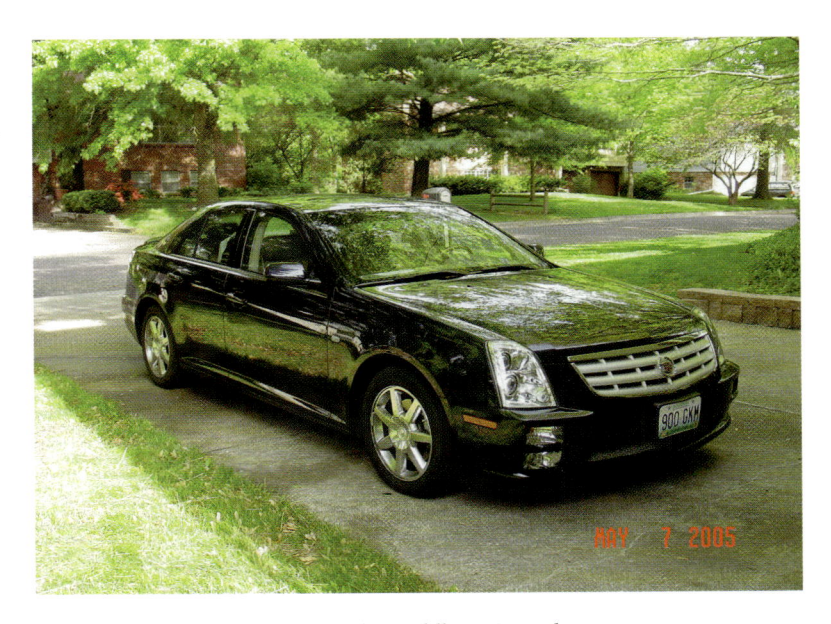

Figure 257. The Cadillac STS ready to go.

in Effingham, Illinois, but the hotel was not shown on the map or on GPS because it was a relatively new building (two years old: Is that new?). We had to ask locals for directions, something hard to swallow for me. We attended 5 pm Mass in the Sacred Heart Church in Effingham and then went for dinner at Ruby Tuesday Restaurant.

The following day, starting from Effingham, we drove 309 miles, mostly on the I-70 through Indianapolis, Indiana, to the Country Inn & Suites on 1155 Evans Way Court in Columbus, Ohio. We had a rest stop in Bedford County on the way, so we covered the distance in about six hours. On Monday we continued on the I-70 to the Best Western at 4517 Business 220 in Bedford, Pennsylvania, a distance of 278 miles, which we covered in six hours with a one-hour rest stop. In Bedford we visited a bakery in the Espy House (Fig. 258), which was built in 1771. It was the headquarters of George Washington in October 1794, when he came to Bedford to review troops assembled here to quell the Whiskey Rebellion[41] in the western part of the state.

---

41. The Whiskey Rebellion was a violent protest in the western part of the U.S. in the 1790s against the excise tax on whiskey that was a central grievance of the westerners. The resistance collapsed before the arrival of the army.

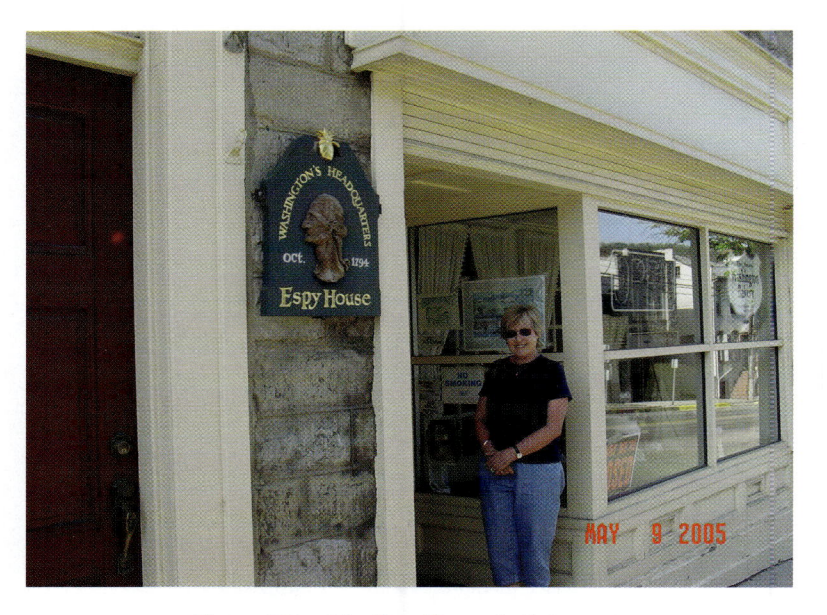

Figure 258. The Espy House, built in 1771.

On May 10 we started at 9 am as we wanted to arrive early in Washington, D.C. It was supposed to be less than 140 miles, which could be covered in less than two-and-a-half hours. However, it turned out that I made at least two mistakes and arrived later than planned. First, I was caught speeding on Route 220, doing 65 mph instead of the allowed 55 mph, which lost us some time — and US$125. Then, instead of taking the Pennsylvania Turnpike east, I went west and drove the wrong way for 20 miles. In spite of these mishaps we arrived shortly after 11 am at the Washington Cathedral, which is situated at Massachusetts and Wisconsin Avenues in the northwest quadrant of the U.S. capital. Officially named the Cathedral Church of Saint Peter and Saint Paul, it is the seat of both the presiding Bishop of the Episcopal Church and the Bishop of the Diocese of Washington and is designated by the Congress as the "National House of Prayer." In 1893, the Protestant Episcopal Cathedral Foundation of the District of Columbia was granted a charter from Congress to establish the cathedral. Construction began on September 29, 1907, when the foundation stone was laid in the presence of President Theodore Roosevelt, and was completed 83 years later when the last finial (crowning ornament) was placed in the presence of President George H. W. Bush in 1990. An impressive construction in a neo-Gothic style, not only is it the fourth tallest building in Washington, D.C., but it is also the sixth largest cathedral in the world. After praying, we admired the stained glass windows, including the famous Space Window honoring man's landing on the Moon, which includes a fragment of lunar rock at its center. The most impressive parts for us were the apse with the high altar called the Jerusalem Altar, built from 12 stones brought from Solomon's Quarry in Jerusalem, and the carved stone screen behind the altar called the Ter Sanctus (Thrice Holy) reredos, which features 110 carved figures surrounding the central figure of Jesus (Fig. 259). We also spent some time in the beautiful gardens surrounding the cathedral and then checked in to the Hotel Rouge at 1315 16th Street NW. In the afternoon we went to the International Spy Museum at 901 F Street NW, the only spy museum in the U.S. that showcases more than 200 gadgets, weapons, bugs, buttonhole cameras, vehicles and technologies used for espionage

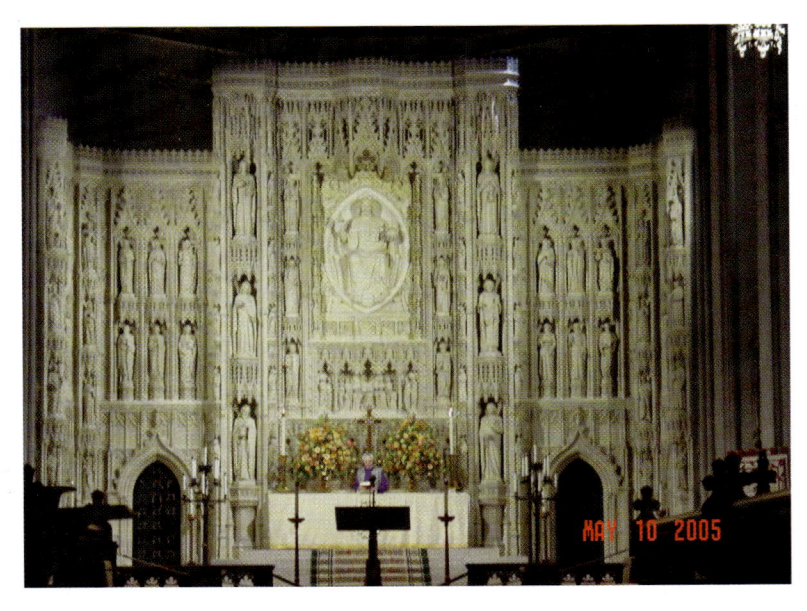

Figure 259. The high altar in the National Cathedral, Washington, D.C.

throughout the world. We were very pleased to see that the role of Polish cryptographers in deciphering the Enigma was presented correctly in the museum. In December 1932, Polish mathematicians from the University of Poznań, Marian Rajewski, Jerzy Różycki and Henryk Zygalski, were the first to break Germany's Enigma ciphers. Five weeks before the outbreak of WWII, on July 25, 1939, the Polish Cipher Bureau (Polskie Biuro Szyfrów) in Warsaw gave Enigma decryption techniques and equipment to French and British military intelligence. Using the information, Allied code breakers were able to decrypt many messages that had been enciphered using the Enigma. For a long time the role of these Polish cryptographers remained largely neglected, so we were happy to see the whole story being presented at the museum.

On Wednesday morning we visited the Pope John Paul II Catholic Cultural Center at 3900 Harewood Road NE (Fig. 260). The concept for the center began at a meeting between Pope John Paul II and then-Bishop Adam Maida in 1988. The building is adjacent to the Catholic University of America and the Basilica of the National Shrine

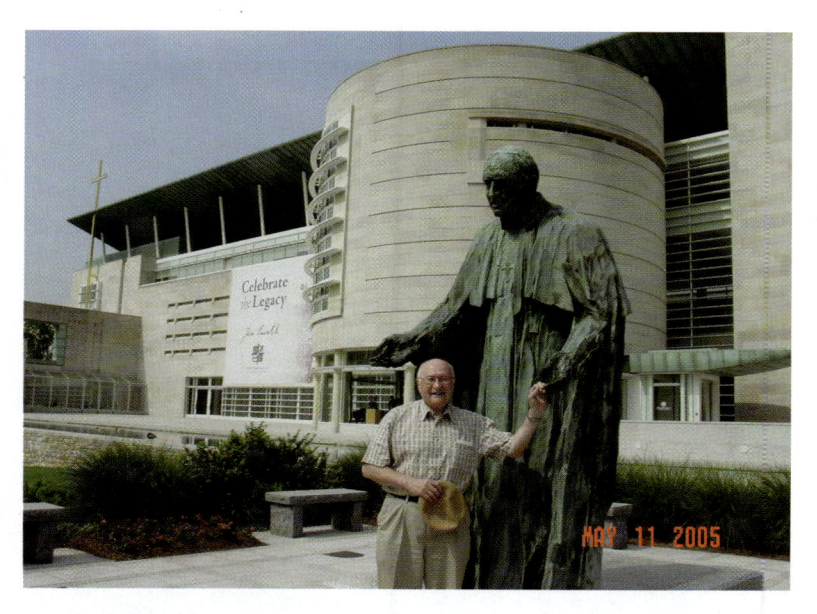

Figure 260. The statue of Pope John Paul II at the entrance to the Catholic Cultural Center.

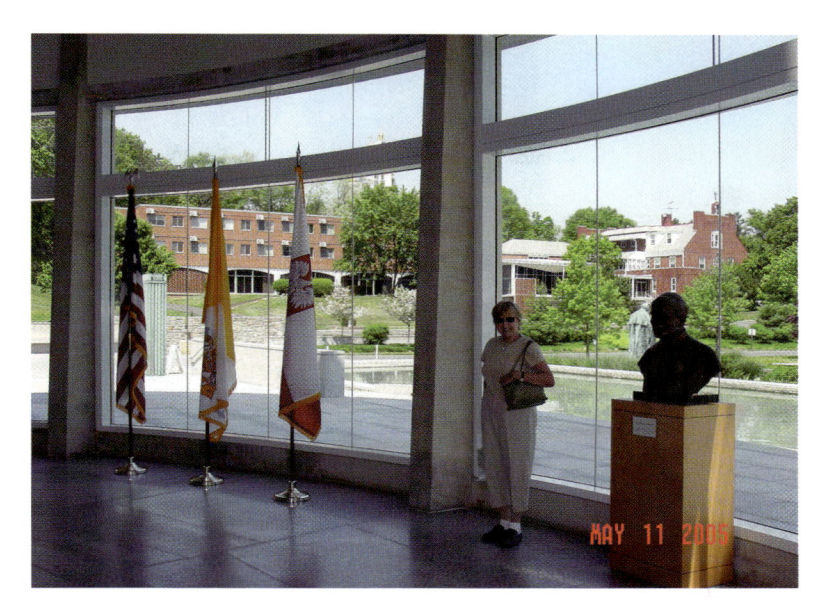

Figure 261. Flags of the U.S., the Vatican and Poland in the rotunda.

of the Immaculate Conception. The center was opened to the public in a ceremony in March 2001 attended by President George W. Bush. The center's original purpose was to explore the intersection of faith and culture through interactive displays, academic discussion and research, and museum exhibits. In the rotunda stand flags of the U.S., the Vatican and Poland (Fig. 261). Halina is a supporting member of the center (Nr 50580 J11JE53). That evening I paid my speeding ticket of US$125 with a money order at the post office on Rhode Island Ave. It is hard for me to say whether speeding a little is dangerous — since I have never had an accident while driving above the speed limit[42] — but it is definitely a time-consuming business being stopped by police and then having to trudge to a post office to pay the fine!

The next day we drove northeast, mostly on the I-95 bypassing Baltimore to Philadelphia, Pennsylvania. The distance was only 140 miles, which we covered in less than three hours. First we visited the Liberty Bell Center located in the block bordered by Market Street,

---

42. As I mentioned in Chap. 12, the only accident I have ever had in the U.S. was in Warrenton, Missouri, in 1991 — when I was driving very slowly and we were hit from behind by a speeding vehicle.

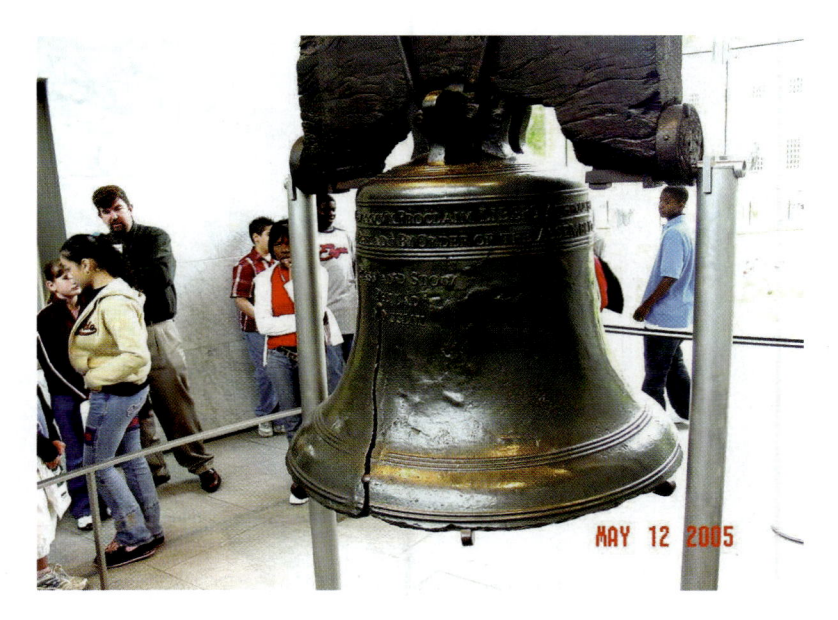

Figure 262. The Liberty Bell, an iconic symbol of American Independence.

Chestnut Street, S. 5th Street and S. 6th Street. The center had been opened only two years earlier. We saw a video presentation and exhibits on the Liberty Bell, focusing on its origins and its history. We were there in May, but we learned that on every Fourth of July, children who are descendants of the signers of the Declaration symbolically tap the Liberty Bell 13 times while bells across the nation also ring 13 times in honor of the patriots from the original 13 states. The Liberty Bell itself is displayed in a magnificent glass chamber with Independence Hall in the background (Fig. 262). It hangs from its original yoke, made from American elm, also known as slippery elm. The bell is inscribed with the words of Leviticus 25:10: "Proclaim liberty throughout all the land unto all the inhabitants thereof." The inscription also reveals that the bell was made "By Order of the Assembly of the Province of Pensylvania for the State House in Philada."[43] The bell was cast in London, England, in 1751, but cracked soon after arriving in Philadelphia. Local craftsmen John Pass and John Stow cast a new bell in 1753 (see the inscription on the bell: "Pass and Stow, Philada,

---

43. Pennsylvania and Philada were the original spellings of Pennsylvania and Philadelphia.

MDCCLIII") using metal from the English bell. In 1846, when a thin crack began to affect the sound of the bell, it was repaired, but when it was rung for a celebration of the birth of George Washington, it cracked again. It has not been rung since. No one knows why the bell cracked either time. The old State House bell was first called the "Liberty Bell" by a group trying to outlaw slavery. The abolitionists remembered the words on the bell and, in the 1830s, adopted it as the symbol of their cause.

After leaving the center we decided to take a city tour around Philadelphia. We went to see Benjamin Franklin's grave, the Philadelphia Convention Center, Chinatown, and Philadelphia skyline. On Benjamin Franklin Parkway we passed the Statue of Kopernik (Copernicus), the Rodin Museum, a Thaddeus Kosciuszko monument in front of the Embassy Suites, the Clip Sculpture and the Philadelphia Museum of Art (Fig. 263), with its stairs made famous by the *Rocky* movies. During our stay, there was an exhibition of Salvatore Dali paintings. The Parkway is lined with flags of countries from around the world, and although we drove by quite fast, I managed to take a

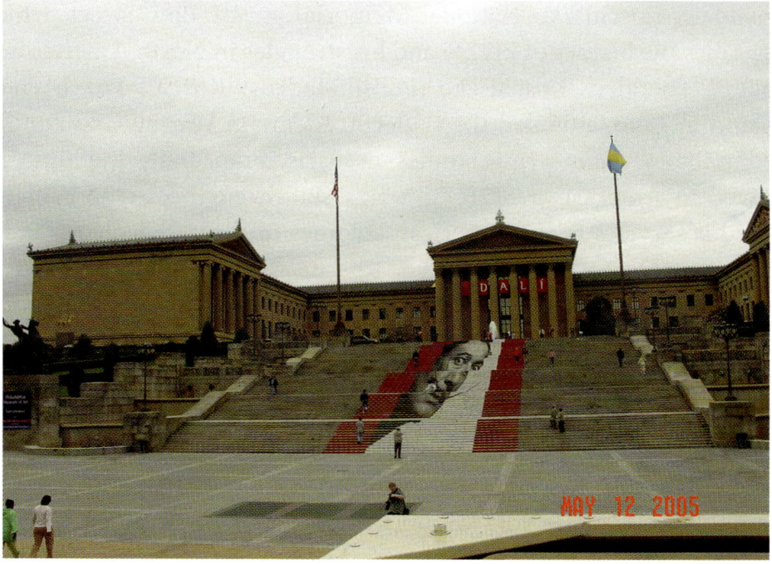

Figure 263. The famous stairs from the movie *Rocky Balboa* at the Philadelphia Museum of Art.

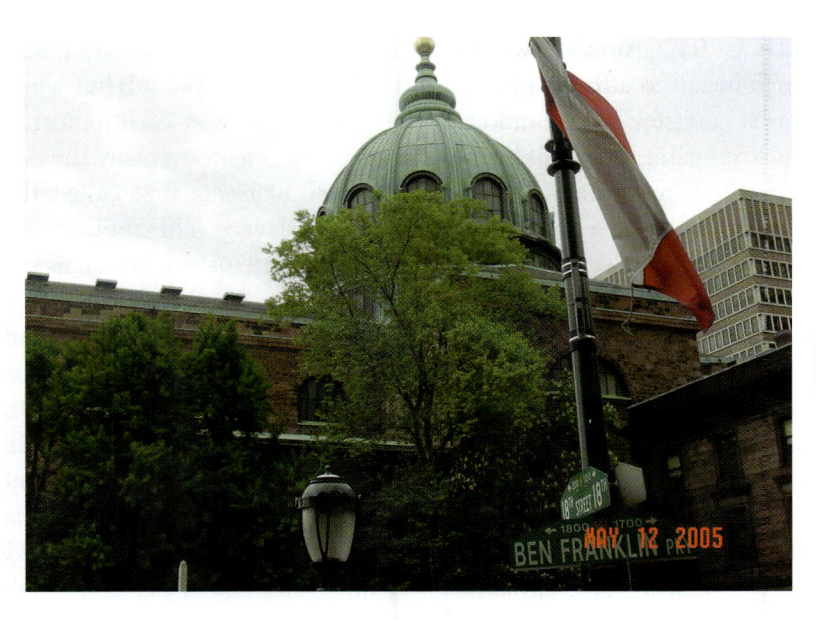

Figure 264. A reminder of home on the Parkway.

picture of the Polish flag (Fig. 264). After the tour we went to the Thaddeus Kosciuszko National Memorial at 301 Pine Street, which describes the history of his life and his struggles in North America and Poland. Thaddeus Kosciuszko (Polish: Tadeusz Kościuszko), born in Poland in 1746, attended the Cadet Academy in Warsaw and continued military engineering studies in Paris, France. By the time he arrived in America in 1776, he was a skilled engineer who came to offer his services to the American colonies in their struggle for independence. On October 18, 1776, Kosciuszko was commissioned as Colonel of Engineers by the Continental Congress and began his outstanding service of fortifying battle sites, many of which became turning points in America's fight for independence from the British. In the early days of the war, Kosciuszko helped to fortify the Philadelphia waterfront at Fort Mercer. Shortly after, he was transferred to New York, where he helped with fortifications along the Hudson and planned the defense for Saratoga. The Battle of Saratoga became known as one of military history's most famous struggles for independence and proved to be a turning point in the war. In 1778, Kosciuszko was made chief engineer of West Point, New York. This fortification became known as the American Gibraltar because it could not be penetrated by the British Army. Eventually West Point became a military academy. As chief of engineers, Kosciuszko twice rescued the army of General Nathanael Greene by directing river crossings. He also directed the blockade of Charleston, S.C. In 1783, he was appointed Brigadier General and awarded the Cincinnati Order Medal by General George Washington, Commander-in-Chief of the Continental Army. Washington also presented Kosciuszko with two pistols and a sword as gifts for his outstanding service to America. In recognition of his many services, the following year the Continental Congress made Kosciuszko a citizen of the U.S. and awarded him a land grant.

After the colonies won their independence, Kosciuszko returned to Poland in 1784 to help his own country defend independence, this time as a major general of the Polish army in defense of his native land against the Russians. Kosciuszko was the national hero of the 1794 insurrection, leading a victorious, if brief, uprising of the Poles. After the successful battle of Racławice on April 4, 1794, first Warsaw and then Wilno were liberated from enemy occupation. However, Kosciuszko was wounded, captured and sent to St. Petersburg, where he was imprisoned. Released and exiled in 1796, he traveled to several European countries before returning to a hero's welcome in America in 1797. He lived in the house on Pine Street, the site of the present-day memorial, from November 1797 to May 1798. He later moved to Switzerland, where he died in 1817. He is buried at Wawel Castle in Kraków among the tombs of the Polish Kings. The Kosciuszko Mound, modeled after prehistoric mounds of Prince Krak and Princess Wanda, was erected in 1823. Many soldiers in the Kosciuszko insurrection were peasants and their motto was *Żywią y Bronią* ("They Feed and Defend"). A banner bearing this motto was granted to the scythe bearer detachment by Kosciuszko on August 16, 1794. The original banner is in the Polish Army Museum in Warsaw, while the copy is in Philadelphia[44] (Fig. 265). After visiting the memorial we

---

44. *Żywią y Bronią* is the original spelling of the motto from 18th century when "*y*" was used instead of "*i*" (and). As Fig. 265 shows, the banner features a scythe crossed with a lance behind a sheaf of wheat.

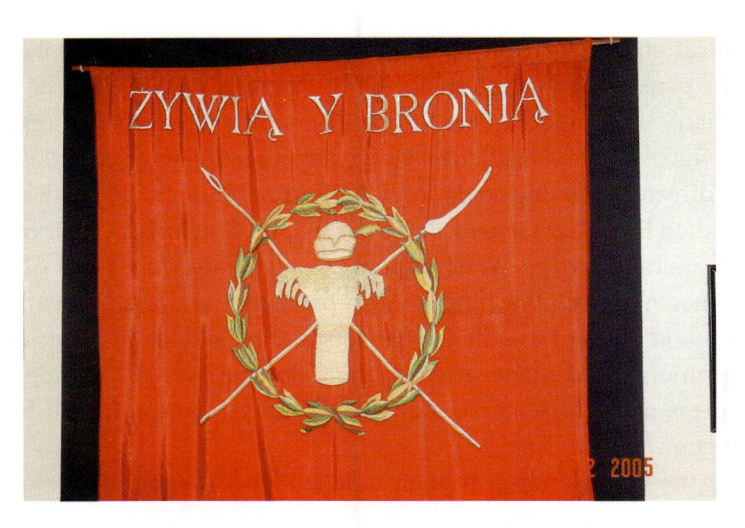

Figure 265. A banner with the motto "They Feed and Defend."

took the I-95 to Morrisville and stayed overnight in the Holiday Inn Express at 7 South Pennsylvania.

On May 13 we drove from Morrisville to Trenton, then the New Jersey Turnpike, the New England Thruway and the Connecticut Turnpike/Governor John Davis Lodge Turnpike to Norwalk. We covered the 119 miles in less than three hours. Norwalk is in the southwestern corner of Connecticut. Our travel agent, Lynn Schwartze, had recommended a historic country inn in Norwalk called Silvermine Tavern. Located in a nice wooded neighborhood next to a waterfall on the Silvermine River, it occupies several historic buildings dating back about 200 years and includes a country store (Fig. 266). Silvermine was long an art colony and remains the home of the Silvermine Guild Arts Center. The name "Silvermine" comes from old legends of a silver mine in the area, although, according to locals, no silver has ever been found. The inn itself was quintessential New England style complete with creaky wooden floor, authentic antiques, claw foot bathtub, canopy bed, fireplace and old paintings on the walls. In the evening we had a very nice "Romantic Dinner" in the tavern.

On following day we started on the I-95, then Hwy 138, through Jamestown Bridge and Newport Bridge, stopped at Newport City Hall

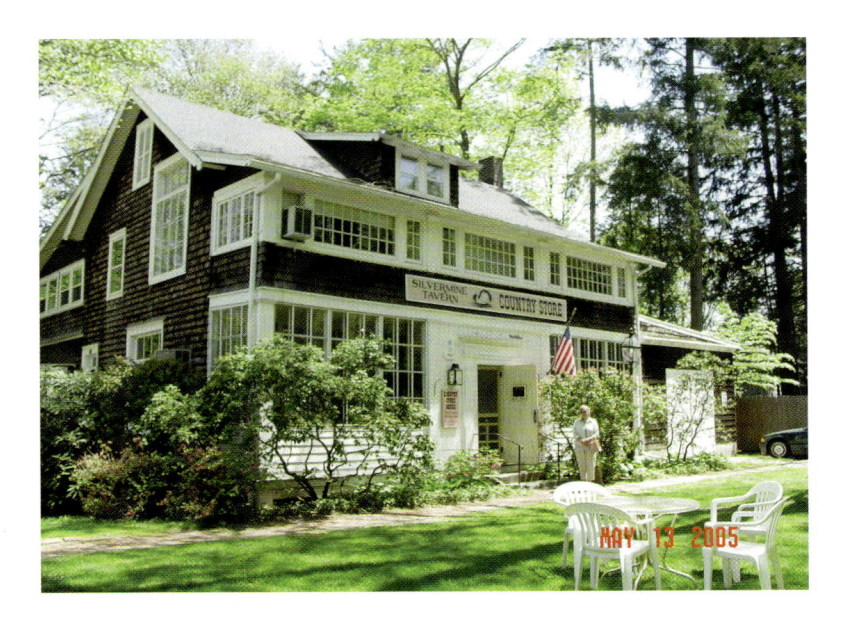

Figure 266. The Silvermine Tavern and Country Store.

and went to the Brenton Point State Park to see a monument that honors Portuguese navigators of the golden age of maritime exploration. We took pictures of the World Sphere and the Interpretative Plaque, both sponsored by the Portuguese American Federation and the Division of Parks and Recreation of Rhode Island and dedicated on June 10, 1988. We continued on Hwy 138, Hwy 24, the I-195 and I-495 (Blue Star Memorial Highway), and through the Scenic Highway north of the Cape Cod Canal. We stopped and took a picture of a plaque on a rock with the inscription: "In Memory of August Belmont (February 18, 1853–December 10, 1934) whose vision initiative and indomitable courage made possible the first complete construction of the Cape Cod Canal Connecting Buzzards Bay and Cape Cod Bay which was officially open for traffic July 29, 1914." We then continued across Sagamore Bridge and took the Mid-Cape Hwy to South Yarmouth, Massachusetts, and the hotel where we stayed the night, Best Western Blue Water, 291 South Shore Dr. Although it was only around 230 miles, it took us about six hours to get there with our stops along the way. In the evening we attended Mass at the Saint Pius X Church on Barbara Street in South Yarmouth.

The next day we were back on the I-495, then the I-95, and finally the I-93 to Boston. We drove through an impressive tunnel in Boston built during a pork barrel project secured from federal funds by Massachusetts Senator Ted Kennedy. There is no question that the billions of dollars Kennedy funneled to the state helped him achieve multiple reelection. Back on the I-95, we crossed the border with New Hampshire, continued on the New Hampshire Turnpike, passed Portsmouth, crossed the bridge on the Piscataqua River, the border between New Hampshire and Maine, and on to Kittery, Maine. Kittery was where our neighbor Miles McCoy lived before coming to Columbia. After joining Route 1, we had a break for lunch and then stopped in Kennebunkport, situated along the Atlantic Ocean and Kennebunk River. Settled in the 1600s, the village was a longtime shipbuilding mecca and is now a popular summer destination. In fact, it is famous for being the location of the Bush Compound, a summer retreat belonging to the Bush family. We skipped the compound and instead visited Dock Square and enjoyed a walk on Goose Rocks Beach. Later in the afternoon we drove to our hotel, the Hampton Inn at 48 Industrial Park Road in Saco. That day we clocked up only 170 miles, but with stops it took us almost six hours. We had arrived in Maine, a state that gained statehood at about the same time as Missouri. Missouri applied for statehood in 1818, but as a "slave state" it was not accepted. Ultimately, the so-called Missouri Compromise was achieved: Maine was separated from Massachusetts as a free state on March 1, 1820, with Missouri as a slave state to keep the balance between free and slave states.

On May 16, we started driving before 8 am. Back on the I-94, we passed Portland, Yarmouth, Gardiner, Augusta and Pittsfield, and then hit the I-395 bound for Bar Harbor, Maine. Our room for the night was in the Holiday Inn Sunspree, 123 Eden Street, which is located on Mount Desert Island, the largest island off the coast of Maine. We covered the distance of 187 miles in three-and-a-half hours. After lunch we went to Oli's Trolley Gift Shop at 1 West Street in the Harbor Place Building to buy tickets for a two-and-a-half-hour tour of Acadia National Park and Bar Harbor. It turned out that we were the only ones who signed up for the tour (Fig. 267). Our guide was very knowledgeable and shared lots of details about the national

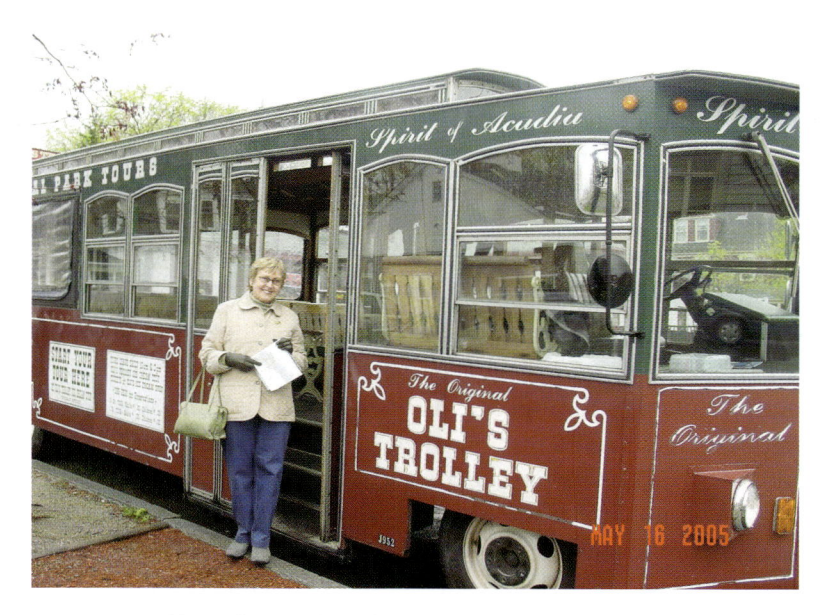

Figure 267. Oli's Trolley — "The fun way to see Mount Desert Island and Bar Harbor."

park. The island was spotted in 1604 by Samuel de Champlain, who called them île de Monts Déserts, literally "Island of Barren Mountains." The island was settled by Jesuit priests in 1613 and was part of the province of Acadia.[45] Millions of years ago, the Earth's tectonic and volcanic forces pushed the land upward to form the mountains on the island, and during the ice ages that followed, huge mile-high, slow-moving glaciers sheared off the tops, leaving the rounded off appearance seen today. Our trolley bus ascended Park Loop Road, which winds its way to the top of Cadillac Mountain,[46] passing the pink

---

45. Acadia (French: Acadie) was the name given to lands of the French Colonial Empire in northeastern America that included parts of eastern Quebec and modern-day New England. People living in Acadia, and sometimes former residents and their descendants, are called Acadians, and Cajuns after resettlement to Louisiana.

46. Antoine Laumet de La Mothe, sieur de Cadillac (1658–1730) was a French explorer and adventurer in Acadia. Rising from modest beginnings, he achieved various positions of political importance in the colony. In 1701, he founded Fort Pontchartrain du Détroit, the beginnings of modern Detroit, and he was the governor of Louisiana from 1710 to 1716. The founders of the Cadillac auto company adopted his name and his armorial bearings as its emblem in 1902. Various places in North America bear his name, including Cadillac Mountain.

granite rocks and boulders once carried by the glaciers. The rounded boulders transported and deposited by glaciers are called erratics; they are different in composition from local bedrock. We passed one huge erratic boulder stranded on the precipice of the South Bubble mountain that (according to a roadside poster entitled "Glacial Freight") was carried from a granite ledge more than 20 miles (30 km) to the northwest.

At the top of Cadillac Mountain, we dropped by the souvenir shop. The mountain lived up to its status as the highest mountain on the east coast: we could see very little but fog — or should we say cloud? While descending, the visibility markedly improved and we could see Frenchman's Bay. We then passed a beaver dam in Jordan Pond, which serves as the water supply for the nearby village of Seal Harbor. Our guide also showed us a palace (Fig. 268) built in 1912 by Princeton professor Rudolph Brunnow for his bride-to-be. As a wedding gift he bought her a blue diamond. Unfortunately, the lady tragically went down with the *Titanic* that same year. More tragic still, while looking out for the coming of his bride on the Precipice Trail situated on the east face of Champlain Mountain, he fell to his death. According to our guide, a blue diamond was waiting for her in the palace, but the ultimate fate of the stone is unknown. Further down we were shown Thunder Hole, a small inlet naturally carved out of the

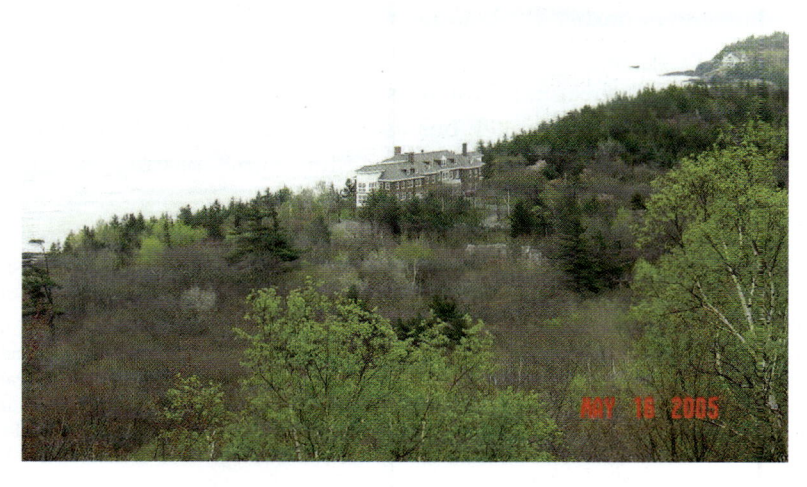

Figure 268.   Rudolph Brunnow's palace.

rocks into which the waves roll. Low down at the end of the inlet is a small cavern where, when the rush of the wave arrives, air and water is forced out like a clap of distant thunder — hence the name. The water spouts as high as 40 feet (12 meters) with a thunderous roar. Nearby was Sand Beach, another natural phenomenon unique to the island. From a distance the beach seems to be covered by sand, but on closer inspection it is actually ground up shells. All in all, we were very impressed with the tour and learned a tremendous amount about the region from our guide.

On May 17, we drove north through Bangor, then west at Newport and on State Road 2 to Jefferson, N.H., for our overnight stay at Jefferson Inn, 6 Renaissance Lane, a very nice inn in a small town. We covered the distance of 215 miles in less than two-and-a-half hours. As we got there, we went for a walk along the Starr King Trail and up to the Waumbek Golf Course to admire the view of the White Mountains. We turned in early as we expected the following day to be rather busy.

The next day, we took the I-93, then I-89, and finally State Road 4 to Coolidge State Park in Plymouth, Vermont. It was only 123 miles and took us less than two-and-a-half hours. I have always admired President Calvin Coolidge for his respect for the founding principles of the U.S. enshrined in the Declaration of Independence and in the Constitution. He gained a reputation as a rather consistent defender of limited government and entrepreneurial freedom, but among presidents he is one of the least appreciated by the country's academic elite, whose political orientation tilts rather noticeably to the left.[47] His reputation underwent a renaissance during the Ronald Reagan Administration when I came to the U.S. in 1981. I think I will always remember this quote from Coolidge: "Nothing in the world can take the place of persistence. Talent will not; nothing is more common than unsuccessful men with talent. Genius will not; unrewarded genius is almost a proverb. Education will not; the world is full of educated derelicts. Persistence and determination alone are omnipotent."

---

47. In Sarah Palin's book *America by Heart*, which I recently read, the author cites Coolidge's speech on the 150th anniversary of the Declaration of Independence in 1926. Here is a thought-provoking excerpt: "If all men are created equal, that is final. If they are endowed with inalienable rights, that is final. If governments derive their power from the consent of the governed, that is final. No advance, no progress can be made beyond these propositions."

Interestingly, in his private life, Coolidge is remembered as being laconic and was therefore commonly referred to as "Silent Cal." According to one well-known story, his wife was unable to attend church one Sunday so Coolidge went alone. After he returned, she asked him whether he enjoyed the sermon. "Yes," he answered. "And what was it about?" she asked. "Sin," he replied. "But what did he say?" she persisted. "He was against it," said Coolidge. At one White House dinner, an opera singer was invited, but her performance was not too good. One of the President's aids asked him, "Mr. President, what do you think about this lady's execution?" The President answered, "I am all for it." Another story, of somewhat doubtful authenticity, has it that a lady seated next to him at a dinner told him, "Mr. Coolidge, I've made a bet against a fellow who said it was impossible to get more than two words out of you." His famous reply: "You lose."

Unfortunately, Coolidge State Park was closed for the season, but we could still see the house where he was born (Fig. 269) and the house where he was sworn in as President by his father (a public notary) on August 3, 1923, after the death of President Harding (Fig. 270). (Coolidge was reelected in 1924, but refused to run in 1928.)

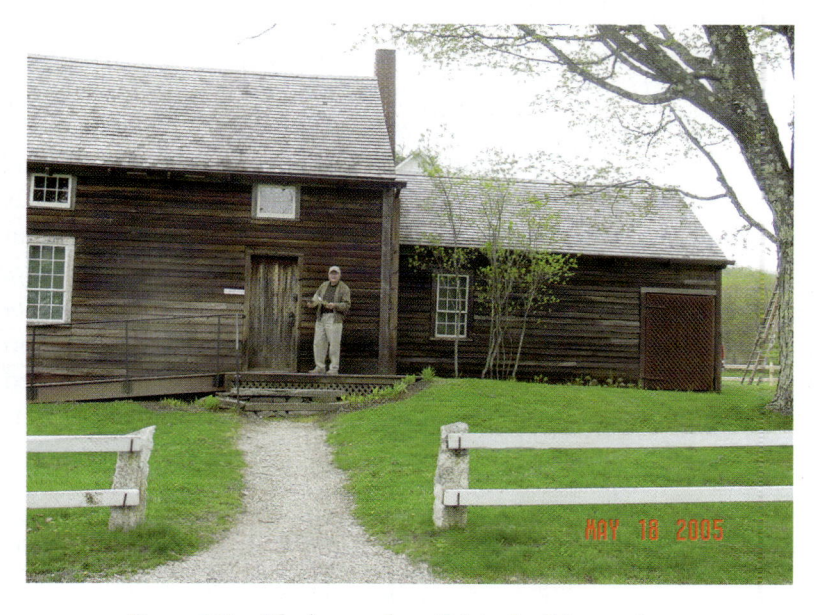

Figure 269. The house where Calvin Coolidge was born.

496   Around the World with Nephrology

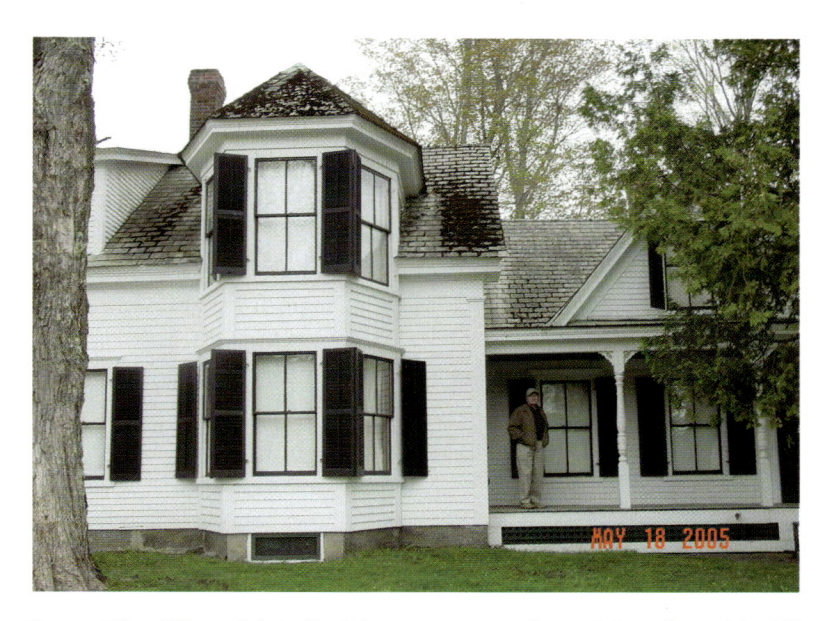

Figure 270. Where Calvin Coolidge was sworn as the 30th President of the U.S.

We also visited a memorial for the veterans of WWI. The Aldrich House, which houses the Regional Administrative Office of the Vermont Division for Historic Preservation for the Plymouth Notch Historic District, was unfortunately closed. At 10:30 am we started out on Coolidge Memorial Road, then the VT-100, and Route 7 through Bennington, Vermont, and Troy, N.Y., before arriving in Latham, N.Y., and checking in to our hotel, the Ramada Inn on 946 New Loudon Road. The stretch was only 97 miles and we covered it in two hours and 15 minutes. After checking in, we took a trip to Albany, capital of the state of New York, only about 12 miles away. We went to Lincoln Park and the Empire State Plaza to see the Military Women Memorial, the Korean War Memorial (Fig. 271) at Madison Avenue (close to the New York State Museum), the WWII Memorial, and the Cathedral of the Immaculate Conception (which unfortunately was closed).

Leaving Latham on May 19, we headed for East Syracuse, N.Y., driving mostly on the I-90 and taking two-and-a-half hours to go 135 miles. Our overnight accommodation was the Hampton Inn at Carrier Circle on 6605 S. Old Collamer Road. After checking in, we

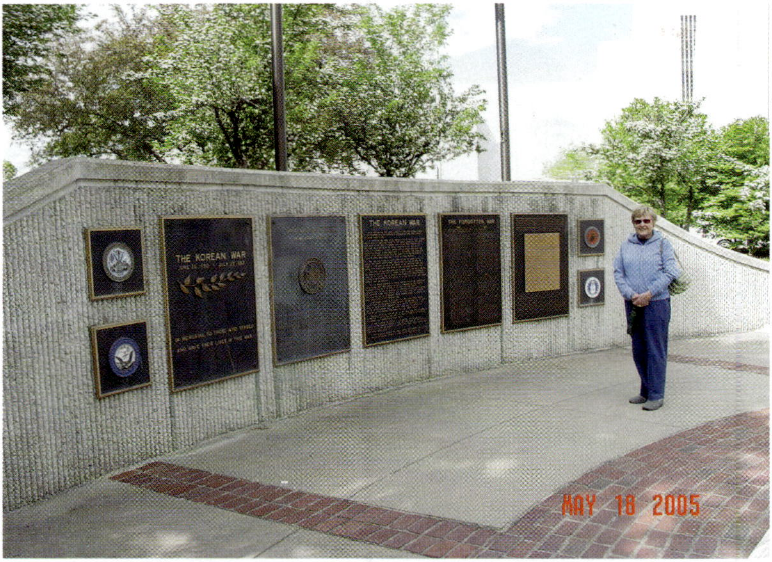

Figure 271. The Korean War Memorial in Albany.

went to see the city, though there is not a great deal to see in Syracuse. We went to "Armory Square, an Historic Business District,"[48] and then to Clinton Square, the historic center of Syracuse named in honor of New York Governor De Witt Clinton, leader in the development of the Erie Canal (Fig. 272).

On May 20, we started at 9 am and drove 163 miles on the I-90, arriving at noon at the Hampton Inn on 501 Rainbow Blvd in Niagara Falls, N.Y. Niagara River flows north from Lake Erie to Lake Ontario. It splits around Great Island, joints again and flows west, then splits again at Goat Island and the Three Sisters Islands, which are on the American side of the U.S.-Canadian border. About 90 percent of the water in the left channel turns into Horseshoe Rapids and then creates the bigger Canadian or Horseshoe Falls between Terrapin Point of Goat Island and Table Rock, where the channel angles about 90 degrees to the Lower Niagara River. The remaining 10 percent of water runs through the steeper American Rapids, creating the smaller American Falls between Prospect Point and Luna Island, and the smallest, the Bridal Veil Falls, between Luna Island and Goat Island. The water from both

---

48. Original spelling on the board.

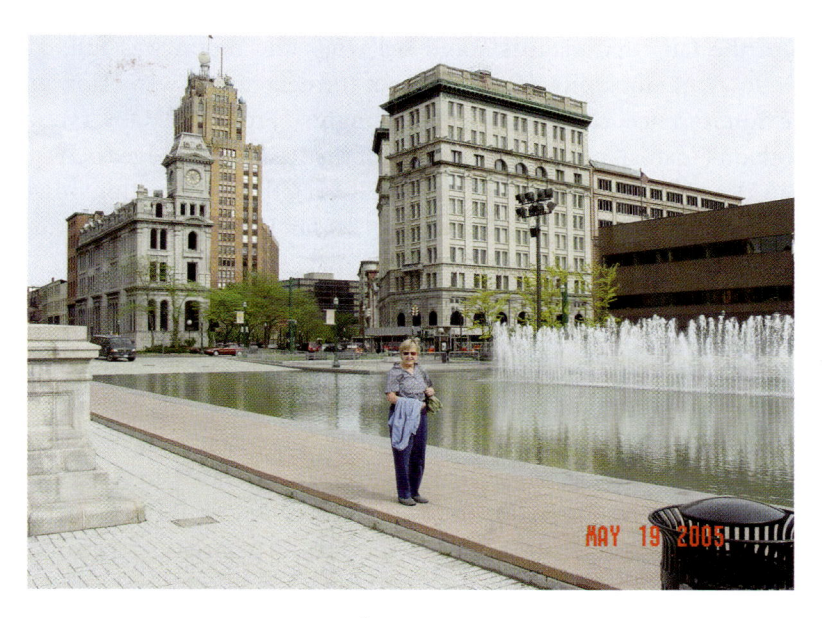

Figure 272. Clinton Square in Syracuse.

falls unites in the Lower Niagara River, which flows north to Lake Ontario.

In the afternoon we went to Goat Island by the way of the pedestrian bridge. The island was in the possession of the British and was cared for by a settler called John Stedman. During one very harsh winter, all his animals died except for one goat. Impressed by the hardiness of his goat, he gave the island the name Goat Island. From Goat Island we went to the Three Sisters Islands, on the west side of Goat Island. According to a board at the entrance to the three islands, they were named for the daughters of Parkhurst Whitney, a local businessman and a decorated veteran of the War of 1812: "In the spring of 1816 when ice jams in the shallow rapids created natural bridges between the islands, Whitney took his three daughters on a walk to the farthest island. Whitney was so proud of the success that he convinced Augustus Porter, the islands' new owner to name them after his daughters. The nearest was called Asenath, the next Angeline, and the farthest Celinda Eliza. The island adjacent to Celinda Eliza is called 'Little Brother' after the Whitney daughters' brother Solon." Next we went over a bridge to Luna Island, which was named in the 19th century for the beautiful moonlit rainbows made by the mist from the falls that visitors could see when the moon was full. The rainbows are not seen today because of the decrease in water flow and the interference caused by artificial lights. From the Observation Deck on Goat Island, I took a picture of the Rainbow Bridge (between the U.S. and Canada over the Niagara River), the Observation Tower, the American Falls, Luna Island, the Bridal Veil Falls and a bridge leading to Luna Island (Fig. 273).

The following day we headed for the Visitor Center on Prospect Point to take a tour with Gray Line. Our guide Sam told us that the name "Niagara" is derived from the Iroquois Indian word *Onguiaahra*, which means "thundering waters," but other sources suggest that this word means "the strait" or "the throat." Sam first took us to the Schoelkopf Hydroelectric Power Station, inaugurated in 1881, and more recently transformed into the Niagara Power Project, located about 4.5 miles downstream from the falls. It consists of two main facilities: the Robert Moses Niagara Power Plant, boasting 13 turbines, and the Lewiston Pump-Generating Plant, with 12 pump-turbines. Between the two plants is a forebay capable of holding about 740 million gallons (2.8 billion liters) of water; behind the Lewiston plant, a

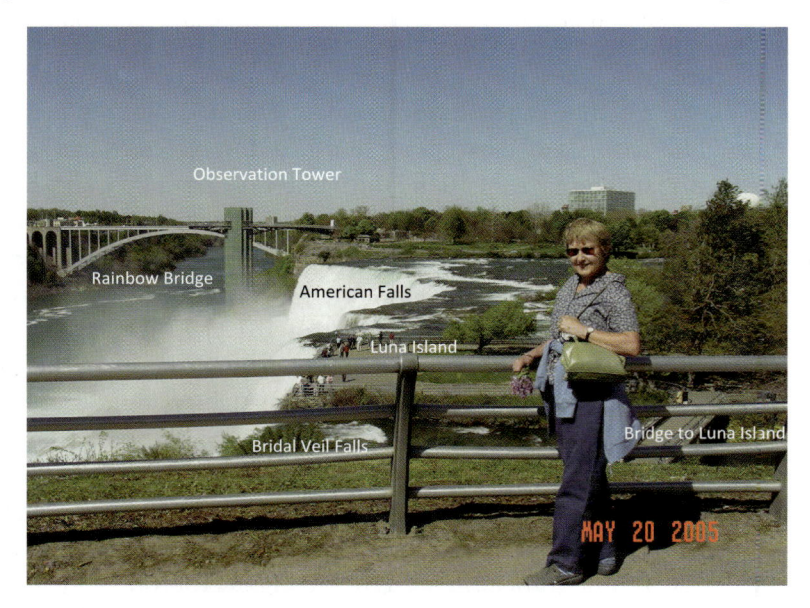

Figure 273. A picture taken from the Observation Deck on Goat Island in the Niagara River.

1,900-acre (770-ha) reservoir holds additional supplies of water. As I understood it, the water is diverted from the Niagara River and conveyed through conduits under the city of Niagara Falls to Lewiston. From there the water is taken to power generating turbines. Water is pumped at night when demand for electricity is low; the Lewiston units operate as pumps, transporting water from the forebay up to the plant's reservoir. Pumping water at night is a strategy used in many hydroelectric power plants; I was surprised that this method was not used in the Hoover Dam power plant, as I mentioned previously. It was explained to me at the time that Lake Mead has a surplus of water and that such a trick is not needed. After seeing the power plant, we went to the Observation Tower, where all three falls are visible (Fig. 274).

Next on our itinerary was the *Maid of the Mist* boat cruise from the U.S. side. As I mentioned, we had previously taken a similar cruise from the Canadian side. According to our guide, the name of the cruise is derived from the Indian legend of Lelawala, which means "Maid of the Mist." Legend has it that a beautiful girl lost her husband at a young age and out of desperation decided to take her own life. She got in her canoe and paddled down the Niagara River singing a death song to herself. The canoe hurtled toward the falls and as it pitched

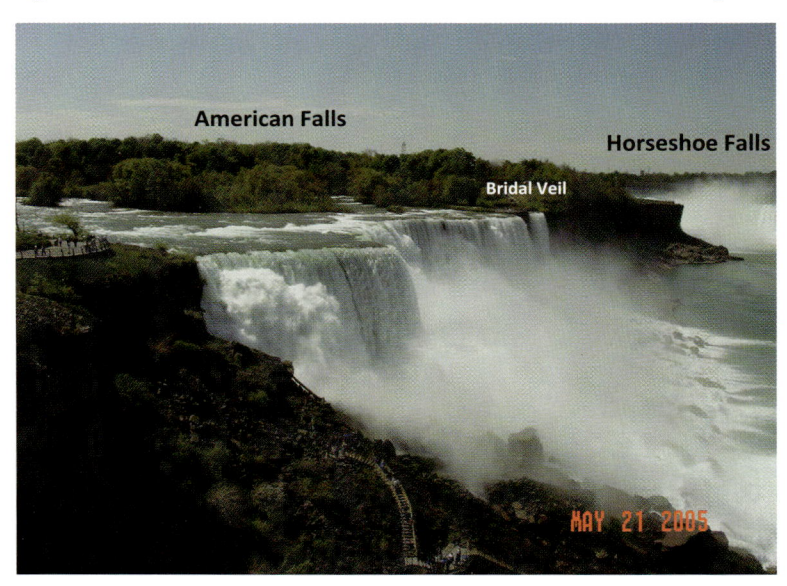

Figure 274. A view of the Niagara Falls from the Observation Tower.

she fell. But Heno, the god of thunder who lived in the falls, caught her gently in his arms and carried her to his home beneath the thundering veil of water. After the cruise we went to the Cave of the Winds, which is on Goat Island near the Bridal Veil Falls. Very close to its entrance is a monument to Nikola Tesla (Fig. 275), who designed the first hydroelectric power plant in Niagara Falls. On the monument is a plaque that reads: "Nikola Tesla, 1856–1943, inventor of alternating current induction motor." A gift from the Yugoslavian Government in 1976, the monument is the work of Croatian sculptor Frano Kršinić. On the other side of the monument is another plaque that states: "Nikola Tesla, Inventor — 10 July 1856 — Smiljan, Yugoslavia — 7 January 1943 — New York." After returning from the tour we checked out of the Hampton Inn and headed for Independence, Ohio, taking the I-190 through Buffalo, N.Y., and then the I-90 parallel to Lake Erie past Erie, Pennsylvania. Our overnight stay was in the Comfort Inn on 6191 Quarry Lane in Independence. We covered the distance of 217 miles in three-and-a-half hours.

On Sunday morning, May 22, we attended Mass at St. Michael's Catholic Church on 6540 Breksville Road. The next day we took the

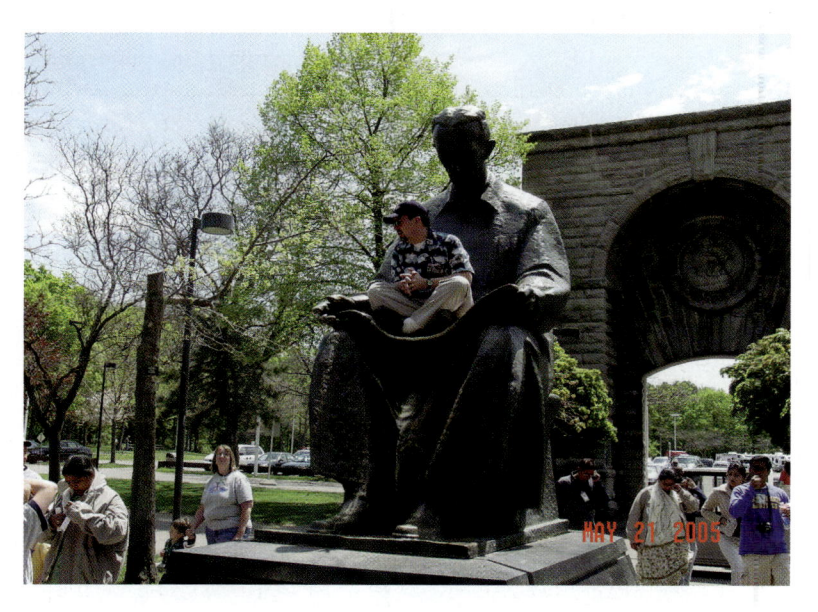

Figure 275. A monument to Serbian-American electrical engineer Nikola Tesla.

I-71 to Columbus, Ohio, and then the I-70 to Huber Heights, Ohio, where we checked in to the Holiday Inn Express at 5612 Merily Way. We covered 187 miles in less than three-and-a-half hours. The day after, we continued on to Terre Haute, Indiana, taking the I-70 through Indianapolis, and it took us less than three hours to drive the 186 miles. In Terre Haute, we stayed at Drury Inn on 3040 South US Hwy 41. On the last day of our tour, we drove through Illinois to our home in Columbia, which was 290 miles in about five hours, mostly on the I-70. The total distance covered during the tour was 3,282 miles. We learned a great deal about the history and geography of New England.

That year we went to Poland on July 1. Adam came for a visit on July 19, and it was quite a busy time. We drove to Wadowice, the Sanctuary of Divine Mercy in Łagiewniki, Zakopane, the monastery in Czerna, Pieskowa Skała Castle, and the monastery in Częstochowa. We biked with Adam on the Vistula Boulevard and once went to the monastery in Tyniec, which is about 7 miles (11 km) from our apartment on Smocza Street in Kraków. Ludwik Kotliński, Adam's other grandfather, visited us in Kraków. We then visited Ludwik in Puławy, and from there we went to Warsaw, where we stayed at the Courtyard by Marriott, close to Okęcie Airport.

During the Warsaw visit, our itinerary was packed. We visited Lazienki, the Royal Castle, the Old Town Square, and the Barbican. Among the churches we visited were St. John's, St. Anna's, the Capucines, and the Paulines. We also spent time on two of Warsaw's great streets, Ulica Nowy Świat (New World Street) and Krakowskie Przedmiescie, stopping at numerous monuments. Starting from Stare Miasto (Old Town) and heading to Castle Square, we stopped at Sigismund's Column, the oldest secular memorial in Warsaw. It is dedicated to King Zygmunt III Waza (Sigismund III Vasa), who transferred his residence from Kraków to Warsaw in 1596 to be closer to Sweden. The column was erected in 1644 on the orders of his son, King Władysław (Vladislav) IV. Although the column is appreciated in Warsaw, some Cracovians do not like it, as they believe that the drawn-out decline of Poland started in 1596 with the transfer of the Polish capital to Warsaw. We then went to Park Łazienkowski (literally "Baths Park") and stopped at a monument to King John III Sobieski on Agrykola Bridge (Fig. 276); the king is

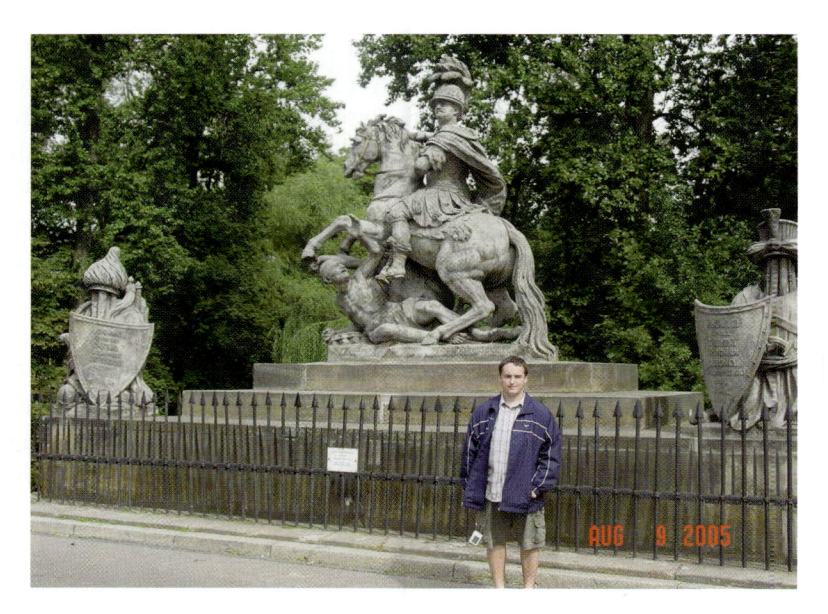

Figure 276. Adam in front of the John III Sobieski monument in Warsaw.

wearing Roman-style armor according to the artistic conventions of the time and his horse is trampling a Turk. The monument honors Sobieski's victories over the Turkish Army in the late 1670s and under the command of Kara Mustafa at Vienna in 1683, this being a decisive victory as it prevented Turkish expansion into Europe. A military genius, he was known by the Turks as the "Lion of Lechistan" and was honored as savior of European Christendom by the Pope. The monument was erected by Poland's last king, Stanisław August Poniatowski, in 1788.

In Park Łazienkowski we saw the monument to Frédéric Chopin. It was erected in 1926, destroyed by the Germans during the wartime occupation of Warsaw, and reconstructed in 1958 (Fig. 277). We also stopped at monuments honoring Nicolaus Copernicus, Warsaw's mermaid, Marshal Józef Piłsudski[49] and Jan Kiliński.[50] There was no monument to Tadeusz Kościuszko in Warsaw. I found this surprising given the number of other places he is honored: at the entrance to the Wawel

---

49. Józef Piłsudski played an instrumental role in the regaining of independence by Poland after 123 years of partitions. He successfully defended Poland against Soviet invasion in 1920.

50. A cobbler by trade was one of the commanders of the Kościuszko Uprising against Russia in 1794. He was promoted to the rank of colonel by Kościuszko.

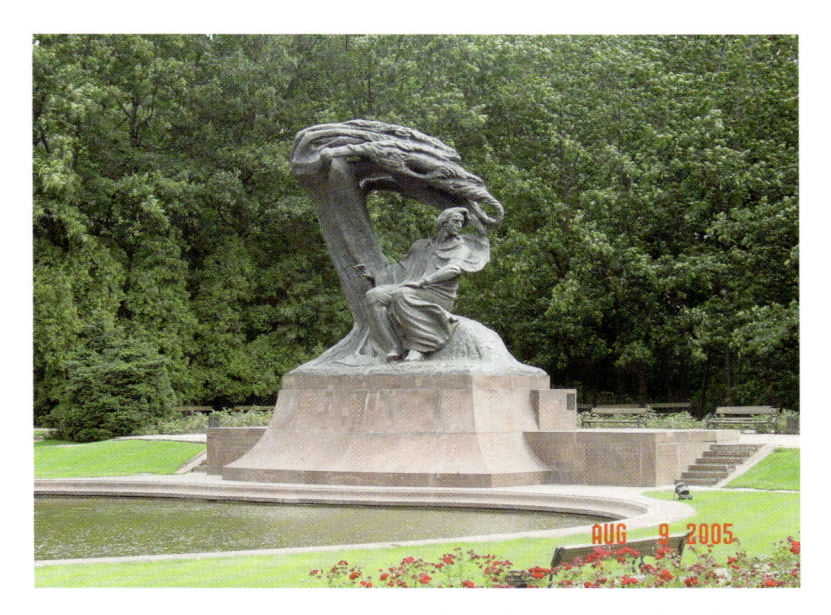

Figure 277. A monument to Frédéric Chopin in Łazienki Park.

Castle in Kraków; in Philadelphia, as mentioned previously; at West Point; at Boston Public Garden; at Lafayette Park across from the White House; and in Milwaukee, Chicago, Cleveland, Detroit and St. Petersburg, Florida. In Poland, besides Kraków, there are Kościuszko monuments in Łódź and Poznań. There are only two monuments of foreign persons in Warsaw. The first is that of Charles de Gaulle, who served as an instructor of Polish infantry during its war against Soviet Russia from 1919 to 1921. Only recently, on November 20, 2011, a second monument of a foreign person, Ronald Reagan, was unveiled by Lech Wałęsa in Warsaw. Ronald Reagan is highly respected in Poland and particularly by Lech Wałęsa, the leader of Solidarity movement, for having helped the fall of the Iron Curtain in Eastern Europe. After the ceremony, Lech Wałęsa said: "I wonder if the current Poland, Europe and the world would look the same without President Reagan, As a participant in these events, I must say that it is inconceivable. We returned very late to our hotel after the tour. The next day Adam left for Bismarck, North Dakota.

Przemek and Kasia arrived on September 4 and spent two weeks with us. On September 28, we returned to Columbia. That year we went to Bismarck to celebrate Thanksgiving with our older son Radek and his family. Leaving on Tuesday, November 22, we drove from home in Columbia to our hotel in Sioux Falls, South Dakota (Best Western Ramkota Hotel on 3200 West Maple Street), and then to Bismarck the following day. After our stay with Radek's family, we left early on Sunday, November 27, intending to get to the Ramkota Hotel by evening, stay overnight, and then leave again the next morning. Unfortunately, this plan completely changed when a blizzard hit North Dakota. On our way from Bismarck on the I-94, a few miles before Fargo, freezing rain caught us by surprise and within a few seconds the windshield of our Cadillac STS was completely iced over. I could not see anything and I tried to slow down, but we skidded off the road. Luckily, there was no ditch on the I-94, but rather a gradual slope, and we came to a stop well away from the road. There were at least five cars close by. Our car was rear wheel drive and I was unable to get it back onto the road. I called OnStar, but they could only provide assistance within two hours at the soonest. Fortunately, there were two enterprising guys in a car with a winch helping people to get their vehicles back onto the tarmac for a small fee of US$75. Afterwards, I drove very slowly, only about 20 to 40 mph, depending on the road surface. We turned on to the I-29 and it was still risky to drive any faster. Two cars overtook me and immediately skidded off the road. Gradually conditions improved, and we could go up to 50 mph as we approached Sioux Falls. We finally arrived very late at the hotel and checked the forecast. A blizzard was on its way, so we decided to keep driving after taking a two-hour nap. As we started again, the temperature was 34°F (1°C), so I was constantly checking the outside temperature to make sure it did not fall below freezing. At one point it was 32°F (0°C), and it looked like the blizzard from the northwest was going to catch us. Fortunately, we managed to outrun the blizzard, and when we reached Kansas City, the temperature was over 40°F (4°C). We eventually arrived safely in Columbia after a 20-hour drive.

We spent the Christmas holiday with Przemek and Kasia in Pasadena. But I had learned a lesson after the disappointing performance of our STS on the slippery winter roads, so we did not drive. Instead, we took a MoX (minibus) to Kansas City for a Southwest Airlines flight to Los Angeles.

2006 — Adam and Ania in Kraków, Zamość, Puławy

In 2006 we arrived in Kraków in May and then went to Vicenza, Italy, for a meeting, which I described earlier. Adam and Ania came to Kraków on July 4, and on July 14 we went to Puławy to see Ludwik, Ania and Adam's other grandpa. I planned to go to Shatsk (Polish: Szack), the place where I was born, which is presently located in Ukraine. On July 15 we attempted to drive across the border at Dorohusk, with the plan to get to Szack via Starovoitove, Rymachi, Kotsury, Vyshniv, Luboml, Kusnyscha and Zghorany. But when we came within a couple of kilometers of the border crossing, we spotted a line of waiting cars. We found out that it would take us about two days to make it into Ukraine, so we decided to scrap the trip to Szack that year and delay it for another year — or figure out a faster way of getting there. Originally, we had predicted that the whole drive from Dorohusk to Szack (68 miles or 110 km) would take one-and-a-half hours; we had planned to spend about 3 or 4 hours in Szack and come back in the afternoon. We already had a hotel reservation in Hotel Orbis on Kołłątaja Street in Zamość, so we decided to go to Zamość immediately.

We had never been to Zamość before, but we were aware of the fascinating history of the town and its fortress. Zamość was founded in 1580 by Jan Zamoyski (also spelled Zamojski), Chancellor of the Polish Crown and Hetman (head of the army of the Polish-Lithuanian Commonwealth), on the trade route linking western and northern Europe with the Black Sea. It was modeled on Italian trading cities and is a perfect example of a Renaissance town of the late 16th century blended with fortifications. At that time Zamość Fortress was one of the most impressive fortresses belted with powerful bastion fortifications. Its defensive value was tested twice in the 17th century during sieges of Cossacks under Bogdan Chmielnicki (Bohdan Khmielnytsky) in 1648 and during the Swedish Deluge in 1656 that failed to capture the city. Only during the Great Northern War at the beginning of 18th century was Zamość occupied by the Swedish and Saxon troops. During the Polish Soviet War of 1920, the Soviet army surrounded the city but failed to capture it. In the interwar period, Zamość enjoyed a time of rapid economic development. During WWII the city and surrounding area were slated for colonization by the Germans; Polish citizens were taken to concentration camps or taken for slave labor in the Nazi Third Reich. Children, if racially "clean" (i.e., with physical characteristics deemed "Germanic"), were sent for Germanization with German families. The colonization was not successful, due to Polish resistance and because not many Germans were eager to move. These families had to go back to Germany later during the war. Zamość is the birthplace of former German President Horst Köhler, who was in the area when it was intended for German colonization.

In Zamość we visited the Great Market, the cathedral in which Zamoyski is buried, and a prominent monument to Zamoyski. We also visited the city's remaining bastion (Fig. 278). The next day we returned to Puławy and visited Czartoryski's Palace, which was acquired by Prince Adam Kazimierz Czartoryski and his wife Izabela Czartoryska in 1784. Under their stewardship, and after the loss of Polish Independence in 1795, the palace became a museum of Polish national memorabilia and a major cultural and political center. Tadeusz Kościuszko visited this palace before the uprising of 1794 (Fig. 279). In the afternoon we returned to Kraków, and Adam and Ania left for Bismarck. We flew back to Columbia on September 27.

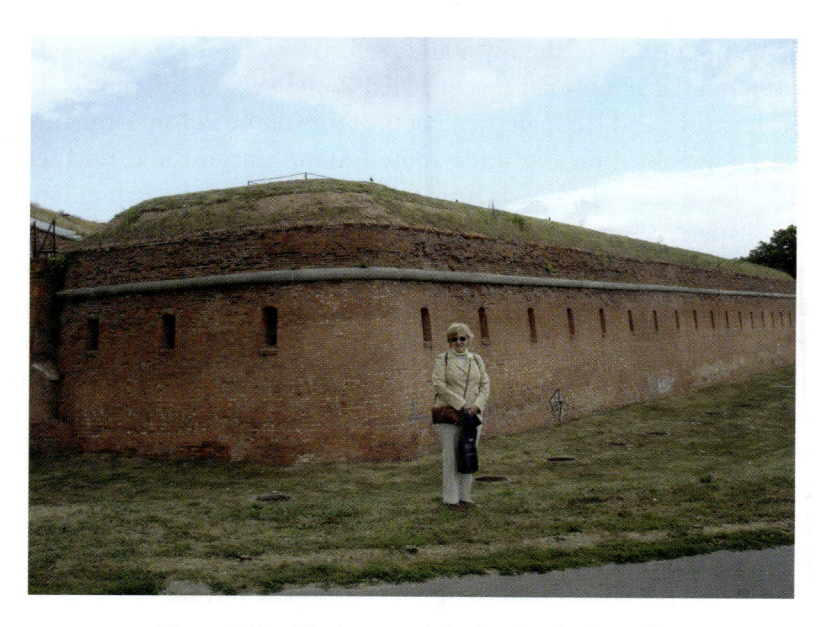

Figure 278.   The last remaining bastion in Zamość.

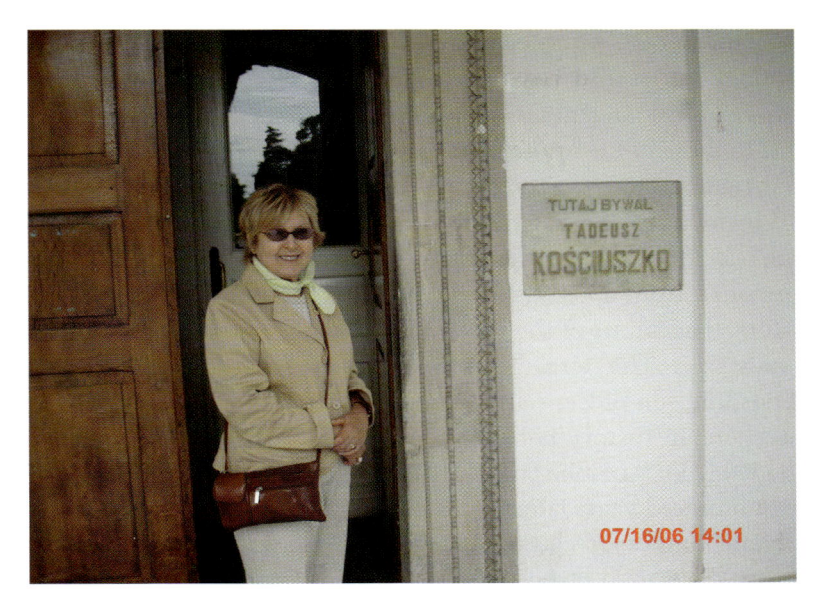

Figure 279. Prince Czartoryski's Palace in Puławy; Thaddeus Kosciuszko visited this palace.

That year we decided to go to Bismarck earlier, between October 5 and 9, to avoid inclement road conditions.

2007 — Crete, Peru tour

In 2007 I had a meeting in Austin, Texas, entitled "Advances in CKD," as already described. On January 30, four days after returning from the meeting, we traveled to Kraków for the funeral of Jola, a close friend of Halina's, and returned to Columbia on February 6. Later in February we had our annual conference, and in early May, before going to Poland, I was also in Istanbul for work. Later that month our son Przemek came for one day and then went to Lublin to celebrate the 25th anniversary of his graduation from high school. From May 18 to 20, I participated in the 5th International Congress of Uremic Research and Toxicity combined with the 7th Baltic Meeting on Nephrology. During the meeting I co-presided over the Free Communication Session with Vytautas Razukas from Lithuania and Zofia Wankowicz from Warsaw.

On June 30 we traveled with Basia, Halina's sister, to Crete, a popular tourist and vacation destination. Crete was the centre of Europe's most ancient civilization, the Minoan, and is considered to be the cradle of European civilization. Little is known about the rise of ancient Cretan society, because very few written records remain, and many of them are written in the undeciphered script known as Linear A. Knossos was the center of the Minoan civilization, which flourished from approximately 2700 to 1450 BC. There are no real historical accounts of the civilization; what is known is mostly from excavations. The term "Minoan" comes from the mythic King Minos, the son of Zeus and Europa according to Greek mythology. Later Cretan history is better understood. It is thought Crete was invaded from Anatolia (modern Turkey) in about 1700 BC. Around three hundred years later it was overrun by Mycenaean Greeks and remained under Greek influence until 69 BC when it was conquered by Rome. Rome suspected Crete of backing Mithridates VI of Pontus and sent Quintus Caecilius Metellus with three legions to the island. After a ferocious three-year campaign, Crete was conquered, earning Metellus the agnomen *Creticus*. Crete continued to be part of the Eastern Roman or Byzantine Empire until 824 when it fell into the hands of the Arabs, who established an emirate on the island. In 960 Nicephorus Phocas took back Crete for the Byzantines, who held it until 1204 when the Venetians took over at the time of the Fourth Crusade. The Venetians retained it until 1669 when the Ottoman Turks took possession of the island. Ultimately, Crete became a part of the independent Greece in the 1830s. It is a convoluted history that left traces in towns, buildings and archeological excavations.

We stayed in the Creta Maris Hotel in Hersonissos (Chersonissos). After a few days at the beach and swimming in the Aegean Sea, we decided to visit some places of interest. We took a tour to Knossos with Polish (Paweł) and Greek guides, both of which were very knowledgeable about the history of Crete and Greek mythology. Knossos was excavated at the beginning of the 20th century by British archeologist Sir Arthur Evans. It was apparently supposed to have been built by Daedalus on the order of King Minos. Only a few ruins are left, and some have been restored. The most interesting

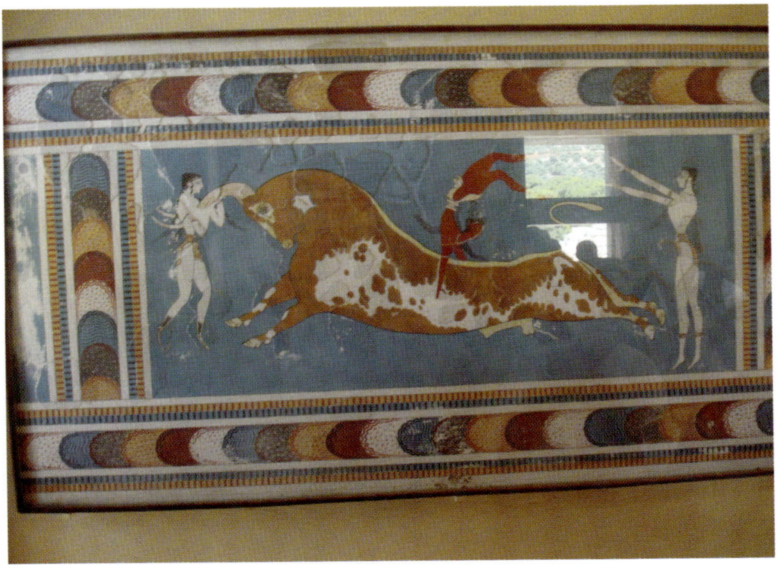

Figure 280. A copy of the Bull-Leaping Fresco in room 19 of the West Wing of the Knossos Palace; the original is in the Heraklion Archaeological Museum.

aspects of the site for us were the ruined theater and the many beautiful frescoes (Fig. 280). The Bull-Leaping Fresco does not depict a bullfight in the modern sense, since the bull was a sacred animal, and the contest can be considered a ritual act. The contestant (boy or girl) grasped the horns of a bull, made a double somersault on its back and leapt to the ground; according to our guide, not many could do it without serious injury. Almost every visitor wants to see the Throne Room, with the small gypsum throne of King Minos (Fig. 281). It takes about half an hour standing in line to see the throne. Judging by its size, he was probably less than five feet tall. A replica of the throne is in the UN International Court in The Hague. There are also well-preserved *pithoi* (Fig. 282), large jars of a characteristic shape made of heated clay that were used for storing oil, wine and cereals.

There are very interesting myths associated with King Minos, Knossos and Greece, which were related to us by our guides. (Our Greek guide told us that Greek mythology is an important course in

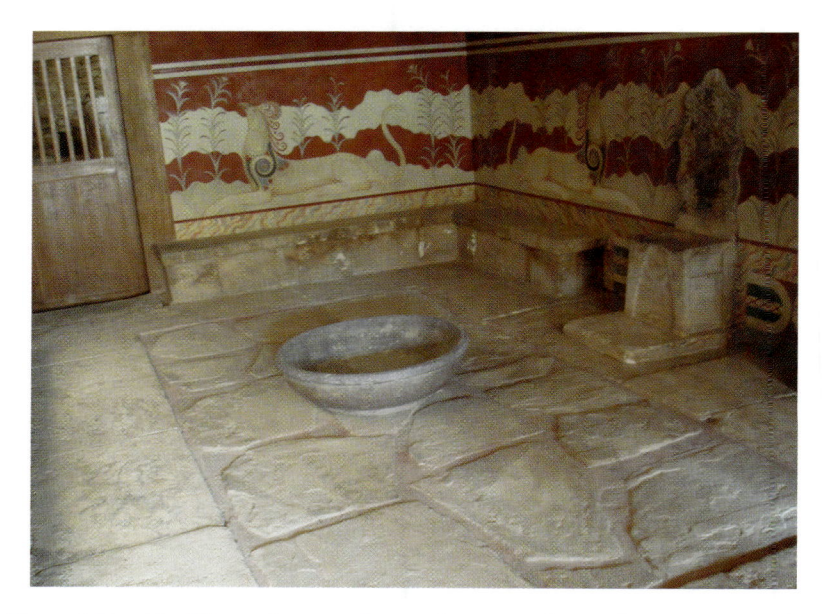

Figure 281. The Throne Room with a small gypsum throne that was preserved in the position it still occupies today. A lustral basin in front of the throne was probably for ritual purification. Note the griffins in the reed-like vegetation. A replica of the throne is in the Peace Palace in The Hague, which houses the International Court of Justice.

high school and graduates have to pass their final examination on the subject.) Although Minos was the son of Zeus, he had to struggle with his brothers for the right to rule Crete. They story is that he prayed to Poseidon to send him a snow-white bull as a sign of the gods' approval. He was to sacrifice the bull in honor of Poseidon but decided to keep it instead because of its beauty. However, the goddess Aphrodite did not support him and made Pasiphaë, Minos' wife, fall madly in love with the bull. She had the archetypal craftsman Daedalus make a hollow wooden cow for her, and Pasiphaë climbed into the wooden cow in order to copulate with the white bull. Their offspring was the monstrous Minotaur, half man and half bull. Pasiphaë nursed him in his infancy, but he became ferocious as he grew. Being the unnatural offspring of man and beast, he had no natural source of nourishment and thus devoured man for sustenance. After getting advice from the oracle at Delphi, Minos had Daedalus

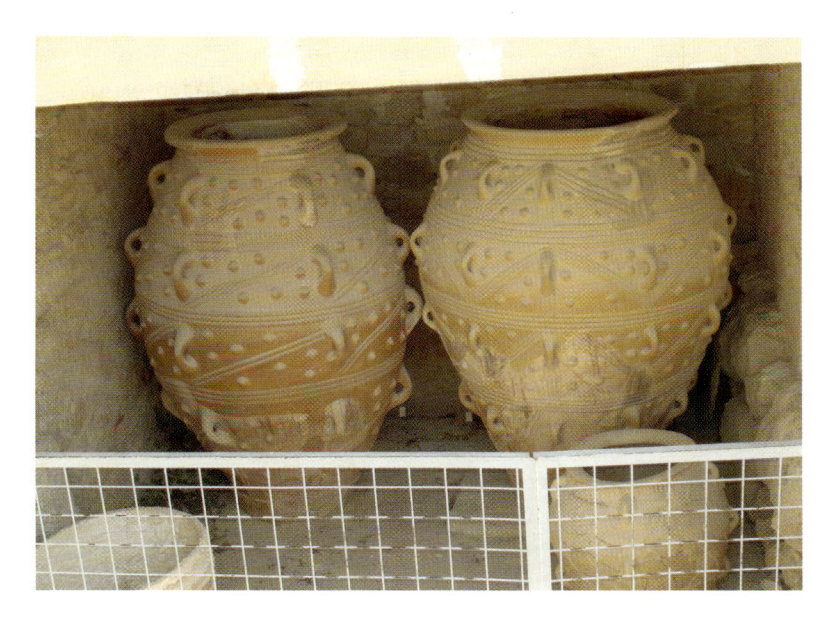

Figure 282.   Clay *pithoi* were used for storing oil, wine and cereals.

construct the gigantic Labyrinth to hold the Minotaur. The labyrinth was located in Knossos.[51]

King Minos' son Androgeus had been killed by the Athenians. Following tradition, Minos waged a war to avenge the death of his son. After emerging victorious, Minos required that seven Athenian youths and seven maidens, drawn by lots, be sent every year to be devoured by the Minotaur. When the third sacrifice approached, Theseus volunteered to slay the monster. He promised his father, Aegeus, that he would put up a white sail on his journey back home if he was successful and would have the crew put up black sails if he was killed. On his arrival on Crete, Ariadne, King Minos' daughter, fell in

---

51. There is another myth related to the Labyrinth and Daedalus. To prevent the spread of knowledge regarding the Labyrinth to the public, King Minos made sure Daedalus could not escape the island by keeping a strict watch on all vessels leaving by sea. Daedalus (in Greek Δαίδαλος, which means "cunning worker"), a genius craftsman and artisan, decided to construct wings for himself and his son so that they could leave Crete by air. Daedalus was able to reach a small island south of Samos, but his son Icarus flew too close to the Sun, which melted the wax holding his wings together, and he fell into the sea and drowned. His father called the island Icaria, and it has this name to this day.

love with Theseus and helped him navigate the labyrinth, which had a single path to the center. In most accounts she gave him a ball of thread, allowing him to retrace his path. Theseus killed the Minotaur with the sword of Aegeus and led the other Athenians back out of the labyrinth. On the way back Theseus forgot to change his ship's sails from black to white, and when his father thought that he had been killed, he committed suicide by drowning in the sea. Another famous, but apparently historical rather than mythical, person living in Knossos in the sixth century BC was Epimenides, known for his paradox.[52]

We also visited Heraklion (Iraklio), the capital of Crete. The original name given by the Saracens was Khandaq, which means "moat," and this was corrupted by the Venetians to Candia and then named Ηράκλειον by the Greeks. Heraklion has been developing quickly since becoming the capital in 1973. There are remnants from Venetian rule, like the Church of Saint Titus and Morosini Fountain (Lion's Fountain), and there is also a monument to Sir Arthur Evans in Heraklion. Doménikos Theotokópoulos, better known by his nickname "El Greco," was born in a village nearby. As mentioned earlier, we admired a painting of his when we were in Madrid for a meeting and visited various places in the area.

The next day, July 7, we rented a Chevrolet Matiz in Chersonissos. While settling the paperwork at the rental company, I started talking to the clerk about Greek mythology, and he also told me that he had been obliged to pass an exam on the subject before graduating. He informed me that you did hear several versions of the myths depending on the region of Greece you were in. I asked him about the myth of Theseus. He confirmed the story but said that the end of the story, as accepted on Crete, is slightly different and is related to a small island, Dia Nisida, north of Heraklion and Chersonissos. In this version, on the way back to Athens, Theseus was passing Dia Nisida, which was devoted to Zeus. On the island lived Dionysos, son of Zeus and Semele, daughter of King Kadmos. Theseus stopped at the island

---

52. In one of his poems Epimenides, himself a Cretan, said, "The Cretans [are] always liars." Was the statement true or false? If he was a Cretan and he said that they always lie, was he then lying? If he was not lying, he was telling the truth, and therefore Cretans do not always lie. Thus, since the assertion cannot be true and it cannot be false, the statement turns back on itself. This is the origin of the so-called Epimenides paradox.

(called Naxos at that time) and Ariadne went with him to Athens. Dionysos fell in love with Ariadne and asked Theseus to leave her on the island. He did so, leaving in a hurry early in the morning and forgetting to change the sails from black to white. His father, Aegeus, thought that Theseus had been killed and in despair jumped to his death in the sea, named the Aegean Sea after him. Taking the E-75 parallel to the Aegean Sea to Rethymnon (Rethymno), which is about 70 miles (100 km) west of Chersonissos, we stopped to take a photo of Dia Nisida on the way. Unfortunately, the island was not clearly visible because of fog. The most interesting thing in Rethymno was the old city with the Rimondi Fountain and the Venetian-era Castro Fortezza (Fig. 283). On July 8, after our thoroughly enjoyable time on Crete, we returned to Kraków on Central Wings flight CO0484. We did not go anywhere else until our return to Columbia on September 23.

In November and December we decided to tour Peru. At the time I had been to many countries in South America but never to Peru. My interest in the country had been stimulated after reading about Inca civilization and the *conquista* by Pizarro as well as about

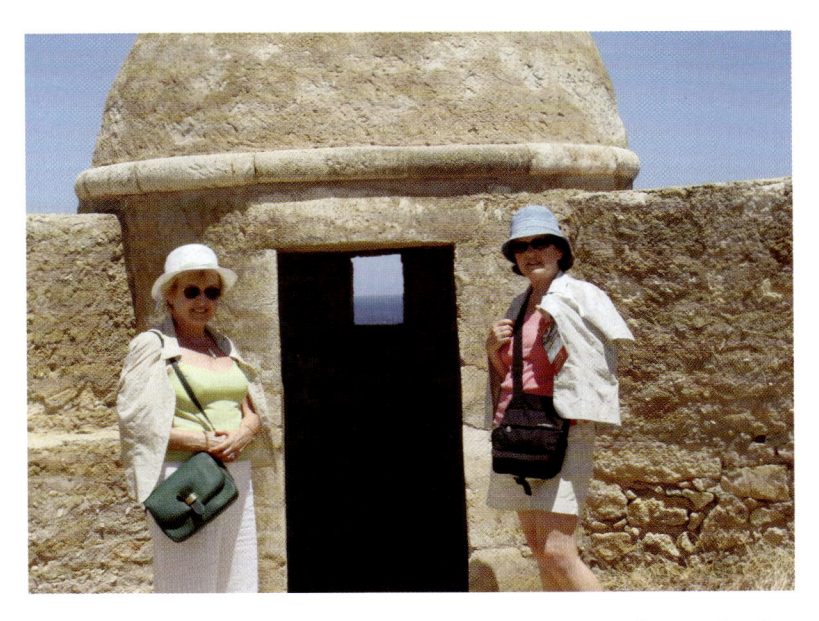

Figure 283. A view of the Aegean Sea through a turret window in the Castro Fortezza in Rethymno.

some Polish links with Peru.[53] Halina was initially not very eager to go as she had some concerns about mountain sickness, and I advised her to take acetazolamide over several days before going, which helps with the acclimatization process and relieves symptoms. She advised me to do the same, but I was so confident about my excellent cardiopulmonary health that I did not take any precautions. I will describe later how things turned out as we reached higher altitudes.

Although there are disputes about when and how many groups of people arrived in America, there is general agreement that they arrived through Beringia[54] and populated both Americas. The first traces of human presence in Peruvian territory date between 9,000 and 12,000 years ago. The oldest known complex society in Peru, the Norte Chico civilization, flourished along the coast of the Pacific Ocean between 3000 BC and 1800 BC. These early developments were followed by Andean cultures such as the Paracas, the Nazca, the Ica, and others. In the 15th century, the Incas emerged as a powerful state that, in the span of a century, formed the largest empire in pre-Columbian America. Andean societies were based on agriculture, using techniques such as irrigation and terracing; camelid husbandry and fishing were also important. In the 1520s there was a civil war between the heirs to the Inca throne, Atahualpa and Huascar, each of whom was seeking to control the empire. The war was concluded in Atahualpa's favor, but the empire was markedly weakened by the war. In 1532, a group of about 180 *conquistadors* led by Francisco Pizarro defeated and captured Atahualpa. The Spaniards met Atahualpa, the victor in the civil war, and his army at a prearranged conference at Cajamarca in 1532. When Atahualpa arrived, the Spaniards ambushed and seized him, killing thousands of his followers. Although Atahualpa paid the most fabulous ransom known in history — a room full of gold and another full of

---

53. The Polish engineer, Ernest Adam Malinowski (born in Poland in 1818, died in Lima in 1899), was the originator and builder of the highest altitude railroad in the world. After the fall of the November Uprising (1831), he left Poland for France, where he graduated from the elite Ecole des Ponts et des Chaussees and subsequently, in 1852, moved to Peru as an expert in the field of railroad construction. The railroad project he suggested would facilitate the transport of minerals and valuable types of wood across High Andes to the Peruvian capital. The project began in 1872, and already in spring of the next year it reached the Ticlio Pass at an altitude of 4,818 meters (15,806 ft), the highest railway spot in the world at that time. In 1999 a monument to his honor was erected at the Ticlio Pass.

54. Beringia was the landmass that connected northeast Siberia to Alaska during the last ice age. The Bering Strait currently separates Russia and the U.S.

silver — for his freedom, the Spaniards murdered him in 1533. By November that year Cuzco fell with little resistance. The Spanish destroyed many of the irrigation projects and the north-south roads that had knit the empire together, speeding its disintegration. The primary reason only a handful of Spaniards managed to conquer this vast empire was that their horses and guns — unknown to the Incas till then — inspired terror among the populace. Members of the Inca dynasty took refuge in the mountains and were able to resist the Spaniards for about four decades. However, by 1572, the Spaniards had executed the last Inca ruler, Tupac Amaru, along with his advisers and his family.

We wanted to take a tour with our regular travel company, Trafalgar Tours, but at the time they did not have any. On the advice of Lynne Schwartze from AAA in Columbia, we decided to take the Peru Explorer Tour with Peruvian company Coltur Peru (Fig. 284). We started from Columbia at 7:30 am on November 30, taking the MoX minibus to St. Louis, flying to Atlanta on Delta 4704, and then to Lima on Delta 335. Arriving at 11:30 pm, we were transferred from the airport by car to San Agustin Exclusive Hotel, Calle San Martin 550, Miraflores, Lima 18. The next morning a Coltur car took us to the very nice Las Dunas Hotel in Ica. In the early afternoon the travel company had arranged an overflight of the Nazca Lines, which were made about 1,500 years ago. Although they are referred to as "lines in the sand" and the surface looks like sand

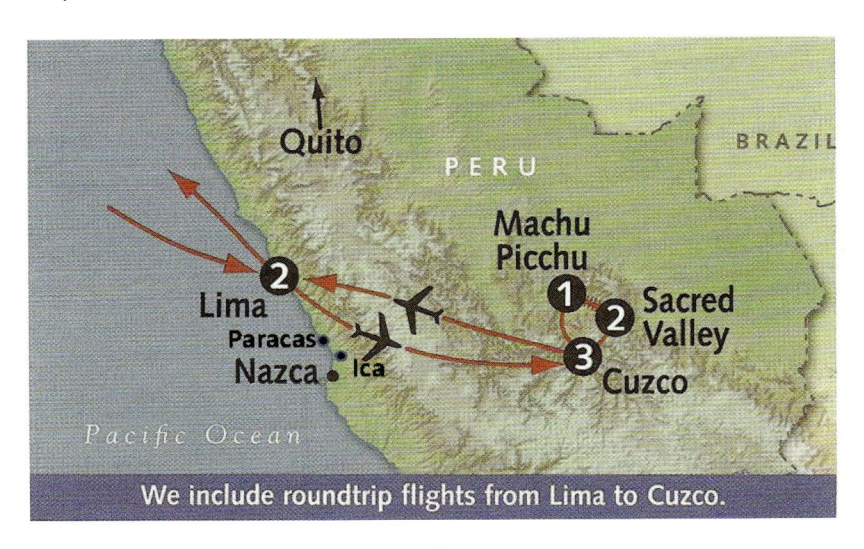

Figure 284. A map showing our Peru tour.

from above, in reality it is clay covered with iron oxide coated pebbles. This is one of the reasons that the lines have not eroded for thousands of years. It is also significant that the Nazca Desert is one of the driest places on Earth and maintains a consistent temperature of around 77°F (25°C) all year round. There are lines showing a geometrical figure resembling a landing field, and various figures like a condor, spider, hummingbird, monkey and pelican, as well as some enigmatic figure like an "astronaut" (a man with an owl head). Next our guide, Diego, took us to the town of Cachicha, close to Ica. He showed us a statue of witches and the "seven-headed palm tree." The eighth head is cut off, if it appears, as legend has it that if it is left to grow, Cachicha will be destroyed. Our next stop was Huacachina Oasis, a lagoon in the middle of the desert. The medicinal properties of the lagoon's waters were discovered by Italian Angela Perotti. Diego pointed out some people climbing the dunes in the distance who had come for sandboarding; I had a camera with 15X optical zoom, so I managed to take a good picture of them (Fig. 285). He also told us about the production of Peru's wine and its national drink, pisco — a strong, colorless grape brandy named after the town of Pisco on the Peruvian coast. The country's iconic cocktail, pisco sour, is made by adding lemon juice, egg whites, and *amargo de*

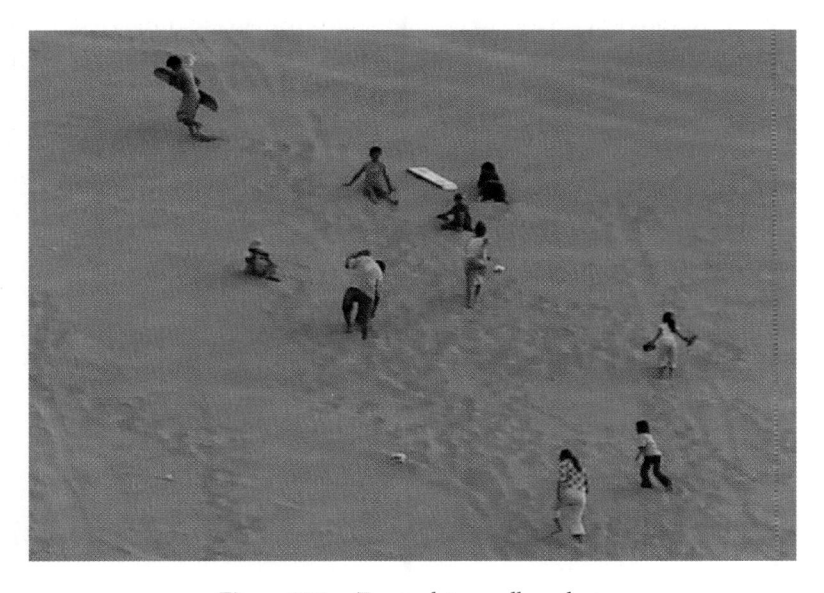

Figure 285. Zoomed-in sandboarders.

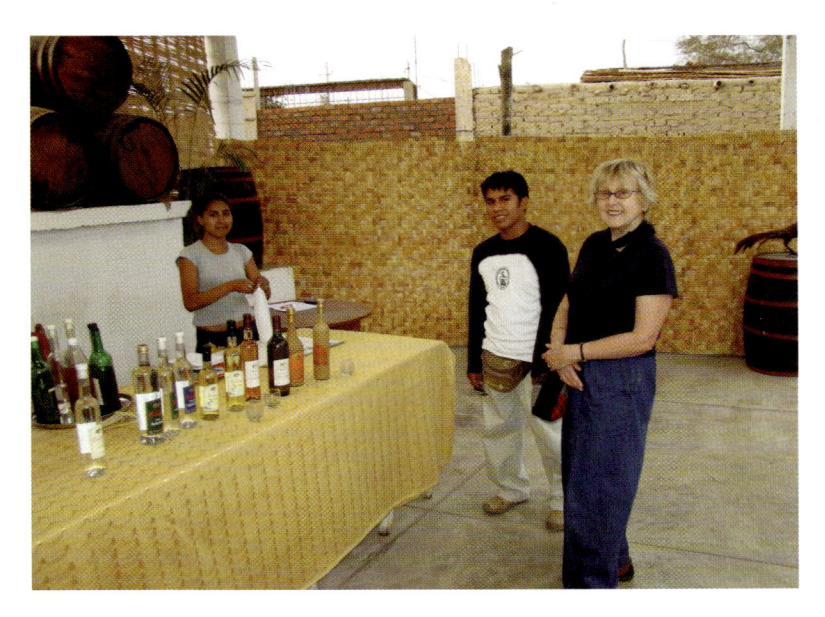

Figure 286. Diego and Halina in the Tres Generaciones winery.

angostura, which gives a slightly bitter taste. We ended the day at the Tres Generaciones winery, where both wine and pisco were on sale (Fig. 286).

The next morning we went to the wharf at Pisco port for a Ballestas Islands excursion. Sonya and Julio were our tour guides on board, and we were the only passengers. The boat sailed through Paracas Bay, initially along the Paracas Peninsula, and passed the Paracas Candelabra carved into the side of a cliff (Fig. 287). According to our guides, it is speculated that the giant prehistoric geoglyph depicts either a cactus or the Southern Cross Constellation. Probably used as a navigation landmark, it indicates the direction of Nazca city. The Paracas Candelabra has no connection with the Nazca Lines, however, since it was created by the Paracas people and predates the latter by about 700 years. Within a few minutes of passing the peninsula, our boat approached the Ballestas Islands, or islands with arches (Fig. 288); Sonya pronounced the name of the islands "Vayestas." We saw all of the principal creatures found on the islands: South American fur seals, sea lions, Peruvian pelicans, Guanay cormorants, Peruvian boobies, Humboldt penguins and gulls. Guano, the excrement of seabirds and seals, is harvested and deposited on special decks before being transported to the fields to be used as fertilizer. It is a

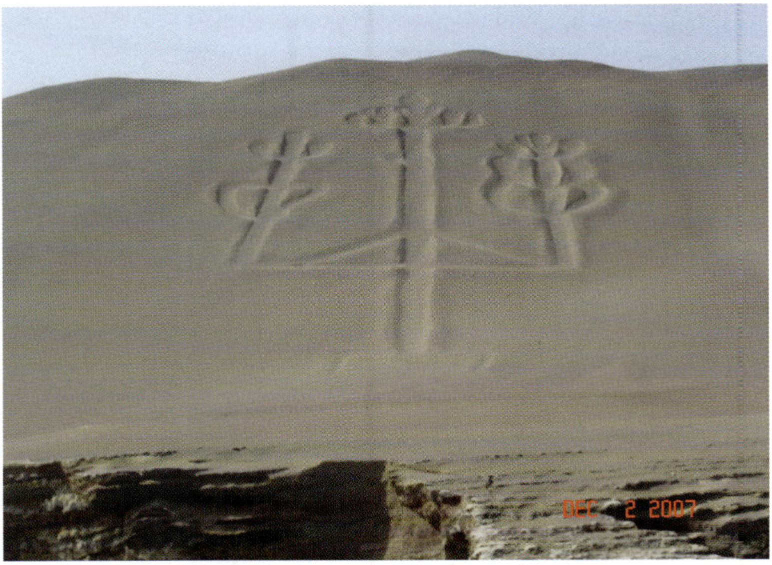

Figure 287. A candelabrum carved into the cliff of Paracas Peninsula.

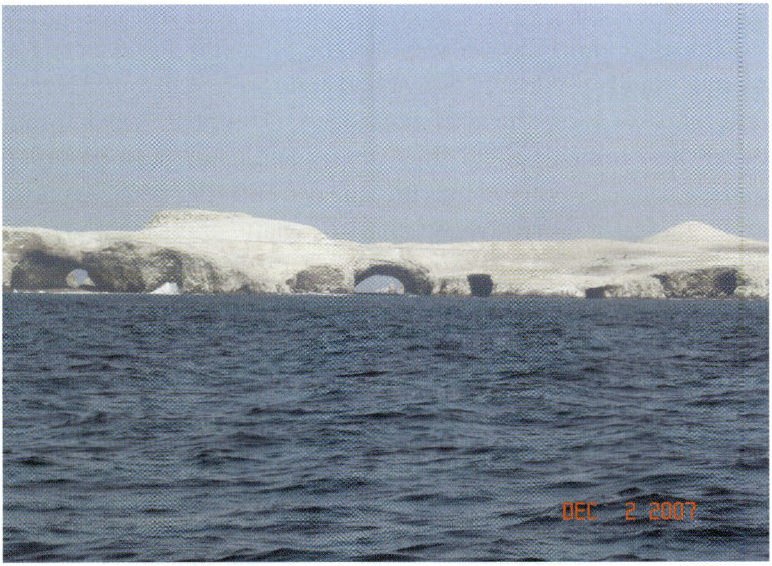

Figure 288. The Ballestas Islands.

520   Around the World with Nephrology

fascinating landscape and we took lots of pictures; too many to include here. Later that afternoon Alex, our new guide, drove us back to Lima. On the way we stopped in Chincha for dinner at El Pilot Restaurant and saw the damage caused to various buildings after the severe earthquake in August of that year. Afterwards Alex took us back to the San Agustin Exclusive Hotel in Miraflores, and that evening we attended Mass in La Virgen Milagrosa (Miraculous Virgin) church. There was a replica of the famous painting depicting Christ's divine mercy in the Sanctuary of the Divine Mercy in Łagiewniki, Kraków (Fig. 289).

December 3 was dedicated to visiting Lima, the sprawling Peruvian capital. The name of the city was initially Ciudad de los Reyes (City of the Kings) because it was founded on January 6, the Feast of the Epiphany. However, Lima, the original native name, persisted. It is uncertain where this name originated; it may derive from the Quechuan *rimaq*, meaning "talking." In the oldest Spanish maps of Peru, Lima and Ciudad de los Reyes can be seen together as names of the city. The river that feeds Lima is still called Rímac, the Quechua word for "Talking River." Located in the valley of the Rímac River, on the coast

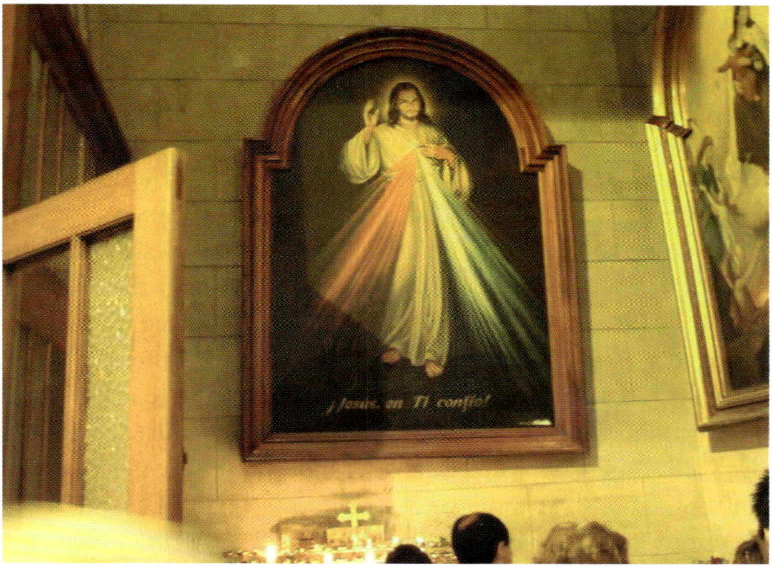

Figure 289. "Jesus I trust in you" — a painting in the Iglesia Virgen Milagrosa in Miraflores.

overlooking the Pacific Ocean, Lima forms a contiguous urban area with the seaport of Callao. Its first university, Saint Mark University, was established in 1551 and its first printing press in 1584. It also became an important religious center: a Roman Catholic diocese was established in 1541 and converted to an archdiocese five years later. It became the most important city in the Spanish Viceroyalty of Peru and, after the Peruvian War of Independence, the capital of the Republic of Peru. Today's Lima ranks as the 19th most populous city in the world, with the number of people living in the metropolitan area fast approaching 9 million, around one-third of the country's total population.

The sightseeing started early the following morning. Again we were impressed with the skill of our bus driver, José, and the knowledge of our guide, Sheila. Our first stop was at Parque del Amor (Park of Love) in Miraflores overlooking the Pacific Ocean. A sculpture of a couple kissing and mosaic walls with love inscriptions added to the romantic atmosphere. Next we drove by the Huaca Huallamarca Ruins, located in the San Isidro District. Built in 200 BC by the Hualla ethnic group using thousands of handmade adobe bricks, the pyramid served as a temple and a burial site. Spaniard conquistadores called it the "sugarloaf ruins." Afterwards we drove through the Miraflores District with its beautiful, expensive-looking houses. Miraflores, originally founded as San Miguel de Miraflores, was established as a district in 1857 and is one of the wealthiest residential areas in Lima. As a result of the Battle of Miraflores in 1881, fought during the War of the Pacific, Miraflores was referred to as Ciudad Heroica (Heroic City). Lima was occupied by Chilean forces during the war.

Next we were taken to Bolívar Plaza, with its equestrian statue of Simón Bolívar, liberator of Peru from Spanish rule in the 1820s. We visited the Museum of the Inquisition, which is situated on the plaza. The Spanish Inquisition was established in 1478 by Catholic monarchs Ferdinand and Isabella of Castile to maintain Catholic orthodoxy in their kingdoms and was under the direct control of the Spanish monarchy with Tomás de Torquemada as Inquisitor General. It was not definitively abolished until 1834, during the reign of Isabel II. The Museum in Lima is housed in the building that was the home of the Inquisition from 1570 to 1820 when it was abolished after Peru gained independence. Inside, we saw numerous sculptural depictions of various methods of torture, which were often designed to inflict pain in

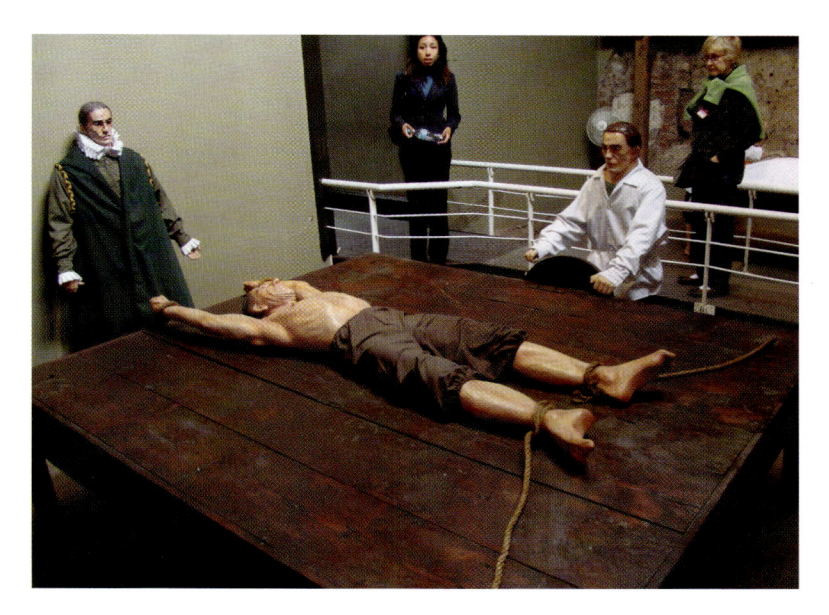

Figure 290. Sheila and Halina observe the gradual stretching that results in the systematic dislocation of every joint in the body.

different parts of the body simultaneously (Fig. 290). Our next stops were the Santo Domingo Convent and the San Francisco de Asis Church, which was founded by Francisco Pizarro in 1535, destroyed in 1656 and reconstructed in 1674. We entered the eerie catacombs beneath the church, where the remains of tens of thousands of people are held, but we only spent a short time there as the air was far from fresh. We also stopped at the old train station, which had been restored and converted into the cultural exhibition space.

Our next stop was Plaza Mayor, the birthplace and the core of the city as well as the location of various important buildings. The first place we visited there was the Basilica Cathedral of Lima, founded at the same time as Lima itself on January 6, 1535. Initially under the patronage of Our Lady of Assumption, it was recognized as a cathedral by the Pope Paul II in 1541 and placed under the patronage of John the Evangelist. We also saw the Government Palace, the famous Bronze Fountain designed by Spanish sculptor Pedro de Nogueras in the 17th century, and the Archbishop's Palace, which was constructed in 1924 and is adorned with Moorish style balconies. A few blocks from Plaza Mayor is Plaza San Marco with the bronze equestrian statue of General San Martin erected in 1921 to celebrate the first centenary of Peruvian Independence.

Next we traveled through the poorer parts of Lima and arrived at the Museo Rafael Larco Herrera, founded by a Peruvian archeologist in 1926 with the aim of showcasing remarkable chronological galleries and providing an excellent overview of 3,000 years pre-Columbian Peruvian history. Among the many exhibits we focused on the ceramics, sculptures, golden ceremonial costumes of Chimú (Fig. 291), and the erotic gallery. I already knew that no early cultures in America used the wheel, so it was very interesting for me to see circular objects. As there were no axles in the center of those objects, the invention of the wheel had evidently not been achieved. Our last stop was the Parque Salazar with its monument commemorating Alfredo Salazar Southwell, an aviator celebrated as a national hero. We stopped at the shopping center in the park and went to a very nice restaurant called Mangos.

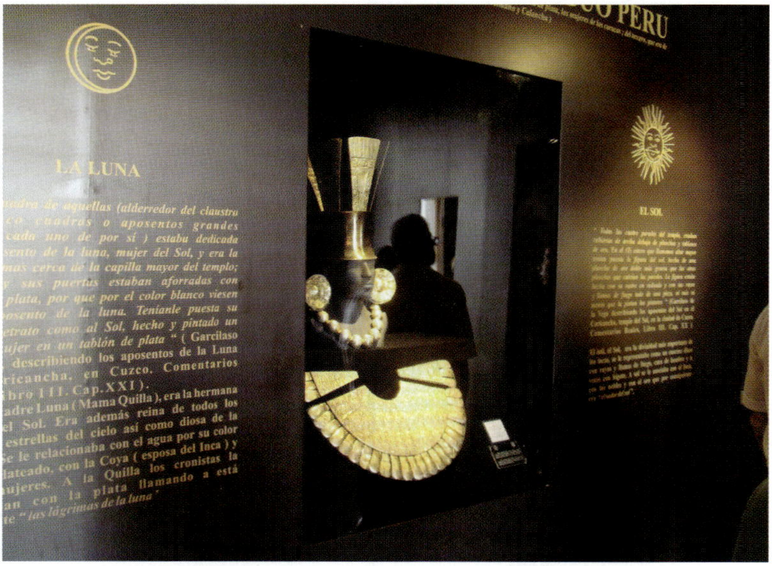

Figure 291. Ceremonial costumes of Chimú from around 1300 BC at the Larco Museum: a circular crown with four feathers, earrings, a bead necklace, a pair of epaulets and a repoussé pectoral. They belonged to an important person and were probably worn for rituals and ceremonies.

On Tuesday, December 4, we made our way to the Lima Aeroporto Internacional Jorge Chávez for our Lan Peru 023 flight to Cusco. At the airport, for the first time I saw a collection of items confiscated by security forces. After a short flight we arrived at Cusco's Alejandro Velasco Astete International Airport, named after the Peruvian pilot who was the first person to fly over the Andes in 1925, and who used the airport. Cusco (also spelled Cuzco, and in the native Quechua language *Qusqu*) is a city in southeastern Peru, near the Urubamba Valley (Sacred Valley) of the Andes mountain range. It is the capital of the Cusco region as well as Cusco Province. The altitude of the city, located on the eastern end of the Knot of Cusco, is around 11,500 feet (3,500 meters). In 2006 it was found that this historic capital of the sun-worshiping Inca Empire has the highest ultraviolet light level of any spot on Earth.

After a short break in the airport we started our tour to the town of Urubamba through the Urubamba Valley (Fig. 292). On the way we stopped at an Awanacancha farm to see its resident llama and alpaca. Our next stop was at Pisac Village and Market, which are at an altitude of 9,750 feet (2,970 meters). The village is best known for its Sunday market, which draws hundreds of tourists each week, but there are smaller markets on both Tuesday and Thursday; our visit was on a Tuesday. In spite of its popularity, the market retains much of its local charm, at least in the part where villagers from miles around gather to

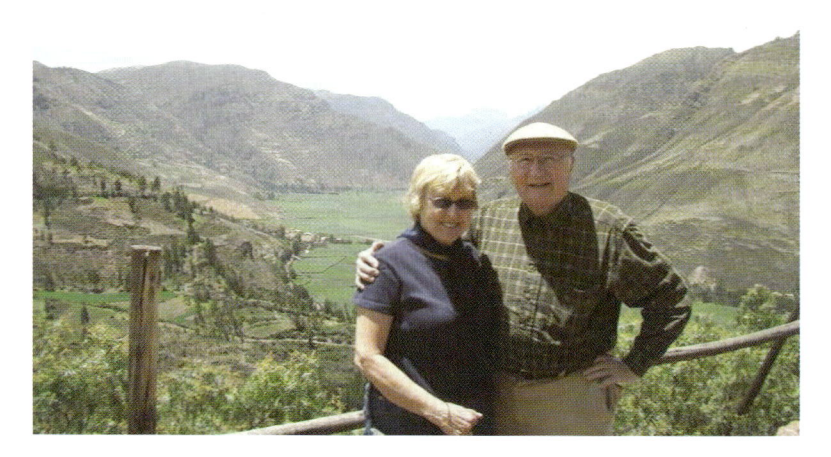

Figure 292. The Urubamba Valley in the Andes.

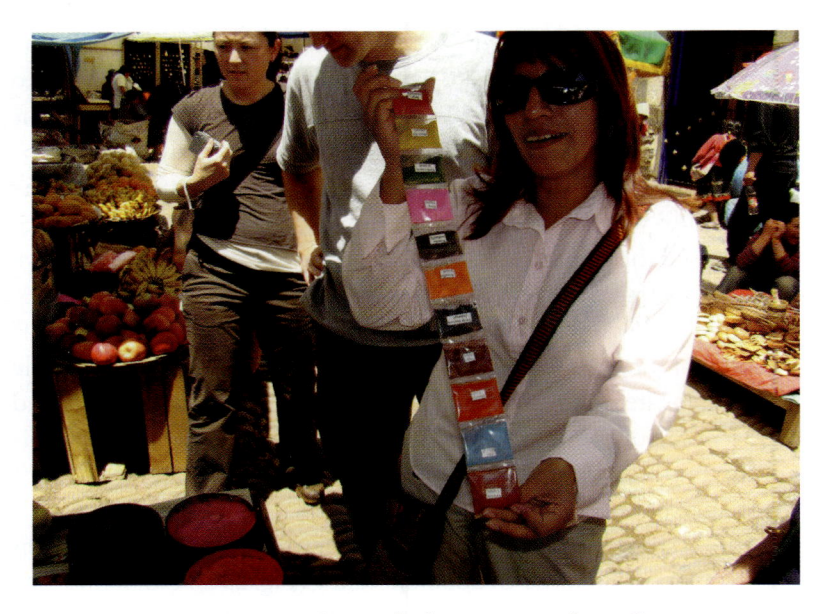

Figure 293. Our guide shows us some dyestuffs.

barter and sell their produce. Our guide, Milusca, showed us various handicrafts, which you can buy from the tourist section of the market, including excellent dyestuffs for wool (Fig. 293). The market also sells guinea pigs (*cui* in local language), which are bred for food. Our next stop was San Agustin Hotel in Urubamba, where we were to stay the night. On the way Milusca drew our attention to *illia*, a common sight on homes in former Inca lands. It embodies the description of upcountry Peruvians as "pagan Christians" in that it comprises a cross flanked by two bulls — the cross to ward off evil and the bulls to bring fertility and prosperity. It also contains two bottles, one for wine and the other for beer (Fig. 294). After dinner we went to see Urubamba and then participated in the Pago a la Tierra (Tribute to the Earth) to the Pachamama, meaning "Mother Earth" and referring to a goddess of fertility. The celebration was conducted in Studio Alpaca by a local shaman, Altomisanio (the Highest Priest). The final ritual performed by the shaman was the burning of fruits of the Earth, and the end of ceremony was the *arrascasca* (loosely translated as "dancing with drinks"), though we were only offered pisco without music to dance to.

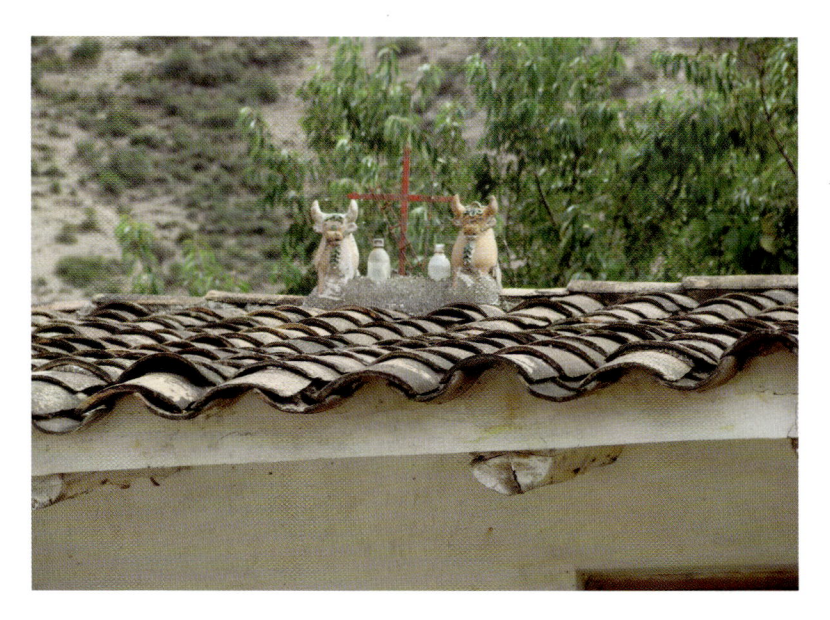

Figure 294. *Illia*, a common sight on homes in former Inca lands.

We left early the following morning for the town of Ollantaytambo, which is about 40 miles (60 km) to the northeast of Cusco and is situated at an altitude of 9,164 feet (2,792 meters) above sea level. The name is derived from the Quechua word *Ollantay*, an Incan general, whose love story is known throughout the literature,[55] and the word *tambo*, a Spanish derivation of the word *tampu,* which means city that offers lodging, food and comforts. Our goal was mostly to see the ruins of Ollantaytambo Fortress. Because of its strategic location in the Sacred Valley, Ollantaytambo became a prime center within the Inca Empire, and it was generally reserved for the elite. Ollantaytambo is located at place called Temple Hill and the name "fortress" is a misnomer since the site was first and foremost a place of worship. The Fortress also served as a place for the study of astronomy. On one part of the slope are ruins known as Inca Misanca, believed to have been a small temple or observatory, and a series of seats and niches have been carved out of the cliff. Among the Ollantaytambo ruins that are the most visually spectacular are the rising terrace walls, which served as

---

55. Markham CR. (2007) *Apu Ollantay: A Drama of the Time of the Incas*. BiblioBazaar.

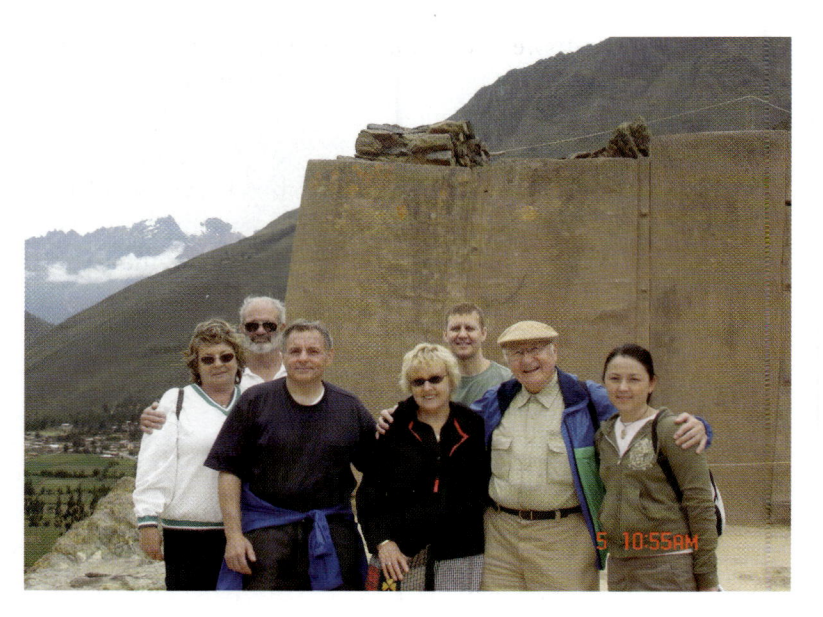

Figure 295. Our group in front of the gigantic Wall of the Six Monoliths, which are part of the Sun Temple; the picture was taken by our guide.

an integral means of defense. The temple sector is constructed from cut and fitted stones. The gigantic stones began their journey from the quarry of Kachiqhata (Cachicata) located at 4 miles (6 km) away on the left side of the Vilcanota River. The rock was partially carved at the hewn stones and then they were brought down to the valley. That these huge stones were transported uphill long distances is impressive (Fig. 295), especially given that the Incas did not have wheels as they had not invented the axle. Milusca told us that they created an artificial channel parallel to the river and transported them to the bottom of the slope. They then used instruments such as log rollers, rolling stones, camelide-leather ropes and levers — and the strength of thousands of men. The defensive value of the Fortress was proven when Inca emperor Manco defeated the Spaniards under the command of Hernando, the younger brother of Francisco Pizarro. It was the only place that the Incas were able to resist the Spanish attacks.

After coming down from the Temple Hill, we went to a *chicheria* (an Inca bar) called Aja Huasi, whose owner was Mercedes. The alcoholic beverage sold there, *chicha*, is distilled from corn and comes in two kinds: bitter and sweet. Our guide wanted to show us how this local beverage is prepared and, of course, wanted us to try it. We dutifully did, but it turned out not to be a good idea, as I will get into later. We then went to the Sonesta Posades del Inca Hotel, located in the middle of the Sacred Valley, in Yucay, Urubamba Province, 3,330 feet (1,000 meters) below Cusco. The hotel was converted from a 300-year-old monastery. We had lunch there and then headed to a nearby trout farm in Arariwa. We then visited the Pablo and Marilu Seminario, home of artisans who have devoted 20 years to the study of Pre-Colombian pottery techniques and designs, incorporating these ancient traditions into their own beautiful works. We bought a very nice wooden chair there. In addition to their works, they had a lovely garden brimming with flowers and they also kept llamas and alpacas. Most of the ceramics were made of red clay found in the valley. At the entrance to the studio we found a sculpture that appeared to be made of scrap, but I have to confess that my knowledge of modern art is rather superficial (Fig. 296). We spent the night at San Agustin Hotel in Urubamba.

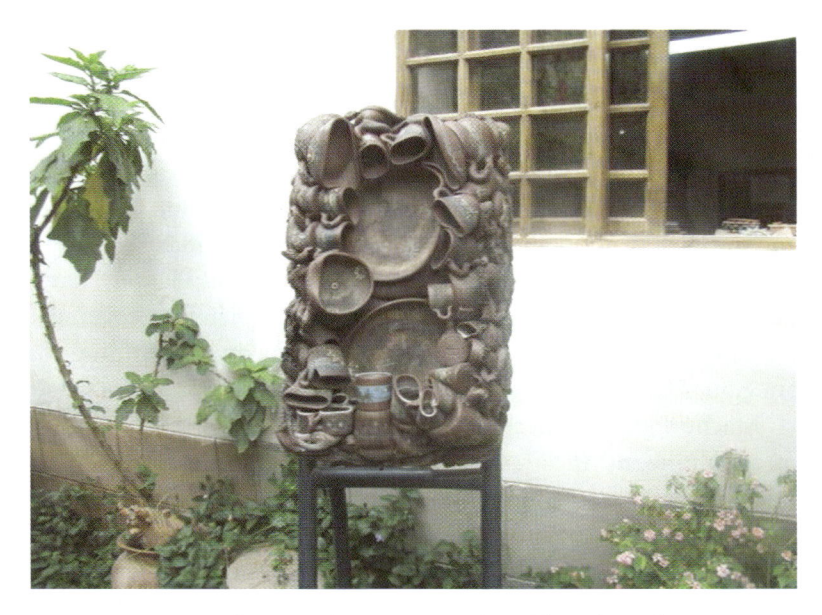

Figure 296. A sculpture at the entrance to the Pablo and Marilu Seminario.

Our experiments with the local liquor, however, turned that night into a nightmare. Everyone in our group drank the *chicha*, but only three of us got sick. Halina suffered the most, with constant vomiting and diarrhea keeping us up most of the night. We woke at 5 am the next morning, December 6, and Halina was very dehydrated. Unfortunately, we did not have any suitable medication to relieve her discomfort, but luckily by the time we were on the train to Aquas Calientes, the diarrhea had stopped. The tourist train from Ollantaytambo took us through the Urubamba River Valley, through tunnels and past Indian villages and terraced fields, with magnificent vistas of snow-capped Andean peaks. Along its 30-mile (47-km) course through the Machu Picchu sanctuary the Urubamba River undergoes a vertical drop of 3,300 feet (1,000 meters), creating spectacular whitewater rapids. The Urubamba (Quechua: *Willkamayu*, meaning "sacred river") is a tributary of the Amazon River.

Arriving at Hatuchay Hotel at 9 am, we asked for a doctor. A very pleasant local doctor called Dr. Gary Molero Tejeira prescribed Nifurat, which contains nifuroxazida (an antibiotic), activated attapulgite (an absorbent), metoclopramide (an antiemetic), Panadol (acetaminophen), and Electroral (electrolyte solution) for oral rehydration; it was the standard treatment for gastroenteritis in Peru. We had planned to join our tour to Machu Picchu in the afternoon, but it was obvious that Halina could not go (and two others were also unable to). The issue was whether Halina would be able to go the next day. It would have been very unfortunate to be unable to see Machu Picchu, as it was very much the highlight of Peru. But Dr. Tejeira came in the afternoon and was optimistic about Halina's recovery, so we booked a tour for four with a guide called Dimas. Happily, having taken the medication, Halina had almost completely recovered by next morning, so we were ready to take the bus on the winding road from Aquas Calientes to Machu Picchu (Fig. 297).

Machu Picchu (Quechua: *Machu Pikchu*, meaning "old peak") is a pre-Columbian Inca city located at an altitude of 7,970 feet (2,430 meters) on a mountain ridge above the Urubamba Valley, about 44 miles (70 km) northwest of Cusco. Probably the most familiar symbol of the Inca Empire, Machu Picchu is often referred to as "The Lost City of the Incas." UNESCO designated it a World Heritage

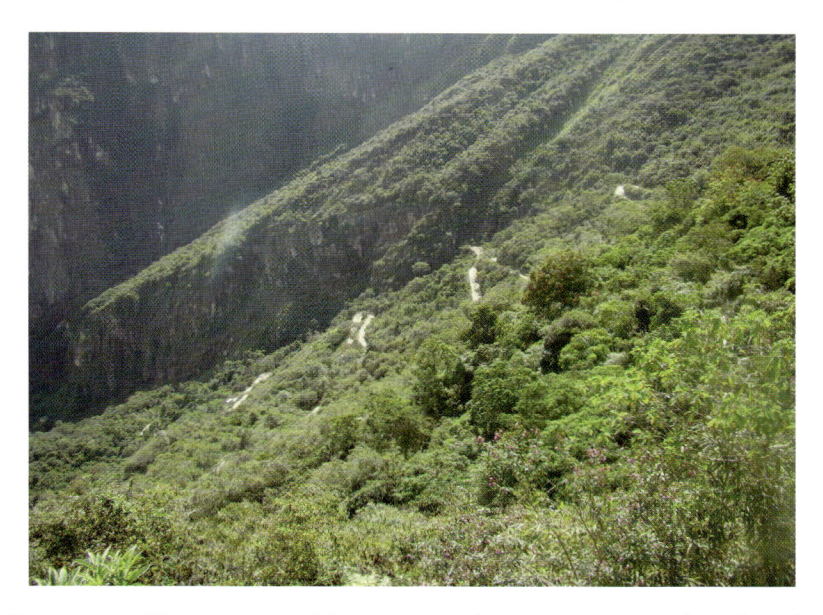

Figure 297. The twisting road from Aquas Calientes to Machu Picchu, where the picture was taken.

Site in 1983, calling it "an absolute masterpiece of architecture and a unique testimony to the Inca civilization." Machu Picchu was constructed around 1450, at the height of the Inca Empire, and was abandoned less than 100 years later, as the empire collapsed under Spanish conquest. Although the citadel is located only about 50 miles from Cusco, the Inca capital, it was never found and destroyed by the Spanish, as were many other Inca sites. Over the centuries, the surrounding jungle grew to enshroud the site, and few knew of its existence. In 1911, Yale historian and explorer Hiram Bingham brought the "lost" city to the world's attention.

According to the archeologists, the urban sector of Machu Picchu was divided into three great districts: the Sacred District, the Popular District, to the south, and the District of the Priests and the Nobility, or the Royalty Zone (Fig. 298). Located in the first zone are the primary archeological treasures: the Intihuatana, the Temple of the Sun, and the Room of the Three Windows. These were dedicated to Inti, the sun god and the Incas' greatest deity. The Popular District, or Residential District, is the place where the lower-class people lived,

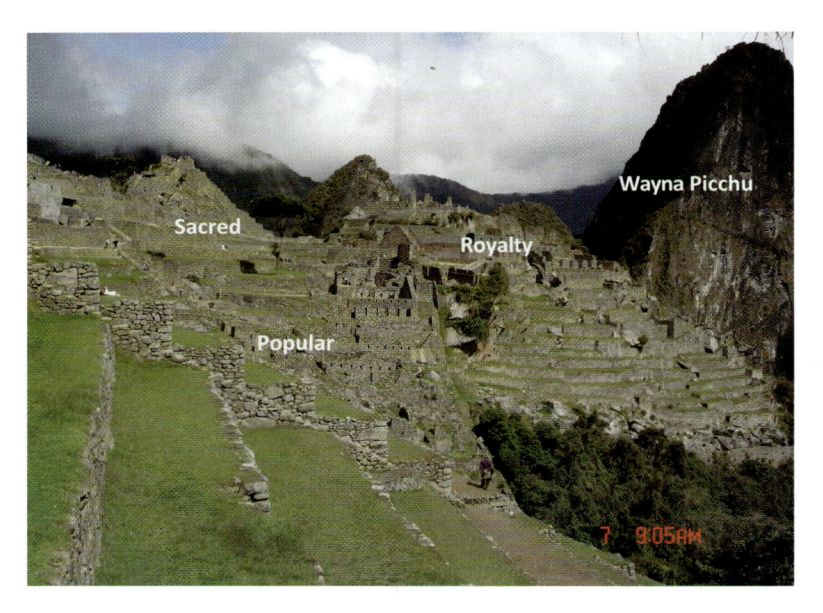

Figure 298. The various districts of Machu Picchu and Wayna Picchu.

and it includes storage buildings and simple houses. In the Royalty Zone there is a group of houses located in rows over a slope. The residence of the Amautas (wise men) was characterized by its reddish walls, and the zone of the Ñustas (princesses) had trapezoid-shaped rooms.

Our guide, Dimas, took us through all the districts (Fig. 299). I was impressed with the Incas' stonework in the Temple of the Sun (Fig. 300). Inca architecture was among the finest prehistoric architecture in the world. The building style is characterized by exquisitely cut masonry placed together completely without mortar. The raw material was granite worked by stone and sand into irregular shapes that fit together like a gigantic puzzle. Some stones have as many as thirty faces worked into the surface, and as a result, the faces of the stone fit together so tightly that a needle would not fit between them (Fig. 301). Rooms were built with sloped windows and walls as protection against the effects of earthquakes (Fig. 302). The stone quarry was situated above the area, and boulders were partly hewn there before being finished on-site. The photo in Fig. 303 shows how the boulders were split: wooden wedges were soaked in water before being driven

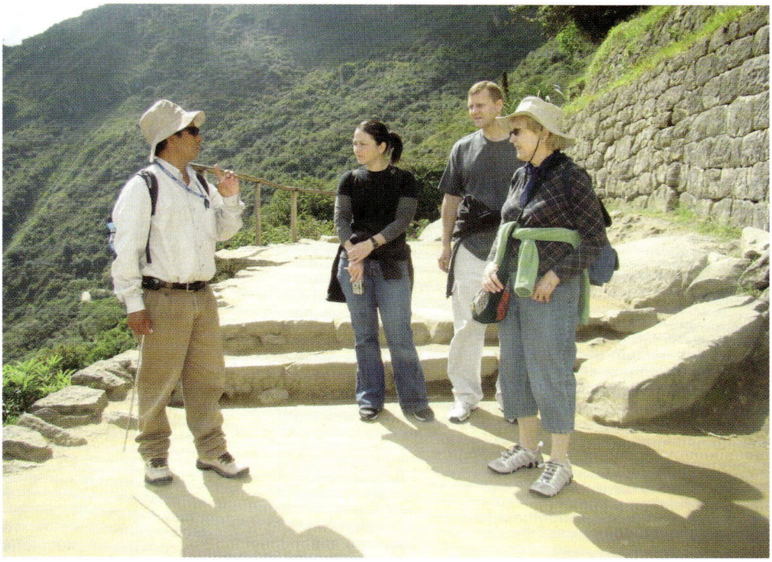

Figure 299. Three convalescents and our guide, Dimas; picture taken by a healthy person.

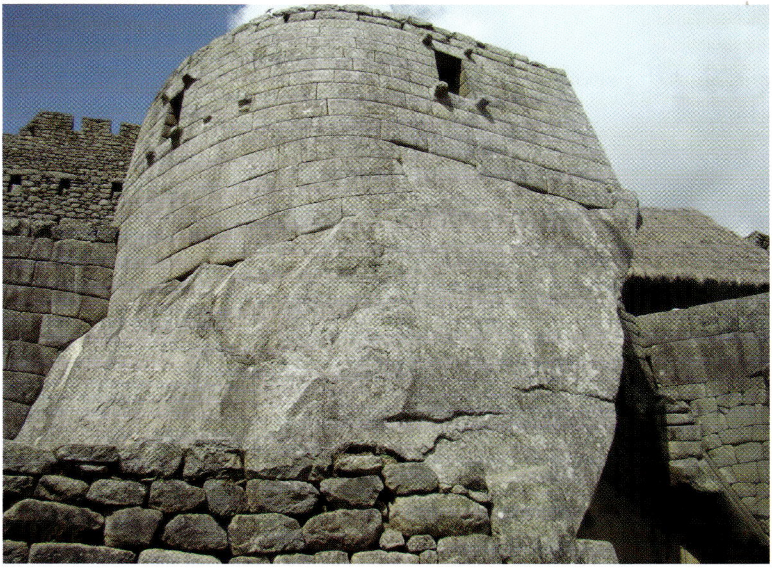

Figure 300. Machu Picchu's Temple of the Sun.

Vacations and Travel Unrelated to Business

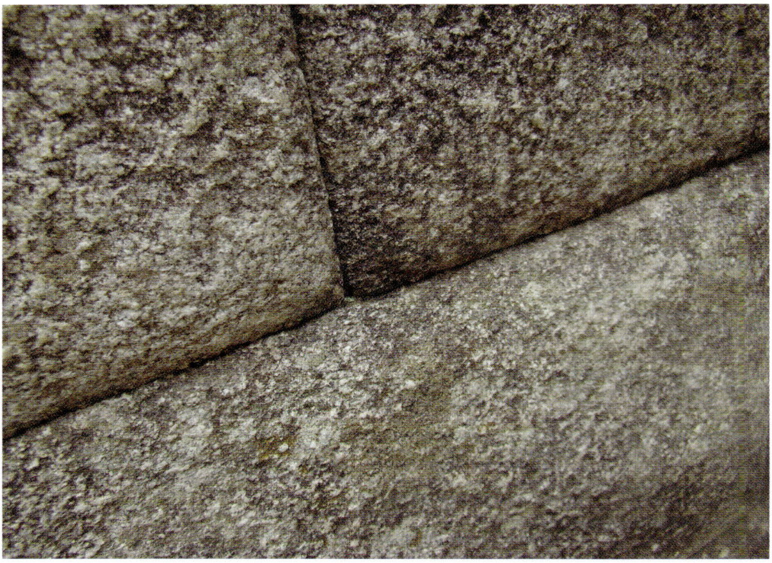

Figure 301. The Incas' impressively close-fitting stones.

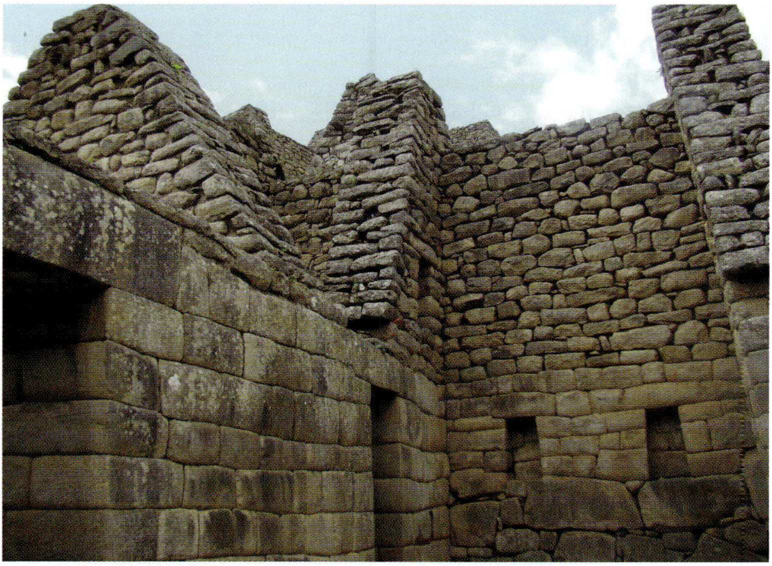

Figure 302. Windows and walls in Inca structures were typically sloped to mitigate the effects of earthquakes.

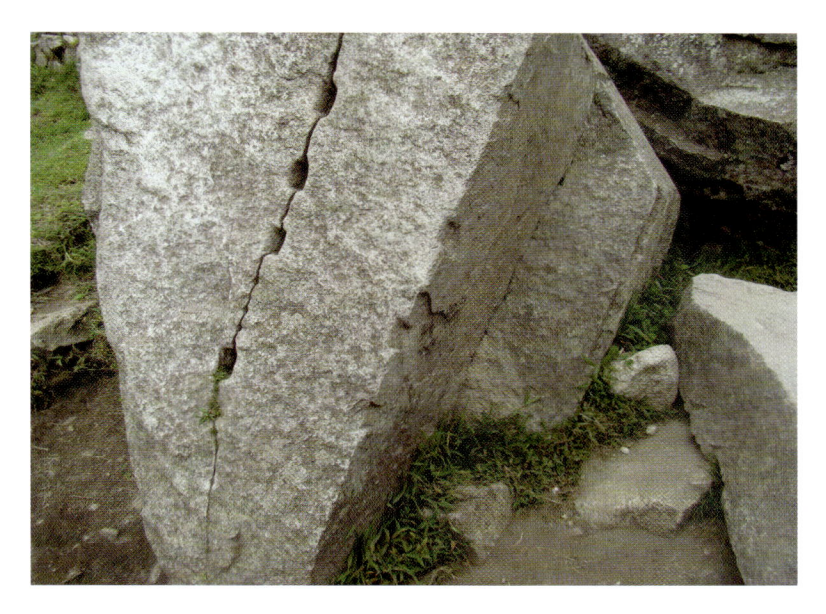

Figure 303. A method for splitting boulders: wedges of wood soaked in water and inserted into holes in the rock.

into holes made in the stone; the wedges would swell sufficiently to force the blocks to split. There were also some so-called "tired stones," large cut blocks that were abandoned en route to the site. We also saw the Intihuatana, or "Hitching Post of the Sun" (Fig. 304). Legend has it that the Incas would ritually "tie" the sun to pillars like this one on the solstice to bring the sun back. This was called Intiwatana ("tying of the sun"). The Incas used astronomy extensively for agricultural purposes. One of the last objects we saw was a "sacred rock" described as an "echo" of the peak behind. Unfortunately, because of clouds covering the peak, we could not appreciate its resemblance to the rock. Some believe that by touching the Sacred Rock, strength and vigor enters the body; Halina certainly needed to touch the Sacred Rock that day (Fig. 305). There is a trail built by the Incas that leads up the side of Wayna Picchu, or Huayna Pikchu ("Young Peak"), which rises over Machu Picchu, but we gave that a miss.

From Machu Picchu we returned by bus to Aquas Calientes. On the way we spotted high voltage power lines along the Urubamba River carrying electricity from the hydroelectric power

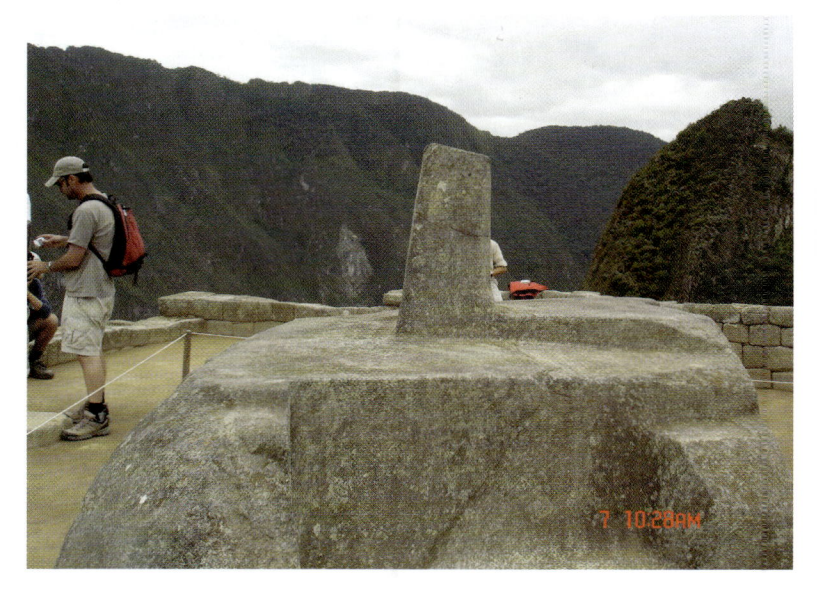

Figure 304. Intihuatana, meaning "Hitching Post of the Sun," one of three main structures at Machu Picchu.

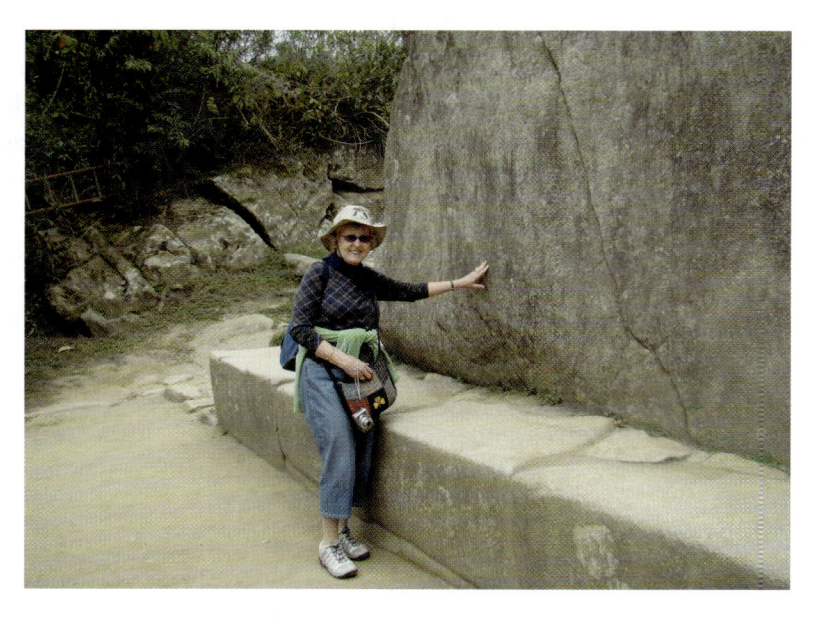

Figure 305. Halina receives energy through the Sacred Rock.

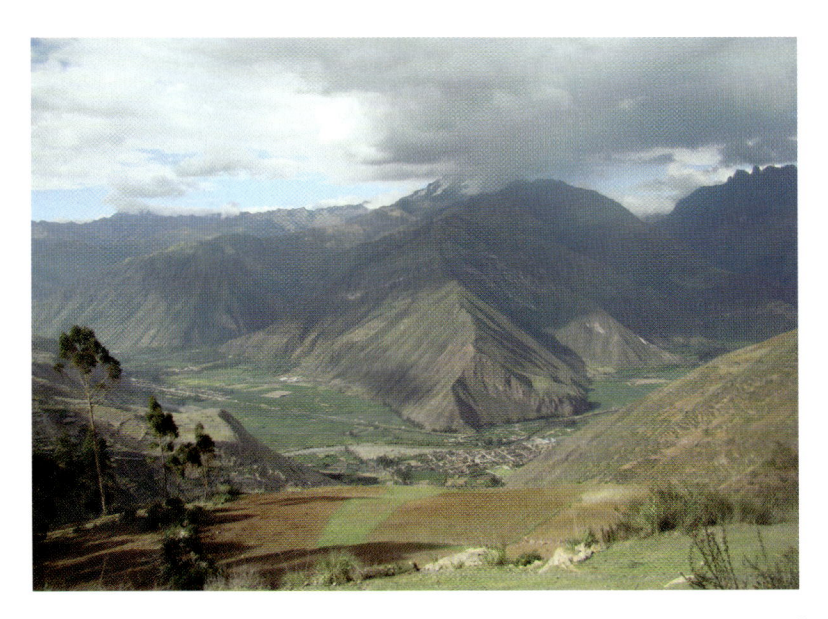

Figure 306. The small village of Chinchero viewed from the highest point on the road between Urubamba and Cusco.

station. The rest of our group, who had spent two days at Machu Picchu, met up with us at Aquas Calientes, and we took the train to Ollantaytambo, and then went by bus to Cusco. We made a stop at the highest point, about 12,800 feet (3,900 meters) above sea level, between Urubamba and Cusco, and took a picture of Chinchero, a small village perched on the high plains (Fig. 306). Chinchero is situated at too high an altitude for farmers to raise corn, lettuce or fruits, but they can grow potatoes and grain. The village was an early Inca center built by Emperor Tupa Inca as his country estate. During Inca reign, textiles were woven and offered to mark special occasions. For the people of this region, weaving is a way of life, as important for preserving ancient traditions as it is for earning a livelihood. Children grow up playing with their mother's spindle and loom. By age six or seven, most have learned to weave by watching their elders. We admired their craft when we visited Chinchero's weaving factory (Fig. 307), and Halina bought a scarf made of baby alpaca wool. Extremely fine and soft, the yarn has a diameter of just 21 to 23 microns.

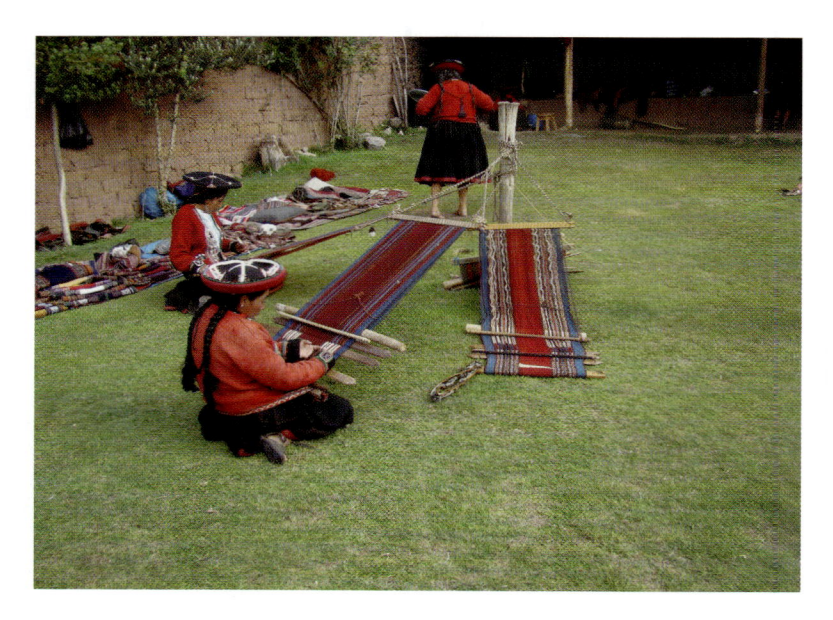

Figure 307. A weaving factory in Chinchero.

In Cusco we stayed at the San Agustin El Dorado hotel at Avenida Sol. That night I was punished for my cockiness and for not listening to my wife. Unlike Halina, who had taken acetazolamide over several days before going to Peru and advised me to do the same, I was so confident about my excellent cardiopulmonary health that I did not take any precautions. That night I could not fall asleep and felt short of breath; I had bradyarrhythmia and my pulse was below 40, sometimes only slightly above 30. In fact, my pulse had always been slow since my training as a runner, but it was usually in the mid-40s. As mentioned previously, I would sometimes have ventricular arrhythmia with rapid changes in time zone, but this time it was worse. I could feel my irregular heartbeat — and sometimes there was no heartbeat for as long as four seconds. With these very upsetting symptoms, it was impossible to fall asleep. The symptoms were somewhat atypical for altitude sickness, but I could see no other reason.

I did not sleep at all that night; most of the time I had to sit upright. It was obviously too late for acetazolamide; there was *mate de coca* (coca tea) but that did not work for me. There was also some oxygen at reception that could be taken for 10 minutes, but I decided not to try it. By morning I had come to the conclusion that I needed to treat the bradycardia by blocking the parasympathetic system with atropine. We found a pharmacy near our hotel, and with some difficulty because of the language barrier, I managed to buy antispasmodic tablets containing atropine and papaverine. I took one tablet in the morning and my pulse increased to almost 50. The arrhythmia disappeared and I felt OK. Staying in Cusco, I took one tablet three times daily and had no further problems the following nights. I am still not sure whether I really had altitude sickness or something else, but it did not matter. The most important thing was that by blocking the parasympathetic receptors the atropine worked its magic on me.

Cusco was the capital of the Inca Empire. Many believe that the city was planned to be shaped like a puma. According to Inca legend, Sapa Inca Pachacuti transformed the Kingdom of Cusco from a sleepy city-state into a vast empire. Cusco also has a rich history of Incan art. Ceramic objects made and used in Cusco are known under the rubric of the Cusco Inca style. Pottery was considered a prestige ware and was closely associated with the fine craftsmanship and status of the capital. The first Spaniards arrived in the city on November 15, 1533, but the date of the official discovery by Francisco Pizarro is recorded as March 23, 1534. He named it the "very noble and great city of Cusco." The many buildings constructed after the Spanish conquest, including the Santa Clara and San Blas barrios, are a mix of Inca architecture and Spanish influence. In essence, the Spanish undertook the construction of a new city on the foundations of the old Inca city, replacing temples with churches and palaces with mansions for the *conquistadors*. During the period of colonization, Cusco was very prosperous thanks to agriculture, cattle raising, mining and trade with Spain. This allowed the construction of many churches and convents, and even a cathedral, a university and an archbishopric. Often, Spanish buildings were juxtaposed atop the massive stone walls built by the Inca. Cusco has several sister cities, including New Jersey, Santa Barbara and Kraków, Poland.

On the morning of December 8, we had some free time so we did some sightseeing in Cusco. We went to the Plaza de Armas (Market Square), visited Cusco Cathedral and Iglesia de la Compañia de Jesús (the Jesuit Church), and walked through Rio Mantas and other streets

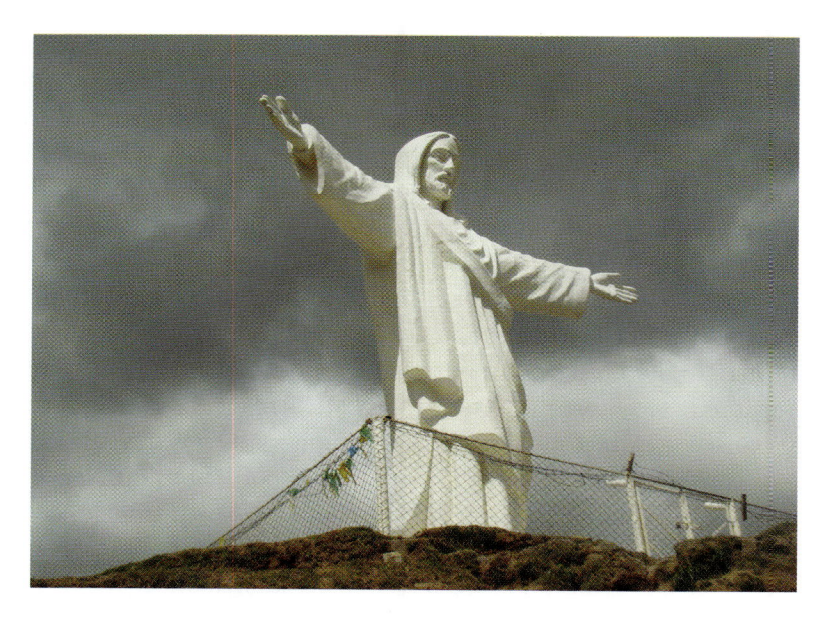

Figure 308. A statue of Christ overlooking Cusco.

in the city. We found out that Mass in the local Jesuit Church was at 6 and 7 pm. In the early afternoon our tour bus took us to Sacsayhuamán (also known as Saqsaywaman, Sacsahuaman or Saxahuaman, and pronounced "sexy woman," according to our guide), a nearby walled complex. The site, which is situated at an altitude of 12,140 feet (3,700 meters), was added to the UNESCO World Heritage List in 1983. I was again impressed with the Incas' stonework. The stones were fitted tightly within the walls, but they were semicircular in shape, for some reason, on the outside. Near the fortress is a huge white statue of Christ overlooking Cusco (Fig. 308).

Our next stop was the oldest parish in Cusco, San Blas Church, which was built in 1563. The San Blas barrio is a mixture of old Inca buildings and Spanish mansions. On the way, we dropped into Sumac Alpaca, a shop selling traditional baby alpaca products, and Halina bought a very nice sweater. The San Blas Church's most impressive feature is a pulpit carved from a single piece of wood; its creator, Diego Tomas de Cerda, worked on it for 20 years. Unfortunately, it was not possible to take photos inside the church. Afterwards, we visited the Santo Domingo Convent, which was built on top of the

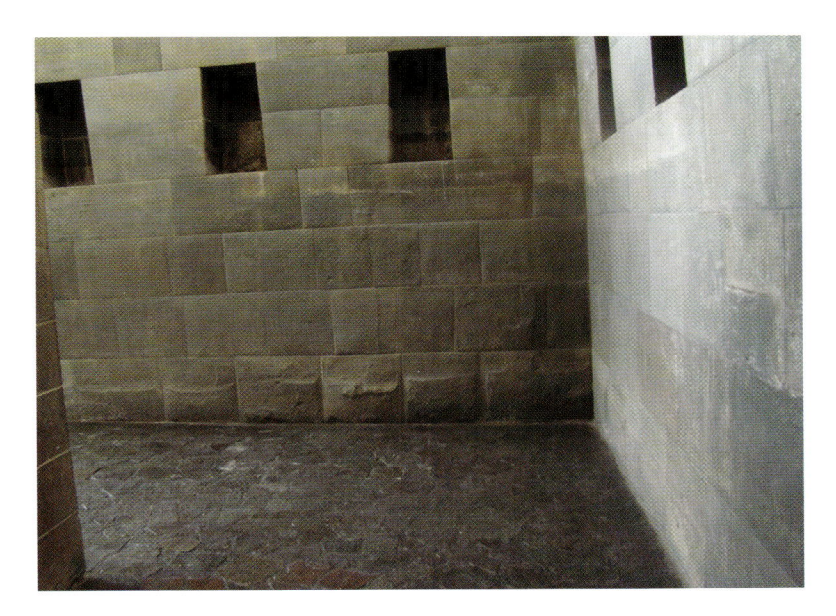

Figure 309. The large square-cut stones of the Coricancha.

Coricancha, or Qorikancha (Temple of the Sun). When the Spaniards conquered the Inca Empire, they used the fine Inca stonework to form the base of the Church of Santo Domingo. The Coricancha is a fine example of how the fusion of Inca and colonial styles evolved into the unique architecture of Cusco today. It was built mostly by means of ashlar or dressed blocks, rectangular blocks with smooth faces (Fig. 309). We first went to the cloister and then to the Coricancha. Similar to what we saw in Machu Picchu, the walls here were sloped. A major earthquake in 1950 seriously damaged the Dominican Priory and Church of Santo Domingo, but the masonry of the Coricancha survived unscathed. The rooms were once adorned with elaborate gold ceremonial objects. Immediately after conquering Cusco, the Spaniards started stripping the gold from the temples and melting it down. It is said that it took three months to cart all of the gold out of the temple. Only one huge gold disc, considered sacred, was not destroyed (Fig. 310). Our last stop that day was a Catholic orphanage that was doing a wonderful job of taking care of and educating orphaned children. As our guide, Miluska, had clearly intended by making the visit, we made some donations. We got back to our hotel

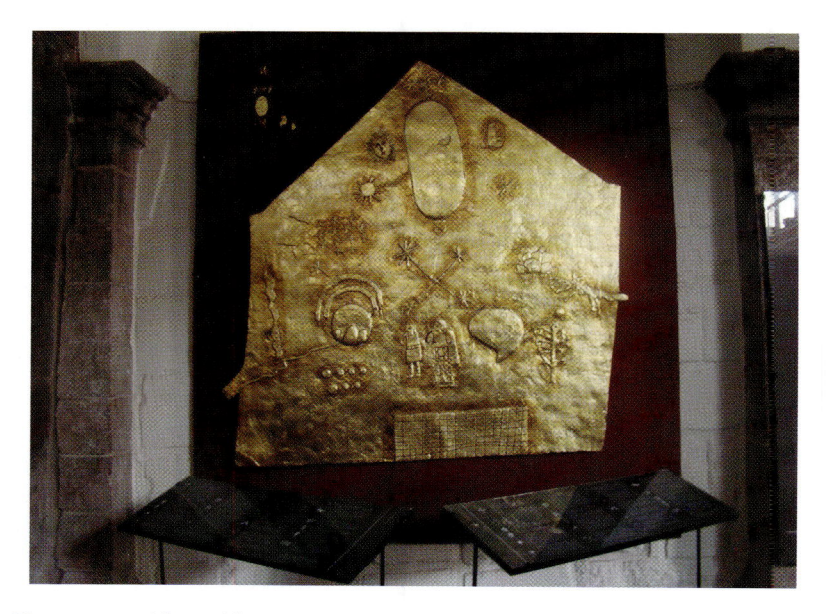

Figure 310. The Golden Sun Disk, a sacred object of the Incas in the Coricancha.

at around 6 pm so we were able to attend Mass an hour later at the Jesuit Church.

On Sunday, December 9, we first stopped at San Pedro de Andahuaylillas, 22 miles (36 km) from Cusco, en route to Puno. Built in 1580, the Catholic church was constructed on the site of an ancient Inca temple. Despite its rather modest external architecture, it is considered by some to be the "Sistine Chapel of the Americas"[56] because of the beauty of its mural painting. One of the murals, which was created by Luis de Riaño at the beginning of 17th century, represents the path to glory and the path to hell. He was also said to be the creator of an important oil painting of the archangel San Miguel. There is a painting by the Spanish painter Esteban Murillo called *La Asunción de la Virgen*. The church also contains a magnificent piano, baroque altars and numerous canvases of the Academy of Cusco. Photos of the interior were not allowed.

---

56. We visited the Sistine Chapel in the Vatican 20 years ago, and in my opinion, this cognomen of the San Pedro Church is an exaggeration. When we saw the Sistine Chapel, the famous frescoes had only been partly restored, but what we did see was absolutely breathtaking.

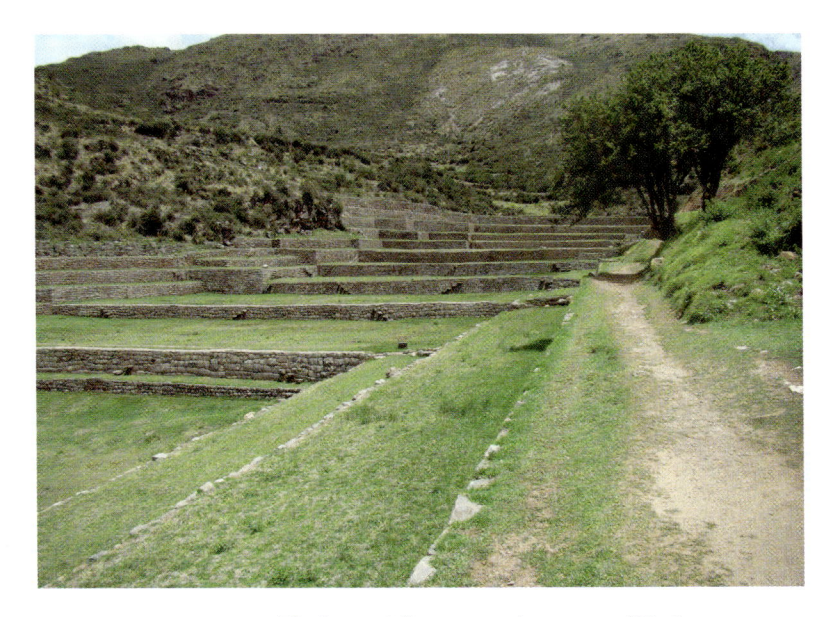

Figure 311. The beautifully preserved terraces of Tipón.

Later that morning we went to Tipón, an Incan site with elaborate agricultural terraces that ascend the steep and narrow valley, irrigated in ancient times by an aqueduct from the mountaintop. This old town is located 15 miles (23 km) southeast of Cusco at a height of 11,684 feet (3,560 meters) above sea level; the highest area of the park is found at the pass of Ranraq'asa above 12,487 feet (3,800 meters). The amazing site is located over a very irregular surface: with no available flatlands, the inhabitants had to create terraces suitable for agriculture (Fig. 311). The Incas achieved an impressive level of architectural development, especially with regard to their hydraulic constructions. Every complex featured elaborately designed canals that channeled water around the site (Fig. 312), and some of the canals are still used today to provide the inhabitants of the area with water. In addition to terraces and aqueducts, there are remnants of walls and houses. The stonework was not as precise as in the temples so mortar was used (Fig. 313). The next day we had some free time, so we wandered around Cusco, and in the evening we had a dinner organized by Coltur at the Tunupa

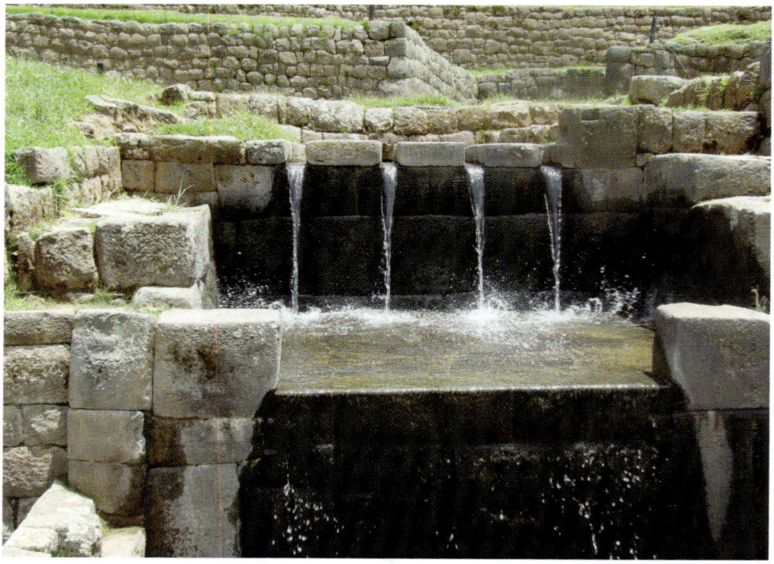

Figure 312. According to historian Luis Antonio Pardo, the name Tipón may come from the Quechua word *Timpuj*, meaning "to be boiling," which relates to the water flowing from the mountains as if the liquid were boiling.

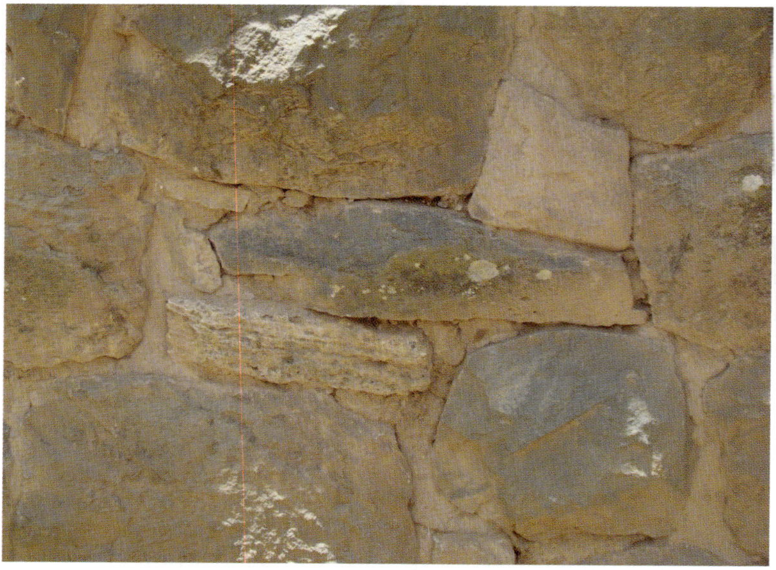

Figure 313. Mortar was used where the stonework was less precise.

Restaurant that included Andean music and dance. Our journey back to the U.S. began on December 11 with our return flight to Lima, where we had a day-use room at the San Agustin Exclusive Hotel. At 10 pm we were taken to the airport to catch our 1:30 am flight to Atlanta, followed by another flight to St. Louis and finally the MoX minibus to Columbia, arriving at 2:30 pm the next day. Altogether, it was a satisfying tour and a thoroughly enjoyable time in Peru.

2008 — Adam and his friends in Kraków, touring London, our golden wedding anniversary, and a pilgrimage to Turkey

In 2008 we arrived in Kraków on May 21. Shortly after, on July 2, Adam and his friends Thomas Johnson and Clay Feldner came to visit. This time we did not go sightseeing with them, as we had already seen the various places of interest several times. Instead, Adam did his turn as a guide on their visits to the Wieliczka Salt Mine, the Auschwitz-Birkenau State Museum, Nowa Huta, and Warsaw. At the time I was going for regular bike rides on the Vistula Boulevard, and they decided to cycle with me to the Benedictine Abbey in Tyniec, situated on the right bank of the Vistula River, about 7.5 miles (12 km) from our apartment near Wawel Castle. The abbey, founded in 1044 by Prince Casimir I the Restorer, then ruler of Poland, is beautifully located on a limestone hill with the Vistula River below. Throughout history the abbey was destroyed and rebuilt many times. Mongols burnt it down in the 12th century, Swedes in the 17th century, and Russians in the 18th century, when the abbey was a crucial stronghold of the first Polish national uprising under the command of Thaddeus Kosciuszko. The abbey has recently been renovated and it now hosts concerts in the summer. There is a little store where you can buy wonderful products manufactured by the friars, like jams (cherries and rum, "fruits of the forest" with vodka, black currant), very good beer, and mead made of fermented honey. The boys returned to Bismarck on July 14.

On July 29, we went to London for a couple of days, departing at 11:40 am from Kraków on BA2775. Arriving at 13:10 pm at London Gatwick, we checked in to the nearby Hotel Sofitel. The next day we went by train to Harrods, the U.K. capital's famous department store on Brompton Road in Knightsbridge that specializes in luxury goods. By the following day, we were already back in Kraków. The reason for going to London was because of the issue of staying in Poland on U.S. passports for more than 90 days. We could not go to Slovakia as we had previously, because by that time the country was part of the Schengen Area (which represents that part of Europe, then 26 countries, for which there are border controls for those traveling in and out of the area, but with no internal border controls). The U.K. is outside that area, so going there allowed us to get new stamps in our passports. This turned out to be the last time we would make such a trip, because we found out that one may arrive in Poland on a Polish passport and return to the U.S. on an American one. We could obtain Polish passports based on our previous passports issued by the Consulate General of the Republic of Poland and our *dowody osobiste* (Polish identity cards).

We decided we would celebrate our golden wedding anniversary — 50 years of marriage — more than once, as we had been apart for our silver wedding anniversary. At that time, in 1983, I had to be in Columbia, while Halina was in Kraków. This time, another 25 years on, we were together. On August 9, friends joined us for Mass at the Church of St. Nicholas, where we were married. We then invited our friends to the wonderful Wierzynek Restaurant in the heart of Kraków's Old Town. The second celebration, on August 31, was for family, including our son Przemek and his wife, Kasia, her parents, my brother and his family, and Halina's family. We again attended Mass in the St. Nicholas Church and again went to the Wierzynek Restaurant. The atmosphere was jovial and good-humored. My brother's wife, Marysia, told a joke about a couple that died after their 50th wedding anniversary (Fig. 314). The wife passed away first, and when her husband died, he went to heaven and started to look for her. He first looked among the saints, but she was not there, so he looked among the blessed, and then among the pious and the devout, but to no avail. So he asked St. Peter where his wife could be. "How many years were you married?" asked St. Peter. "50 years," came the answer. St. Peter responded, "So you must look among the martyrs!" I also recited one of Adam Mickiewicz's famous ballads, *Pani Twardowska*

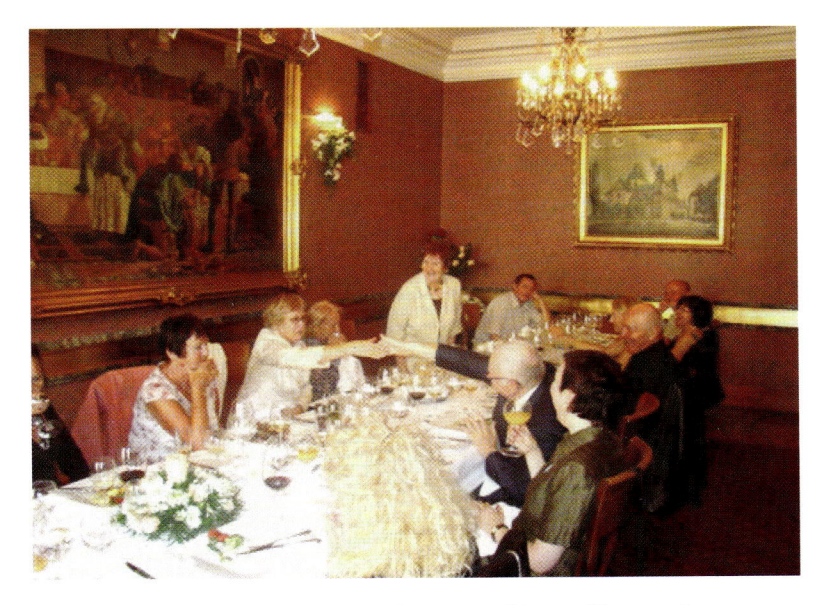

Figure 314. Marysia relates a joke at our golden wedding anniversary.

(Mrs. Twardowska),[57] which could be considered an allusion to my wife, but everybody knew that I was joking and that Halina bore no resemblance to the wife of Mr. Twardowski, the magician (Fig. 315). It is not too difficult to imagine that the restaurant bill was a little higher than the US$20 it had cost two decades earlier.

From September 8 to 19 we went on a pilgrimage to Turkey called "In the Footsteps of St. Paul and St. John," which was organized by the La Salette Pilgrimage Ministry. From Warsaw-Okęcie Airport, we flew to Atatürk International Airport and checked in to the Crystal Hotel in Istanbul. Traveling by bus, we were to visit Istanbul, Ankara, Cappadocia, Antioch, Antalya, Pamukkale, Ephesus, Miletus and

---

57. The story has it that Mrs. Twardowska was a terrible wife. In the ballad, when Mephistopheles came to an inn called "Rzym" to claim his soul, Mr. Twardowski presented a contract in which it was clearly stated that the soul might be taken on the condition that three difficult tasks be fulfilled. The first, to change a painting of a horse into a real horse, was a simple matter for the Devil. The second was markedly tougher: to bathe in holy water, but the Devil did it. The third task was the toughest of all: the Devil had to live with Mrs. Twardowska as husband and wife for one whole year. The final task turned out to be beyond the Devil's ability; he escaped and Mr. Twardowski saved his soul.

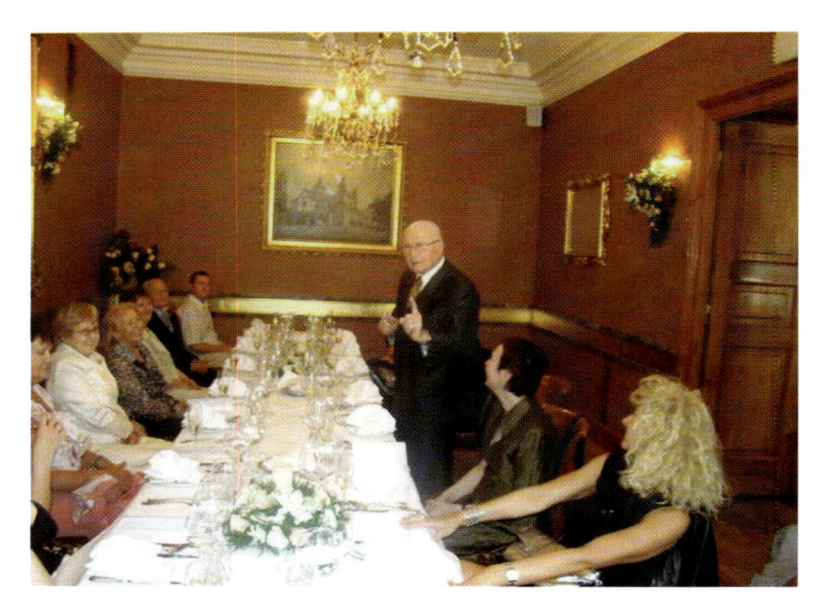

Figure 315. The author recites the ballad *Pani Twardowska*.

Çanakkale, before returning to Istanbul (Fig. 316). The European part of Turkey is called Rumelia (Turkish: *Rumeli*, meaning "land of the Romans"). Each morning began with Mass and thereafter we visited places of interest. I already described many of these when I talked about my visit to Istanbul in May 2007. This time we visited fewer places than I saw previously. As is typical for tours, we started with the Hippodrome and then went to the Hagia Sophia (Fig. 317), the Blue Mosque and the Basilica Cistern. The Topkapi Palace was closed that day. The following day, after Mass and breakfast, we drove to Ankara to see the Museum of Anatolian Civilizations and then to the Hotel Perissia in Ürgüp, a little town in the center of Cappadocia.

The Asian part of Turkey was referred to as "Anatolia" by the Greeks, and that name has been retained to this day. The Romans called it "Asia Minor" (Lesser Asia). A broad peninsula surrounded by the Mediterranean, Black Sea and Aegean Sea, it is also bordered by the Dardanelles strait, the Sea of Marmara and the Bosporus strait to the northwest. The history of Anatolia is just as convoluted as all the other regions of the Middle East. The people known as the Hattis are amongst the first settlers in Anatolian history. They ruled Central

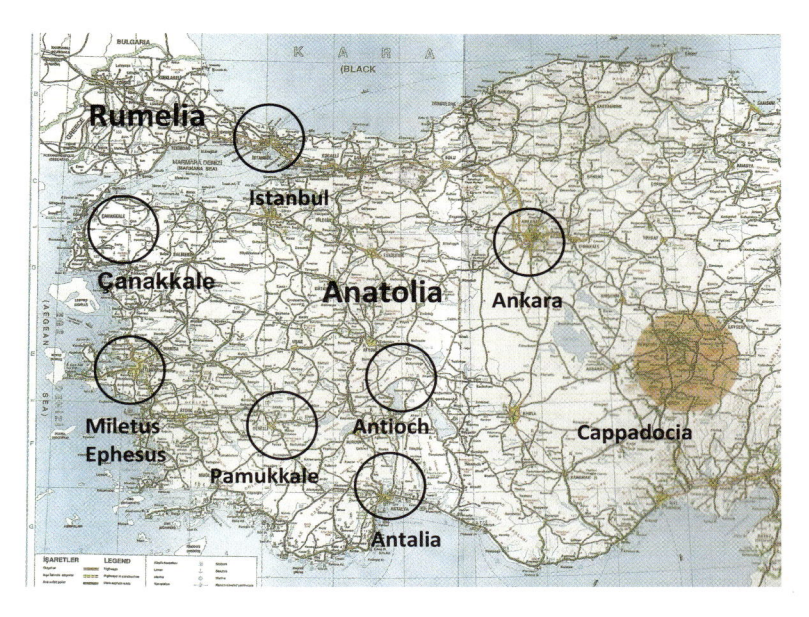

Figure 316. The itinerary for our pilgrimage to Turkey.

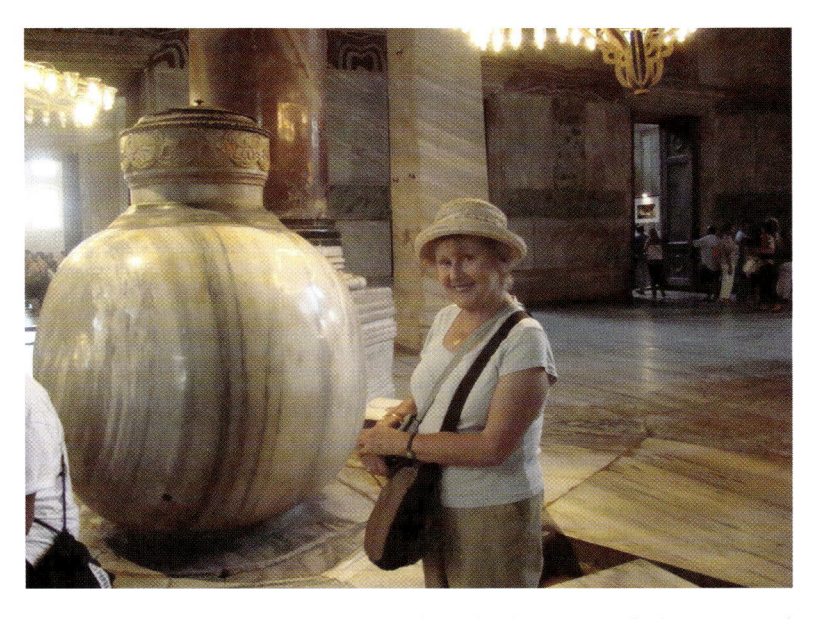

Figure 317. Carved from a single block of marble, this vase inside the Hagia Sophia was brought from Pergamum during the reign of Murat III (1576–1595).

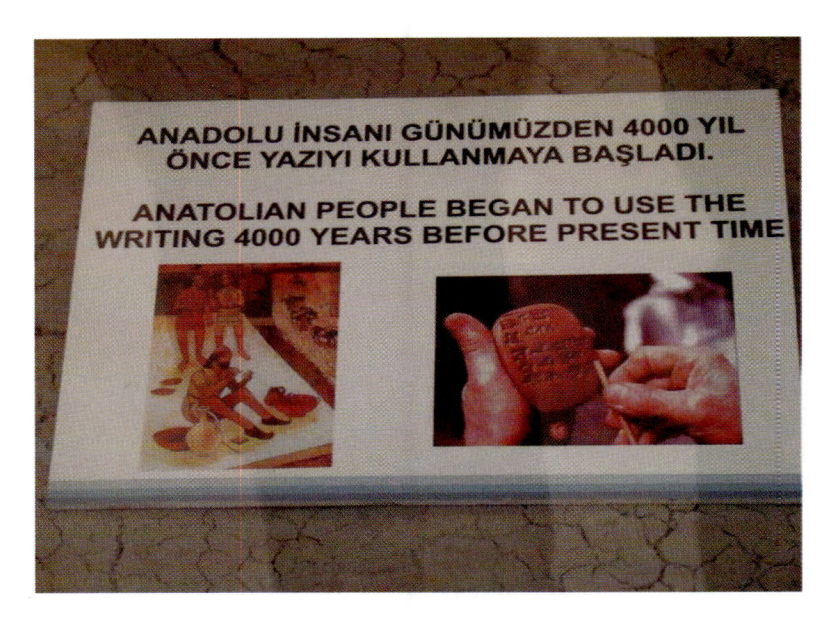

Figure 318.   Cuneiform writing.

Anatolia from 2500 BC to 2000 BC. There are signs of Mesopotamian influence on Hatti art and culture. Cuneiform writing, which is on display in the Museum of Anatolian Civilizations (Fig. 318), also came from Mesopotamia. The ancient Anatolians believed in a number of gods representing various acts of Nature in the form of animals, such as the bull and the stag. Of great importance was Earth Mother (Cybele, Kubaba or Hebat), similar to the Greek Gaia or the Incan Panchamama.

In about 2000 BC, a large-scale migration took place mainly from cold Europe to the mild weathered south, mainly through the area east of the Black Sea. The Hittites, one of the dominant groups of Indo-European people, settled alongside the existing people and in time established their own settlements. Instead of seeking to destroy the existing people and their cities, they mixed with the Hattis and other peoples of Anatolia. They even shared their gods, goddesses, art, culture, writing and a large proportion of words from their language. Their civilization would eventually rival that of the Egyptians and Babylonians. In the 12th century BC their empire fell to the Assyrians from the east. In the west, close to the Aegean Sea, small seaboard states sprang up, settled by the Greeks, who colonized the entire coast by around the 8th century BC. In 560 BC, Croesus, who was known for his wealth, mounted the throne of Lydia on the Mediterranean Sea coast and soon brought all the Greek colonies under his rule. He was overthrown by Cyrus the Great of Persia after just 13 years of rule, and it would be another two hundred years before Alexander the Great would again spread Greek influence over the peninsula. After its conquest by Rome in the second century BC, Anatolia enjoyed centuries of peace. During the Middle Ages, as a part of the Byzantine Empire, it became a center of Christianity and the guardian of Greek and Roman culture. It was mainly for this reason that we undertook this pilgrimage. As the power of the Empire declined, Arabs and Mongols invaded. In the 11th century, the Seljuk Turks came from Central Asia through Persia and established a government in Central Anatolia. In the 13th century the Ottoman Turks, also from Persia, started to take control of the peninsula and by the 15th century they had made Istanbul — then known as Constantinople — the capital. The Ottoman Empire became one of the largest and longest lasting empires in history, and it was not until 1923 that Anatolia became the larger part of the Turkish Republic. Kemal Atatürk, president of the newly minted state, set up his government in Ankara, which subsequently became the new capital.

On the morning of September 11, we enjoyed the amazing panorama of Cappadocia and the natural rock citadel of Uçhisar (Fig. 319), which is the area's highest point. Between two and ten million years ago, lava flows from the region's active volcanoes formed layers of tuff composed of ignimbrite, soft tufa, lahar (mudflow), ash (silica), clay (aluminum silicate), sandstone (silicon dioxide), calcium carbonate and basalt. Due to the different hardnesses of these materials, over the millennia the action of rainwater carved the rocks into a multitude of astonishing shapes, like chimneys (Fig. 320) and mushrooms. The Göreme Open Air Museum in the Göreme Valley (Fig. 321), where we went next, is famous for its rock-cut churches and colorful frescoes. The churches followed the rules laid down by St. Basil the Great, the Bishop of Caesarea Mazaca in the 4th century. Afterwards, we went to see an onyx factory, which produced various carved items and jewellery from the semiprecious stone, a form of quartz that comes in a whole host of different colors. In this particular factory, they were

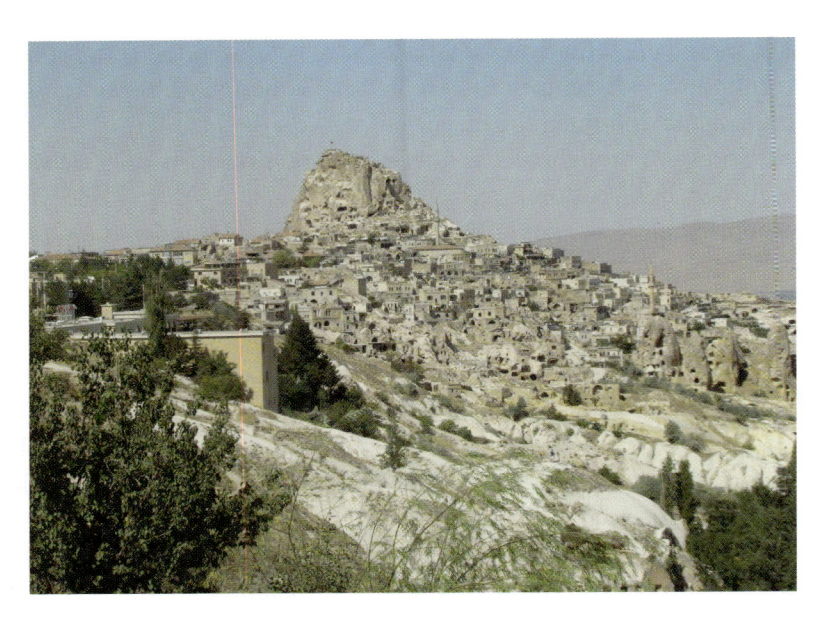

Figure 319. The natural rock citadel of Uçhisar.

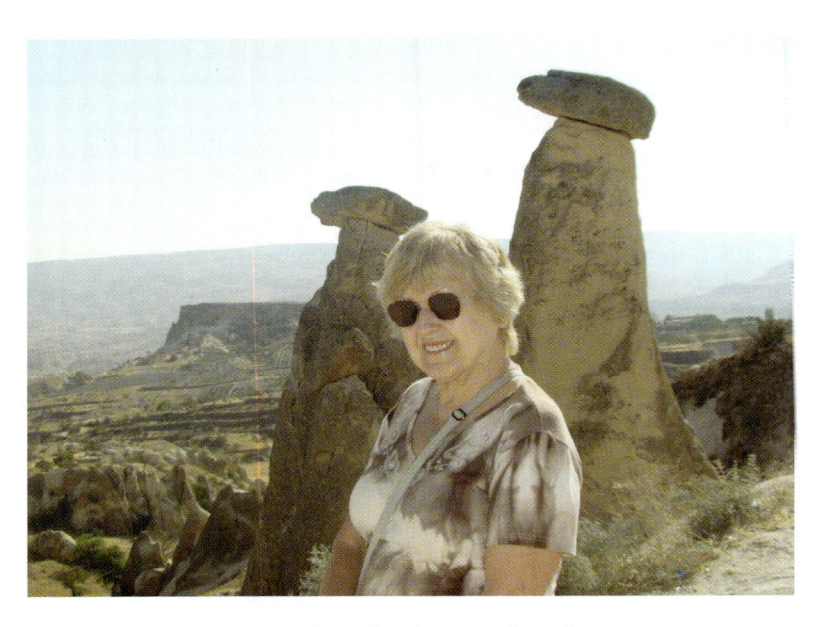

Figure 320. Cappadocia's strange fairy chimneys.

552 Around the World with Nephrology

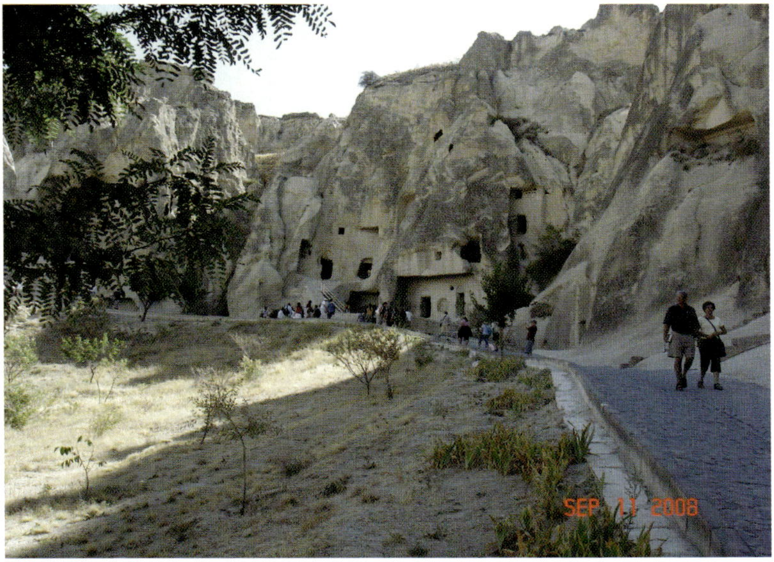

Figure 321. The Göreme Open Air Museum, famous for its rock-cut churches.

working with white onyx, and we were shown how onyx eggs were produced. We were given the opportunity to win an egg if we answered a question correctly. The question was: *What is the capital of Turkey?* With the question being in English — and being one of the few English speakers in the group — I quickly answered, "Ankara!" It was evidently supposed to be a trick question, as many tourists think that the capital is Istanbul. In any event, I won the prize (Fig. 322). After our little quiz, we headed to Paşabağı, or Monks Valley, five minutes by bus from Göreme. As well as mushroom shaped fairy-chimneys (Fig. 323), Paşabağı has a chapel dedicated to a 5th-century hermit named St. Simeon (Simon), who fashioned a shelter for himself by carving into the rock. In the evening we returned to our hotel in Ürgüp.

The next day, we drove to Antalya. On the way we stopped at the Pisidian Antioch, which was founded by Seleucus I Nicator and named in honor of his father, Antiochus. It is situated in Phrygia, not far from Pisidia, and was therefore called Pisidian Antioch to distinguish it from the other cities of the same name. Paul and Barnabas preached in the synagogue there on their first missionary journey; but

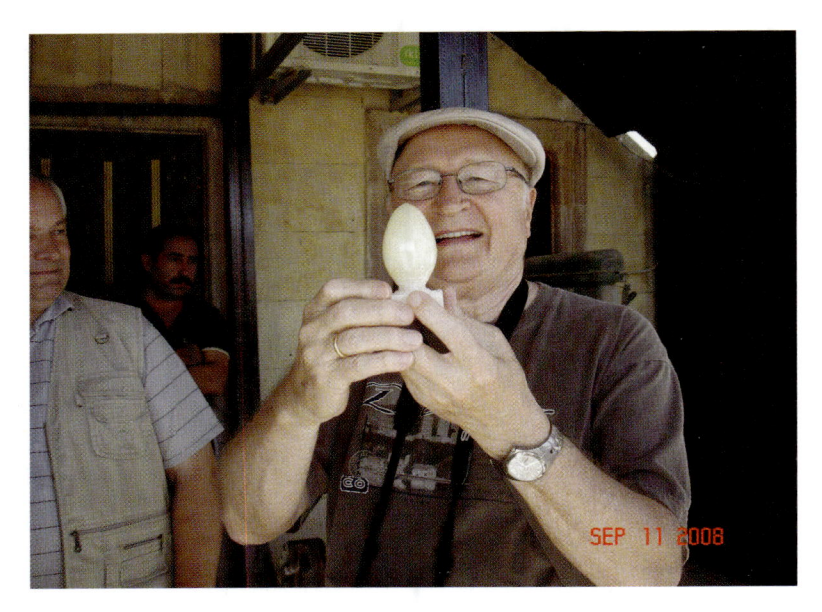

Figure 322. The winner of an onyx egg.

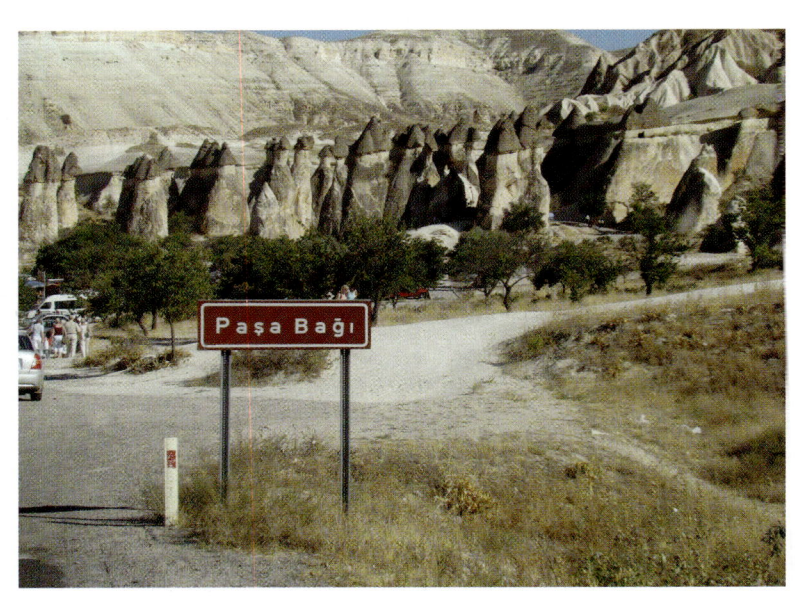

Figure 323. Mushroom shaped fairy chimneys in Paşabağı.

the Jews, resentful of the many conversions of Gentiles, drove the missionaries from the city to Iconium and followed them even to Lystra (Acts 13:14–14:19). In Antioch we visited the ruins of the Great Basilica (St. Bassus Church), which was built in 4th century. We also stopped at Lake Eğirdir, the second largest freshwater lake in the country, before reaching in Antalya in the evening. Situated at the Mediterranean coast of southwestern Turkey, Antalya is the capital city of Antalya Province. In 150 BC Attalos II, King of Pergamum, founded the city he called Attalia as a base for his powerful naval fleet. In 133 BC it became part of the Roman Republic with the death of King Attalos III of Pergamum, who left his kingdom to Rome in his will. The city grew and prospered in the Ancient Roman period. Paul of Tarsus visited Antalya, as recorded in the Acts of the Apostles (Acts 14:25–26), wherein it is referred to as Attalia. St. Paul and St. Barnabas went to Antalya and from there to Antioch after preaching in Pisidia and Pamphylia. Christianity started to spread in the region after the second century.

The next day we visited the nearby sites of Perge, Aspendos and Side. Perga, now commonly spelled "Perge" and pronounced *per-geh*, was the capital of a region called Pamphylia, meaning "land of the tribes." Today it is a large site of ancient ruins on the coastal plains, about 9 miles (15 km) east of Antalya. In the 12th century BC, there was a large wave of Greek migration from northern Anatolia to an area that came to be known as Pamphylia, the modern-day Antalya Province. Four great cities eventually rose to prominence in Pamphylia: Perga, Sillyon, Aspendos and Side. Located nearly 12 miles (20 km) inland, Perga was situated inland as a defensive measure in order to avoid the pirate bands that terrorized this stretch of the Mediterranean. In 546 BC, the Achaemenid Persians defeated the local powers and gained control of the region. Two hundred years later, in 333 BC, the armies of Alexander the Great arrived in Perga during his war of conquest against the Persians. The citizens of Perga sent out guides to lead his army into the city. Alexander's was followed by the Diadoch Empire of the Seleucids. Roman rule began in 188 BC, and most of the surviving ruins today date from this period. After the collapse of the Roman Empire, Perga remained inhabited until Seljuk times, before being gradually abandoned. A notable historical figure who visited Perga was

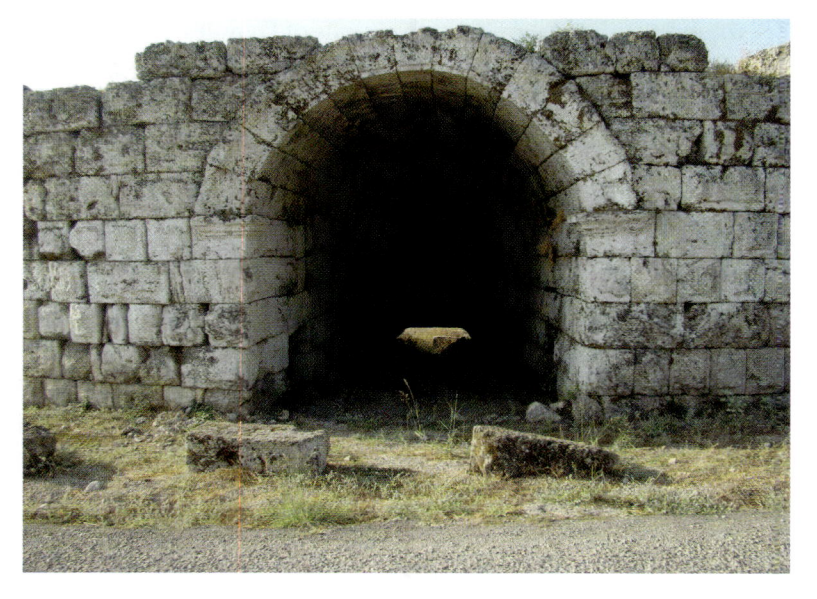

Figure 324. The entrance to the Stadium, a typical Roman arch in Perge.

St. Paul the Apostle and his companion St. Barnabas, as recorded in the Acts of the Apostles (Acts 13:13–14 and 14:25), during their first missionary journey, where they "preached the word" (Acts 14:25) before heading through Attalia (modern-day Antalya city) to Antioch.

The Perge of today is an archeological treasure and a major tourist attraction. Some of the ruins we visited included the Theater, the Stadium (Fig. 324), the Hellenistic Gate, the Roman Gate and the Agora (Fig. 325). We also saw the ancient city's colonnaded street, which has the Nympheum at one end and the Acropolis above, divided by a canal that supplied the water needs of its citizens. Our next stop was Aspendos, whose history is similar to that of Perga. Aspendos is known for having one of the best-preserved ancient theaters on the Mediterranean. Built in 155 AD by the Greek architect Zenon, a citizen of Aspendos, during the rule of Marcus Aurelius, the theater provided seating for 7,000 and had a diameter of some 315 feet (96 meters). It was periodically repaired by the Seljuks, who used it as a caravanserai. In order to keep with Hellenistic traditions, a small part of the theater was built so that it leaned against the hill, while the remainder was built on vaulted arches (Fig. 326). For me the most

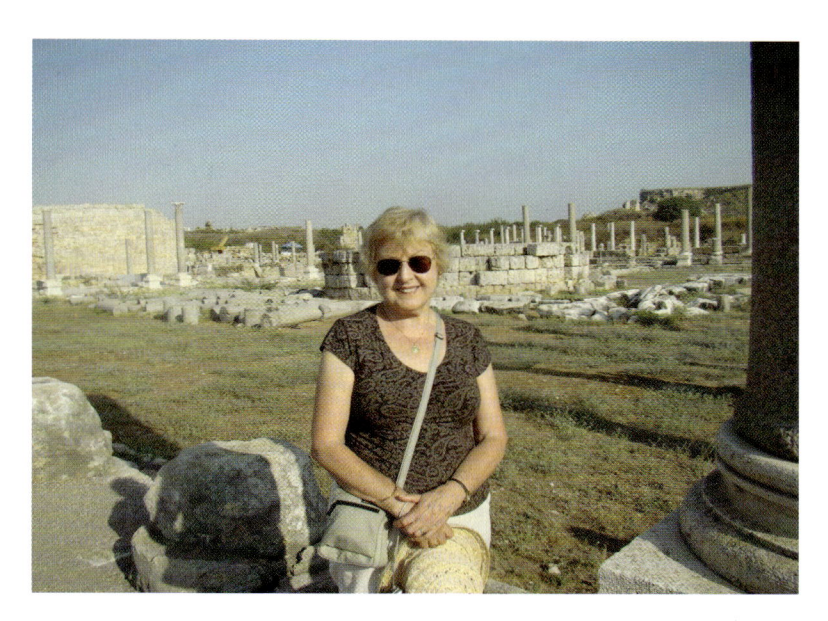

Figure 325. A round structure in the Agora is dedicated to Hermes (the god of trade) or Tyche (the goddess of fortune).

amazing feature was the acoustics, which was typical for Roman theaters: a whisper on the stage could be heard under the vault. The final stop that day was Side, whose early history was similar to that of Perge and Aspendos. Side, however, was a port and in the first century BC misfortune overtook Side in the form of Cilician pirates, who seized the city and turned it into a naval base and slave market. The people of Side apparently tolerated the pirates because of the highly profitable nature of their trade, but the activities gave the city a bad name in the region. Rome tolerated Side's pirates for some time, but they eventually began disrupting commerce in the Mediterranean and the delivery of grain to Rome. Ultimately, the Roman Senate decided to deal with the pirates. In 67 BC the famous Roman general Pompey was sent to end the reign of the pirates in Side and Cilicia. He duly did so, and statues and monuments were erected in his honor. Some say that by honoring Pompey, the people of Side were attempting to erase the city's bad name. We entered the city through a gate with columns of emperors Vespasian and Titus of the Flavian family, known for the construction of many buildings, including the Colosseum, but also for

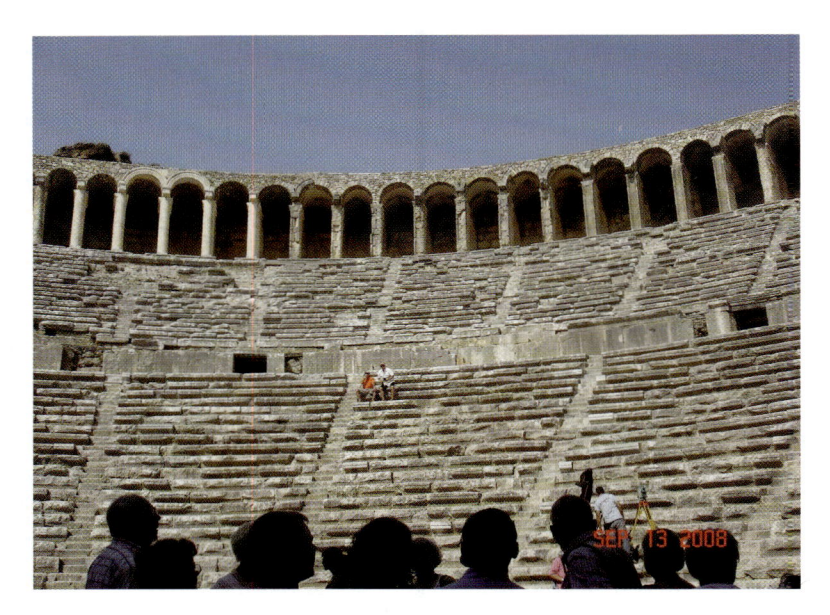

Figure 326. The theater at Aspendos.

the famous exchange between them that ended in an adage "*Pecunia non olet, Tite*" (Money does not stink, Titus).[58] We also saw Side's Theater. There were no monuments of Pompey to be seen. Our guide told us that, over the ages, they had all been destroyed.

The next day we drove to the Lycus River Valley area called Pamukkale (meaning "Cotton Castle" in Turkish), home to the three cities of Colossae, Laodycea and Hierapolis. When we arrived at Colossae, I set out to look for some giant monuments, as I thought that the name came from some colossus like that of Rhodes or a huge building like the Colosseum. But there was nothing like that, so I assumed that they had been destroyed during the earthquake that hit in the first century during the reign of Nero. To my great surprise, I learned that the name comes from the purple color (*colossinus*)

---

58. Emperor Vespasian levied a tax upon the distribution of urine. It applied to all public toilets within Rome's now famous Cloaca Maxima (great sewer) system. The lower classes of Roman society urinated into pots, which were emptied into cesspools. The liquid was then collected from public latrines, where it was sold and served as the valuable raw material for a number of chemical processes. The Roman historian Suetonius reported that when Vespasian's son Titus complained to him about the stinky nature of the tax, his father held up a gold coin and told him this adage.

made from the juice of the madder root and used to dye wool. Later, however, I found a text by Antonio Telesio of Cosenza from 1524 stating that the color "[c]olossinus is named after the Trojan city of Colossae, where wool is dyed in a way that recalls the cyclamen flower." Thus, it is not entirely clear which name came first, but there were certainly no giant statues to be found there.

St. Paul had never visited Colossae when he composed his Epistle to the Colossians, but he did imply that Epaphras founded the church, along with those at Laodicea and Hierapolis (Colossians 1:7–8). The Christianization of the region was also attributed to the efforts of Timothy and Filemon. Laodicea was founded in the third century BC by the Seleucid King Antiochus II and named for his wife Laodike. The Church in Laodicea was one of the Seven Churches of Revelation. In John's message to the Laodicean church (Revelation 3:14–22), he speaks of the lukewarmness of Laodicea, that they were "neither cold nor hot." This local allusion would have been clear to citizens of Laodicea, who knew of the cold, pure waters of nearby Colossae, and the hot springs of Hierapolis. We visited the ruins of the church, which was destroyed during an earthquake in the fifth century, and then we went to Hierapolis, on the other side of the Lycus River. Named after Hiera, the wife of Telephus (son of Heracles), the mythical founder of Pergamum, Hierapolis was ceded to Rome in 133 BC along with the rest of the Pergamum Kingdom and became part of the Roman province of Asia. Hierapolis is famous for its hot springs. The water in Hierapolis is about 35° C (95° F) and is rich in calcium and carbon dioxide; after cooling, calcium carbonate precipitates and forms chalky deposits of a beautiful white color ("cotton castle") (Fig. 327). We also visited Hierapolis' Theater and later went to the Necropolis through the Gate of Domitian, built in 83 AD. Hierapolis had a significant Jewish population in ancient times, as is evidenced by numerous inscriptions on tombs and elsewhere in the city. This was probably the basis for the Christian conversion of some residents of Hierapolis, recorded in Colossians 4:13. Finally, we visited the third-century Roman baths converted to a church in sixth century. We spent that night in the Hierapolis Thermal Hotel.

On Monday, September 15, we went to Miletus. According to legend, the city was founded by Neleus, son of King Codrus of Athens. Neleus came to settle with his men and killed the resident males and

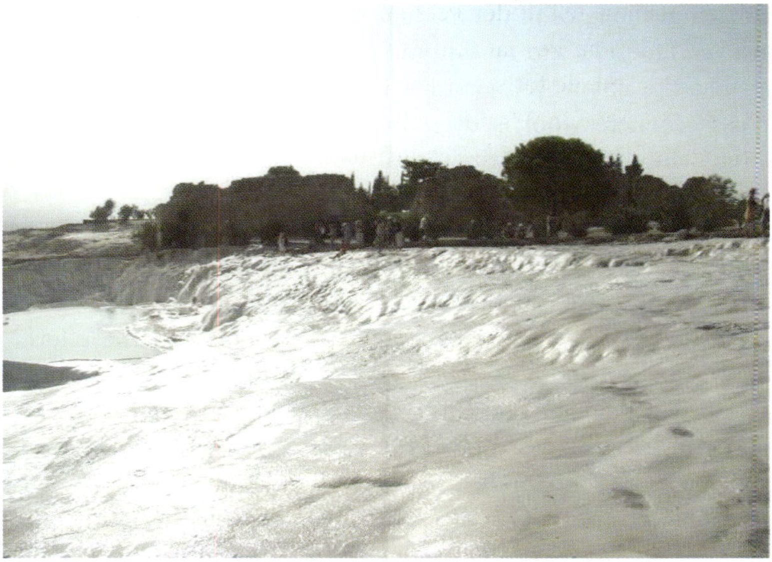

Figure 327. Chalky deposits with a beautiful white color ("cotton castle") at Hierapolis.

forced the women to marry the newcomers.[59] In the 11th century BC, Ionians came to Miletus, and by the seventh century BC, Miletus was at its peak, a period of prosperity that was to last for more than two centuries. Tyrants ruled during this period, and one of the most successful was Thrasybulus.[60] When Cyrus of Persia defeated Croesus

---

59. The killing of men and marrying of women by invaders was a typical practice in ancient times. You may recall the abduction of Sabines and the slaughter of males in Babylon by the Persians under Cyrus. The Israelites also slaughtered all the inhabitants of Jericho, including women and children (Joshua 6:21). I always wondered why they did this and started to speculate that killing women was in accordance with their belief that only a child of an Israeli woman could be considered a Jew. But this remains my speculation, as I have never found such an explanation.

60. The tyrant Cypselus died after 30 years of bloody rule in Corinth. His inexperienced replacement, his son Periander, wanted to know what the best method of maintaining power was, and he sent a messenger to Thrasybulus, a tyrant of Miletus, to ask him how to keep people in fear and subjugation. Thrasybulus took the messenger into a field of corn. He cut any corn ear that was higher than the others, until he had destroyed the best part of the field. He did not say a word to the messenger and sent him back. The messenger described the encounter, surprised why Periander had sent him to a mad person who destroyed his own goods. However, Periander understood the message immediately and proceeded to systematically murder all citizens who were outstanding in influence and ability. [Herodotus. (2003) *The Histories*, revised edition. Penguin Books; p. 348.] The method was emulated by modern tyrants such as Joseph Stalin, Adolf Hitler and Saddam Hussein.

of Lydia, Miletus fell under Persian rule. In 479 BC, the Greeks decisively defeated the Persians at the Greek mainland, and Miletus was freed of Persian rule for some time. It was captured by Alexander the Great after a siege in 334 BC and was ruled by the Seleucid Dynasty in the years that followed. Between the second century BC and the third century AD, Miletus was under Roman rule. During the Byzantine period (4th–11th centuries AD), it became a residence for archbishops. Seljuk Turks settled in 12th century and Ottoman Turks in the 14th century. Many famous people lived in Miletus, including Thales (circa 624–546 BC), Anaximander (circa 610–546 BC), Anaximenes (circa 585–525 BC), the writer Aristides (circa 530–468 BC), the historian Hecateus (circa 550–476 BC), and Isidore (6th century AD), one of the builders of the Hagia Sophia. Miletus was a major port city located on a peninsula with four harbors. Paul visited Miletus for a day or two as he waited for his messengers to return with the Ephesian elders (Acts 20:15–17). With the silting of the Büyük Menderes River (or Meander River), today the ruins of the ancient city are a few kilometers from the sea.

In the morning we first looked at the ruins of the theater, which was built in the fourth century BC after Alexander the Great defeated the Persians who controlled the city. In its first phase during the Hellenistic period, the theater could seat 5,300; after being enlarged during the Roman period, it held some 25,000. From the top of the theater hill we could see the caravansary, an inn with a large courtyard for the overnight accommodation of caravans. The inn, which has a lower floor for animals and an upper one for people, was constructed in the 15th century from stones taken from the theater. Next, we went to the Delphinium, a Hellenistic open-air shrine surrounded by stoas[61] on four sides with an altar in the center from the sixth century BC. Only the Ionic Stoa on the south of Delphinium is preserved in a reasonable condition (Fig. 328). We then visited the Bath of Faustina, which was built by Faustina, Marcus Aurelius' wife, who usually accompanied her husband on his journeys through the Empire. Like all Roman bathhouses, this bathhouse had an apodyterium (dressing room), a frigidarium (cold room), a tepidarium (warm

---

61. Stoa is an ancient Greek portico usually walled at the back with a front colonnade designed to offer a sheltered promenade.

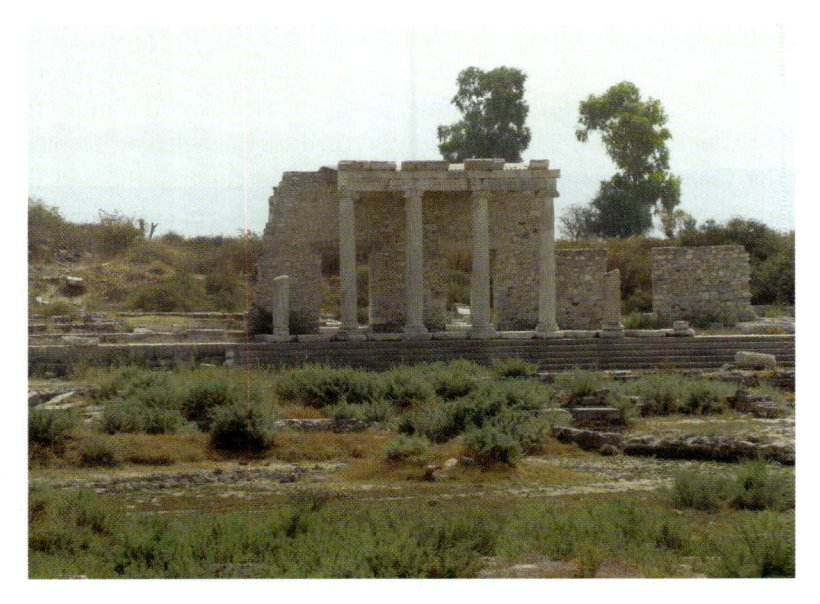

Figure 328. Miletus' ruined Ionic Stoa (colonnade) on the south of the Delphinium parallel to the processional road with shops behind the columns.

room) and a caldarium (steam room). The frigidarium had a reclining statue of the river god probably personifying the Meander River. (The river really was meandering, hence the word.)

On our way to the Basilica of St. John, we passed the well-preserved grand fortress of Selçuk on Ayasoluk Hill, built during the Byzantium period. The basilica is on the slopes of the hill, just below the fortress, and is only a couple of miles from Ephesus. Constructed by Emperor Justinian in the sixth century, the basilica stands over what is believed to be the burial site of St. John (d. 98 AD), apostle, evangelist (author of the Fourth Gospel) and prophet (author of Revelation). While we were there, we stopped at St. John's tomb and the Baptismal Font, which has seven steps down, one for each cardinal sin (Fig. 329). In Latin these sins create the acronym *SALIGIA*: *superbia* (pride), *avaritia* (greed), *luxuria* (lust), *ira* (wrath), *gula* (gluttony), *invidia* (envy) and *acedia* (sloth). The last two are the basis of socialism; the others are also important in this system. "Baptism" comes from the Greek βαπτειν (*baptein*): to dip, immerse or submerge. In the past, baptism was always performed with submersion in water.

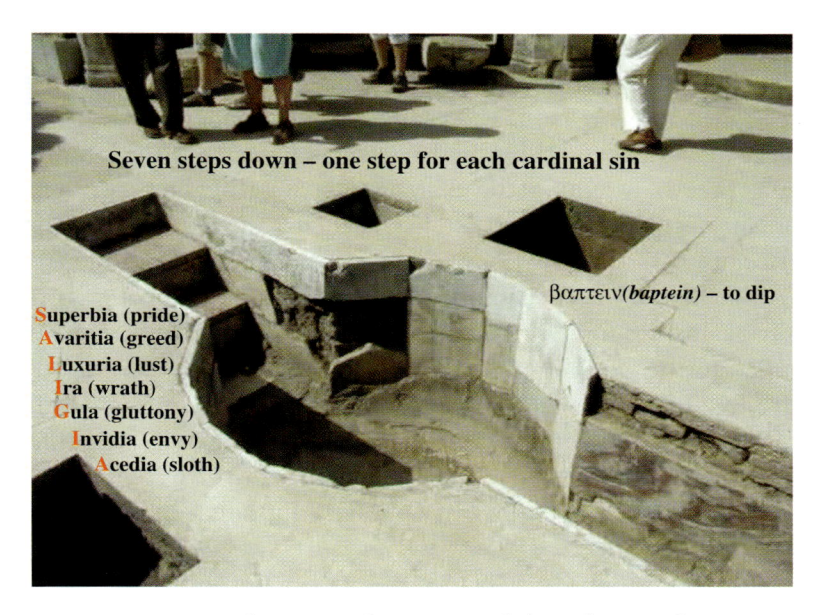

Figure 329. The Baptismal Font in St. John's Basilica in Miletus.

(Labels on image: Seven steps down – one step for each cardinal sin; Superbia (pride), Avaritia (greed), Luxuria (lust), Ira (wrath), Gula (gluttony), Invidia (envy), Acedia (sloth); βαπτειν(baptein) – to dip)

The following day we went to Ephesus, which is located close to Miletus in Izmir Province. The histories of the two ancient cities are quite similar. The Ephesus region was inhabited during the Bronze Age by the Mycenaeans, Achaeans and Hittites. Ephesus itself was founded by the Ionians in the 10th century BC, and it was conquered by the Lydians under Croesus around 560 BC. Many important people hailed from Ephesus, including the pre-Socratic philosopher Heraclitus, who is famous for his expression *panta rhei* (Πάντα ῥεῖ, meaning "everything flows"; everything is in a state of flux).[62] The Greek goddess Artemis and the great Anatolian goddess Cybele were identified together as Artemis of Ephesus. The goddess was venerated in the Temple of Artemis, financed by Croesus, which became one of the Seven Wonders of the World and the largest building of the ancient world. Cyrus of Persia conquered western Anatolia, including Ephesus, in about 500 BC. In 479 BC, the Greeks decisively defeated the Persians at the Greek mainland, and Ephesus (like Miletus) was

---

62. Heraclitus may be considered the father of the theory of evolution of everything that exists in the Universe.

freed of Persian rule for some time. On July 21, 356 BC, one day after Alexander the Great was born, Herostratus,[63] in his quest for fame, set fire to the temple. Ephesus was captured by Alexander the Great after a siege in 334 BC and ruled by the Seleucid Dynasty in the following years. In 190 BC the battle of Magnesia was fought between the Romans — led by the consul Scipio (Asiaticus) and his brother, Scipio Africanus, with their ally Eumenes II of Pergamum — and the army of Antiochus III the Great of the Seleucid Empire. Hannibal was once more against Rome. The resulting decisive Roman victory ended the conflict for the control of Greece.[64] Between the second century BC and the third century AD, Ephesus was under Roman rule. During the Byzantine period (4th–11th centuries AD), it initially flourished, but later declined. Seljuk Turks settled in the 12th century and Ottoman Turks in 14th. Most of Ephesus' ruins are from the Roman period.

We first stopped at the State Agora. Close by is the Odeon (Bouleterion), which served two purposes, hosting concerts (Odeon) and *boule*, or city council, meetings (Bouleterion). We passed the Memmius Monument with sculptures of Memmius, his father Caius, and his grandfather Sulla (138–78 BC), then the Domitian Temple, and through the Heracles Gate to Kurets Street, which leads to the Library of Celsus. On the way to the library, passing the Trajan Fountain (built 102–114 AD), we stopped at Skolastikia Bath. Originally a Roman structure from the first century AD, it deteriorated with time, and renovations and modifications were made by a Christian woman named Skolastikia in the fourth century; there is a headless statue of Skolastikia at the site. The bath was built in the style of other Roman baths; public toilets (*latrina*) were built close by. We

---

63. Herostratus proudly claimed credit in an attempt to immortalise his name in history. To dissuade similar-minded fame-seekers, the Ephesean authorities not only executed him, but also condemned him to a legacy of obscurity by forbidding the mention of his name under penalty of death. This did not stop Herostratus from achieving his goal, as the ancient historian Theopompus recorded the event and its perpetrator in his *Hellenics*. Nobody has ever been executed, so I am not afraid to mention his name.

64. According to Plutarch, after the Battle of Magnesia, Scipio Africanus met with Hannibal, and during their conversation he asked him who was the greatest commander. Hannibal answered that Alexander was the greatest, Pyrrus was second, and himself third. Scipio smiled at this and asked, "What would be the order if you were not defeated by me at Zama?" Hannibal's answer was: "I would be the greatest."

also passed the Temple of Hadrian, which was completed in 138 AD. Hadrian visited Ephesus in 128 AD and gave permission to build a temple in his name. We finally arrived at the Library of Celsus. I initially thought that this library was associated in some way with Aulus Cornelius Celsus, the author of the book *De Medicina*, but I quickly learned that this was not the case. It was actually built in honor of Tibrius Julius Celsus Polemaeanus, a Roman senator and governor of the Province of Asia — and a great lover of books — by his son, and completed in 135 AD (Fig. 330). In front of the library are statues representing the virtues of Celsus: *sophia* (sagacity, wisdom), *arete* (character), *ennoia* (judgment) and *episteme* (knowledge). Our final stop before lunch was the Great Theater and the Harbor Street. Ephesus is now separated from the Aegean Sea by silt from the Caystros River, so the Harbor Street ends a few miles from the sea.

In the afternoon we visited Meryemana Evi (Turkish for "Mother Mary's House"). Catholics believe that Jesus' mother Mary lived in Ephesus from shortly after the crucifixion and resurrection until her assumption to heaven. This belief comes from the Gospel of John. When Jesus was on the cross, he spoke to the apostle John, apparently

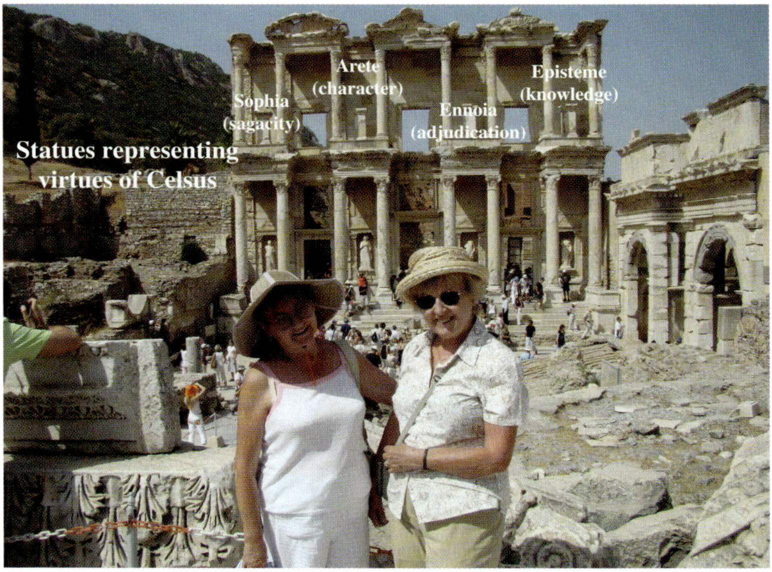

Figure 330.   The Celsus Library in Ephesus.

the youngest of all his apostles, and charged him with taking care of Mary: "*When Jesus therefore saw his mother, and the disciple standing by, whom he loved, he saith unto his mother, Woman, behold thy son! Then saith he to the disciple, Behold thy mother! And from that hour that disciple took her unto his own home.*"[65] There is considerable evidence to suggest that John moved to Ephesus almost immediately (soon after 30 AD) and spent the rest of his life in that region. The main Christian church in Ephesus, built in the fourth century and used for a long time, was called the Basilica of the Virgin Mary. Church doctrine during that time required that a church designated a "basilica" had to be named after someone who had lived in the immediate vicinity. The Third Ecumenical Council took place in 431 in that basilica in Ephesus and the title "Mother of God" was formally applied to Mary. Some speculate that the emphasis on Mary may have been placed to include a comfortably familiar major mother figure (Artemis of Ephesus) and thereby make Christianity more attractive to the local people in what was then one of the top three cities in the empire. In the 1800s a stigmatized invalid German nun named Anna Catherine Emmerich[66] wrote down her visions of Mary's life, including detailed descriptions of her home and its surroundings. In 1891 a French priest used Emmerich's writings to explore the area. He discovered what has since been identified as the ruins of a chapel from about 300 AD, built on top of an earlier structure. The suggestion is that Mary lived here, and by the beginning of the fourth century a chapel had been built over her home. Sometime within the next century, a larger church was built about 100 yards away. The last restoration was in 1951. On the way to the shrine we passed signs in various languages, including English (NOTICE ABOUT THE SHRINE) and Polish (*NOTATKA HISTORYCZNA O SANKTUARIUM*) (Fig. 331), and just behind the signs is the Statue of the Virgin Mary at the entrance to the shrine (Fig. 332). Afterwards, we visited Meryemana Evi itself (Fig. 333). There is also an outdoor chapel where weddings frequently take place; as we were leaving, we saw a British couple's wedding. In the evening we went to Kuşadası (meaning "Bird Island" in

---

65. John 19:26–27.

66. Hollywood actor Mel Gibson is a devotee of Emmerich. He included some of her non-canonical details (that is, not included in officially accepted writings) in his movie *The Passion of the Christ*.

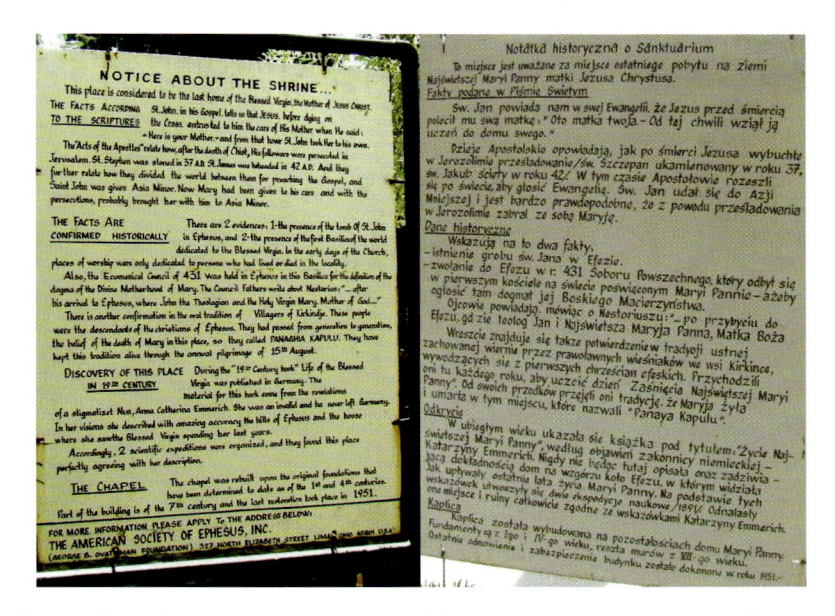

Figure 331. Posters in English and Polish on the way to Meryemana Evi near Ephesus.

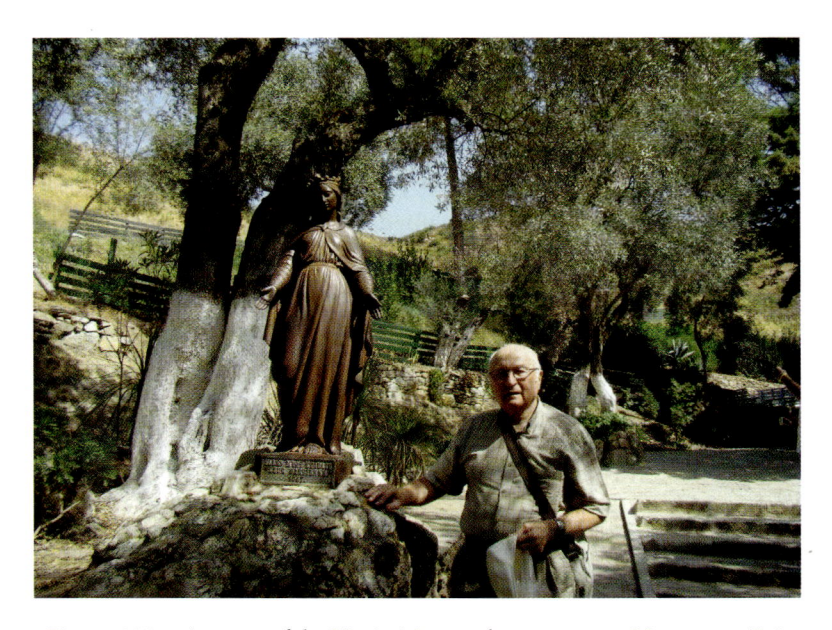

Figure 332. A statue of the Virgin Mary at the entrance to Meryemana Evi.

Vacations and Travel Unrelated to Business 567

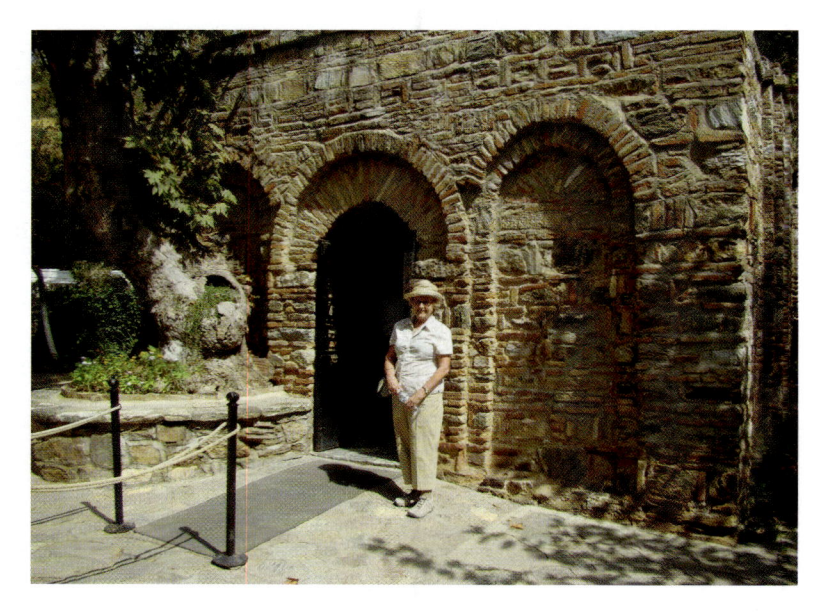

Figure 333. The front of Mother Mary's House, Meryemana Evi.

Turkish) and watched a presentation on leatherwear, for which the resort town is known, and checked in to the Tatlises Hotel.

The next morning we drove through Izmir and stopped at Pergamum. A very important kingdom during the second century BC, Pergamum grew from the city-state captured by Alexander the Great to become the capital of the Kingdom of Pergamum. After the battle of Magnesia, Eumenes II allied with the Romans and became the most powerful ruler in Anatolia. He founded Asclepion, an ancient medical center, which became famous under Galen (131–210 AD) two centuries later. Under Attalus, the kingdom's power declined and in 129 BC became the Roman Province of Asia. Roman Pergamum was still a rich, important city with many important buildings, including the Traianeum (Temple of Trajan), the Library and the Asclepion. Our first stop in Pergamum was the ruins of the Basilica of St. John. Then we went to a shop (Fig. 334) selling various pictures and inscriptions on parchment. The Acropolis of Pergamum, which we did not see, is also the location of the Pergamum Library, which was one of the most important libraries in the ancient world. In fact, the Egyptian king Ptolemy was so envious of the library that he halted the export of

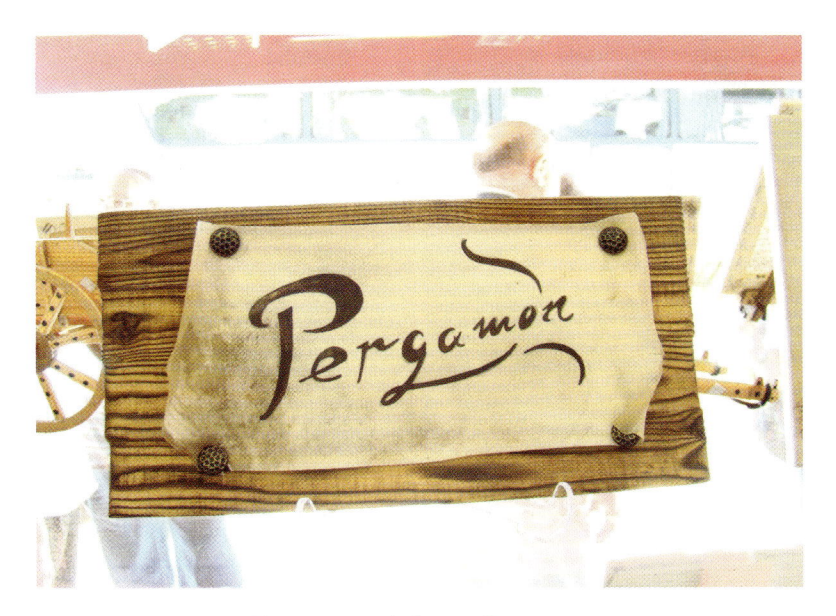

Figure 334. A shop in Pergamum.

papyrus from Alexandria to squeeze the competition. In response, the Pergamenes invented a new material for writing, called *pergaminus* or *pergamena* (parchment) after the city, which was made of fine calfskin, a predecessor of vellum. The Library of Pergamum was believed to contain 200,000 volumes, the entirety of which, legend has it, Mark Antony later gave to Cleopatra as a wedding present. Placed in the Alexandria Library, the collection was finally totally destroyed in the 7th century AD on the order of Caliph Omar, who said of the library holdings: "They will either contradict the Koran, in which case they are heresy, or they will agree with it, so they are superfluous." It is reported that it took at least six months to burn all books.

From Pergamum we drove to the ruins of Troy, which were initially excavated by the English archeologist Frank Calvert in 1865. He bought a field from a local farmer at Hisarlik and first trial trenches showed that the ruins were indeed there. In 1868, more excavations were done by a wealthy German businessman and archeologist Heinrich Schliemann, who met Frank Calvert by chance in Çanakkale. At the entrance to the excavations is a sign in Turkish and English (Fig. 335) indicating that we were entering the Historic National Park

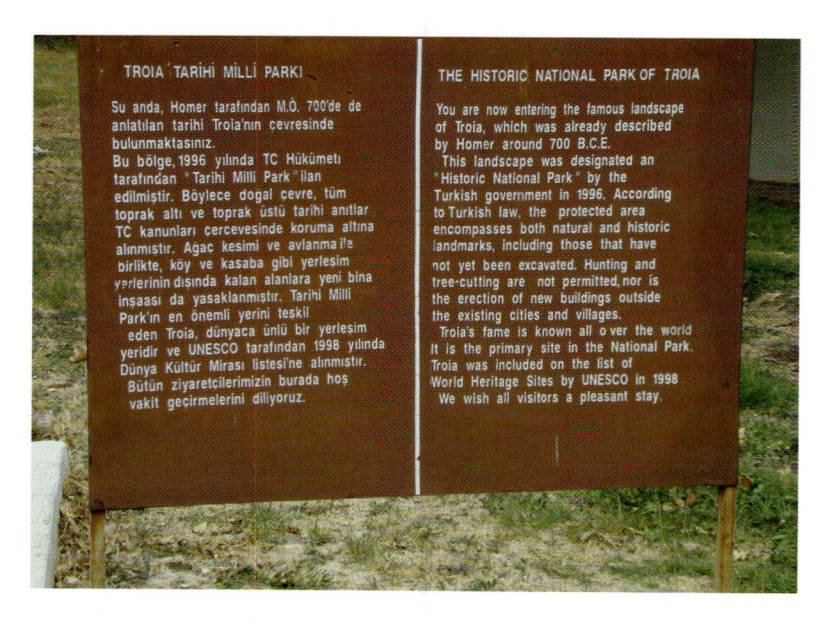

Figure 335. Signs in Turkish and English at the entrance to Troy.

of Troia. Our first stop was, naturally, a fun reconstruction of the famous Trojan horse (Fig. 336), which allowed the Greeks to enter the city and end the Trojan War. The excavations of consecutive layers in the citadel at Hisarlik are numbered Troy I–IX. Troy VII, which has been dated to the mid- to late-13th century BC, is the most often-cited candidate for the Troy of Homer. The best preserved are Troy VIII and IX from Roman times with the Odeon and Bouleterion, and the Sanctuary. We stayed the night in the Kolin Hotel in Çanakkale.

During ancient Greek times the strait connecting the Aegean Sea with the Sea of Marmara was called Hellespont. The Byzantine name for the Çanakkale region and the strait was Δαρδανέλλια (*Dardanellia*), from which the English name Dardanelles is derived. Çanakkale was an Ottoman fortress called Kale-i Sultaniye, or Sultaniye kalesi (Fortress of the Sultan). It later became known for its pottery — hence the later name *Çanak kalesi*, "pot fortress" or Çanakka. The real history of Çanakkale started with Troy. By the eighth century BC, the Aeolians had settled on that important land and established many trade colonies in the region called Aeolis. In ancient times Abydos was located where the city of Çanakkale is now situated. The Lydians took

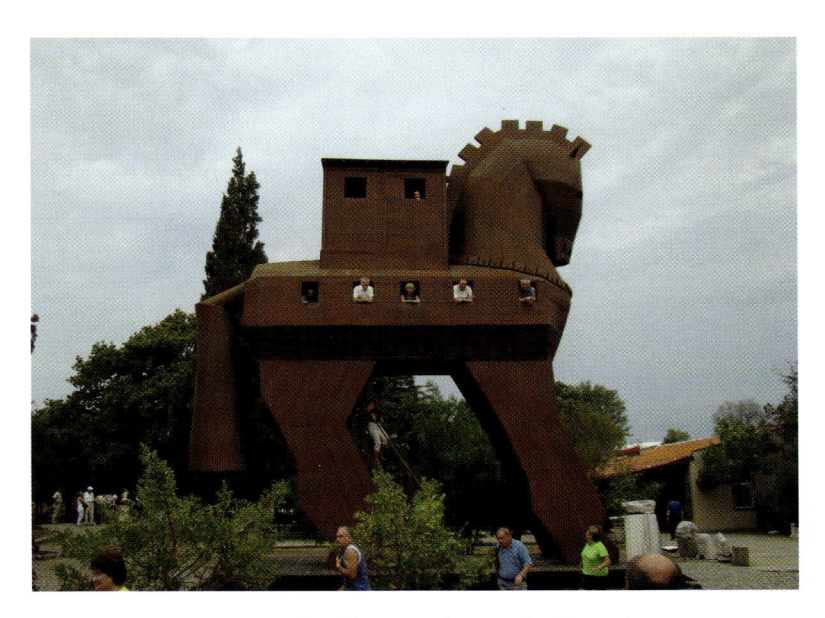

Figure 336. The obligatory photo in the Trojan horse.

control of the region in the seventh century BC and then the Persians in the sixth century BC. When Alexander the Great defeated the Persians at the Granicus River in 334 BC, Aeolis came under the control of the Macedonians. By the second century BC, the region was controlled by the Kingdom of Pergamum and was allied with the Roman Empire. It was not until 1367 AD that the Ottomans gained control. The region, the meeting point of two great continents, is rich in historical events (Fig. 337). Herodotus tells of Xerxes I, son of Darius, who in 482 BC built two bridges across the width of the Hellespont at Abydos in order that his huge army could cross from Anatolia into Greece. One bridge was built by the Phoenicians using flax cables and the other by Egyptians using papyrus cables. Both bridges were destroyed by a storm, which made Xerxes furious. He "gave orders that the Hellespont should receive three hundred lashes and have a pair of fetters thrown into it."[67] Alexander the Great had no

---

67. Herodotus also mentioned that he instructed the men with whips to utter: "You salt and bitter stream, your master lays this punishment upon you for injuring him, who never injured you. But Xerxes the King will cross you with or without your permission." [Herodotus. (2003) *The Histories*, revised edition. Penguin Books; p. 429.]

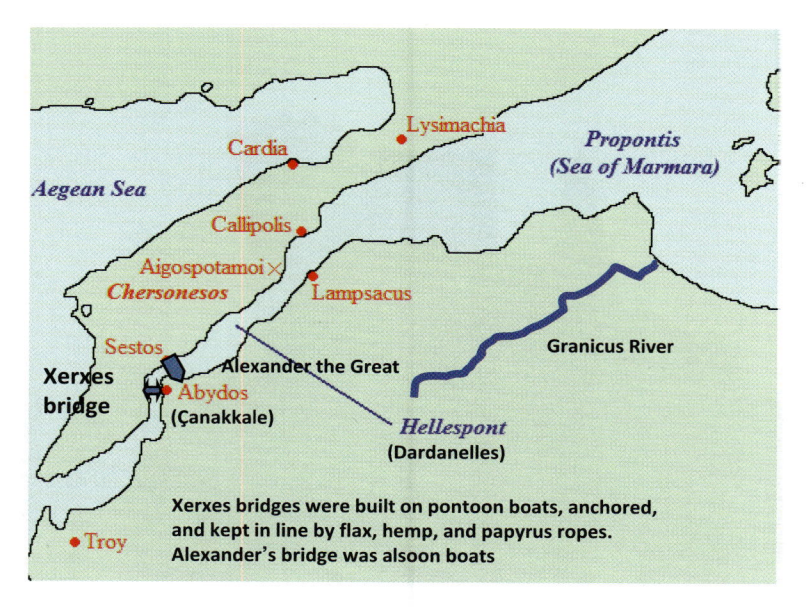

Figure 337. A historical map of Hellespont, now known as the Dardanelles.

such difficulties crossing Hellespont before the battle at Granicus River.

On the morning of September 18, we drove to Bursa, an industrial center in northern Turkey. We only visited the Green Mosque (again the name is from the color of the tiles) and the Muradiye Complex, or the Complex of Murat II, the Ottoman sultan who ruled from 1421–1451. He was the last of the Ottoman sultans to reign in the original Ottoman capital of Bursa, prior to the conquest of Constantinople in 1453. Thereafter, we drove close to İzmit (Byzantine Nicea), the place where the Council of Nicea[68] was held in 325. I tried to talk our organizers into visiting İzmit, but as it was not on the program, it was difficult to accommodate due to the lack of time.

---

68. It was quite a surprise to discover that the Council of Nicea was to the east of the Sea of Marmara. Prior to our pilgrimage, I had always thought that this Council was held in Nice, France (Latin: Nicaea), not knowing about any other Nicea. The Council of Nicea dealt with the problem of whether Jesus was with the father homoousian (ὁμοούσον, *consubstantialis*), meaning of the same substance ("one in being with the father"), or homoiousian (ὁμοιούσον, *similis substantiae*), meaning of similar substance. The expression "not one iota of difference" comes from this controversy: the smallest Greek letter but a very important difference.

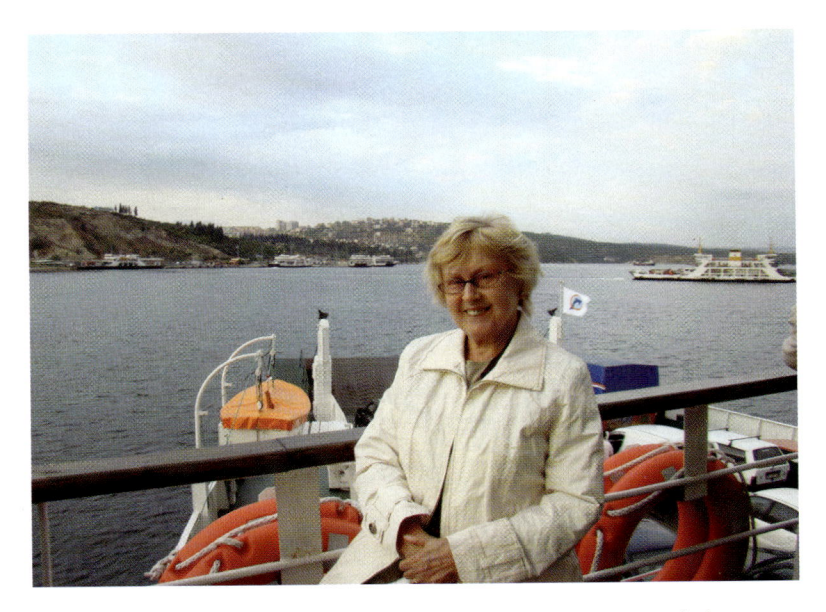

Figure 338. The ferry across the Sea of Marmara to Istanbul.

We soon found ourselves on the ferry to Istanbul traversing the Sea of Marmara (Fig. 338), and the following day was our flight to Warsaw and our bus home to Kraków.

We returned to Columbia on September 26. Our older son Radek and his family had not been able to come to Kraków for our 50th wedding anniversary, so he decided to organize a celebration in Minneapolis one day before the exact day of our wedding anniversary, Friday, October 10. Radek and our younger son Przemek organized everything, including travel, hotel rooms and a dinner at the Hyatt Regency on Nicollet Mall in the center of Minneapolis. In addition to our sons (Fig. 339) and their wives, the dinner was attended by our grandchildren Ania, Adam and Alek, as well as Ania's husband-to-be, Sean (Fig. 340). The following day we went to the Mall of America and for Mass at the Basilicae Sanctae Mariae Minneapolitanae. On Sunday, October 12, we returned to Columbia. For Thanksgiving we drove to Muskogee, Oklahoma, where Radek worked in a Veterans Affairs hospital. It was nice to see the annual Garden of Lights in the bushes and byways of Honor Heights. We had two further celebrations of our golden wedding anniversary with our Columbia friends, Georgia and

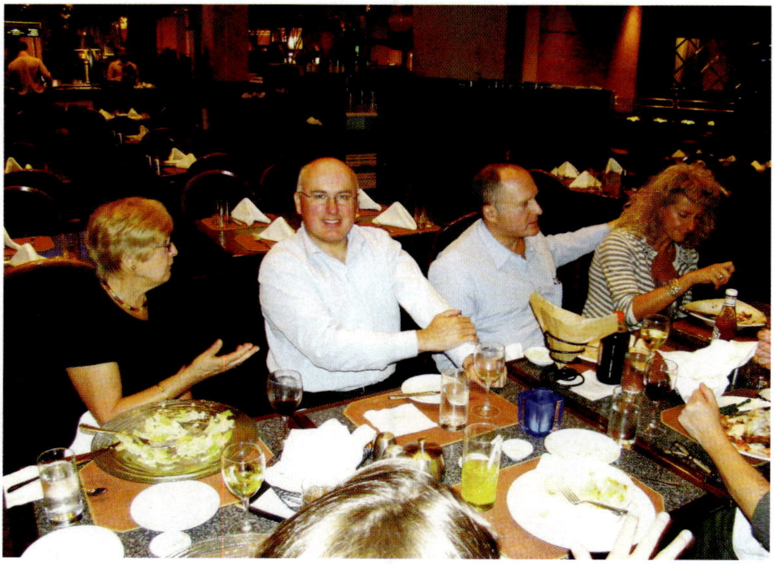

Figure 339. Dinner in Minneapolis: Halina, Radek, Przemek and Kasia.

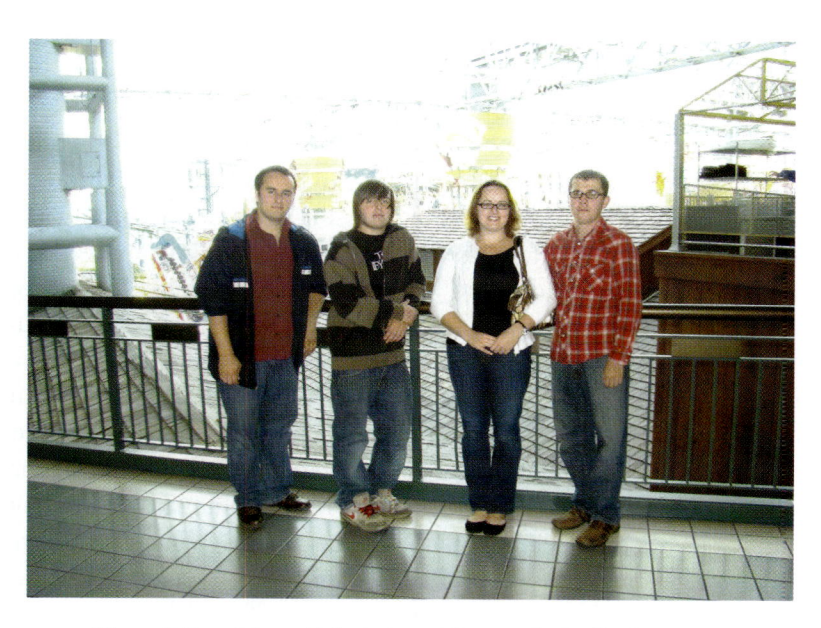

Figure 340. Adam, Alek, Ania and Sean in the Mall of America.

Karl Nolph, Pushpa and Ramesh Khanna, and Shamita and Madhukar Misra. One was organized by our friends in the Misras' home at 4804 Silver Clif Drive on Oxtober 18 and the other was in our home on December 13.

2009 — Ania's wedding in Minneapolis

In 2009 we went to Poland on May 2. In addition to traveling for presentations in Warsaw and Turkey, which I have already described, we went to Minneapolis for the wedding of our granddaughter Ania. On June 18 we flew via Chicago to Minneapolis, checking in to the Holiday Inn at 3 Appletree Square. The wedding was on June 20 at the Church of Christ the King on 5029 Zenith Avenue South. Adam, Ania's brother, played *Ave Maria* on a violin constructed by Halina's grandfather. The wedding was attended by family from both sides (Figs. 341 and 342). We returned to Kraków on June 22, and Ania and Sean came to Kraków on July 31 for their honeymoon. It was Sean's turn to see the various places of interest in and around Kraków.

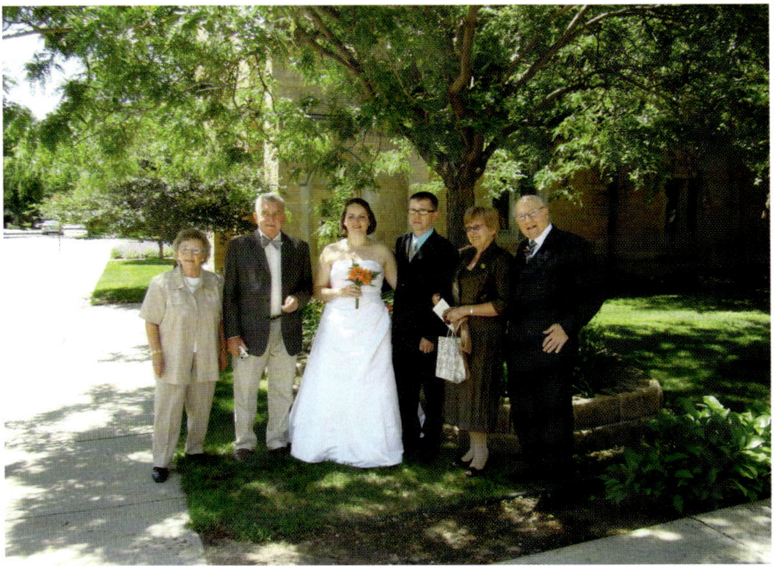

Figure 341. Sean's grandma, Ania's maternal grandpa (Ludwig), Ania, Sean, and Ania's paternal grandma (Halina) and grandpa (the author).

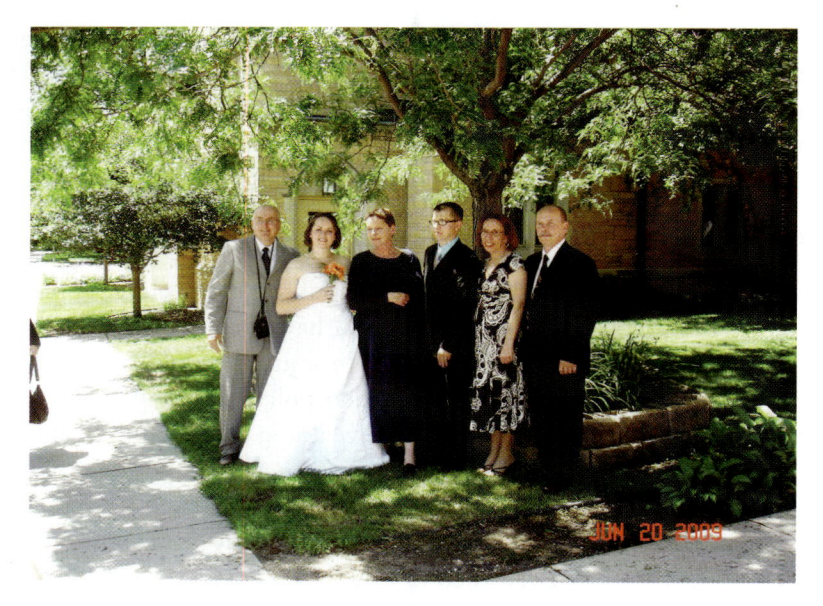

Figure 342.   Radek (Ania's father), Ania, Gosia (Ania's mother), Sean and his parents.

On September 9, Wiesław Tlałka, our colleague from the medical school and a board member of the Stowarzyszenie Bochniaków (Association Bochniaków) organized a conference honoring my professional achievements (Fig. 343). I talked about my carreer and my ties with Bochnia County. As a son of parents born in Bochnia County and a student in Bochnia School, I was accepted as an honorary member of the Association. We returned to Columbia on September 20.

2010 — Bieszczady

I decided to buy a Toyota Prius, a hybrid car with nearly unrivaled fuel consumption (60 mpg or 3.9 L/100 km). We arranged the purchase through the Internet at Toyota ANWA in Kraków and expected to retrieve the car in May. We were supposed to arrive in Kraków on April 20, but because of the eruption of Icelandic volcano Eyjafjallajökull, our flight was postponed eight days. I picked up our new Prius on May 25. In the middle of June we traveled to Tours,

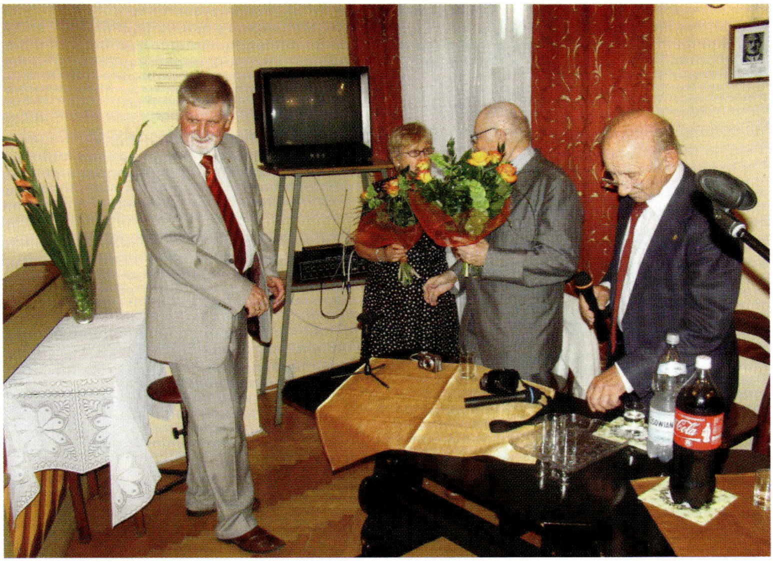

Figure 343. After a conference honoring the author's professional achievements: Stanisław Kobiela, President of the Association Bochniaków (*left*); Dr. Wiesław Tlałka (*right*).

France, for a meeting, as I have already described. On July 2, Adam visited and we decided to go to Bieszczady, a very picturesque part of the extreme southeast of Poland near the borders of Slovakia and Ukraine. Settled in prehistoric times, the region was overrun in pre-Roman times by various tribes, including the Celts, Goths, Vandals, and later by Hungarians and West Slavs. The region subsequently became part of the state of Great Moravia in the ninth century. It was an area that was contested by Kievan Rus and Poland. The first king of Poland, Bolesław Chrobry (Bolesław the Brave or the Valiant), annexed it into Poland in 1018, but it became part of the Rus in 1031. It was Casimir the Great who recovered it for Poland for many centuries. In 1991, the UNESCO East Carpathian Biosphere Reserve was created to encapsulate a large part of the area, which continues into Slovakia and Ukraine.

Like other tourists, we drove to Sanok and checked into Hotel Jagielloński on 49 Jagiellońska Street, which we used as a base to visit a number of attractive places. In Sanok itself, on one of the benches, is

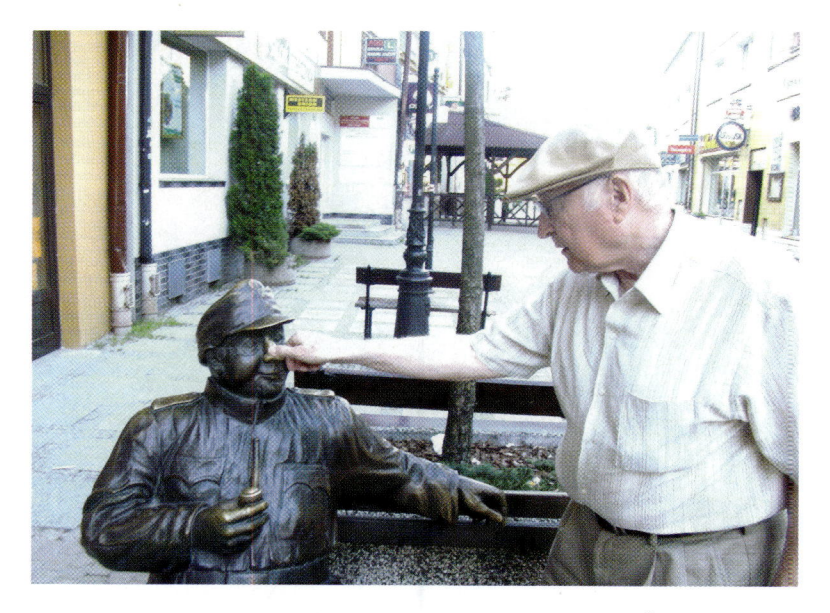

Figure 344. Touching the nose of the Good Soldier Švejk.

a statue of the Good Soldier Švejk, the chief character from the popular novel by Jaroslav Hašek, well known in Poland and all over the world. It is said that people who touch his nose receive good luck, so I did so, just in case it were true (Fig. 344). We also went to Queen Bona Castle to see its collection of pictures by the fantasy artist Ździsław Beksiński. We also visited a nearby antique building museum with old farmhouses, churches and miniature churches from many parts of Bieszczady. The next day we drove to Jezioro Solińskie (Lake Solina), an artificial lake created in 1968 by the construction of the Solina Dam on the San River. As well as its electric power plant, the lake serves as a tourist attraction for boaters and other lovers of water sports. It has been nicknamed the "Bieszczady Sea" because of its great depth, the water's clarity, and the surrounding mountainous scenery. Naturally, we went for a boat cruise on the lake. Finally, we visited the charitable Caritas Center in Myczkowce, which has miniature models of Catholic, Greek Catholic and Orthodox Churches (Fig. 345). From Sanok we drove to Puławy to visit Adam's maternal grandfather. We were back in Kraków on July 11, and Adam departed for Bismarck on July 21.

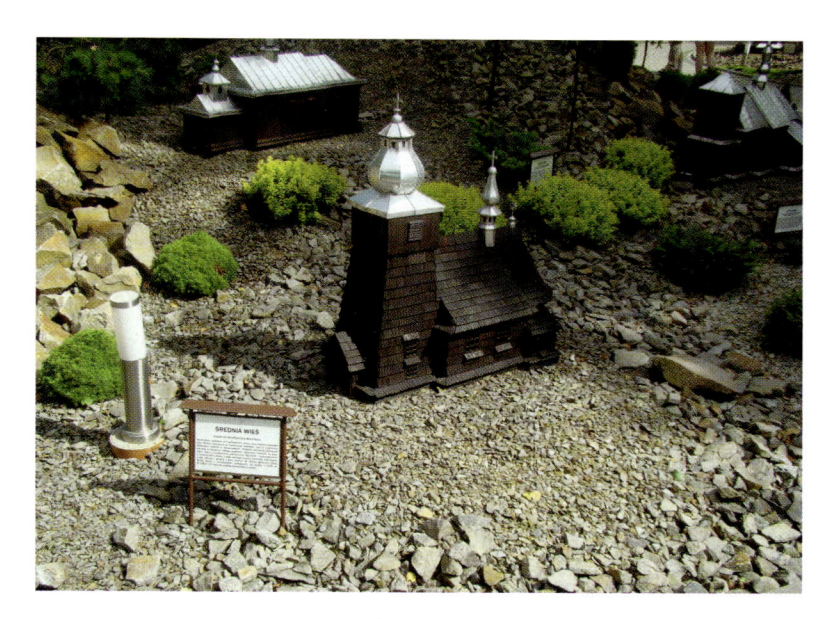

Figure 345. Models of churches in Myczkowce.

During the summer we drove our Prius (half in town) 2,064 miles (3,322 km) and used 55.5 gallons (210 L) of gas. Thus, our mileage was 37.2 mpg (6.32 L/100 km), lower than that indicated by Toyota, but still very good. According to the Toyota dealer the Prius Prestige should not be left for seven months without occasional use, and the battery could not be disconnected. As we did not have anybody to drive our Prius during our stay in Columbia, the dealer suggested taking it for storage at their ANWA plant, which was free of charge. I was very happy to accept their offer.

We returned to Columbia on September 20. On October 6 we went to Pasadena to visit our younger son, Przemek, and his wife, Kasia. The next day Przemek took us to their beach house in Oxnard, California, where we spent four days bodysurfing or if the waves were not good, swimming in the pool in nearby Ventura. We were back in Columbia on October 11. On November 2 we drove to Kansas City to hear a performance by the orchestra of Concordia College in Moorhead, Minnesota, in which Adam plays the violin. We had booked a room at the Hyatt Regency Crown Center at 2345 McGee

Street, where the members of the orchestra were also staying. They gave a very nice performance at Olathe East High School at 14545 W. 127th Street in Olathe, Kansas. Adam told us that their orchestra organizes such trips to entice high school students to study at Concordia College.

2011 — Adam and Gosia in Kraków, and a trip to Ukraine

In 2011 we came to Kraków on April 30. We had to fly via Warsaw as for some reason direct flights from Chicago to Kraków had been discontinued — in spite of high demand. On May 2 I retrieved our Prius, which was in excellent shape, having only been driven 47 miles over seven months. Gosia and Adam arrived on July 15 and we visited a few places in Kraków. The most interesting was an exhibit under the Main Square. In 2005, as part of preparations for repaving the eastern part of the Main Market Square, it was discovered that there were relics suitable for exhibition. Over the following six years the exhibition was prepared and is now available for public viewing. In addition to exhibits, there are movies discussing the history of Kraków, its role as the capital of Poland and the importance of the Main Market Square for trade and the development of the city. The city was founded by Krak, a legendary Polish prince, at the beginning of the eighth century, and it became the capital of Poland in 1058 during the reign of Kazimierz Odnowiciel (Casimir the Restorer). I learned for the first time that Kraków belonged to the Hanseatic League as early as the second half of the 14th century and was located further from the sea than any other member of the League.

In August we went for a trip to Ukraine. I wanted to see my place of birth, but also to visit Lviv (Polish: Lwów), a city that belonged to Poland for centuries and has many monuments from that period. Recalling our futile effort to cross the Ukrainian border at Dorohusk in 2006, we decided to find somebody familiar with the Ukrainian system to help us with the trip. On the recommendation of Zbigniew Wawszczak, our younger son's father-in-law, we asked Mr. Antoni Bosiak of the MOTO Company in Zamość, which organizes foreign tours, including to Ukraine. He proposed that we go to Chełm, near the Ukrainian border, and then he would take us in his van across the

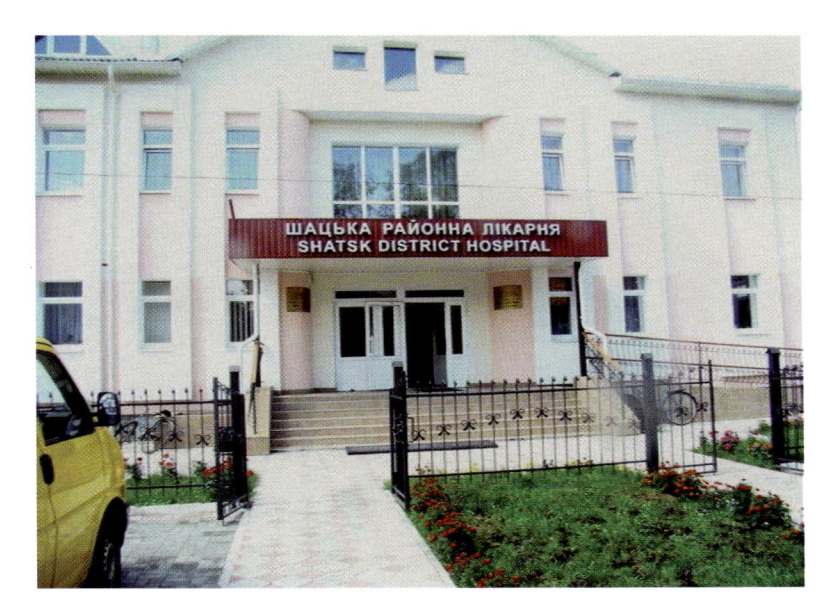

Figure 346. Shatsk District Hospital, too new to be the building where I was born.

border to Shatsk (Szack), Lviv and back to Chełm. So on Monday, August 8, we drove to Chełm — taking Halina's sisters, Joanna and Barbara, with us — and stayed a night at Hotel Kozak on 37 Hrubieszowska Street. (This time we got excellent mileage: 47.1 mpg or 5 L/100 km.) In the morning Mr. Bosiak picked us up in his van and took us through the Dorohusk border crossing. This time, for some unknown reason, there was a very short line, and we crossed the border in about half an hour, arriving in Szack about an hour later. The difficult part would be trying to find the old hospital where I was born, a building from the first half of the 19th century. We stopped by the Shatsk District Hospital (Fig. 346), but it was soon obvious that the hospital was new. However, the hospital administrator, Nickolas Dudko, told us that there was an old hospital about 10 minutes' walk away and that he would take us there. Apparently, it only had two departments, internal medicine and pediatrics, and the buildings were slated to be demolished later that year, or the following year, to make way for a new hospital. As I was only about a year old when my parents left, I had no memory of anything in Szack. My brother, Lesław, who was four at the time, had some vague recollection that the

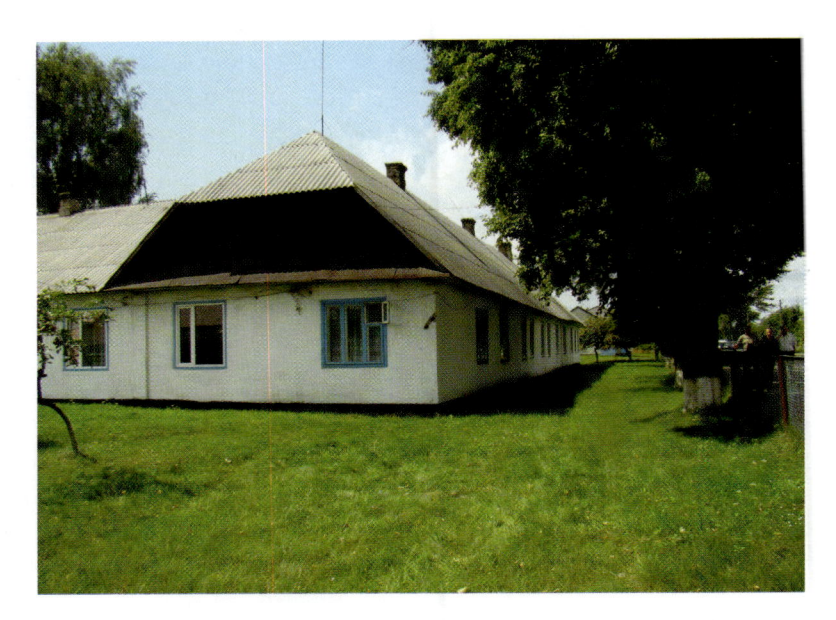

Figure 347. The left wing and front of the hospital where I was born.

hospital building was long and that the staff quarters were in the left-hand corner. He remembered that when leaving the staff quarters, the hospital was on your left and that the entrances to the quarters and to the hospital were from the backyard. I took a photo of the hospital from the front, close to the street (Fig. 347) and from the backyard (Fig. 348). It was wonderful to see the building where I was born, and I was very happy that we had decided to go given that there was a good chance the building would be gone by the following year.

On the way to Lviv, we passed Svitiaź Lake in Shatsk National Nature Park, Luboml and Volodymyr-Volynsky (Polish: Włodzimierz Wołyński), and we stopped in Zhovkva (Polish: Żółkiew). The condition of the roads was horrible. The terrain is largely steppe, with a very small percentage of cultivated land. We only saw a single cornfield, which had very tall stalks and large ears as grown on chernozem (black earth); I was astonished that this fertile land was not cultivated. Apparently, agriculture in the region was destroyed during Soviet rule, and people do not own the land and do not have proper tools. The road from Zhovkva to Lviv was much better, as preparations were ongoing for the European Cup in 2012. In Lviv we stayed at the Opera

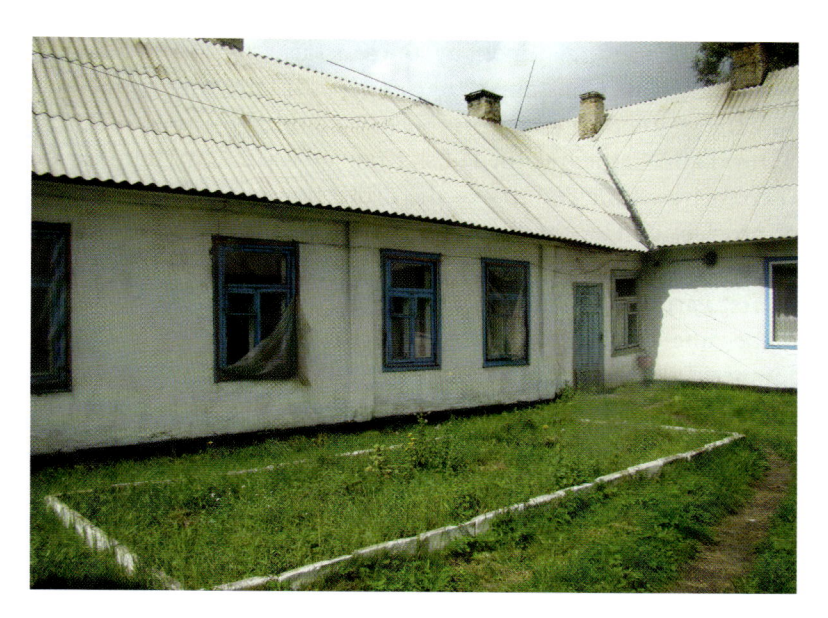

Figure 348. A view from the backyard: the staff quarters with the entrance door.

Hotel, which is very nice, but pricey. The following night Antoni managed to secure rooms at the Natalia Hotel, equally nice but much less expensive. As we were enquiring about rooms at the Natalia Hotel and were talking in Polish, a young man approached us and offered to show us some places in Lviv. His name was Włodek Kurżyński and he was a first year medical student. His father was Ukrainian, but his mother, grandmother and great grandmother were all Polish. His Polish was excellent and marked with a melodious Lvivian accent, which I liked very much.

Our new Polish-Ukrainian guide took us to Prospekt Svobody (Freedom Square) and Rynok Square (Polish: Rynek we Lwowie) with its town hall, and he told us a little about the city's history. He knew the history and the monuments of Lviv inside out. The city was founded by the King of Ruthenia (*Rex Rutheniae*), Daniel I of Galicia, in 1256. To honor his son, Lev (lion), he named it Lviv (Lion City). In 1349 the King of Poland, Casimir the Great, attached these territories to Poland and made Lviv (Polish: Lwów) the capital of the Ruthenian Voivodeship. Lwów was part of Poland and then the Polish-Lithuanian Commonwealth. In the 17th century, Lwów was besieged unsuccessfully several times: by the Cossacks in 1649 and by the Swedes in 1655. Constant struggles against invading armies gave Lwów the motto *Semper Fidelis* ("Always faithful"). On April 1, 1656, at Lwów Latin Cathedral, the Polish King Jan Kazimierz (John Casimir III) consecrated the country to the protection of the Mother of God and proclaimed Her the Patron and Queen of the lands in his kingdom. The king went on to found a university in Lwów in 1661. During the First Partition of Poland in 1772, the city was annexed by Austria and became the capital of the Austrian Kingdom of Galicia and Lodomeria under the name Lemberg. At the end of WWI, the city was proclaimed the capital of independent Ukraine, but its predominantly Polish citizens successfully rebelled and western Ukraine became part of independent Poland. The city was again unsuccessfully attacked by Soviet troops during the Soviet-Polish War of 1920, and after the signing of the Riga Treaty the city remained in Poland as the capital of the Lwów Voivodeship. The city developed rapidly. The university was named John Casimir University in honor of its founder and became the third most important institute of higher education in Poland, with five departments. The Department of Mathematics was strengthened by its resident mathematical genius, Stefan Banach. When the Nazis occupied the city and closed the university, Banach was given work feeding lice in a German institute dealing with infectious diseases, infinitely preferable to the concentration camps where many other university professors were sent. After WWII, western Ukraine became the Soviet Ukrainian Republic until the demise of the Soviet Union, when Ukrainian Independence was proclaimed on July 16, 1990.

The next day a guide took us around Lviv. Among the many places we visited were the Latin Cathedral (Fig. 349), the Main Square with the Town Hall, and the Opera, which was built by Zygmunt Gorgolewski between 1897 and 1900. We wanted to visit the Opera to see the curtain painted by Henryk Siemiradzki, the same artist responsible for the painted curtain in the Słowacki Theater in Kraków. Unfortunately, the curtain is not displayed during every premiere, only some of them. In the afternoon we went to Lychakiv Cemetery (Polish: Cmentarz Łyczakowski), which boasts the tombs of many famous citizens of Lviv — Stefan Banach, Zygmunt Gorgolewski and Maria Konopnicka among them. Of course, we also visited the Cemetery of the Defenders of Lwów (Polish: Cmentarz Orląt, or "Cemetery of

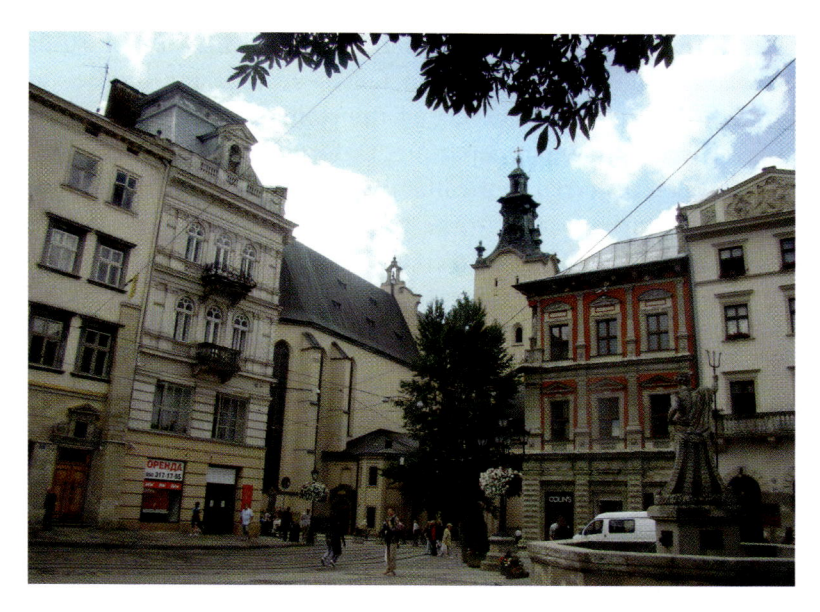

Figure 349. Lviv's Latin Cathedral, viewed from the Main Square.

Eaglets"), a memorial and burial place for the brave Poles and their allies who died in Lviv in the tumultuous years after WWI during the hostilities of the Polish-Ukrainian War of 1918–19 and the Polish-Soviet War of 1919–21. The inscription on the entrance gate reads: *Mortui sunt ut liberi vivamus* ("They died so we could live free").

We headed back to Poland the following day, this time with Antoni taking us across the border at Rava Ruska/Hrebenne. As we approached the border, we saw a line of cars about a mile long. Luckily for us, we had Antoni's unorthodox skills at our disposal; otherwise we would probably have waited two days or more to cross. He got us through in about four-and-a-half hours using methods typical for communist regimes (i.e., bribery), which still work in Ukraine. After crossing the border, we were struck by the stark contrast between Poland and Ukraine in the quality of the roads, fields and houses; Ukraine seemed about 30 years behind Poland in terms of economic development. We arrived at Chełm in the evening and spent one more night in Hotel Kozak, returning to Kraków on August 12. We had airline tickets booked to Columbia for September 18 and on September,

3rd my brother, Lesław, planned to celebrate his 80th birthday. This planned birthday celebration failed, because my brother was admitted to hospital for surgery of the stomach. He was to be discharged a week before our departure. Unfortunately, due to complications he was transferred to the intensive care unit. His condition was very serious, but appeared to be to getting better, and we went to Columbia as planned. Lesław died two weeks after our departure. We returned to Kraków on October 2. His funeral was held on October 4, and was attended by almost all the Twardowskis. That year we got back to Columbia on September 18.

Epilogue

Most of my adult life was devoted to academia, including patient care, teaching and research. My main field of interest was related to the treatment of renal failure, both acute and chronic, but mostly to the treatment of chronic renal failure by dialysis. My most widely accepted contributions to the development of dialysis techniques were the peritoneal equilibration test, which is used for multiple purposes, and the constant site (buttonhole) method of needle insertion into arteriovenous fistula for hemodialysis. My publications related to these discoveries have been cited in numerous publications. These discoveries could not be patented and therefore never resulted in royalties, but they were the principal reason I was invited to give so many presentations around the world. My most successful patents were associated with an artificial kidney for daily (frequent) hemodialysis as well as with intravenous catheters for hemodialysis. Less successful patents were for the Swan Neck peritoneal dialysis catheter and a method of reusing coil dialyzers. Many of my patents have not resulted in any royalties but have been valuable from a theoretical point of view.

I am convinced about the importance of my work on capillary artificial kidneys. Although I was not able to build it in Poland at the time, the theoretical basis for the work was sound and was later confirmed by others. I am particularly certain about the value of the conclusions in my habilitation thesis, which indicated that longer and more frequent hemodialyses are associated with beneficial clinical outcomes. It is very disappointing that short and infrequent (thrice-weekly) dialysis is still accepted as adequate treatment. I believe that the length of dialysis, particularly in the U.S. (less than 240 minutes in a thrice-weekly schedule), remains entirely insufficient, particularly in patients with poor urine output. However, it is encouraging that more and more centers are introducing longer hemodialysis sessions. The conclusion in my thesis concerning the advantages of more frequent hemodialysis sessions fares better, and there are growing numbers of patients on a dialysis schedule more frequent than thrice weekly. A very time-consuming study on exit site classification and treatment has not been widely accepted. However, I am convinced of the study's value and hope that it will be rediscovered in the future. All in all, I am happy with my contributions to progress in dialysis therapy.

My life's achievements would not have been possible were it not for the good fortune with which I have been endowed. I had exemplary parents, aunts and uncles, who both inspired and encouraged. The long distances I traveled to different schools and the long hours of work in the fields in my youth contributed to a lifetime of good health. I have also enjoyed a very happy marriage to Halina, who has always supported me in every possible way in my career. As well, Halina's parents and my own mother and father helped us enormously in the early years of our marriage.

Nearly all of the schools I attended were excellent and did an adequate job of preparing me for my professional life. Choosing dialysis therapy was unplanned, but it turned out to be a good choice. I started working as a department head very early in life, which was unnerving at first but ultimately made the process of learning and thinking independently easier. Many of my discoveries were serendipitous. My contribution to these discoveries was that I did not reject them out of hand but proceeded to prove or disprove them. I was fortunate to cooperate with Prof. Franciszek Kokot, the patron of my habilitation thesis. Moving to Columbia, Missouri, was an essential ingredient of my professional success: I found excellent working conditions and a superb team, particularly Karl D. Nolph, MD, Ramesh Khanna, MD, Barbara F. Prowant, BSN, RN, MSN, CNN, and Harold F. Moore, MA, BS, BSE. Although I conceived many of my ideas in Poland, the communist system in place at the time made it impossible to realize them; that could only happen when I came to the U.S.

Predicting the Future of Chronic Renal Failure Treatment

As Danish physicist Niels Bohr, baseball-playing philosopher Yogi Berra and humorist Mark Twain have all been quoted as saying: "Prediction is very difficult, especially about the future." And who can forget the quote frequently (and accurately, one can only hope) attributed to poor Charles H. Duell, one time commissioner of the U.S. Patent and Trademark Office, who is purported to have said in 1899: "Everything that can be invented has been invented."

In spite of the well-known perils of prediction, let me say a few words about how I see the future of renal failure treatment in the first half of this century. First of all, I do not expect improvements in treatment results only as the consequence of technical progress in the construction of dialyzers: their efficiency is sufficient and the real limitation of efficiency is intercompartmental transport. On the other hand, major progress will be made by rejecting the Kt/V_{urea} index as a measure of dialysis quality. Progress will also be made by returning to the conclusions of my habilitation thesis, which clearly show that longer dialysis sessions produce beneficial results. Longer dialysis time will allow a reduction in dialyzer blood flow, which will improve blood access outcome.

I predict that frequent home hemodialysis patients may grow to 20 percent of the entire chronic hemodialysis population. I am very optimistic that a machine based on my patents will be the most popular in this group of patients. I expect that most of these patients will use the buttonhole method of needle insertion into arteriovenous fistulas and that most of the fistulas will be created on the forearm, as the dialyzer blood flow will be kept below 250 mL/min. In those patients who do not have suitable vessels for arteriovenous fistula, the intravenous catheter will be used. I believe that there is some room for improvement in the results with intravenous catheters: prevention of clot formation and infections through better design, improved locking solution, and better exit site care. I am pessimistic about the possibility of a wearable artificial kidney, particularly because of the problems with continuous anticoagulation. However, I am more optimistic about a peritoneal-based automated wearable artificial kidney. This is also based on a sorbent system, but it does not require continuous anticoagulation, as peritoneal capillaries serve as the "dialyzer." Whether this kind of wearable artificial kidney will be used, depends on the cost and the complexity of procedure. As a matter of fact, CAPD is a kind of wearable artificial kidney

At the same time, I am pessimistic regarding the possibility of increasing peritoneal dialysis efficiency. I believe my peritoneal equilibration test (or its modifications) will always be used to select the most appropriate peritoneal dialysis technique for a patient and for other diagnostic purposes. I do not think that more than 10 percent of patients requiring dialysis will be on peritoneal dialysis. As the efficiency of peritoneal dialysis is unlikely to improve, patients losing residual renal function will be transferred to hemodialysis. Most of these patients will leave peritoneal dialysis within five to ten years from the start of dialysis and likely switch to home hemodialysis or undergo renal transplant.

I believe there is a good chance that there will be major advances in transplantation, while dialysis will not be widely used for the treatment of chronic renal failure, except for a short time. The transplantation of kidneys "grown" from one's own stem cells may well replace chronic dialysis one day. But only time will tell whether this happens in my lifetime. Although the signs are encouraging, I fear it may not even happen before 2050.

Letters to the Editor

Le 1 Twardowski ZJ. (1977) Abatement of psoriasis and repeated dialysis. *Ann Intern Med* **86**: 509–510.

Le 2 Twardowski ZJ, Nolph KD. (1984) Continuous hemofiltration. *Ann Intern Med* **101**: 145–147.

Le 3 Twardowski ZJ. (1984) Treatment of pericardial effusion with local corticosteroid injections. *J Am Med Assoc* **252**: 1283.

Le 4 Twardowski ZJ, Nolph KD, Khanna R. (1984) Absorption of insulin to the surface of peritoneal dialysis solution containers. *Am J Kidney Dis* **4**: 209–210.

Le 5 Twardowski ZJ, Khanna R. (1984) Insulin and the peridex filters. *Perit Dial Bull* **4**: 184–185.

Le 6 Mactier R, Khanna R, Twardowski Z, Nolph KD. (1988) Estimation of lymphatic absorption and intraperitoneal volume during hypertonic peritoneal dialysis. *Trans Am Soc Artif Intern Organs* **34**: 82–84.

Le 7 Twardowski ZJ. (1988) Peritoneal equilibration test. Reply to the letter of Drs. Chandran and Flynn. *Perit Dial Int* **8**: 59–60.

Le 8 Twardowski ZJ. (1988) Peritoneal dialysis glossary II. Reply to Dr. Golper. *Perit Dial Int* **8**: 223.

Le 9 Twardowski ZJ. (1989) CAPD catheters: Solving problems through better design. *Renalife* **4**(1): 14–15.

Le 10 Nolph KD, Khanna R, Mactier R, Twardowski ZJ. (1989) Reply to the letter of Flessner, Dedrick, and Rippe. *Trans Am Soc Artif Intern Organs* **35**: 178–181.

Le 11 Twardowski ZJ. (1990) Malposition and poor drainage of peritoneal catheters. *Semin Dial* **3**: 57.

Le 12 Twardowski ZJ. (1990) Ultrafiltration failure despite normal peritoneal permeability. *Semin Dial* **3**: 192–193.

Le 13 Schmidt LM, Craig PC, Prowant BF, Twardowski ZJ. (1990) A simple method of preventing accidental disconnection at the peritoneal catheter adapter junction. *Perit Dial Int* **10**: 309–310.

Le 14 Prowant BF, Twardowski ZJ, Schmidt LM. (1991) Connectology problems with Swan Neck peritoneal dialysis catheters. *Int J Artif Organs* **14**: 189.

Le 15 Twardowski ZJ, Pasley K. (1994) Reversed one-way obstruction of the peritoneal catheter (the accordion clot). *Perit Dial Int* **14**: 296–297.

Le 16 Twardowski ZJ, Keshaviah P, Nolph KD. (1994) Ascitic fluid albumin and water flows. *J Lab Clin Med* **124**: 455–456.

Le 17   Ersoy FF, Twardowski ZJ, Satalowich RJ, Ketchersid T. (1994) A retrospective analysis of catheter position and function in 91 CAPD patients. *Perit Dial Int* **14**: 409–410.
Le 18   Twardowski ZJ, Khanna R, Nolph KD. (1995) Limitations of the peritoneal equilibration test. *Nephrol Dial Transplant* **10**: 2160–2161.
Le 19   Twardowski ZJ, Khanna R, Nolph KD, Prowant BF. (1996) Comparisons of the Swan Neck and Tenckhoff catheters. *Perit Dial Int* **16**: 189–190.
Le 20   Twardowski ZJ, Khanna, Nolph KD. (1996) "PD Plus": Is it a new concept? *Am J Kidney Dis* **28**: 156–158.
Le 21   Park SE, Twardowski ZJ, Moore HL. (1997) Stability of iron concentrations in peritoneal dialysis solution bags. *Perit Dial Int* **17**(2): 210–211.
Le 22   Twardowski ZJ. (1997) Chronic administration of iron dextran into the peritoneal cavity of rats. *Perit Dial Int* **17**(6): 616–617.
Le 23   Twardowski ZJ. (2000) Urokinase and dialysis therapy. *Kidney Int* **57**: 345.
Le 24   Twardowski ZJ. (2000) Safety of high venous and arterial line pressures during hemodialysis. *Semin Dial* **13**(5): 336–337.
Le 25   Moore HL, Twardowski ZJ. (2004) Reply to letter on diffusion study. *Hemodial Int* **8**(3): 306. [Reply to the letter by Polaschegg H-D. (2004) Diffusion study. *Hemodial Int* **8**(3): 304–305.]
Le 26   Twardowski ZJ. (2009) Glucose in the dialysate. *Hemodial Int* **13**: 86–88.

Patents

Pa I. Dialyzer

1. Twardowski ZJ. Sztuczna nerka kapilarna. (Capillary artificial kidney.) **Polish Patent No. 49 137, granted February 19, 1965.** Application P 103 449, filed January 11, 1964. Expiration February 11, 1984.
2. Twardowski ZJ. Sztuczna nerka kapilarna. (Capillary artificial kidney.) **Polish Patent No. 52 235, granted January 3, 1967.** Application No. P 108 615, filed April 30, 1965. Division of Polish patent number 49 137. Expiration April 30, 1985.
3. Twardowski ZJ, Lebek R. Sposób przygotowania hemodializatora zwojowego do wielokrotnego użycia. (A method of preparing coil dialyzer for repeated use.) **Polish Patent No. 74 878, granted May 30, 1973.** Application No. P 153 334, filed February 7, 1972. Expiration May 30, 1978.

Pa II. Gelatin

1. Twardowski ZJ, Nolph KD. Dialysis solutions containing cross-linked gelatin. Assignee: Curators of the University of Missouri. **USA Patent No. 4,604,379, granted August 5, 1986.** Application No. 621,392, filed June 18, 1984. Abandoned July 31, 1989.

    a) **Canadian Patent No. 1,247,006, granted December 20, 1988.** Application No. 484,204. Abandoned July 31, 1989.
    b) **South Africa Patent No. 85/42654, granted January 29, 1986.** Filed May 6, 1985. Abandoned July 31, 1989.
    c) **Danish Patent. Application No. 745/86.** Filed April 15, 1986. Abandoned July 31, 1989.
    d) **European Patent. Application No. 85902847.4.** Filed April 15, 1986. Abandoned July 31, 1989.

Pa III. Peritoneal Dialysis Catheters

1. Twardowski ZJ, Nolph KD, Khanna R. Peritoneal dialysis catheter. **US Patent No. 4,687,471, granted on August 18, 1987.** Disclosed in the University Patent and Licensing March 25 1985; UM Disclosure No. 85UMC101. Initial patent attorney, Gerrettson Ellis, then Daniel D. Ryan, then Charles R. Matteson of Baxter. Barbara S. Kitchell of Arnold, White and Durkee, 1900 One American Center, 600 Congress Avenue, Austin, TX 78701-3248, took over in 1991. Case No. ABIO 005B. Assignee: Curators of the University of Missouri. Application

No. 826,823, filed February 6, 1986. Continuation of Ser. No. 729,185, May 1, 1985, abandoned. Expiration May 1, 2005.

2. Twardowski ZJ, Nolph KD. Peritoneal dialysis catheter. **US Patent No. 4,772,269, granted on September 20, 1988.** Disclosed in the University Patent and Licensing; UM Disclosure No. 85UMC101. Initial patent attorney, Daniel D. Ryan, then Charles R. Matteson of Baxter. Barbara S. Kitchell of Arnold, White and Durkee, 1900 One American Center, 600 Congress Avenue, Austin, TX 78701–3248, took over in 1991. Case No. ABIO 005B. Assignee: Curators of the University of Missouri. Application No. 14,161, filed February 11, 1987. Continuation of Ser. No. 729,185, filed on May 1, 1985, abandoned. Expiration September 20, 2005.

   a) **Canadian Patent No. 1,293,897, granted on January 7, 1992.** (One Canadian patent corresponding to US Ser. Nos. 729,185 & 826,823.) Assignee: Curators of the University of Missouri. Application No. 508,152. Expiration January 7, 2009.

   b) **Brazilian Patent No. PI 8606640-4, granted by the Brazilian Patent Office July 6, 1993.** (One Brazilian patent corresponding to US Serial Nos. 729,185 & 826,823.) Assignee: Curators of the University of Missouri. Application No. PI8606640, filed April 4, 1986. Expiration April 4, 2001.

   c) **EPO (European Patent) No. 0220288, granted September 15, 1993.** (One European patent corresponding to US Ser. Nos. 729,185 & 826,823.) Assignee: Curators of the University of Missouri. Application No. 86903088.2, filed April 30, 1986. Expiration June 30, 2006.

   d) **Japanese Patent No. 2120327, granted December 20, 1996.** (One Japanese patent corresponding to US Ser. Nos. 729,185 & 826,823.) Assignee: Curators of the University of Missouri. Application No. 502682/1986, filed April 30, 1986. Expiration April 30, 2006.

   e) **Hong Kong Patent No. HK1007967, granted April 30, 1999.** (One Hong Kong patent corresponding to US Ser. Nos. 729,185 & 826,823.) Assignee: Curators of the University of Missouri. Application No. 98107132.7, filed April 30, 1986. Expiration April 30, 2006.

3. Twardowski ZJ, Nichols WK, Khanna R, Nolph KD. Separable peritoneal dialysis catheter. **US Patent No. 5,171,227, granted December 15, 1992.** Disclosed in the University Patent and Licensing Office on December 21, 1990; No. 91-UMC-017. Case No. 632 P 008 in the offices of Gerstman & Ellis, Ltd., Two N. LaSalle Street, Suite 2010, Chicago, IL 60602. Assignee: Curators of the University of Missouri. Application No. 686,186, filed April 16, 1991. Expiration April 16, 2011.

   a) **European Patent No. 0 509 715 B1, granted December 6, 1995.** Proprietor: The Curators of the University of Missouri. Application No. 92303171.0, filed April 9, 1992. Designated states: CH DE DK ES FR GB IT LI. Priority US/April 16, 1991/US 686186. Expiration April 9, 2012.

b) **German Patent No. 692 06 465 T2, granted May 30, 1996.** Proprietor: The Curators of the University of Missouri. Based on European Application No. 92303171.0, filed April 9, 1992, and European Patent No. 0 509 715 B1, granted December 6, 1995. Priority US/April 16, 1991/US 686186. Expiration April 9, 2012.

c) **Australian Patent No. 646729, granted August 1, 1994.** Assignee: The Curators of the University of Missouri. Application No. AU-B-14911/92, filed April 4, 1992. Expiration April 15, 2008.

d) **Canadian Patent No. 2,065,929, issued January 14, 2003.** Assignee: The Curators of the University of Missouri. Filed April 13, 1992. Expiration April 13, 2012.

e) **Japanese Patent No. 3,182,670, granted March 16, 2001.** Assignee: The Curators of the University of Missouri. Japanese Application No. 124157/92, filed April 15, 1992. Expiration April 16, 2012.

Pa IV. Intravenous Catheters

1. Twardowski ZJ, Van Stone JC, Nichols WK. Multiple lumen catheter for hemodialysis. **US Patent No. 5,209,723, granted May 11, 1993.** Disclosed to the Office of Research and Patent Development as "Swan Neck subclavian catheters," June 7, 1985, and assigned No. 85-UMC-044. Amended as "Swan Neck pigtail double lumen intravenous catheters," July 18, 1988, and assigned number 89UMC003. Case No. 632 P 001 in the offices of Gerstman & Ellis, Ltd., Two N. LaSalle Street, Suite 2010, Chicago, IL 60602. Application No. 461,684, filed January 8, 1990, abandoned. Assignee: the Curators of the University of Missouri. Amended on October 8, 1990, on May 14, 1991, and on February 4, 1993. Application No. 772,613, filed October 8, 1991. Expiration May 1, 2010.

    a) PCT (Patent Cooperation Treaty) Application No. PCTUS91/00071, filed January 4, 1991. Abandoned.

2. Twardowski ZJ, Van Stone JC, Nichols WK. Multiple lumen catheter for hemodialysis. **US Patent No. 5,405,320, granted April 11, 1995.** Case No. 632 P 018 in the offices of Gerstman & Ellis, Ltd., Two N. LaSalle Street, Suite 2010, Chicago, IL 60602. Assignee: Curators of the University of Missouri. Application No. 45,016, filed April 8, 1993. Continuation-in-part of Ser. No. 772,613, October 8, 1991, which is a continuation of Ser. No. 461,684, Jan 8, 1990, abandoned. Expiration April 11, 2012.

3. Twardowski ZJ, Van Stone JC, Nichols WK. Multiple lumen catheter for hemodialysis. **US Patent No. 7,695,450, granted April 13, 2010.** Case of Barbara C. McCurdy, Esq., and Lara C. Kelley, Esq., from the Law Firm of Finnegan,

Henderson, Farabow, Garrett & Dunner, LLP, 901 New York Avenue, NW, Washington, D.C., 20001–4413. Assignee: Curators of the University of Missouri. Application No. 08/412,114, filed March 28, 1995. Continuation of Ser. No. 08/045,016, filed April 8, 1993, now US Patent No. 5,405,320, which is a continuation-in-part of application Ser. No. 07/772,613, filed October 8, 1991, now US Patent No. 5,209,723, which is a continuation of application Ser. No. 07/461,684, filed January 8, 1990, now abandoned. Expiration April 12, 2027.

4. Twardowski ZJ, Van Stone JC, Nichols WK. Multiple lumen catheter for hemodialysis. **US Patent No. 5,509,897, granted April 23, 1996.** Case No. 632 P 020 in the offices of Gerstman & Ellis, Ltd., Two N. LaSalle Street, Suite 2010, Chicago, IL 60602. Assignee: The Curators of the University of Missouri. Application No. 389,283, filed February 15, 1995. Division of Ser. No. 45,016, April 8, 1993, US Patent No. 5,405,320, which is a continuation-in-part of Ser. No. 772,613, October 8, 1991, US Patent No. 5,211,983, which is a continuation of Ser. No. 461,684, January 8, 1990, abandoned. Expiration April 23, 2013.

5. Twardowski ZJ, Nichols WK, Van Stone JC. Clot resistant multiple lumen catheter and method. **US Patent No. 5,569,182, granted October 29, 1996,** in force with maintenance fees paid. Next fee is due on April 17, 2008. Disclosed to the Office of Research and Patent Development as "Multiple lumen catheters for hemodialysis (New tip design of intravenous catheter for hemodialysis)," and assigned No. 94-UMC-036. Submitted through the offices of Gerstman & Ellis, Ltd., Case No. 632 P 021, Two N. LaSalle Street, Suite 2010, Chicago, IL 60602, Garrettson Ellis, Esq. Assignee: Curators of the University of Missouri. Application No. 386,473, February 9, 1995. Continuation-in-part of Ser. No. 45,016, April 8, 1993, Patent No. 5,405,320, which is a continuation-in-part of Ser. No. 772,613, October 8, 1991, US Patent No. 5,209,723, which is a continuation of Ser. No. 461,684, January 8, 1990, abandoned. Expiration October 29, 2013.

   a) PCT (Patent Cooperation Treaty), Application No. PCT/US96/01318. Decided to nationalize June 25, 1997.
   b) **Australian Patent No. 706,109, granted on September 23, 1999.** Applicants: The Curators of the University of Missouri. Application No. 199649113, filed January 31, 1996. Expiration January 31, 2016. Annuities due January 31 of each year.
   c) **Australian Patent No. 723,137 (Divisional of 49113/96).** Application No. 22565/99, filed March 31, 1999. Date of sealing: November 30, 2000. Name of patentee: The Curators of the University of Missouri. Title of invention: Clot resistant multiple lumen catheter. Lodgment 31 March 1999. Expiration 31 January 2016 (20 years). Annuities due January 31 of each year.
   d) Canadian patent. Application No. 2,212,511, filed January 31, 1996 (based on PCT). Patent pending and will expire as a patent, when it gets there, on January 31, 2016. Annuities due January 31 of each year.

e) **Japanese Patent No. 3,763,102.** Application No. 524320/1996, filed January 31, 1996 (based on PCT). Name of patentee: The Curators of the University of Missouri. Title of invention: Clot resistant multiple lumen catheter. Date January 27, 2006. Expiration January 31, 2016 (20 years). Next annuity due January 27, 2009.

f) **European Patent (EP) No. 0 808 188 BI.** Application No. 96 905 313.1, filed on January 31, 1996 (based on PCT). Expiration January 31, 2016. The countries where National Processing took place are UK, Ireland, Italy, France, Spain, and Germany. Annuities due January 31 of each year.

6. Twardowski ZJ, Nichols WK, Van Stone JC: Clot resistant multiple lumen catheter. **US Patent No. 5,685,867, granted November 11, 1997,** in force with maintenance fees paid. Third maintenance fee due on May 1, 2009. Disclosed to the Office of Research and Patent Development as "Multiple lumen catheters for hemodialysis (New tip design of intravenous catheter for hemodialysis)," and assigned No. 94-UMC-036. Submitted through the offices of Gerstman & Ellis, Ltd., Case No. 632 P 023, Two N. LaSalle Street, Suite 2010, Chicago, IL 60602, Garrettson Ellis, Esq. Assignee: Curators of the University of Missouri. Application No. 474,376, filed June 7, 1995. Division of Ser. No. 386,473, February 9, 1995, Patent No. 5,569,182, which is a continuation-in-part of Ser. No. 45,016, April 8, 1993, US Patent No. 5,405,320, which is a continuation-in-part of Ser. No. 772,613, October 8, 1991, US Patent No. 5,209,723, which is a continuation of Ser. No. 461,684, January 8, 1990, abandoned. Expiration November 11, 2014.

7. Twardowski ZJ, Nichols WK, Van Stone JC. Clot resistant multiple lumen catheter. **US Patent No. 5,961,486, granted October 5, 1999.** Divisional patent application for "Clot resistant multiple lumen catheter." Submitted through the offices of Gerstman & Ellis, Ltd., Case No. 632 P 032, Two N. LaSalle Street, Suite 2010, Chicago, IL 60602, Garrettson Ellis, Esq., filed in the United States Patent and Trademark Office, Serial No. 09/187,100, filed on November 5, 1998, Continuation of Application No. 08/891,766, July 14, 1997, which is a division of Application No. 08/474,376, US Patent No. 5,685,867, which is a division of Application No. 08/386,473, US Patent No. 5,569,182. Expiration February 9, 2015.

8. Twardowski ZJ. Double cuffed, single lumen, central-vein catheters. Submitted to Gerstman, Ellis & MacMillin, Ltd., on November 6, 1998, Case No. 646 P 006. Submitted to the United States Department of Commerce, Patent and Trademark Office on October 19, 1998, Application No. 09/174,754. Abandoned December 20, 2000.

a) Submitted for foreign patents in Europe, Japan and Canada, on September 20, 1999. International Application No. PCT/US99/21667. Gerstman, Ellis & MacMillin, Ltd., Case No. 646 P 008. Abandoned December 20, 2000.

Pa V. Artificial Kidneys

1. Twardowski ZJ. Artificial kidney for frequent (daily) hemodialysis. **USA Patent No. 5,336,165, granted August 9, 1994.** Disclosed at the Office of Research Program Services on May 18, 1983, and assigned Disclosure No. 83-P-UMC-027. The University of Missouri waived the rights to invention on June 6, 1990. Submitted, as a private inventor, to the offices of Gerstman & Ellis, Ltd., Case No. 632 P 009, Two N. LaSalle Street, Suite 2010, Chicago, IL 60602 on May 22, 1991, patent application corrected, and declaration and small entity statement executed on August 20, 1991. Application filed August 21, 1991, and assigned US Ser. No. 07/748,036. Amended on October 9, 1992 and April 26, 1993. Patent allowed on July 13, 1993. Expiration August 21, 2011.
2. Twardowski ZJ. Artificial kidney for frequent (daily) hemodialysis. **US Patent No. 5,484,397, granted January 16, 1996.** Submitted as a private inventor through the offices of Gerstman & Ellis, Ltd., Case No. 646 P 002, Two N. LaSalle Street, Suite 2010, Chicago, IL 60602. Application No. 155,993, filed November 22, 1993. Divisional of Ser. No. 748,036, August 21, 1991, US Patent No. 5,336,165. Expiration January 16, 2013.
3. Twardowski ZJ. Artificial kidney for frequent (daily) hemodialysis. **US Patent No. 5,902,476, granted May 11, 1999.** Submitted through the offices of Gerstman & Ellis, Ltd., Case No. 632 P 005, Two N. LaSalle Street, Suite 2010, Chicago, IL 60602. Application No. 08/829,537, March 28, 1997. Division of Application No. 08/335,102, November 7, 1994, which is a division of Application No. 08/155,993, November 22, 1993, Patent No. 5,484,397, which is a division of Application No. 07/748,036, August 21, 1991, US Patent No. 5,336,165. Expiration August 21, 2011.
4. Twardowski ZJ, Kenley RS. Method for flushing and filling of an extracorporeal blood circulation system of a dialysis machine. **US Patent No. 6,132,616, granted October 17, 2000.** Submitted through the offices of Gerstman & Ellis, Ltd., Case No. 632 P 003, Two N. LaSalle Street, Suite 2010, Chicago, IL 60602, Garrettson Ellis, Esq. Application No. 08/335,102, November 7, 1994. Division of Application No. 08/155,993, November 22, 1993, US Patent No. 5,484,397, which is a division of Application No. 07/748,036, August 21, 1991, US Patent No. 5,336,165. Expiration October 17, 2017.
5. Twardowski ZJ. Method of preparing a batch of dialysis solution. **US Patent No. 6,146,536, granted November 14, 2000.** Submitted through offices of McDonnell Boehnen Hulbert & Berghoff, Kala Point Professional Building, Suite 204, 260 Kala Point Drive, Port Townsend, WA 98368, Thomas A Fairchild, Esq., Case No. 96,405-B. Application No. 09/290,151, April 12, 1999. Division of Application No. 08/829,537, March 28, 1997, US Patent No. 5,902,476, which is a division of Application No. 08/335,102, November 7, 1994, which is a division of Application No. 08/155,993, November 22, 1993, US Patent No. 5,484,397, which is a division

of Application No. 07/748,036, August 21, 1991, US Patent No. 5,336,165. Expiration August 21, 2011.

Pa VI. Catheter Lock Method and Apparatus

1. Twardowski ZJ. Method and apparatus for locking of central-vein catheters. **USA Patent No. 6,423,050, granted July 23, 2002.** Seyfarth & Shaw, Attorneys, J. Terry Stratman, Esq., Matter No. 40900. Submitted to the United States Department of Commerce, Patent and Trademark Office on June 16, 2000, Ser. No. 09/595,611. Abandoned.

Pa VII. Catheter Dimensions

1. Twardowski ZJ. Patient-tailored central vein catheter. **US Patent No. 6,592,565 B2, granted July 15, 2003.** Garrettson Ellis of Seafarth & Shaw, Attorneys, Matter No. 646 P 010. Submitted to the United States Department of Commerce, Patent and Trademark Office on April 26, 2001, Ser. No. 09/844,578. Expiration July 15, 2020. Abandoned 2010.

Publications

Pu 1   Hanicki Z, Hawiger J, Hirszel P, Twardowski Z. (1964) On some aspects of the antibodies deficiency syndrome. *Acta Med Pol* **4**: 229–241.

Pu 2   Twardowski Z. (1964) On the advantages and possibility of constructing a capillary artificial kidney. *Acta Med Pol* **5**: 303–329.

Pu 3   Hanicki Z, Pączek Z, Wiernikowski A, et al. (1964) Wyniki działalności ośrodka dializy pozaustrojowej w Krakowie. (The results obtained in Artificial Kidney Center in Cracow.) *Pol Tyg Lek* **19**: 1330–1336.

Pu 4   Kowalski E, Twardowski Z. (1965) Udar maciczno-łożyskowy powikłany ostrą niezapalną niedomogą nerek. (Uteroplacental apoplexy complicated by acute non-inflammatory renal failure.) *Pol Tyg Lek* **20**: 1210–1215.

Pu 5   Bross W, Wiktor Z, Kożuszek W, et al. (1967) Własne spostrzeżenia nad przeszczepem nerek u ludzi. (Observations on renal transplantation in man.) *Pol Tyg Lek* **22**: 899–902.

Pu 6   Gasiński J, Twardowski Z, Łotkowski K, Kokot F. (1968) Przeszczepienie nerki od żywych dawców. (Transplantation of the kidney from living donors.) *Pol Tyg Lek* **23**: 458–460.

Pu 7   Twardowski Z, Kokot F. (1968) Zagadnienie przeszczepienia nerki od żywego spokrewnionego dawcy w świetle obserwowanego przypadku. (Problems of kidney transplantation from living related donor in the light of an observed case.) *Patol Pol* **19**: 451–459.

Pu 7a   Twardowski Z, Kokot F. (1969) Problems of kidney transplantation from living related donor in the light of an observed case. Reprinted in *Pol Med J* **8**: 1949–1956.

Pu 8   Twardowski Z, Orawski L, Hakuba A, et al. (1969) Observations on repeated extracorporeal dialysis in patients with terminal renal insufficiency. *Acta Med Pol* **10**: 31–54.

Pu 9   Migdalska-Kornacka Z, Kazubek K, Twardowski Z, Nowak H. (1970) Napadowa nocna hemoglobinuria powikłana ostrą niewydolnością nerek. (Paroxysmal nocturnal hemoglobinuria complicated with acute renal failure.) *Pol Arch Med Wewn* **45**: 709–714.

Pu 10   Twardowski Z, Lebek R, Hakuba A. (1970) Treatment of chronic irreversible renal insufficiency by means of repeated peritoneal dialysis. *Acta Med Pol* **11**: 343–362.

Pu 11   Twardowska H, Twardowski Z. (1970) Zaburzenia psychiczne w przebiegu przewlekłej niewydolności nerek. (Mental disorders in the course of chronic renal insufficiency.) *Pamiętnik XXX Zjazdu Naukowego Psychiatrów Polskich*, Katowice, pp. 159-163.

Pu 12 Twardowski Z, Lebek R, Baran H. (1971) Czynniki wpływające na wielkość utraty białka w czasie dializ otrzewnowych. (Factors exerting an effect on protein loss during peritoneal dialysis.) *Pol Arch Med Wewn* **46**: 69-74.

Pu 12a Twardowski Z, Lebek R, Baran H. (1971) Factors exerting an effect on protein loss during peritoneal dialysis. Reprinted in *Pol Med J* **10**: 1341-1346.

Pu 13 Lebek R, Twardowski Z. (1971) Zastosowanie neuroleptanalgezji II dla zwalczania bólu w czasie dializ otrzewnowych. (Neuroleptanal-gesia II used for abolition of pain in peritoneal dialysis.) *Wiad Lek* **24**: 1965-1968.

Pu 14 Baran H, Lebek R, Spett K, Twardowski Z. (1971) Kinetyka utraty białka w czasie dializ otrzewnowych. (Kinetics of protein loss during peritoneal dialysis.) *Pol Arch Med Wewn* **46**: 551-556.

Pu 14a Baran H, Lebek R, Spett K, Twardowski Z. (1971) Kinetics of protein loss during peritoneal dialysis. Reprinted in *Pol Med J* **11**: 277-280.

Pu 15 Twardowski Z, Kłosowski B. (1972) Znaczenie profilaktycznych — wczesnych, częstych i wydajnych — dializ w leczeniu zespołu zmiażdżenia. (The significance of prophylactic — early, frequent and efficient — dialyses in the treatment of crush syndrome.) *Pol Tyg Lek* **27**: 166-174.

Pu 16 Twardowski Z, Lebek R, Nowak H, Gajdzik C. (1972) Wielokrotne użycie dializatora — prosty i bezpieczny sposób zmniejszenia kosztów dializy. (Repeated use of dialyzer — A simple and safe method for lowering the cost of dialysis.) *Pol Arch Med Wewn* **48**: 171-176.

Pu 17 Twardowski Z, Bahyrycz M, Lebek R, Spett J. (1973) Zalety płynu dializacyjnego bez glukozy w leczeniu przewlekłej niewydolności nerek. (Advantages of glucose-free dializing fluid for hemodialysis treatment in cases of chronic renal failure.) *Pol Arch Med Wewn* **50**: 1079-1086.

Pu 18 Twardowski Z. (1974) O adekwatności hemodializy w leczeniu przewlekłej niewydolności nerek. (Adequacy of hemodialysis in the treatment of chronic renal insufficiency — Preliminary report.) *Przegl Lek* **31**: 457-460.

Pu 19 Pohorecka-Zagroba L, Twardowski Z. (1974) O nefropatii rodzinnej na podstawie obserwowanych przypadków. (On familial nephropathy in the light of observed cases.) *Pol Tyg Lek* **29**: 1433-1435.

Pu 20 Hakuba A, Twardowski Z. (1974) Mieszane zatrucie tlenkiem węgla i wywoływaczem metolohydrochinonowym. (Mixed poisoning with carbon monoxide and metholo-hydroquinone developer.) *Wiad Lek* **27**: 1589-1592.

Pu 21 Twardowski Z. (1974) The adequacy of haemodialysis in treatment of chronic renal failure. *Acta Med Pol* **15**: 227-243.

Pu 22 Twardowski Z. (1974) Significance of certain measurable parameters in the evaluation of haemodialysis adequacy. *Acta Med Pol* **15**: 245-254.

Pu 23 Twardowski Z. (1975) Effect of long-term increase in the frequency and/or prolongation of dialysis duration on certain clinical manifestations and results of laboratory investigations in patients with chronic renal failure. *Acta Med Pol* **16**: 31–44.

Pu 24 Twardowski Z. (1975) Kryteria doboru optymalnej aparatury do hemodializ dla chorych z przewlekłą niewydolnością nerek. (Criteria for the choice of optimal hemodialysis equipment for patients with chronic renal failure.) *Pol Arch Med Wewn* **53**: 275–286.

Pu 25 Drop R, Hanicki Z, Hirszel P, et al. (1975) Pierwsza transplantacja nerki w Krakowie. (The first renal transplantation in Kraków.) *Przegl Lek* **32**: 892–901.

Pu 26 Lebek R, Sobczyk J, Twardowski Z. (1976) Oznaczanie niektórych wskaźników niewydolności nerek w płynie z jamy brzusznej zamiast w osoczu u chorych leczonych powtarzanymi dializami otrzewnowymi. (Determination of some indices of renal failure in abdominal fluid instead of plasma in patients treated by chronic peritoneal dialysis.) *Pol Arch Med Wewn* **56**: 407–410.

Pu 27 Twardowski Z, Lebek R, Kubara H. (1977) Sześcioletnie kliniczne doświadczenie z wytwarzaniem i użytkowaniem wewnętrznych przetok tętniczo-żylnych u chorych leczonych powtarzanymi hemodializami. (Six-year clinical experience with the creation and use of internal arteriovenous fistulas in patients treated with repeated haemodialysis.) *Pol Arch Med Wewn* **57**: 205–214.

Pu 28 Twardowski Z. (1977) Leczenie hemodializami przewlekłej niewydolności nerek. (Treatment of chronic renal failure with haemodialysis.) *Referaty Naukowe XV Zjazdu Polskiego Towarzystwa Urologicznego (Scientific presentations of the XVth Congress of the Polish Society of Urology)*, Katowice, pp. 214–221.

Pu 29 Nolph KD, Popovich RP, Ghods AJ, Twardowski Z. (1978) Determinants of low clearances of small solutes during peritoneal dialysis. (Editorial Review) *Kidney Int* **13**: 117–123.

Pu 30 Twardowski ZJ, Nolph KD, Rubin J, Anderson PC. (1978) Peritoneal dialysis for psoriasis. An uncontrolled study. *Ann Intern Med* **88**: 349–351.

Pu 31 Popovich RP, Moncrief JW, Nolph KD, et al. (1978) Continuous ambulatory peritoneal dialysis. *Ann Intern Med* **88**: 449–456.

Pu 32 Twardowski Z, Nolph KD, Popovich R, Hopkins CA. (1978) Comparison of polymer, glucose, and hydrostatic pressure induced ultrafiltration in a hollow fiber dialyzer: Effects on convective solute transport. *J Lab Clin Med* **92**: 619–633.

Pu 33 Nolph K, Hopkins C, Rubin J, et al. (1978) Polymer induced ultrafiltration in dialysis: High osmotic pressure due to impermeant polymer sodium. *Trans Am Soc Artif Intern Organs* **24**: 162–168.

Pu 34   Nolph KD, Twardowski ZJ, Hopkins CA, *et al.* (1978) Effects of ultrafiltration on solute clearances in cuprophan and cellulose hollow fiber dialyzers: In vitro and clinical studies. *J Lab Clin Med* **91**: 997–1010.

Pu 35   Nolph KD, Twardowski ZJ, Popovich RP, Rubin J. (1979) Equilibration of peritoneal dialysis solutions during long-dwell exchanges. *J Lab Clin Med* **93**: 245–256.

Pu 36   Twardowski Z. (1979) Leczenie łuszczycy dializą. (Treatment of psoriasis with dialysis.) *Przegl Derm* **66**: 99–102.

Pu 37   Twardowski Z. (1979) Epidermopoetyna-hipotetyczny czynnik wywołujący łuszczycę. (Epidermopoietin-hypothetical psoriatogenic factor.) *Przegl Derm* **66**: 103–108.

Pu 38   Twardowski Z. (1979) Ciągła ambulatoryjna dializa otrzewnowa. (Continuous ambulatory peritoneal dialysis.) (Editorial Review) *Pol Arch Med Wewn* **61**: 165–170.

Pu 39   Miller FN, Nolph KD, Harris PD, *et al.* (1979) Microvascular and clinical effects of altered peritoneal dialysis solutions. *Kidney Int* **15**: 630–639.

Pu 40   Nolph KD, Ghods AJ, Brown PA, Twardowski ZJ. (1979) Effects of intraperitoneal nitroprusside on peritoneal clearances in man with variation of dose, frequency of administration and dwell times. *Nephron* **24**: 114–120.

Pu 41   Twardowski Z, Kubara H. (1979) Different sites versus constant sites of needle insertion into arteriovenous fistulas for treatment by repeated dialysis. *Dial Transplant* **8**: 978–979.

Pu 42   Majdan M, Książek A, Twardowski Z. (1979) Wstrząs septyczny u chorej leczonej powtarzanymi hemodializami. (Septic shock in a patient treated by repeated hemodialysis.) *Wiad Lek* **32**: 1229–1232.

Pu 43   Twardowski Z, Książek A. (1979) Farmakokinetyka leków w niewydolności nerek. (Pharmacokinetics of drugs in renal failure.) *Materiały Sesji Naukowej: XXXV lat Wydziałów Lekarskiego i Farmaceutycznego w Lublinie oraz XX Lat Współpracy ze Zjednoczeniem Przemysłu Farmaceutycznego "Polfa,"* Akademia Medyczna w Lublinie, Lublin, pp. 126–134.

Pu 44   Janicka L, Sokołowska G, Twardowski Z, *et al.* (1979) Przypadek stwardnienia międzywłośniczkowego kłębków nerkowych bez zaburzeń w przemianie węglowodanowej i retinopatii. (Glomerulosclerosis intracapillaris in a patient without carbohydrate disturbances or retinopathy.) *Wiad Lek* **32**: 1393–1398.

Pu 45   Bocheńska-Nowacka E, Żbikowska A, Książek A, Twardowski Z. (1979) Dwa przypadki zespołu hemolityczno-mocznicowego u dorosłych. (Two cases of hemolytic-uremic syndrome in adults.) *Wiad Lek* **32**: 1769–1774.

Pu 46   Janicka L, Sokołowska G, Twardowski Z. (1980) Ostra niezapalna niewydolność nerek po leczeniu ciągłym rifampicyną. (Acute renal failure after continuous treatment with rifampicin.) *Pol Arch Med Wewn* **63**: 91–94.

Pu 47 Twardowski Z, Janicka L, Majdan M. (1980) Ocena kliniczna dializatorów zwojowych Vita-2 HF produkowanych przez LZF "Polfa" na licencji firmy "Bellco." (Clinical evaluation of coil dialyzers Vita-2 HF produced by LZF "Polfa" under the license of "Bellco.") *Pol Arch Med Wewn* **53**: 267–274.

Pu 48 Twardowski Z, Janicka L, Dmoszyńska A, et al. (1980) Badanie funkcji płytek przed i po podaniu dipyridamolu u chorych przewlekle hemodializowanych. (Platelet function before and after dipyridamole administration in patients treated by chronic haemodialysis.) *Pol Arch Med Wewn* **63**: 383–392.

Pu 49 Twardowski Z, Książek A, Majdan M, et al. (1981) Kinetics of continuous ambulatory peritoneal dialysis (CAPD) with four exchanges per day. *Clin Nephrol* **15**: 118–130.

Pu 50 Twardowski Z, Sokołowska G, Bocheńska-Nowacka E. (1981) Kinetyka ciągłej ambulatoryjnej dializy otrzewnowej. I. Ultrafiltracja. (Kinetics of continuous ambulatory peritoneal dialysis. I. Ultrafiltration.) *Pol Arch Med Wewn* **65**: 57–64.

Pu 51 Książek A, Twardowski Z, Janicka L, et al. (1981) Kinetyka ciągłej ambulatoryjnej dializy otrzewnowej. II. Utrata białek i immunoglobulin. (Kinetics of continuous ambulatory peritoneal dialysis. II. Protein and immunoglobulin losses.) *Pol Arch Med Wewn* **65**: 107–114.

Pu 52 Majdan M, Twardowski Z, Milczarska D, et al. (1981) Kinetyka ciągłej ambulatoryjnej dializy otrzewnowej. III. Zachowanie się mocznika, kreatyniny, inuliny, sodu, potasu i fosforu w osoczu i dializacie. (Kinetics of continuous ambulatory peritoneal dialysis. III. Urea, creatinine, inulin, sodium, potassium, and phosphorus in plasma and dialysate.) *Pol Arch Med Wewn* **65**: 131–140.

Pu 53 Twardowski Z, Dmoszyńska A, Janicka L, et al. (1981) Platelet counts in arteriovenous fistula blood are lower than in venous blood. *Dial Transplant* **10**: 422–426.

Pu 54 Twardowski Z, Książek A. (1981) Farmakokinetyka w niewydolności nerek. (Pharmacokinetics in renal failure.) *Pol Arch Med Wewn* **65**: 491–500.

Pu 55 Książek A, Twardowski Z. (1981) Przypadek bólu okolicy lędźwiowej związanego z miesiączką u chorej z przewlekłym odmiedniczkowym zapaleniem nerek. (Lumbar pain associated with menstrual periods in a patient with chronic pyelonephritis.) *Wiad Lek* **34**: 411–413.

Pu 56 Janicka J, Twardowski Z, Sokołowska G. (1981) Wpływ płynu dwuwęglanowego i octanowego na przebieg hemodializy w przewlekłej niewydolności nerek. (Influence of bicarbonate and acetate dialysis solutions on patients treated with repeated hemodialysis.) *Pol Arch Med Wewn* **66**: 93–101.

Pu 57 Twardowski Z, Janicka L. (1981) Three exchanges with a 2.5 liter volume for continuous ambulatory peritoneal dialysis. *Kidney Int* **20**: 281–285.

Pu 58 Twardowski Z, Janicka L, Majdan M, et al. (1981) Efficiency of continuous ambulatory peritoneal dialysis with three 2.5 liter exchanges per day. In: GM Gahl, M Kessel, KD Nolph (eds), *Advances in Peritoneal Dialysis: Proceedings of the 2nd International Symposium on Peritoneal Dialysis*, Berlin, June 16–19. Excerpta Medica, Amsterdam, pp. 111–115.

Pu 59 Nolph KD, Twardowski Z. (1981) Unanswered questions about peritoneal dialysis physiology. (Editorial Review) *Perit Dial Bull* **1**: 114–118.

Pu 60 Janicka L, Żbikowska A, Sokołowska G, Twardowski Z. (1981) Dwa przypadki zapalenia osierdzia o prawdopodobnej etiologii gruźliczej u chorych hemodializowanych. (Two cases of pericarditis of possibly tuberculous aetiology in patients on haemodialysis treatment.) *Pol Arch Med Wewn* **67**: 59–66.

Pu 61 Twardowski Z, Dmoszyńska A, Janicka L, et al. (1982) Platelet counts in blood taken from femoral artery, femoral vein, cubital vein, and arteriovenous fistula. *Nephron* **30**: 378–380.

Pu 62 Twardowski ZJ. (1982) Open Forum: Peritoneal dialysis — What's ahead? *Dial Transplant* **11**: 663–680.

Pu 63 Twardowski ZJ, Nolph KD. (1982) Optimal exchange volume for continuous ambulatory peritoneal dialysis (CAPD). (Editorial Review) *Perit Dial Bull* **2**: 154–158.

Pu 64 Twardowski ZJ. (1982) Clinical experience with polyacrylonitrile membrane dialyzers in Lublin, Poland. In: *Proceedings of the First American AN69 Membrane Scientific Exchange*, Hospal Medical Corporation, Atlantic City, October, pp. 19–22.

Pu 65 Nolph KD, Twardowski ZJ. (1982) Current concepts of the physiology of peritoneal dialysis. State of the art address of peritoneal dialysis. In: *Peritoneal Dialysis — The State of the Art. Edited Proceedings of Canada's First International Symposium on Peritoneal Dialysis*, May 6–7. Communications Media for Education, Inc., New Jersey, pp. 5–6.

Pu 66 Twardowski ZJ, Prowant BF, Nolph KD, et al. (1983) High volume, low frequency continuous ambulatory peritoneal dialysis. *Kidney Int* **23**: 64–70.

Pu 67 Twardowski ZJ, Nolph KD, McGary TJ, et al. (1983) Insulin binding to plastic bags: A methodological study. *Am J Hosp Pharm* **40**: 575–579.

Pu 68 Twardowski ZJ, Nolph KD, McGary TJ, Moore HL. (1983) Nature of insulin binding to plastic bags. *Am J Hosp Pharm* **40**: 579–582.

Pu 69 Twardowski ZJ, Nolph KD, McGary TJ, Moore HL. (1983) Influence of temperature and time on insulin adsorption to plastic bags. *Am J Hosp Pharm* **40**: 583–586.

Pu 70 Twardowski ZJ. (1983) Critical to survival — What form/forms of vascular access do you favor? Why? (Up Front) *Dial Transplant* **12**: 330–339.

Pu 71   Twardowski ZJ, Alpert MA, Gupta RC, *et al.* (1983) Circulating immune complexes: Possible toxins responsible for serositis (pericarditis, pleuritis, and peritonitis) in renal failure. *Nephron* **35**: 190–195.

Pu 72   Twardowski ZJ. (1983) Insulin adsorption to peritoneal dialysis bags. (Editorial Review) *Perit Dial Bull* **3**: 113–116.

Pu 73   Twardowski ZJ, Nolph KD, Prowant BF, Moore HL. (1983) Efficiency of high volume, low frequency continuous ambulatory peritoneal dialysis (CAPD). *Trans Am Soc Artif Intern Organs* **29**: 53–57.

Pu 74   Twardowski ZJ, Nolph KD, McGary TJ, Moore HL. (1983) Polyanions and glucose as osmotic agents in simulated peritoneal dialysis. *Artif Organs* **7**: 420–427.

Pu 75   Twardowski ZJ, Nolph KD. (1984) Blood purification in acute renal failure. (Editorial Review) *Ann Intern Med* **100**: 447–449.

Pu 76   Twardowski ZJ. (1984) Ostra niewydolność nerek (Acute renal failure). In: T Widomska-Czekajska (ed), *Internistyczna Intensywna Terapia i Opieka Pielęgniarska — Podstawy Teoretyczne i Praktyka* (*Medical Intensive Therapy and Nursing Care — Theoretical Background and Practice*). Państwowy Zakład Wydawnictw Lekarskich, Warszawa, Chap. 16, pp. 166–192.

Pu 77   Twardowski ZJ. (1984) Individualized dialysis for CAPD patients: A review of the experience at the University of Missouri. *Uremia Invest* **8**(1): 35–43.

Pu 78   Twardowski ZJ, Tully RJ, Nichols WK, Sunderrajan S. (1984) Computerized tomography (CT) in the diagnosis of subcutaneous leak sites during continuous ambulatory peritoneal dialysis (CAPD). *Perit Dial Bull* **4**: 163–166.

Pu 79   Twardowski ZJ. (1984) New and old catheters — Which to choose? *Perit Dial Bull* **4**(Suppl 3): S98–S99.

Pu 80   Twardowski ZJ, Ryan LP, Kennedy JM. (1984) Catheter break-in for continuous ambulatory peritoneal dialysis — University of Missouri experience. *Perit Dial Bull* **4**(Suppl 3): S110–S111.

Pu 81   Twardowski ZJ, Moore HL, McGary TJ, *et al.* (1984) Polymers as osmotic agents for peritoneal dialysis. *Perit Dial Bull* **4**(Suppl 3): S125–S131.

Pu 82   Twardowski ZJ, Burrows L, Prowant BF. (1984) Individualization of exchange volume. *Perit Dial Bull* **4**(Suppl 3): S134–S136.

Pu 83   Khanna R, Nolph KD, Prowant BF, Twardowski ZJ. (1984) Choosing a dialysis therapy: Introduction to mini-symposium. *Am J Kidney Dis* **3**: 217.

Pu 84   Ruder M, Alpert M, Van Stone J, Twardowski Z. (1984) Comparative effects of hemodialysis with acetate and bicarbonate on left ventricular performance. Life Support Systems. *Proceedings XI Annual Meeting ESAO* **2**(Suppl 1): 217–219.

Pu 85   Nolph KD, Ryan L, Prowant B, Twardowski Z. (1984) A cross sectional assessment of serum vitamin D and triglyceride concentrations in a CAPD population. *Perit Dial Bull* **4**: 232–237.

Pu 86   Twardowski ZJ, Nolph KD. (1984) USA CAPD Registry with special emphasis on diabetes mellitus. In: W Weimar, MWJA Fieren, PPNM Diderich, CT Hoek op de (eds), *Proceedings of the Fourth Benelux Symposium on Continuous Ambulatory Peritoneal Dialysis*, Rotterdam, The Netherlands, November 24, pp. 40-57.

Pu 87   Nolph KD, Twardowski ZJ. (1985) The peritoneal dialysis system. In: KD Nolph (ed), *Peritoneal Dialysis*, 2nd ed. Martinus Nijhoff Publishers, Boston, Chap. 2, pp. 23-50.

Pu 88   Twardowski ZJ, Anderson PC. (1985) Continuous ambulatory peritoneal dialysis for psoriasis. *Missouri Med* **82**(1): 15-17.

Pu 89   Alpert MA, Van Stone J, Twardowski ZJ, et al. (1985) Comparative effects of hemodialysis and continuous ambulatory peritoneal dialysis on left ventricular volume and performance. *Prog Artif Organs* **2**: 511-516.

Pu 90   Twardowski ZJ, Nolph KD, Khanna R, et al. (1985) Peritonitis management in the CAPD program at the University of Missouri, Columbia, November 1983-October 1984. In: *Proceedings of the National CAPD Conference*, University of Toronto Press, pp. 61-65.

Pu 91   Twardowski ZJ. (1985) Intraperitoneal therapy in renal failure. *Semin Oncol* **12**(3) (Suppl 4): 81-89.

Pu 92   Twardowski ZJ, Nolph KD, Khanna R, et al. (1985) The need for a "Swan Neck" permanently bent, arcuate peritoneal dialysis catheter. *Perit Dial Bull* **5**: 219-223.

Pu 93   Twardowski ZJ, Khanna R, Nolph KD. (1986) Osmotic agents and ultrafiltration in peritoneal dialysis. (Editorial Review) *Nephron* **42**: 93-101.

Pu 94   Twardowski ZJ, Hain H, McGary TJ, et al. (1986) Sustained UF with gelatin dialysis solution during long dwell dialysis exchanges in rats. In: JF Maher, JF Winchester (eds), *Frontiers in Peritoneal Dialysis: Proceedings of the 3rd International Symposium on Peritoneal Dialysis*, Washington DC Field, Rich & Assoc., Inc., New York, pp. 249-254.

Pu 95   Twardowski ZJ, Khanna R, Burrows LM, et al. (1986) Two years experience with high volume, low frequency CAPD. In: JF Maher, JF Winchester (eds), *Frontiers in Peritoneal Dialysis: Proceedings of the 3rd International Symposium on Peritoneal Dialysis*, Washington, DC Field, Rich & Assoc., Inc., New York, pp. 378-381.

Pu 96   Reams GP, Young M, Sorkin M, et al. (1986) Effects of dipyridamole on peritoneal clearances. *Uremia Invest* **9**(1): 27-33.

Pu 97   Alpert MA, Van Stone J, Twardowski ZJ, et al. (1986) Comparative cardiac effects of hemodialysis and continuous ambulatory peritoneal dialysis. *Clin Cardiol* **9**: 52-60.

Pu 98   Twardowski ZJ. (1986) Apparently inadequate peritoneal membrane function for solute removal. In: AR Nissenson, RN Fine (eds), *Dialysis Therapy*.

Hanley & Belfus, Inc., Philadelphia, The C.V. Mosby Company, St. Louis, pp. 134–137.

Pu 99   Twardowski ZJ, Lempert KD, Lankhorst BJ, et al. (1986) Continuous ambulatory peritoneal dialysis for psoriasis. A report of four cases. *Arch Intern Med* **146**: 1177–1179.

Pu 100   Prowant B, Nolph KD, Ryan LP, et al. (1986) Peritonitis in continuous ambulatory peritoneal dialysis. Analysis of an 8-year experience. *Nephron* **43**: 105–109.

Pu 101   Twardowski ZJ, Nichols WK, Khanna R, Nolph KD. (1986) Swan Neck peritoneal dialysis catheters — Design, features, sterilizing, insertion and break-in. (Instruction Manual) Accurate Surgical Instruments Corp. Toronto, Ontario, pp. 1–8.

Pu 102   Twardowski ZJ, Khanna R, Nolph KD, et al. (1986) Intraabdominal pressures during natural activities in patients treated with continuous ambulatory peritoneal dialysis. *Nephron* **44**: 129–135.

Pu 103   Nolph KD, Twardowski ZJ, Khanna R. (1986) Clinical pathology conference: Peritoneal dialysis. *Trans Am Soc Artif Intern Organs* **32**: 11–16.

Pu 104   Twardowski ZJ, Khanna R, Nolph KD, et al. (1986) Preliminary experience with the Swan Neck peritoneal dialysis catheters. *Trans Am Soc Artif Intern Organs* **32**: 64–67.

Pu 105   Franklin JO, Alpert MA, Twardowski ZJ, Khanna R. (1986) Effect of intraperitoneal infusion volume and posture on left ventricular systolic function in patients on continuous ambulatory peritoneal dialysis. *Trans Am Soc Artif Intern Organs* **32**: 554–556.

Pu 106   Twardowski ZJ, Nolph KD, Khanna R, et al. (1986) Daily clearances with continuous ambulatory peritoneal dialysis and nightly peritoneal dialysis. *Trans Am Soc Artif Intern Organs* **32**: 575–580.

Pu 107   Lampainen E, Khanna R, Schaefer R, et al. (1986) Is air under the diaphragm a significant finding in CAPD patients? *Trans Am Soc Artif Intern Organs* **32**: 581–582.

Pu 108   Khanna R, Mactier R, Twardowski ZJ, Nolph KD. (1986) Peritoneal cavity lymphatics. (Editorial Review) *Perit Dial Bull* **6**: 113–121.

Pu 109   Lal SM, Twardowski ZJ, Van Stone J, et al. (1986) Benign intracranial hypertension: A complication of subclavian vein catheterization and arteriovenous fistula. *Am J Kidney Dis* **8**: 262–264.

Pu 110   Twardowski ZJ, Nolph KD, Khanna R, et al. (1986) Charged polymers as osmotic agents for peritoneal dialysis. *Mater Res Soc Symp Proc* **55**: 319–326.

Pu 111   Twardowski ZJ, Prowant BF. (1986) Can new catheter design eliminate exit-site and tunnel infections? *Perspect Perit Dial* **4**(2): 5–9.

Pu 112   Khanna R, Twardowski ZJ, Oreopoulos DG. (1986) Osmotic agents for peritoneal dialysis. *Int J Artif Organs* **9**: 387–390.

Pu 113   Mactier RA, Nolph KD, Khanna R, Twardowski ZJ. (1986) Risk factors for hyperaluminemia in continuous ambulatory peritoneal dialysis. *Perit Dial Bull* **6**: 188-193.

Pu 114   Levin TN, Rigden LB, Nielsen LH, *et al.* (1987) Maximum ultrafiltration rates during peritoneal dialysis in rats. *Kidney Int* **31**: 731-735.

Pu 115   Lal SM, Nolph KD, Hain H, *et al.* (1987) Total creatine kinase and isoenzyme fractions in chronic dialysis patients. *Int J Artif Organs* **10**: 72-76.

Pu 116   Mactier RA, Khanna R, Twardowski ZJ, Nolph KD. (1987) Role of peritoneal cavity lymphatic absorption in peritoneal dialysis. (Editorial Review) *Kidney Int* **32**: 165-172.

Pu 117   Nolph KD, Mactier R, Khanna R, *et al.* (1987) The kinetics of ultrafiltration during peritoneal dialysis: The role of lymphatics. *Kidney Int* **32**: 219-226.

Pu 118   Colbert C, Twardowski ZJ, Van Stone JC, *et al.* (1987) The influence of parathyroidectomy on bone mineral density and serum chemistries in dialysis patients. In: R Khanna, KD Nolph, BF Prowant, *et al.* (eds), *Advances in Continuous Ambulatory Peritoneal Dialysis. Proceedings of the Seventh Annual CAPD Conference*, Kansas City, Missouri, February. Peritoneal Dialysis Bulletin, Inc., Toronto, pp. 31-37.

Pu 119   Twardowski ZJ, Khanna R, Nolph KD. (1987) Peritoneal dialysis modifications to avoid CAPD drop-out. In: R Khanna, KD Nolph, BF Prowant, *et al.* (eds), *Advances in Continuous Ambulatory Peritoneal Dialysis. Proceedings of the Seventh Annual CAPD Conference*, Kansas City, Missouri, February. Peritoneal Dialysis Bulletin, Inc., Toronto, pp. 171-178.

Pu 120   Oreopoulos DG, Helfrich GB, Khanna R, *et al.* (1987) Peritoneal catheters and exit-site practices: Current recommendations. *Perit Dial Bull* **7**: 130-138.

Pu 121   Twardowski ZJ, Nolph KD, Khanna R, *et al.* (1987) Peritoneal equilibration test. *Perit Dial Bull* **7**: 138-147.

Pu 122   Mactier RA, Khanna R, Twardowski ZJ, *et al.* (1987) Contribution of lymphatic absorption to loss of ultrafiltration and solute clearances in continuous ambulatory peritoneal dialysis. *J Clin Invest* **80**: 1311-1316.

Pu 123   Mactier RA, Van Stone J, Cox A, *et al.* (1987) Calcium carbonate is an effective phosphate binder when dialysate calcium concentration is adjusted to control hypercalcemia. *Clin Nephrol* **28**: 222-226.

Pu 124   Mactier RA, Khanna R, Twardowski ZJ, Nolph KD. (1987) Ultrafiltration failure in continuous ambulatory peritoneal dialysis due to excessive peritoneal cavity lymphatic absorption. *Am J Kidney Dis* **10**: 461-466.

Pu 125   Janicka L, Książek A, Twardowski Z, Kokot F. (1987) Some hormones, minerals and vitamin D in continuous ambulatory peritoneal dialysis. *Int Urol Nephrol* **19**: 453-459.

Pu 126 Mactier RA, Twardowski ZJ. (1988) Influence of dwell time, osmolality, and volume of exchanges on solute mass transfer and ultrafiltration in peritoneal dialysis. *Semin Dial* **1**: 40–49.

Pu 127 Nolph KD, Mactier R, Khanna R, *et al.* (1988) The role of lymphatics in the kinetics of net ultrafiltration during peritoneal dialysis. In: G La Greca, S Chiaramonte, A Fabris, *et al.* (eds), *Peritoneal Dialysis. Proceedings of Third International Course on Peritoneal Dialysis*, Vicenza. Wichtig Editore, Milano, pp. 19–22.

Pu 128 Mactier RA, Khanna R, Moore H, *et al.* (1988) Reduction of lymphatic absorption from the peritoneal cavity with intraperitoneal neostigmine, phosphatidylcholine and other drugs. In: G La Greca, S Chiaramonte, A Fabris, *et al.* (eds), *Peritoneal Dialysis. Proceedings of Third International Course on Peritoneal Dialysis*, Vicenza. Wichtig Editore, Milano, pp. 41–44.

Pu 129 Twardowski ZJ, Nolph KD. (1988) Opinion: Peritoneal dialysis — How much is enough? *Semin Dial* **1**: 75–76.

Pu 130 Twardowski ZJ. (1988) Peritoneal dialysis glossary II. *Perit Dial Int* **8**: 15–17.

Pu 131 Prowant BF, Schmidt LM, Twardowski ZJ, *et al.* (1988) Peritoneal dialysis catheter exit site care. *Am Nephrol Nurs Assoc J* **15**: 219–222.

Pu 132 Khanna R, Twardowski ZJ. (1988) Peritoneal catheter exit site. (Editorial) *Perit Dial Int* **8**: 119–123.

Pu 133 Mactier RA, Khanna R, Moore H, *et al.* (1988) Pharmacological reduction of lymphatic absorption from the peritoneal cavity increases net ultrafiltration and solute clearances in peritoneal dialysis. *Nephron* **50**: 229–232.

Pu 134 Franklin JO, Alpert MA, Twardowski ZJ, *et al.* (1988) Effect of increasing intraabdominal pressure and volume on left ventricular function in continuous ambulatory peritoneal dialysis (CAPD). *Am J Kidney Dis* **12**: 291–298.

Pu 135 Mactier RA, Khanna R, Twardowski ZJ, *et al.* (1988) Influence of phosphatidylcholine on lymphatic absorption during peritoneal dialysis in the rat. *Perit Dial Int* **8**: 179–186.

Pu 136 Kantrowitz A, Daly BDT, Herman VM, *et al.* (1988) Development of a new long-term access device for continuous ambulatory peritoneal dialysis. *Trans Am Soc Artif Intern Organs* **34**: 930–931.

Pu 137 Twardowski ZJ. (1988) Peritoneal catheter development: Currently used catheters — Advantages/disadvantages/complications, and catheter tunnel morphology in humans. *Trans Am Soc Artif Intern Organs* **34**: 937–940.

Pu 138 Nolph KD, Twardowski ZJ. (1989) The peritoneal dialysis system. In: KD Nolph (ed), *Peritoneal Dialysis*, 3rd ed. Kluwer Academic Publishers B.V., Dordrecht, Chap. 2, pp. 13–27.

Pu 139 Twardowski ZJ. (1989) New approaches to intermittent peritoneal dialysis therapies. In: KD Nolph (ed), *Peritoneal Dialysis*, 3rd ed. Kluwer Academic Publishers B.V., Dordrecht, Chap. 8, pp. 133–151.

Pu 140   Khanna R, Twardowski ZJ. (1989) Peritoneal dialysis access. In: KD Nolph (ed), *Peritoneal Dialysis*, 3rd ed. Kluwer Academic Publishers B.V., Dordrecht, Chap. 16, pp. 319–342.

Pu 141   Twardowski ZJ. (1989) Continuous cyclic peritoneal dialysis: New developments. In: S Bengmark (ed), *The Peritoneum and Peritoneal Access*. Butterworth & Co Ltd, London, Chap. 22, pp. 241–264.

Pu 142   Twardowski ZJ. (1989) Peritoneal dialysis: Current technology and techniques. *Postgrad Med* **85**: 161–182.

Pu 143   Nolph KD, Moore HL, Khanna R, Twardowski ZJ. (1989) Pentoxifylline does not influence maximum ultrafiltration rates and peritoneal transport in rats. *Perit Dial Int* **9**: 131–134.

Pu 144   Twardowski ZJ. (1989) Clinical value of standardized equilibration tests in CAPD patients. *Blood Purif* **7**: 95–108.

Pu 145   Twardowski ZJ, Khanna R. (1989) Swan Neck peritoneal dialysis catheters. In: VE Andreucci (ed), *Vascular and Peritoneal Access for Dialysis*. Kluwer Academic Publishers B.V., Boston, Chap. 16, pp. 271–289.

Pu 146   Twardowski ZJ, Nolph KD, Van Stone JC. (1989) Renal replacement in the next decade. (D&T providers look ahead). *Dial Transplant* **18**: 688–689.

Pu 147   Krutak-Król H, Mace C, Nichols WK, *et al.* (1989) Diagnostic dilemma of an unsuspected hyperfunctioning accessory parathyroid gland after total parathyroidectomy with autotransplantation in a peritoneal dialysis patient. *Am J Nephrol* **9**: 495–498.

Pu 148   Dedhia NM, Schmidt LM, Twardowski ZJ, *et al.* (1989) Long-term increase in peritoneal membrane transport rates following incidental intraperitoneal sodium hypochlorite infusion. *Int J Artif Organs* **12**: 711–714.

Pu 149   Twardowski ZJ. (1990) Physiology of peritoneal dialysis. In: AR Nissenson, RN Fine, DE Gentile (eds), *Clinical Dialysis*, 2nd ed. Appleton & Lange, Norwalk, Connecticut, Chap. 12, pp. 240–255.

Pu 150   Twardowski ZJ. (1990) Nightly peritoneal dialysis: Why, who, how, and when? *Trans Am Soc Artif Intern Organs* **36**: 8–16.

Pu 151   Twardowski ZJ. (1990) Dialysis adequacy and new cycler techniques. In: ZJ Twardowski, R Khanna, KD Nolph, *et al.* (eds), *Contemporary Issues in Nephrology*. Churchill Livingstone, New York, Chap. 4, pp. 67–100.

Pu 152   Nolph KD, Twardowski ZJ, Khanna R, *et al.* (1990) Tidal peritoneal dialysis with racemic or L-lactate solutions. *Perit Dial Int* **10**: 161–164.

Pu 153   Twardowski ZJ. (1990) Peritoneal Dialysis Glossary III. *Perit Dial Int* **10**: 173–175.

Pu 154   Twardowski ZJ, Tully RJ, Ersoy FF, Dedhia NM. (1990) Computerized tomography with and without intraperitoneal contrast for determination of intraabdominal fluid distribution and diagnosis of complications in peritoneal dialysis patients. *Trans Am Soc Artif Intern Organs* **36**: 95–103.

Pu 155 Twardowski ZJ. (1990) The fast peritoneal equilibration test. *Semin Dial* **3**: 141–142.

Pu 156 Twardowski ZJ, Prowant BF, Khanna R, *et al.* (1990) Long-term experience with Swan Neck Missouri catheters. *Trans Am Soc Artif Intern Organs* **36**: M491–M494.

Pu 157 Twardowski ZJ, Prowant BF, Nolph KD, *et al.* (1990) Chronic nightly tidal peritoneal dialysis. *Trans Am Soc Artif Intern Organs* **36**: M584–M588.

Pu 158 Twardowski ZJ. (1990) Peritoneal Dialysis Glossary III. Reprinted in: R Khanna, KD Nolph, BF Prowant, *et al.* (eds), *Advances in Continuous Ambulatory Peritoneal Dialysis. Proceedings of the Tenth Annual CAPD Conference*, Vol. 6, Dallas, Texas, February. Peritoneal Dialysis Bulletin, Inc., Toronto, pp. 47–49.

Pu 159 Keshaviah PR, Nolph KD, Prowant BF, *et al.* (1990) Defining adequacy of CAPD with urea kinetics. In: R Khanna, KD Nolph, BF Prowant, *et al.* (eds), *Advances in Continuous Ambulatory Peritoneal Dialysis. Proceedings of the Tenth Annual CAPD Conference*, Vol. 6, Dallas, Texas, February. Peritoneal Dialysis Bulletin, Inc., Toronto, pp. 173–177.

Pu 160 Twardowski ZJ. (1990) PET — A simpler approach for determining prescriptions for adequate dialysis therapy. In: R Khanna, KD Nolph, BF Prowant, *et al.* (eds), *Advances in Continuous Ambulatory Peritoneal Dialysis. Proceedings of the Tenth Annual CAPD Conference*, Vol. 6, Dallas, Texas, February. Peritoneal Dialysis Bulletin, Inc., Toronto, pp. 186–191.

Pu 161 Mactier RA, Khanna R, Nolph KD, *et al.* (1990) Neostigmine increases net ultrafiltration and solute clearances in peritoneal dialysis by reducing lymphatic absorption. In: MM Avram, C Giordano (eds), *Ambulatory Peritoneal Dialysis — Proceedings of the IVth Congress of the International Society for Peritoneal Dialysis*, Venice, Italy, June 29–July 2. Plenum Publishing Corporation, New York, pp. 36–39.

Pu 162 Mactier RA, Khanna R, Twardowski Z, Nolph KD. (1990) Lymphatic absorption in continuous ambulatory peritoneal dialysis patients with normal and high transperitoneal glucose transport. In: MM Avram, C Giordano (eds), *Ambulatory Peritoneal Dialysis — Proceedings of the IVth Congress of the International Society for Peritoneal Dialysis*, Venice, Italy, June 29–July 2. Plenum Publishing Corporation, New York, pp. 71–75.

Pu 163 Nolph KD, Mactier RA, Khanna R, *et al.* (1990) Kinetics of peritoneal ultrafiltration (UF): The role of lymphatics. In: MM Avram, C Giordano (eds), *Ambulatory Peritoneal Dialysis — Proceedings of the IVth Congress of the International Society for Peritoneal Dialysis*, Venice, Italy, June 29–July 2. Plenum Publishing Corporation, New York, pp. 76–78.

Pu 164 Colbert C, Bachtell R, Schloeder FX, *et al.* (1990) Renal osteodystrophy: Bone mineral density loss and recovery with treatment. In: MM Avram, C Giordano (eds), *Ambulatory Peritoneal Dialysis — Proceedings of the IVth*

Congress of the International Society for Peritoneal Dialysis, Venice, Italy, June 29-July 2. Plenum Publishing Corporation, New York, pp. 124-128.

Pu 165 Twardowski ZJ, Khanna R, Nichols WK, *et al.* (1990) One year experience with Swan-Neck Missouri 2 catheter. In: MM Avram, C Giordano (eds), *Ambulatory Peritoneal Dialysis — Proceedings of the IVth Congress of the International Society for Peritoneal Dialysis*, Venice, Italy, June 29-July 2. Plenum Publishing Corporation, New York, pp. 139-142.

Pu 166 Twardowski ZJ, Nolph KD, Khanna R, *et al.* (1990) Tidal peritoneal dialysis. In: MM Avram, C Giordano (eds), *Ambulatory Peritoneal Dialysis — Proceedings of the IVth Congress of the International Society for Peritoneal Dialysis*, Venice, Italy, June 29-July 2. Plenum Publishing Corporation, New York, pp. 145-149.

Pu 167 Cheek TR, Twardowski ZJ, Moore HL, Nolph KD. (1990) Absorption of inulin and high-molecular-weight gelatin isocyanate solutions from peritoneal cavity of rats. In: MM Avram, C Giordano (eds), *Ambulatory Peritoneal Dialysis — Proceedings of the IVth Congress of the International Society for Peritoneal Dialysis*, Venice, Italy, June 29-July 2. Plenum Publishing Corporation, New York, pp. 149-152.

Pu 168 Prowant BF, Schmidt LM, Twardowski ZJ, *et al.* (1990) Use of exudate smears for diagnosis of peritoneal catheter exit site infection. In: MM Avram, C Giordano (eds), *Ambulatory Peritoneal Dialysis — Proceedings of the IVth Congress of the International Society for Peritoneal Dialysis*, Venice, Italy, June 29-July 2. Plenum Publishing Corporation, New York, pp. 220-222.

Pu 169 Alpert MA, Franklin JO, Twardowski ZJ, *et al.* (1990) Impact of increasing intraperitoneal volume on left ventricular function in continuous ambulatory peritoneal dialysis. In: MM Avram, C Giordano (eds), *Ambulatory Peritoneal Dialysis — Proceedings of the IVth Congress of the International Society for Peritoneal Dialysis*, Venice, Italy, June 29-July 2. Plenum Publishing Corporation, New York, pp. 256-259.

Pu 170 Nolph KD, Twardowski ZJ. (1990) Achieving adequate peritoneal dialysis. *Nefrologia* **10**(Suppl 3): 82-85.

Pu 171 Khanna R., Nolph KD, Twardowski ZJ. (1990) Pharmacological alteration of ultrafiltration. In: GA Coles, M Davies, JD Williams (eds), *CAPD: Host Defense, Nutrition and Ultrafiltration*. Karger, Basel, pp. 150-158.

Pu 172 Twardowski ZJ. (1990) Tidal peritoneal dialysis — Acute and chronic studies. *EDTNA/ERCA J* **15**: 4-9.

Pu 173 Twardowski ZJ. (1990) Peritoneal access methods and complications. In: JHM Tordoir, PJEHM Kitslaar, G Kootstra (eds), *Progress in Access Surgery, Proceedings of the 2nd International Congress on Access Surgery*. Maastricht, The Netherlands, November 16. Datawyse, Maastricht, pp. 186-189.

Pu 174 Twardowski ZJ. (1991) Peritoneal equilibration test: Meaning and relevance. In: G La Greca, C Ronco, M Feriani, et al. (eds), *Peritoneal Dialysis: Proceedings of Fourth International Course on Peritoneal Dialysis*, Vicenza, May 21–24. Wichtig Editore, Milano, pp. 101–107.

Pu 175 Twardowski ZJ. (1991) Exit site infection. In: G La Greca, C Ronco, M Feriani, et al. (eds), *Peritoneal Dialysis: Proceedings of Fourth International Course on Peritoneal Dialysis*, Vicenza, May 21–24. Wichtig Editore, Milano, pp. 241–245.

Pu 176 Twardowski ZJ, Dobbie JW, Moore HL, et al. (1991) Morphology of peritoneal dialysis catheter tunnel: Macroscopy and light microscopy. *Perit Dial Int* **11**: 237–251.

Pu 177 Twardowski ZJ. (1991) Opinion: How will chronic dialysis change over the next decade? *Semin Dial* **4**: 231–232.

Pu 178 Khanna R, Nolph KD, Twardowski ZJ. (1991) Pharmacological alteration of ultrafiltration. In: M Hatano (ed), *Nephrology: Proceedings of the XIth International Congress of Nephrology*, Vol. II. Springer-Verlag, Tokyo, pp. 1581–1591.

Pu 179 Chen T-W, Khanna R, Moore H, et al. (1991) Sieving and reflection coefficients for sodium salts and glucose during peritoneal dialysis in rats. *J Am Soc Nephrol* **2**: 1092–1100.

Pu 180 Twardowski ZJ, Schreiber MJ. (1992) Peritoneal Dialysis Case Forum: A 55-year-old man with hematuria and blood-tinged dialysate. *Perit Dial Int* **12**: 61–71.

Pu 181 Nolph KD, Twardowski ZJ, Keshaviah PK. (1992) Weekly clearances of urea and creatinine on CAPD and NIPD. *Perit Dial Int* **12**: 298–303.

Pu 182 Twardowski ZJ, Nichols WK, Nolph KD, Khanna R. (1992) Swan Neck presternal ("bath tub") catheter for peritoneal dialysis. In: R Khanna, KD Nolph, BF Prowant, et al. (eds), *Advances in Peritoneal Dialysis. Selected Papers from the Twelfth Annual Conference on Peritoneal Dialysis*, Vol. 8, Seattle, Washington, February. Peritoneal Dialysis Bulletin, Inc., Toronto, pp. 316–324.

Pu 183 Twardowski ZJ. (1992) Peritoneal dialysis catheter exit site infections: Prevention, diagnosis, treatment, and future directions. *Semin Dial* **5**: 305–315.

Pu 184 Twardowski ZJ, Prowant BF, Nichols WK, et al. (1992) Six-year experience with swan neck catheter. *Perit Dial Int* **12**: 384–389.

Pu 185 Nolph KD, Moore HL, Twardowski ZJ, et al. (1992) Cross-sectional assessment of weekly urea and creatinine clearances in patients on Continuous Ambulatory Peritoneal Dialysis. *Am Soc Artif Intern Organs J* **38**: M139–M142.

Pu 186 Twardowski ZJ. (1993) Tidal peritoneal dialysis. In: AR Nissenson, RN Fine (eds), *Dialysis Therapy*. Hanley & Belfus, Inc., Philadelphia, pp. 153–156.

Pu 187 Twardowski ZJ. (1993) Peritoneal catheter exit-site and tunnel infection. In: AR Nissenson, RN Fine (eds), *Dialysis Therapy*. Hanley & Belfus, Inc., Philadelphia, pp. 165–168.

Pu 188 Twardowski ZJ. (1993) Apparently inadequate peritoneal membrane function for solute removal. In: AR Nissenson, RN Fine (eds), *Dialysis Therapy*. Hanley & Belfus, Inc., Philadelphia, pp. 173–176.

Pu 189 Twardowski ZJ. (1993) Practical issues in prescribing peritoneal dialysis. In: Andreucci VE, Fine LG (eds), *International Yearbook of Nephrology 1993*. Springer-Verlag, London, pp. 287–310.

Pu 190 Gokal R, Ash SR, Helfrich GB, et al. (1993) Peritoneal catheters and exit-site practices: Toward optimum peritoneal access. *Perit Dial Int* **13**: 29–39.

Pu 191 Twardowski ZJ, Van Stone JC, Jones ME, et al. (1993) Blood recirculation in intravenous catheters for hemodialysis. *J Am Soc Nephrol* **3**: 1978–1981.

Pu 192 Nolph KD, Moore HL, Prowant BF, et al. (1993) Cross-sectional assessment of weekly urea and creatinine clearances and indices of nutrition in continuous ambulatory peritoneal dialysis patients. *Perit Dial Int* **13**: 178–183.

Pu 193 Twardowski ZJ, Nichols WK, Nolph KD, Khanna R. (1993) Swan Neck presternal peritoneal dialysis catheter. Selected topics from the VIth ISPD Congress, Thessaloniki, Greece, October 1–4, 1992. *Perit Dial Int* **13**(Suppl 2): S130–S132.

Pu 194 Twardowski ZJ, Prowant BF. (1993) *Staphylococcus aureus* nasal carriage is not associated with an increased incidence of exit-site infection with the same organism. Selected topics from the VIth ISPD Congress, Thessaloniki, Greece, October 1–4, 1992. *Perit Dial Int* **13**(Suppl 2): S306–S309.

Pu 195 Nolph KD, Moore HL, Prowant BF, et al. (1993) Continuous ambulatory peritoneal dialysis with a high flux membrane. *Am Soc Artif Intern Organs J* **39**: M566–M568.

Pu 196 Nolph KD, Moore HL, Prowant BF, et al. (1993) Age and indices of adequacy and nutrition in CAPD patients. In: R Khanna, KD Nolph, BF Prowant, et al. (eds), *Advances in Peritoneal Dialysis. Selected Papers from the Thirteenth Annual Conference on Peritoneal Dialysis*, Vol. 9, San Diego, California, March. Peritoneal Dialysis Bulletin, Inc., Toronto, pp. 87–91.

Pu 197 Twardowski ZJ. (1993) Recurrent peritoneal catheter exit-site infections: II. *Semin Dial* **6**: 406–408.

Pu 198 Nolph KD, Moore HL, Prowant B, et al. (1993) Continuous ambulatory peritoneal dialysis with a high flux membrane. *Am Soc Artif Intern Organs J* **39**(4): 904–909.

Pu 199 Jensen RA, Nolph KD, Moore HL, et al. (1994) Weight limitations for adequate therapy using commonly performed CAPD and NIPD regimens. *Semin Dial* **7**(1): 61–64.

Pu 200 Lo W-K, Brendolan A, Prowant BF, et al. (1994) Changes in the peritoneal equilibration test in selected chronic peritoneal dialysis patients. *J Am Soc Nephrol* **4**: 1466–1474.

Pu 201 Keshaviah PR, Nolph KD, Moore HL, et al. (1994) Lean body mass estimation by creatinine kinetics. *J Am Soc Nephrol* **4**: 1475–1485.

Pu 202 Twardowski ZJ. (1994) Classification of PD catheter exit sites. In: *Proceedings of the Third Annual Spring Clinical Nephrology Meeting of the National Kidney Foundation*, Chicago, IL, April 7–10. National Kidney Foundation, New York, pp. 233–236.

Pu 203 Twardowski ZJ. (1994) Exit-site care in peritoneal dialysis patients. *Perit Dial Int* **14**(Suppl 3): S39–S42.

Pu 204 Vassa N, Twardowski ZJ, Campbell J. (1994) Hyperbaric oxygen therapy in calciphylaxis-induced skin necrosis in peritoneal dialysis patient. *Am J Kidney Dis* **23**: 878–881.

Pu 205 Nolph KD, Khanna R, Twardowski ZJ, Prowant BF. (1994) Computer interaction: Demographics, adequacy, and nutrition. *Adv Perit Dial* **10**: 3–10.

Pu 206 Twardowski ZJ, Nolph KD, Khanna R, Prowant BF. (1994) Computer interaction: Catheters. *Adv Perit Dial* **10**: 11–18.

Pu 207 Khanna R, Nolph KD, Prowant BF, Twardowski ZJ. (1994) Computer interaction: Peritonitis. *Adv Perit Dial* **10**: 19–21.

Pu 208 Prowant BF, Khanna R, Nolph KD, Twardowski ZJ. (1994) Computer interaction: Instructions to home dialysis patients regarding disposal of peritoneal dialysis waste. *Adv Perit Dial* **10**: 22–24.

Pu 209 Wieczorowska K, Khanna R, Moore HL, et al. (1994) Reproducibility of peritoneal equilibration test (PET) in rats. *Adv Perit Dial* **10**: 33–37.

Pu 210 Suzuki K, Twardowski ZJ, Moore HL, Nolph KD. (1994) Absorption of iron from peritoneal cavity of rats. *Adv Perit Dial* **10**: 42–43.

Pu 211 Trivedi HS, Twardowski ZJ. (1994) Long-term successful nocturnal intermittent peritoneal dialysis: A ten-year case study. *Adv Perit Dial* **10**: 81–84.

Pu 212 Nolph KD, Jensen R, Khanna, Twardowski ZJ. (1994) Weight limitations for weekly urea clearances using various exchange volumes in continuous ambulatory peritoneal dialysis. *Perit Dial Int* **14**: 261–264.

Pu 213 Dobbie JW, Krediet RT, Twardowski ZJ, Nichols KW. (1994) Peritoneal Dialysis Case Forum: A 39-year-old man with loss of ultrafiltration. *Perit Dial Int* **14**: 384–394.

Pu 214 Twardowski ZJ, Khanna R. (1994) Peritoneal dialysis access and exit site care. In: R Gokal, KD Nolph (eds), *The Textbook of Peritoneal Dialysis*. Kluwer Academic Publishers, Dordrecht, pp. 271–314.

Pu 215 Prowant BF, Nolph KD, Twardowski ZJ, et al. (1994) Quality systems in the dialysis center: Peritoneal dialysis. In: LW Henderson, RS Tuma (eds),

Quality Assurance in Dialysis. Kluwer Academic Publishers, Dordrecht, pp. 23–45.

Pu 216 Alpert MA, Hüting J, Twardowski ZJ, et al. (1995) Continuous ambulatory peritoneal dialysis and the heart. *Perit Dial Int* **15**: 6–11.

Pu 217 Nolph KD, Twardowski ZJ, Khanna R, et al. (1995) Predicted and measured daily creatinine production in CAPD: Identifying noncompliance. *Perit Dial Int* **15**: 22–25.

Pu 218 Twardowski ZJ. (1995) Physiology of peritoneal dialysis. In: AR Nissenson, RN Fine, DE Gentile (eds), *Clinical Dialysis*, 3rd ed. Appleton & Large, Norwalk, Connecticut, Chap. 15, pp. 322–342.

Pu 219 Twardowski ZJ. (1995) Peritoneal dialysis case forum popular with conference attendees. In: *Peritoneal Dialysis Today. Highlights of the 15th Annual Conference of Peritoneal Dialysis*, Vol. 1, Baltimore, Maryland, February, p. 6.

Pu 220 Twardowski ZJ. (1995) "Do not remove the catheter during the acute phase of severe peritonitis," advocates Alain Slingeneyer from France. In: *Peritoneal Dialysis Today. Highlights of the 15th Annual Conference of Peritoneal Dialysis*, Vol. 1, Baltimore, Maryland, February, pp. 7–8.

Pu 221 Twardowski ZJ. (1995) Initial improvement following therapy could be misleading in polymicrobial peritonitis. In: *Peritoneal Dialysis Today. Highlights of the 15th Annual Conference of Peritoneal Dialysis*, Vol. 1, Baltimore, Maryland, February, p. 9.

Pu 222 Twardowski ZJ. (1995) A treatment paradox is on the verge of being solved at the First International Symposium on daily home hemodialysis. In: *Peritoneal Dialysis Today. Highlights of the 15th Annual Conference of Peritoneal Dialysis*, Vol. 1, Baltimore, Maryland, February, p. 10.

Pu 223 Vassa N, Nolph KD, Prowant BF, et al. (1995) Leukocyte kinetics in patients with peritonitis on long-term peritoneal dialysis. *Am Soc Artif Intern Organs J* **41**: 194–197.

Pu 224 Twardowski ZJ. (1995) Percutaneous blood access for hemodialysis. *Semin Dial* **8**: 175–186.

Pu 225 Suzuki K, Khanna R, Nolph KD, et al. (1995) Expected white blood cell counts and differentials in a rat model of peritoneal dialysis. *Perit Dial Int* **15**: 142–146.

Pu 226 Twardowski ZJ. (1995) Constant site (buttonhole) method of needle insertion for hemodialysis. *Dial Transplant* **24**: 559–560, 576.

Pu 227 Twardowski ZJ. (1995) Will daily home hemodialysis be an important future therapy for end-stage renal disease? *Semin Dial* **8**(5): 263–265.

Pu 228 Nolph KD, Keshaviah P, Emerson P, et al. (1995) A new approach to optimizing urea clearances in hemodialysis and continuous ambulatory peritoneal dialysis. *Am Soc Artif Intern Organs J* **41**: M446–M451.

Pu 229 Goel S, Nolph KD, Moore HL, et al. (1995) A prospective study of the effect of noncompliance on small solute removal in continuous ambulatory peritoneal dialysis. *Am Soc Artif Intern Organs J* **41**: M452–M456.

Pu 230 Wieczorowska K, Khanna R, Moore HL, et al. (1995) Rat model of peritoneal fibrosis: Preliminary observations. In: R Khanna (ed), *Advances in Peritoneal Dialysis*. Multimed Inc., Toronto, Ontario, pp. 48–51.

Pu 231 Suzuki K, Khanna R, Nolph KD, et al. (1995) Spontaneous peritonitis and peritoneal fibrosis in rats on peritoneal dialysis for nine weeks. In: R Khanna (ed), *Advances in Peritoneal Dialysis*. Multimed Inc., Toronto, Ontario, pp. 52–56.

Pu 232 Suzuki K, Twardowski ZJ, Nolph KD, et al. (1995) Absorption of iron dextran from the peritoneal cavity of rats. In: R Khanna (ed), *Advances in Peritoneal Dialysis*. Multimed Inc., Toronto, Ontario, pp. 57–59.

Pu 233 Twardowski ZJ. (1995) Advantages and limits of the jugular catheter approach. *Nephrol Dial Transplant* **10**: 2178–2182.

Pu 234 Bhatla B, Khanna R, Twardowski ZJ. (1994) Peritoneal access. *J Postgrad Med* **40**(3): 170–178. [Inadvertently omitted from Scientific Publications Volume IV.]

Pu 235 Twardowski ZJ, Prowant BF, Pickett B, et al. (1996) Four-year experience with Swan Neck presternal peritoneal dialysis catheter. *Am J Kidney Dis* **27**(1): 99–105.

Pu 236 Twardowski ZJ, Nolph KD. (1996) Is peritoneal dialysis feasible once a large muscular patient becomes anuric? *Perit Dial Int* **16**: 20–23.

Pu 237 Twardowski ZJ, Prowant BF. (1996) Exit-site study methods and results. *Perit Dial Int* **16**(Suppl 3): S6–S31.

Pu 238 Twardowski ZJ, Prowant BF. (1996) Classification of normal and diseased exit sites. *Perit Dial Int* **16**(Suppl 3): S32–S50.

Pu 239 Twardowski ZJ, Prowant BF. (1996) Exit-site healing post catheter implantation. *Perit Dial Int* **16**(Suppl 3): S51–S70.

Pu 240 Twardowski ZJ, Prowant BF. (1996) Appearance and classification of healing peritoneal catheter exit sites. *Perit Dial Int* **16**(Suppl 3): S71–S93.

Pu 241 Prowant BF, Twardowski ZJ. (1996) Recommendations for exit care. *Perit Dial Int* **16**(Suppl 3): S94–S99.

Pu 242 Khanna R, Twardowski ZJ. (1996) Recommendations for treatment of exit-site pathology. *Perit Dial Int* **16**(Suppl 3): S100–S104.

Pu 243 Prowant BF, Khanna R, Twardowski ZJ. (1996) Case reports for independent study. *Perit Dial Int* **16**(Suppl 3): S105–S114.

Pu 244 Nolph KD, Twardowski ZJ, Prowant BF, Khanna R. (1996) How to monitor and report exit/tunnel infections. *Perit Dial Int* **16**(Suppl 3): S115–S117.

Pu 245 Twardowski ZJ. (1996) Daily home hemodialysis: A hybrid of hemodialysis and peritoneal dialysis. *Adv Renal Replace Ther* **3**(2): 124–132.

Pu 246   Twardowski ZJ. (1996) Peritoneal Dialysis Case Forum. In: *Peritoneal Dialysis Today. Highlights of the 16th Annual Conference of Peritoneal Dialysis*, Vol. 2(1), Seattle, Washington, February, p. 10.

Pu 247   Suzuki K, Khanna R, Nolph KD, et al. (1996) Effects of bicarbonate dialysis solution on peritoneal transport in rats. *Adv Perit Dial* **12**: 24–26.

Pu 248   Kathuria P, Moore HL, Mehrotra R, et al. (1996) Evaluation of healing and external tunnel histology of silver-coated peritoneal catheters in rats. *Adv Perit Dial* **12**: 203–208.

Pu 249   Twardowski ZJ. (1996) What is the role of permanent central vein access in hemodialysis patients? *Semin Dial* **9**(5): 39–395.

Pu 250   Ponferrada LP, Prowant BF, Rackers JA, et al. (1996) A cluster of gram-negative peritonitis episodes associated with reuse of homechoice cycler cassettes and drain lines. *Perit Dial Int* **16**(6): 636–638.

Pu 251   Park SE, Twardowski ZJ, Moore HL, et al. (1997) Chronic administration of iron dextran into the peritoneal cavity of rats. *Perit Dial Int* **17**(2): 179–185.

Pu 252   Twardowski ZJ, Prowant BF. (1997) Current approach to exit site infections in patients on peritoneal dialysis. *Nephrol Dial Transplant* **12**(6): 1284–1295.

Pu 253   Twardowski ZJ. (1997) Grundlagen und Möglichkeiten der Durchführbarkeit der täglichen Heimhämodialyse. *J Nephrologische Team* **2**: S57–S60.

Pu 254   Mehrotra R, Khanna R, Yang TCK, et al. (1997) Calculation of 6 hour D/P creatinine ratio from the 4 hour peritoneal equilibration test: The effect of dwell duration on the results. *Perit Dial Int* **17**(3): 273–278.

Pu 255   Twardowski ZJ, Prowant BF. (1997) *Peritoneal Catheter Exit Site Classification Guide*. Baxter Healthcare Corporation.

Pu 256   Golper TA, Twardowski ZJ, Warady BA, et al. (1997) Dose and adequacy in peritoneal dialysis. *Perit Dial Int* **17**(Suppl 3): S40–S41.

Pu 257   Iman TH, Moore HL, Nolph KD, et al. (1997) Cross-sectional analyses of non-urea nitrogen appearance (NUNA) in a CAPD population. *Perit Dial Int* **17**(3): 303–305.

Pu 258   Kathuria P, Moore HL, Khanna R, et al. (1997) Effect of dialysis modality and membrane transport characteristics on dialysate protein losses of patients on peritoneal dialysis. *Perit Dial Int* **17**(5): 449–454.

Pu 259   Mehrotra R, Saran R, Moore HL, et al. (1997) Toward targets for initiation of chronic dialysis. *Perit Dial Int* **17**(5): 497–508.

Pu 260   Trivedi HS, Twardowski ZJ. (1997) Use of double-lumen dialysis catheters: Loading with locked heparin. *Am Soc Artif Intern Organs J* **43**(6): 900–903.

Pu 261   Twardowski ZJ. (1997) Peritoneal catheter placement and management. In: WN Suki, SG Massry (eds), *Therapy of Renal Diseases and Related Disorders*, 3rd ed. Kluwer Academic Publishers, Chap. 57, pp. 953–979.

Pu 262 Twardowski ZJ. (1997) Patient-tailored prescription of peritoneal dialysis. *EDTNA/ERCA J* **XXIII**(3): 4–13, 33 (English Edition).
Pu 262a Twardowski ZJ. (1997) Εξατομικευμένη επιλογή της περιτοναικής κάθαρσης. *EDTNA/ERCA J* **XXIII**(3): 4–15 (Ελληνική Εκδοση).
Pu 262b Twardowski ZJ. (1997) Prescrizione per la Dialisi Peritoneale. *EDTNA/ERCA J* **XXIII**(3): 5–14 (Edizione Italiana).
Pu 262c Twardowski ZJ. (1997) Patienten angepaßte PD Therapie. *EDTNA/ERCA J* **XXIII**(3): 4–13, 33 (Deutsche Ausgabe).
Pu 262d Twardowski ZJ. (1997) Peritoneaal dialysevoorschrift. *EDTNA/ERCA J* **XXIII**(3): 4–13, 33 (Nederlandstalige Editie).
Pu 262e Twardowski ZJ. (1997) Prescripción individualizada de la diálisis peritoneal. *EDTNA/ERCA J* **XXIII**(3): 4–14 (Edición Española).
Pu 263 Misra M, Twardowski ZJ. (1997) Daily home hemodialysis: Issues and implications. *Nephrol Dial Transplant* **12**(12): 2494–2496.
Pu 264 Twardowski ZJ. (1997) Three ironworkers with abdominal pain and neuropathy. In: KT Weber (ed), *Medical Mysteries*. University of Missouri, Columbia, pp. 235–239.
Pu 265 Gokal R, Alexander S, Ash S, *et al.* (1998) Peritoneal catheters and exit-site practices toward optimum peritoneal access: 1998 update (Official report from the International Society for Peritoneal Dialysis). *Perit Dial Int* **18**(1): 11–33.
Pu 266 Pecoits-Filho RFS, Twardowski ZJ, Khanna R, *et al.* (1998) The effect of antibiotic prophylaxis on the healing of exit sites of peritoneal dialysis catheters in rats. *Perit Dial Int* **18**(1): 60–63.
Pu 267 Pecoits-Filho RFS, Twardowski ZJ, Kim YL, *et al.* (1998) The absence of toxicity in intraperitoneal iron dextran administration: A functional and histological analysis. *Perit Dial Int* **18**(1): 64–70.
Pu 268 Meyer KV, Venkataraman V, Twardowski ZJ. (1998) Creatinine kinetics in peritoneal dialysis. *Semin Dial* **11**(2): 88–94.
Pu 269 Twardowski ZJ. (1998) High-dose intradialytic urokinase to restore the patency of permanent central vein hemodialysis catheters. *Am J Kidney Dis* **31**(5): 841–847.
Pu 270 Twardowski ZJ. (1998) Relationships between creatinine clearances and Kt/V in peritoneal dialysis patients: A critique of the DOQI document. *Perit Dial Int* **18**(3): 252–255.
Pu 271 Twardowski ZJ. (1998) Influence of different automated peritoneal dialysis schedules on solute and water removal. *Nephrol Dial Transplant* **13**(Suppl 6): 103–111.
Pu 272 Twardowski ZJ. (1998) *Laudatio*: Professor Vittorio Bonomini. *Home Hemodial Int* **2**: 1–2.
Pu 273 Twardowski ZJ. (1998) Prevention and treatment of thrombosis associated with long-term hemodialysis catheters. *Home Hemodial Int* **2**: 60–66.

Pu 274 Torigian JI, Twardowski ZJ, Prowant BF. (1998) Home Hemodialysis International, innovation, and the internet. (Editorial) *Home Hemodial Int* **2**: 71.

Pu 275 Usha K, Ponferrada L, Prowant BF, Twardowski ZJ. (1998) Repair of chronic peritoneal dialysis catheter. *Perit Dial Int* **18**(4): 419–423.

Pu 276 Twardowski ZJ. (1998) The clotted central vein catheter for hemodialysis. *Nephrol Dial Transplant* **13**(9): 2203–2206.

Pu 277 Twardowski ZJ, Van Stone JC, Haynie J. (1998) All currently used measurements of recirculation in blood access by chemical methods are flawed due to intradialytic disequilibrium or recirculation at low flow. *Am J Kidney Dis* **32**(6): 1046–1058.

Pu 278 Twardowski ZJ. (1998) The use of urokinase in the treatment of hemodialysis catheter thrombosis. *Contemp Dial Nephrol* **19**(12): 22–25.

Pu 279 Twardowski ZJ, Prowant BF, Nichols WK, *et al.* (1998) Six-year experience with Swan Neck presternal peritoneal dialysis catheter. *Perit Dial Int* **18**(6): 598–602.

Pu 280 Ehrig F, Waller S, Misra M, Twardowski ZJ. (1999) A case of "green urine." *Nephrol Dial Transplant* **14**: 190–192.

Pu 281 Prowant BF, Nolph KD, Ponferrada L, *et al.* (1999) Quality in peritoneal dialysis: Achieving improving outcomes. In: LW Henderson, RS Thuma (eds), *Quality Assurance in Dialysis*, 2nd ed. Kluwer Academic Publishers, Dordrecht.

Pu 282 Pinto AG, Twardowski ZJ, Nolph KD, *et al.* (1999) Longitudinal changes in peritoneal membrane transport kinetics in normal rats. *Perit Dial Int* **19**(1): 72–74.

Pu 283 Popovich RP, Moncrief JW, Nolph KD, *et al.* (1999) Continuous ambulatory peritoneal dialysis. *J Am Soc Nephrol* **10**(4): 901–910.

Pu 284 Twardowski ZJ. (1999) Relationship between creatinine clearance and Kt/V in peritoneal dialysis: A response to the defense of the DOQI document. *Perit Dial Int* **19**: 199–203.

Pu 285 Twardowski ZJ. (1999) Have new materials, shapes, and designs of peritoneal dialysis catheters improved their function? *Semin Dial* **12**(3): 146–148.

Pu 286 Twardowski ZJ. (1999) Paul Teschan, MD, Originator of prophylactic daily hemodialysis. *Home Hemodial Today* **1**(1): 1–3.

Pu 287 Twardowski ZJ, Prowant BF. (1999) Editor's note. *Home Hemodial Today* **1**(1): 1.

Pu 288 Clark WR, Twardowski ZJ. (1999) High blood flow against hydraulic resistance leads to increased hemolysis. *Home Hemodial Today* **1**(1): 3.

Pu 289 Twardowski ZJ. (1999) Primary fistula complications and longevity are better in daily (frequent) hemodialysis than in routine hemodialysis. *Home Hemodial Today* **1**(1): 9.

Pu 290 Twardowski ZJ. (1999) Acute renal failure from the battlefield to the intensive care unit. *Home Hemodial Today* **1**(1): 10.

Pu 291 Twardowski ZJ, Prowant BF. (1999) The 5th International Symposium on Home Hemodialysis bigger than ever. *Home Hemodial Today* **1**(1): 16.

Pu 292 Twardowski ZJ. (1999) *Laudatio*: Professor Paul E. Teschan. *Home Hemodial Int* **3**: 1–4.

Pu 293 Kjellstrand CM, Twardowski ZJ. (1999) Measurement of hemodialysis adequacy in a changing world. *Home Hemodial Int* **3**: 13–15.

Pu 294 Twardowski ZJ, Haynie JD, Moore HM. (1999) Blood flow, negative pressure, and hemolysis during hemodialysis. *Home Hemodial Int* **3**: 45–50.

Pu 295 Twardowski ZJ. (1999) Blood access complications and longevity with frequent (daily) hemodialysis and with routine hemodialysis. *Semin Dial* **12**(6): 451–454.

Pu 296 Twardowski ZJ. (2000) Intravenous catheters for hemodialysis: Historical perspective. *Int J Artif Organs* **23**: 73–76.

Pu 297 Twardowski ZJ, Nichols WK. (2000) Peritoneal dialysis access and exit site care including surgical aspects. In: R Gokal, R Khanna, RT Krediet, KD Nolph (eds), *Peritoneal Dialysis*, 2nd ed. Kluwer Academic Publishers, Dordrecht, Chap. 9, pp. 307–361.

Pu 298 Kathuria P, Twardowski ZJ. (2000) Automated peritoneal dialysis. In: R Gokal, R Khanna, RT Krediet, KD Nolph (eds), *Peritoneal Dialysis*, 2nd ed. Kluwer Academic Publishers, Dordrecht, Chap. 13, pp. 435–463.

Pu 299 Twardowski ZJ. (2000) Carl Kjellstrand, MD, PhD: Architect of the dialysis "Unphysiology" concept. *Home Hemodial Today* **2**(1): 1–2.

Pu 300 Twardowski ZJ, Prowant BF. (2000) Editor's note. *Home Hemodial Today* **2**(1): 1.

Pu 301 Twardowski ZJ. (2000) What went wrong with hemodialysis in the US? *Home Hemodial Today* **2**(1): 5.

Pu 302 Twardowski ZJ. (2000) Intravenous catheters are here to stay. *Home Hemodial Today* **2**(1): 13.

Pu 303 Twardowski ZJ, Prowant BF. (2000) The 6th International Symposium on Home Hemodialysis continues to grow. *Home Hemodial Today* **2**(1): 14.

Pu 304 Twardowski ZJ, Prowant BF. (2000) Society for diagnostic and interventional nephrology founded in San Francisco. *Home Hemodial Today* **2**(1): 14–15.

Pu 305 Twardowski ZJ, Prowant BF. (2000) International society for hemodialysis founded in San Francisco. *Home Hemodial Today* **2**(1): 16.

Pu 306 Twardowski ZJ. (2000) Vascular access for hemodialysis: An historical perspective of intravenous catheters. *J Vasc Access* **1**(2): 42–45.

Pu 307 Twardowski ZJ. (2000) *Laudatio*: Professor Carl Magnus Kjellstrand. *Hemodial Int* **4**: 1–4.

Pu 308 Scribner BH, Twardowski ZJ. (2000) The case for every-other-day dialysis. *Hemodial Int* **4**: 5–7.

Pu 309 Ing TS, Blagg CR, Delano BG, *et al.* (2000) Use of systemic blood urea nitrogen levels obtained 30 minutes before the end of hemodialysis to portray equilibrated, postdialysis blood urea nitrogen values. *Hemodial Int* **4**: 15–17.

Pu 310 Saran R, Venkataraman V, Leavey SF, *et al.* (2000) Outpatient high-dose urokinase infusion improves dialysis catheter longevity: A prospective observational study. *Hemodial Int* **4**: 32–36.

Pu 311 Twardowski ZJ. (2000) Stepwise anticoagulation with warfarin for prevention of intravenous catheter thrombosis. *Hemodial Int* **4**: 37–41.

Pu 312 Twardowski ZJ. (2000) Quotidian hemodialysis: Hemeral and nocturnal. CD-ROM: *1st Congress of Nephrology in Internet*, UNINet, Spanish Society of Nephrology, Sección de Nefrología del Hospital General Yagüe, Burgos, February 15–March 15. www.uninet.edu/cin2000/conferences/zjt/zjt.html.

Pu 313 Misra M, Twardowski ZJ, Khanna R. (2000) Complications of peritoneal access in acute and chronic peritoneal dialysis. In: N Lameire, RL Mehta (eds), *Complications of Dialysis*. Marcel Dekker, Inc., New York, Chap. 8, pp. 133–149.

Pu 314 Lee JH, Reddy DK, Saran R, *et al.* (2000) Advanced glycosylation end-products in diabetic rats on peritoneal dialysis using various solutions. *Perit Dial Int* **20**(6): 643–651.

Pu 315 Twardowski ZJ. (2000) From the rotating drum dialyzer to the personal hemodialysis system: A brief history of hemodialysis technology. *Int J Artif Organs* **23**(12): 791–797.

Pu 316 Twardowski ZJ, Harper G. (1997) The "buttonhole" method of needle insertion takes center stage in the attempt to revive daily home hemodialysis. *Contemp Dial Nephrol* **18**: 18–19.

Pu 317 Lee JH, Reddy DK, Saran R, *et al.* (2000) Peritoneal accumulation of advanced glycosylation end-products in diabetic rats on dialysis with icodextrin. *Perit Dial Int* **20**(Suppl 5): S39–S47.

Pu 318 Reddy DK, Moore HL, Lee JH, *et al.* (2001) Chronic peritoneal dialysis in iron deficient rats with solutions containing iron dextran. *Kidney Int* **59**(2): 764–773.

Pu 319 Twardowski ZJ, Moore HL. (2001) Side holes at the tip of chronic hemodialysis catheters are harmful. *J Vasc Access* **2**(1): 8–16.

Pu 320 Twardowski ZJ, Nichols WK. (2001) Opti-flow catheter tip translocation from the right atrium to the right ventricle. *J Vasc Access* **2**(1): 17–19.

Pu 321 Twardowski ZJ. Bernard Charra MD. (2001) Champion of blood pressure control by slow ultrafiltration. *Hemodial Today* **3**(1): 1–2.

Pu 322 Twardowski ZJ, Prowant BF. (2001) Editor's note. *Hemodial Today* **3**(1): 1.

Pu 323 Twardowski ZJ. (2001) New developments in hemodialysis: Technical and clinical updates. *Hemodial Today* **3**(1): 5.

Pu 324 Twardowski ZJ, Prowant BF. (2001) Update on International Society for Hemodialysis (ISHD). *Hemodial Today* **3**(1): 14.

Pu 325 Twardowski ZJ, Prowant BF. (2001) Update on the American Society for Diagnostic and Interventional Nephrology. *Hemodial Today* **3**(1): 14.

Pu 326 Twardowski ZJ, Prowant BF. (2001) The 7th International Symposium on Hemodialysis bigger than ever. *Hemodial Today* **3**(1): 20.

Pu 327 Twardowski ZJ. (2001) Daily dialysis: Is this a reasonable option for the new millennium? *Nephrol Dial Transplant* **16**(7): 1321–1324.

Pu 328 Twardowski ZJ. (2001) Codzienna hemodializa jest optymalną hemodializą (Daily hemodialysis is the optimal hemodialysis). *Nefrologia Dializ Pol* **5**(Suppl 1): 36–38.

Pu 329 Twardowski ZJ. (2001) *Laudatio*: Dr. Bernard Charra. *Hemodial Int* **5**: 1–5.

Pu 330 Tan SH, Prowant BF, Khanna R, *et al.* (2001) Cardiovascular comorbidity and mortality in patients starting peritoneal dialysis: An American Midwestern center experience. *Adv Perit Dial* **17**: 142–147.

Pu 331 Twardowski ZJ. (2001) Peritoneal dialysis access — Is it time to move up? CD-ROM: *2nd Congress of Nephrology in Internet*, UNINet, Spanish Society of Nephrology, Sección de Nefrología del Hospital General Yagüe, Burgos, November 5–30. Filename: Nuevo/cin2001/conf/Twardowski.

Pu 332 Twardowski ZJ. (2002) Tidal peritoneal dialysis. In: AR Nissenson, RN Fine, *Dialysis Therapy*, 3rd ed. Hanley & Belfus, Inc., Philadelphia, pp. 225–228.

Pu 333 Twardowski ZJ. (2002) Peritoneal catheter exit-site and tunnel infections. In: AR Nissenson, RN Fine, *Dialysis Therapy*, 3rd ed. Hanley & Belfus, Inc., Philadelphia, pp. 239–244.

Pu 334 Twardowski ZJ. (2002) Apparently inadequate peritoneal membrane function for solute removal. In: AR Nissenson, RN Fine, *Dialysis Therapy*, 3rd ed. Hanley & Belfus, Inc., Philadelphia, pp. 253–256.

Pu 335 Twardowski ZJ, Seger RM. (2002) Dimensions of central venous structures in humans measured *in vivo* using magnetic resonance imaging: Implications for central-vein catheter design. *Int J Artif Organs* **25**(2): 107–123.

Pu 335a Twardowski ZJ, Seger RM. (2002) Measuring central venous structures in humans: Implications for central-vein catheter design. *J Vasc Access* **3**(1): 21–37 [reprinted with permission from *Int J Artif Organs* **25**(2): 107–123 (2002)].

Pu 336 Twardowski ZJ, Haynie JD. (2002) Measurements of hemodialysis catheter blood flow *in vivo*. *Int J Artif Organs* **25**(4): 276–280.

Pu 337 Twardowski ZJ. (2002) *Laudatio*: Dr. Belding H. Scribner. *Hemodial Int* **6**: 1–8.

Pu 338 Charra B, Scribner BH, Twardowski ZJ, Bergstrom J. (2002) The middle molecule hypothesis re-visited: Should short, three times weekly hemodialysis be abandoned? *Hemodial Int* **6**: 9–14.

Pu 339　Twardowski ZJ. (2002) Pre-sternal peritoneal access. *Adv Renal Replace Ther* **9**(2): 125–132.

Pu 340　Twardowski ZJ. (2003) PHD®: — The technological solution for daily hemodialysis? *Nephrol Dial Transplant* **18**(1): 19–23.

Pu 341　Twardowski ZJ. (2003) We should strive for optimal hemodialysis: A criticism of the hemodialysis adequacy concept. *Hemodial Int* **7**(1): 5–16.

Pu 342　Twardowski ZJ. (2003) Fallacies of high-speed hemodialysis. *Hemodial Int* **7**(2): 109–117.

Pu 343　Twardowski ZJ, Prowant BF, Moore HL, *et al.* (2003) Short peritoneal equilibration test: Impact of preceding dwell time. *Adv Perit Dial* **19**: 53–58.

Pu 344　Twardowski ZJ. (2003) *Laudatio*: Albert Leslie Babb, PhD, PE. *Hemodial Int* **7**(4): 269–277.

Pu 345　Moore HL, Twardowski ZJ. (2003) The air-bubble method of locking central-vein catheters with acidified NaCl as a bactericidal agent: *In vitro* studies. *Hemodial Int* **7**(4): 311–319.

Pu 346　Twardowski ZJ, Reams G, Prowant B, *et al.* (2003) Air-bubble method of locking central-vein catheters for prevention of hub colonization: A pilot study. *Hemodial Int* **7**(4): 320–325.

Pu 347　Kjellstrand CM, Blagg CR, Twardowski ZJ, Bower J. (2003) Blood access and daily hemodialysis. *Am Soc Artif Intern Organs J* **49**: 645–649.

Pu 348　Twardowski ZJ. (2004) History and development of the access for peritoneal dialysis. In: C Ronco, LW Levin (eds), *Hemodialysis Vascular Access and Peritoneal Dialysis Access*, Contrib Nephrol, Vol. 142. Karger AG, Basel, pp. 387–401.

Pu 349　Twardowski ZJ. (2004) Catheter exit site care in long term. In: C Ronco, LW Levin (eds), *Hemodialysis Vascular Access and Peritoneal Dialysis Access*, Contrib Nephrol, Vol. 142. Karger AG, Basel, pp. 422–434.

Pu 350　Williams AW, Chebrolu SB, Ing TS, *et al.* (2004) Early clinical quality of life and biochemical changes of "daily hemodialysis" (6 dialyses per week). *Am J Kidney Dis* **43**(1): 90–102.

Pu 351　Twardowski ZJ. (2004) Blood access in daily hemodialysis. *Hemodial Int* **8**(1): 70–76.

Pu 352　Twardowski Z. (2004) Effect of long-term increase in the frequency and/or prolongation of dialysis duration on certain clinical manifestations and results of laboratory investigations in patients with chronic renal failure. *Hemodial Int* **8**(1): 30–38 [published in the section: "Historical Milestones in Daily Dialysis." Republished from *Acta Med Pol* **16**: 31–44 (1975)].

Pu 353　Twardowski ZJ. (2004) Short, thrice-weekly hemodialysis is inadequate regardless of small molecule clearance. *Int J Artif Organs* **27**(6): 452–466.

Pu 354　Twardowski ZJ. (2004) *Laudatio*: Prof Claudio Ronco. *Hemodial Int* **8**(4): 309–315.

Pu 355 Kjellstrand CM, Blagg CR, Bower J, Twardowski ZJ. (2004) The Aksys personal hemodialysis system. *Semin Dial* **17**(2): 151–153.

Pu 356 Twardowski ZJ. (2005) What clinical insights from the early days of dialysis are being overlooked today? *Semin Dial* **18**(1): 16–18.

Pu 357 Twardowski ZJ. (2005) Physiology of peritoneal dialysis. In: AR Nissenson, RN Fine (eds), *Clinical Dialysis*, 4th ed. McGraw-Hill, Medical Publishing Division, New York, Chap. 14, pp. 357–384.

Pu 358 Whaley-Connell A, Pavey BS, Satalowich R, *et al.* (2005) Rates of continuous ambulatory peritoneal dialysis-associated peritonitis at the University of Missouri. *Adv Perit Dial* **21**: 72–75.

Pu 359 Twardowski ZJ. (2006) Dialyzer reuse — Part I: Historical perspective. *Semin Dial* **19**(1): 41–53.

Pu 360 Twardowski ZJ. (2006) History of peritoneal access development. *Int J Artif Organs* **29**(1): 2–40.

Pu 361 Twardowski ZJ. (2006) Pathophysiology of peritoneal transport. In: C Ronco (ed), *Peritoneal Dialysis: A Clinical Update*, Contrib Nephrol, Vol. 150. Karger, Basel, pp. 13–19.

Pu 362 Twardowski ZJ. (2006) Peritoneal access: The past, present, and the future. In: C Ronco (ed), *Peritoneal Dialysis: A Clinical Update*, Contrib Nephrol, Vol. 150. Karger, Basel, pp. 195–201.

Pu 363 Saran R, Bragg-Gresham JL, Levin NW, *et al.* (2006) Longer treatment time and slower ultrafiltration in hemodialysis: Associations with reduced mortality in the DOPPS. *Kidney Int* **69**(7): 1222–1228.

Pu 364 Twardowski ZJ. (2006) Dialyzer reuse — Part II: Advantages and disadvantages. *Semin Dial* **19**(3): 217–226.

Pu 365 Twardowski ZJ. (2006) Buttonhole method for fistulas. *Live & Give*, Vol. 2 (Iss. 1), www.rsnhope.org/newsletter/RSNHope_LiveGiveWinter2006.pdf

Pu 366 Negoi D, Prowant BF, Twardowski ZJ. (2006) Current trends in the use of peritoneal dialysis catheters. *Adv Perit Dial* **22**: 147–152.

Pu 367 Odar-Cederlöf I, Bjellerup P, Williams A, *et al.* (2006) Plasma levels of brain natriuretic peptide (BNP) decrease in daily dialysis, suggesting improved left ventricular function. *Hemodial Int* **10**(4): 394–398.

Pu 368 Twardowski ZJ. (2006) Buttonhole method for needle insertion into A-V fistula. *Nephrol Dial Pol* **10**(4): 156–158.

Pu 369 Twardowski ZJ. (2007) Longer hemodialysis is better than shorter hemodialysis. *Kidney Times*, February, www.kidneytimes.com. EasyLink Access #126.

Pu 370 Twardowski ZJ. (2007) Commentary on the article by Verhallen AM *et al.* Utility of the buttonhole cannulation method for hemodialysis patients with arteriovenous fistulas. *Nat Clin Pract Nephrol* **3**(12): 649.

Pu 371 Twardowski ZJ. (2007) Treatment time and ultrafiltration rate are more important in dialysis prescription than small molecule clearance. *Blood Purif* **25**(1): 90–98.

Pu 371a Twardowski ZJ. (2008) Behandlungszeit und Ultrafiltrations rate sind bei der Hämodialyse wichtiger als kleinermolekulare Clearance. (Translated from *Blood Purif* by Dr. med. Michael Gehrkens) *Spektr Nephrol* **21**(1): 19–25.

Pu 371b Twardowski ZJ. (2008) Behandlungszeit und Ultrafiltrations rate sind bei der Dialyseverordnung wichtiger als die Clearance kleiner Moleküle. (Translated from *Blood Purif.* by Dr. med. Michael Gehrkens) *Nieren-Hochdruckkrankheiten* **37**(3): 136–147.

Pu 372 Twardowski ZJ. (2008) Tidal peritoneal dialysis. In: AR Nissenson, RN Fine (eds), *Handbook of Dialysis Therapy*, 4th ed. Saunders Elsevier, Inc., Philadelphia, pp. 549–557.

Pu 373 Twardowski ZJ. (2008) Peritoneal catheter exit-site and tunnel infections. In: AR Nissenson, RN Fine (eds), *Handbook of Dialysis Therapy*, 4th ed. Saunders Elsevier, Inc., Philadelphia, pp. 584–595.

Pu 374 Twardowski ZJ. (2008) Apparently inadequate peritoneal membrane function for solute removal. In: AR Nissenson, RN Fine (eds), *Handbook of Dialysis Therapy*, 4th ed. Saunders Elsevier, Inc., Philadelphia, pp. 617–627.

Pu 375 Twardowski ZJ. (2008) History of hemodialyzers' designs. *Hemodial Int* **12**: 178–210.

Pu 376 Twardowski ZJ. (2008) Sodium, hypertension, and an explanation of the "lag phenomenon" in hemodialysis patients. *Hemodial Int* **12**: 412–425.

Pu 377 Twardowski ZJ. (2009) Sodium and hypertension in hemodialysis patients. (Invited Editorial) *US Nephrol* **4**(1): 65–68.

Pu 378 Kathuria P, Twardowski ZJ. (2009) Automated peritoneal dialysis. In: R Khanna, RT Krediet (eds), *Nolph and Gokal's Peritoneal Dialysis*, 3rd ed. Springer Science + Business Media, LLC, Chap. 2, pp. 303–334.

Pu 379 Kathuria P, Twardowski ZJ, Nichols WK. (2009) Peritoneal dialysis access and exit site care including surgical aspects. In: R Khanna, RT Krediet (eds), *Nolph and Gokal's Peritoneal Dialysis*, 3rd ed. Springer Science + Business Media, LLC, Chap. 14, pp. 371–446.

Pu 380 Twardowski ZJ. (2009) Can chronic volume overload be recognized and prevented in hemodialysis patients? The critical role of treatment time. *Semin Dial* **22**(5): 486–489.

Pu 381 Twardowski ZJ, Moore HL, Prowant BF, Satalowich R. (2009) Long-term follow-up of body size indices, residual renal function and transport characteristics in continuous ambulatory peritoneal dialysis. *Adv Perit Dial* **25**: 155–164.

Pu 382 Prowant BF, Moore HL, Twardowski ZJ, Khanna R. (2010) Understanding discrepancies in peritoneal equilibration test results. *Perit Dial Int* **30**(3): 5–8.

Pu 383 Twardowski ZJ, Misra M. (2010) "Daily" dialysis: Lessons from a randomized, controlled trial. *N Engl J Med* **363**: 2363–2364.

Pu 384 Prowant BF, Moore HL, Satalowich R, Twardowski ZJ. (2010) Peritoneal dialysis survival in relation to body size and peritoneal transport characteristics. *Nephrol Nurs J* **37**(6): 641–646.

Pu 385 Twardowski ZJ. (2011) The buttonhole method spreads "like wildfire." (Commentary) *Dial Transplant* 10: 443.

Pu 386 Twardowski ZJ. (2012) Pionner Editorial: My fortuitous encounter with dialysis therapy. *Artifi organs* 36(4): 327–331.

Pu 387 Twardowski ZJ. Dialyzer Reuse — Invited chapter in: *Dialysis History, Development*, and Promise, edited by Todd S. Ing, Mohamad A. Rahman and Carl M. Kjellstrand.

Pu 388 Twardowski ZJ. Hemodialysis access — Invited chapter in: *Dialysis History, Development, and* Promise, edited by Todd S. Ing, Mohamad A. Rahman, and Carl M. Kjellstrand.

Pu 389 Twardowski ZJ. A story of the first machine for quotidian home hemodialysis — Invited chapter in: *Dialysis History, Development, and Promise*, edited by Todd S, Ing, Mohamad A, Rahman, and Carl M. Kjellstrand.

Selected Abstracts

Ab 1   Twardowski Z, Nolph KD, Popovich RP, Hopkins CA. (1977) Comparison of polymer, glucose, and hydrostatic pressure induced ultrafiltration in a hollow fiber dialyzer: Effects on convective solute transport. Proceedings, *10th Annual Meeting of the American Society of Nephrology*, Vol. 10, p. 40A.

Ab 2   Nolph KD, Hopkins CA, Rubin JE, et al. (1978) Polymer induced ultrafiltration in hollow fiber dialyzer (HFK): High osmotic pressure due to impermeant polymer sodium. Abstracts, *Am Soc Artif Intern Organs* **4**: 41.

Ab 3   Nolph KD, Van Stone JC, Hopkins CA, et al. (1978) Polymer induced ultrafiltration in hollow fiber dialyzers (HFK): High osmotic pressure due to impermeant polymer sodium. *Clin Res* **26**: 471A.

Ab 4   Twardowski Z, Książek A, Majdan M, et al. (1980) Kinetics of continuous ambulatory peritoneal dialysis with four exchanges per day. Abstracts, EDTA, Prague, p. 99.

Ab 5   Twardowski Z, Dmoszyńska A, Janicka L, et al. (1980) Platelet counts in cubital vein, femoral vein, femoral artery, and arteriovenous fistula. Abstracts, EDTA, Prague, p. 100.

Ab 6   Twardowski Z, Janicka L, Majdan M, et al. (1981) Efficiency of continuous ambulatory peritoneal dialysis (CAPD) with three 2.5 L exchanges per day. *Artif Organs* **5**: 4.

Ab 7   Twardowski ZJ, Nolph KD, McGary TJ, Moore HL. (1981) Sustained ultrafiltration with polymer dialysate during long dwell peritoneal dialysis exchanges. Proceedings, *14th Annual Meeting of the American Society of Nephrology*, Vol. 14, p. 54A.

Ab 8   Twardowski ZJ, Nolph KD, McGary T, Moore HL. (1981) Comparison of glucose and polyacrylate as osmotic agents for peritoneal dialysis: *In vitro* and rat studies. *Clin Res* **29**: 874A.

Ab 9   Twardowski Z, Nolph KD, Moore HL, McGary T. (1982) Long dwell peritoneal dialysis exchanges in rats with polyacrylate and glucose as osmotic agents. *Clin Res* **30**: 80A.

Ab 10   Twardowski ZJ, Nolph KD, Prowant BF, et al. (1982) Influence of time on dialysate cell count and differential in samples with and without preservative. *Am Soc Artif Intern Organs* **11**: 69.

Ab 11   Twardowski ZJ, Nolph KD, Prowant BF, et al. (1982) Factors influencing tolerance to 3 L volumes for continuous ambulatory peritoneal dialysis (CAPD). Abstracts, *Am Soc Artif Intern Organs* **11**: 69.

Ab 12   Twardowski ZJ, Alpert MA, Gupta RC, *et al.* (1982) Circulating immune complexes: A possible toxin responsible for serositis (pericarditis, pleuritis, and peritonitis) in renal failure. Proceedings, *IX Annual Meeting ESAO*, pp. 20–23.

Ab 13   Twardowski ZJ, Prowant BF, Nolph KD. (1983) High volume, low frequency continuous ambulatory peritoneal dialysis (CAPD). *Kidney Int* **23**: 153.

Ab 14   Twardowski ZJ, Nolph KD, McGary TJ, Moore HL. (1983) Influence of temperature and time on insulin adsorption to peritoneal dialysis bags. Abstracts, *Am Soc Artif Intern Organs* **12**: 68.

Ab 15   Twardowski ZJ, Nolph KD, Prowant B, Moore HL. (1983) Efficiency of high volume, low frequency continuous ambulatory peritoneal dialysis (CAPD). Abstracts, *Am Soc Artif Intern Organs* **12**: 69.

Ab 16   Khanna R, Nielsen L, Nolph KD, *et al.* (1984) Cross sectional assessment of triglyceride (TG) and cholesterol (C) in a CAPD population. Abstracts, III International Symposium on Peritoneal Dialysis, Washington, D.C., June 17–20. *Perit Dial Bull* **4**(Suppl 2): S32.

Ab 17   Khanna R, Nolph KD, Ryan L, *et al.* (1984) Cross sectional assessment of serum 25 $(OH)D_3$ and 1,25 $(OH)_2D_3$ in a CAPD population. Abstracts, III International Symposium on Peritoneal Dialysis, Washington, D.C, June 17–20. *Perit Dial Bull* **4**(Suppl 2): S32.

Ab 18   Twardowski ZJ, Burrows L. (1984) Two year experience with high volume, low frequency continuous ambulatory peritoneal dialysis. Abstracts, III International Symposium on Peritoneal Dialysis, Washington, D.C., June 17–20. *Perit Dial Bull* **4**(Suppl 2): S67.

Ab 19   Twardowski ZJ, Anderson PC, Prowant BF, Schmidt L. (1984) Continuous ambulatory peritoneal dialysis (CAPD) for psoriasis. Abstracts, III International Symposium on Peritoneal Dialysis, Washington, D.C., June 17–20. *Perit Dial Bull* **4**(Suppl 2): S67.

Ab 20   Twardowski ZJ, Moore HL, McGary TJ, Poskuta M. (1984) Sustained ultrafiltration (UF) with gelatin dialysate during long dwell peritoneal dialysis exchanges in rats. Abstracts, III International Symposium on Peritoneal Dialysis, Washington, D.C., June 17–20. *Perit Dial Bull* **4**(Suppl 2): S67.

Ab 21   Twardowski ZJ, Tully RJ, Nichols WK, Sunderrajan S. (1984) Computerized tomography (CT) in the diagnosis of subcutaneous leak sites during continuous ambulatory peritoneal dialysis (CAPD). Abstracts, III International Symposium on Peritoneal Dialysis, Washington, D.C., June 17–20. *Perit Dial Bull* **4**(Suppl 2): S68.

Ab 22   Janicka L, Książek A, Twardowski Z, Kokot F. (1984) Metabolism of minerals, vitamin D, glucose and some hormones in continuous ambulatory peritoneal dialysis/CAPD. *Kidney Int* **26**: 569.

Ab 23   Twardowski ZJ, Janicka L, Tarkowska A, Jankowska H. (1984) Kinetics of albumin transport in intermittent peritoneal dialysis (IPD) and

Ab 24   continuous ambulatory peritoneal dialysis (CAPD). Abstracts, XXIst Congress of the European Dialysis and Transplant Association-European Renal Association, Florence, Italy, September 23–26. *Kidney Int* **26**: 604.

Ab 24   Twardowski ZJ, Janicka L, Tarkowska A, Jankowska H. (1984) Kinetics of radioactive iodide (^{131}I) transport during intermittent peritoneal dialysis (IPD) and continuous ambulatory peritoneal dialysis (CAPD). Abstracts, XXXIst Congress of the European Dialysis and Transplant Association-European Renal Association, Florence, Italy, September 23–26. *Kidney Int* **26**: 604.

Ab 25   Twardowski ZJ, Nolph KD, Khanna R, *et al.* (1985) Charged polymers as osmotic agents for peritoneal dialysis. Materials Research Society. Fall Meeting Final Program and Abstracts, Publishers Choice Book Mfg. Co., Mars, PA, p. 291.

Ab 26   Khanna R, Twardowski ZJ, Gluck Z, *et al.* (1986) Is daily nightly peritoneal dialysis (NPD) an effective peritoneal dialysis schedule? Abstracts, American Society of Nephrology. *Kidney Int* **29**: 233.

Ab 27   Lampainen E, Khanna R, Schaefer R, *et al.* (1986) Is air under the diaphragm a significant finding in CAPD patients? Abstracts, American Society of Nephrology. *Kidney Int* **29**: 233.

Ab 28   Twardowski ZJ, Nolph KD, Khanna R, *et al.* (1986) The need for Swan Neck tunnel peritoneal dialysis catheter. Abstracts, American Society of Nephrology. *Kidney Int* **29**: 238.

Ab 29   Khanna R, Twardowski ZJ, Gluck Z, *et al.* (1986) Is daily nightly peritoneal dialysis (NPD) an effective peritoneal dialysis schedule? Abstracts, *Am Soc Artif Intern Organs* **15**: 48.

Ab 30   Lampainen E, Khanna R, Schaefer R, *et al.* (1986) Is air under the diaphragm a significant finding in CAPD patients (Pts)? Abstracts, *Am Soc Artif Intern Organs* **15**: 48.

Ab 31   Twardowski ZJ, Khanna R, Nolph KD, *et al.* (1986) Preliminary experience with Swan Neck Tunnel Peritoneal Dialysis Catheters (SNTPDC). Abstracts, *Am Soc Artif Intern Organs* **15**: 49.

Ab 32   Twardowski ZJ, Nolph KD, Khanna R, *et al.* (1986) Daily clearances (C) with continuous ambulatory peritoneal dialysis (CAPD) and nightly peritoneal dialysis (NPD). Abstracts, *Am Soc Artif Intern Organs* **15**: 49.

Ab 33   Franklin JO, Alpert MA, Twardowski ZJ, Khanna R. (1986) Effect of intraperitoneal infusion volume and posture on left ventricular systolic function in patients on continuous ambulatory peritoneal dialysis. Abstracts, *Am Soc Artif Intern Organs* **15**: 49.

Ab 34   Prowant B, Schmidt L, Twardowski ZJ, *et al.* (1986) Use of smears for diagnosis of peritoneal catheter exit site infection. *17th National Symposium of American Nephrology Nurses' Association*, Vol. 13, p. 95.

Ab 35   Prowant B, Ryan L, Twardowski ZJ. (1986) Effect of dialysis solution volume, position and activity on intraabdominal pressure (IAP) in continuous ambulatory peritoneal dialysis (CAPD) patients. *17th National Symposium of American Nephrology Nurses' Association*, Vol. 13, p. 95.

Ab 36   Mactier RA, Van Stone J, Cox A, Twardowski ZJ. (1986) Calcium carbonate ($CaCO_3$) is an effective phosphate binder when hypercalcemia is prevented by lowering dialysate calcium concentration (Ca conc). Program and Abstracts, Annual Scientific Meeting. *Am J Kid Dis*, p. A13.

Ab 37   Colbert C, Twardowski ZJ, Van Stone JC, *et al.* (1986) The influence of parathyroidectomy on bone mineral density and serum chemistries in dialysis patients. Abstracts, VII Annual CAPD Conference. *Perit Dial Bull* **6**(Suppl 4): S4.

Ab 38   Mactier RA, Nolph KD, Khanna R, *et al.* (1987) Lymphatic absorption in peritoneal dialysis in the rat. Abstracts, North American Society of Lymphology, 4th Biennial Meeting. *Lymphology* **20**: 47.

Ab 39   Alpert MA, Franklin JO, Twardowski ZJ, Khanna R. (1987) Effect of increasing intra-abdominal pressure and posture on left ventricular function in patients on CAPD. Abstracts, American Society of Nephrology. *Kidney Int* **31**: 248.

Ab 40   Frock J, Twardowski Z, Nolph K, *et al.* (1987) Tidal peritoneal dialysis (TPD). Abstracts, American Society of Nephrology. *Kidney Int* **31**: 250.

Ab 41   Mactier RA, Khanna R, Twardowski Z, Nolph KD. (1987) Lymphatic absorption in CAPD. Abstracts, American Society of Nephrology. *Kidney Int* **31**: 252.

Ab 42   Nolph KD, Mactier RA, Khanna R, *et al.* (1987) Kinetics of peritoneal ultrafiltration (UF): The role of lymphatics. Abstracts, American Society of Nephrology. *Kidney Int* **31**: 253.

Ab 43   Alpert MA, Franklin JO, Twardowski ZJ, Khanna R. (1987) Impact of increasing intraperitoneal volume on left ventricular function in CAPD patients. Abstracts, IVth Congress of the International Society for Peritoneal Dialysis, Venice, Italy, June 29–July 2. *Perit Dial Bull* **7**(Suppl): S2.

Ab 44   Cheek TR, Twardowski ZJ, Moore HL, Nolph KD. (1987) High molecular weight (MW) gelatin isocyanate absorption from the peritoneal cavity of rats. Abstracts, IVth Congress of the International Society for Peritoneal Dialysis, Venice, Italy, June 29–July 2. *Perit Dial Bull* **7**(Suppl): S16.

Ab 45   Mactier RA, Khanna R, Twardowski Z, Nolph KD. (1987) Lymphatic absorption in CAPD. Abstracts, IVth Congress of the International Society for Peritoneal Dialysis, Venice, Italy, June 29–July 2. *Perit Dial Bull* **7**(Suppl): S50.

Ab 46   Mactier RA, Khanna R, Nolph KD, *et al.* (1987) Neostigmine increases ultrafiltration and solute clearances in peritoneal dialysis by reducing lymphatic drainage. Abstracts, IVth Congress of the International Society

Ab 47 for Peritoneal Dialysis, Venice, Italy, June 29–July 2. *Perit Dial Bull* **7**(Suppl): S50.

Ab 47 Nolph KD, Mactier RA, Khanna R, *et al.* (1987) Kinetics of peritoneal ultrafiltration (UF): The role of lymphatics. Abstracts, IVth Congress of the International Society for Peritoneal Dialysis, Venice, Italy, June 29–July 2. *Perit Dial Bull* **7**(Suppl): S56.

Ab 48 Prowant B, Twardowski Z, Schmidt L, *et al.* (1987) Use of smears for diagnosis of peritoneal catheter exit site (ESO) infection (INF). Abstracts, IVth Congress of the International Society for Peritoneal Dialysis, Venice, Italy, June 29–July 2. *Perit Dial Bull* **7**(Suppl): S60.

Ab 49 Prowant BF, Schmidt LM, Twardowski ZJ, *et al.* (1987) A randomized prospective evaluation of three peritoneal catheter exit site care procedures. Abstracts, IVth Congress of the International Society for Peritoneal Dialysis, Venice, Italy, June 29–July 2. *Perit Dial Bull* **7**(Suppl): S60.

Ab 50 Twardowski Z, Nolph K, Khanna R, *et al.* (1987) Eight hr tidal peritoneal dialysis (TPD) matches 24 hr CAPD and surpasses 8 hr nightly intermittent peritoneal dialysis (NIPD) clearances (C). Abstracts, IVth Congress of the International Society for Peritoneal Dialysis, Venice, Italy, June 29–July 2. *Perit Dial Bull* **7**(Suppl): S79.

Ab 51 Twardowski ZJ, Nolph KD, Khanna R, *et al.* (1987) Choice of peritoneal dialysis regimen based on peritoneal transfer rates (PTR). Abstracts, IVth Congress of the International Society for Peritoneal Dialysis, Venice, Italy, June 29–July 2. *Perit Dial Bull* **7**(Suppl): S79.

Ab 52 Twardowski ZJ, Khanna R, Nichols WK, *et al.* (1987) Low complication rates with Swan Neck Short Tunnel Missouri (SNSTM) peritoneal catheter. Abstracts, IVth Congress of the International Society for Peritoneal Dialysis, Venice, Italy, June 29–July 2. *Perit Dial Bull* **7**(Suppl): S80.

Ab 53 Prowant BF, Schmidt L, Twardowski Z, *et al.* (1987) A randomized prospective evaluation of three procedures for peritoneal dialysis catheter exit site care. *ANNA J* **14**: 149.

Ab 54 Mactier RA, Khanna R, Moore H, *et al.* (1987) Phosphatidylcholine enhances the efficiency of peritoneal dialysis by reducing lymphatic reabsorption. Abstracts and Program, *The American Society of Nephrology, 20th Annual Meeting*, Sheraton-Washington, Washington, D.C., December 13–16, p. 100A. [Reprinted in: *Kidney Int* (1987) **33**: 247.]

Ab 55 McDonald RJ, Early J, Nichols WK, *et al.* (1988) Concomitant surgical illness in CAPD patients. Abstracts of the VIII Annual CAPD Conference. *Perit Dial Int* **8**: 89.

Ab 56 Artis AK, Alpert MA, Van Stone J, *et al.* (1989) Effect of beta blockade on LV systolic function in patients undergoing hemodialysis. Abstracts and Program, *American Society of Nephrology, 21st Annual Meeting*, San

Antonio, TX, December 11–14, Vol. 21, p. 90A. [Reprinted in: *Kidney Int* (1989) **35**: 238.]

Ab 57 Helfrich G, Villano R, Khanna R, *et al.* (1989) Recommendations for successful surgical implantation of PD catheters. Abstracts of the IX Annual Conference on Peritoneal Dialysis. *Perit Dial Int* **9**(Suppl 1): 78.

Ab 58 Khanna R, Moore H, Mactier R, *et al.* (1989) Effect of increased intraperitoneal hydrostatic pressure (HP) on Starling's forces during a peritoneal dialysis exchange (PDEX) in rat. Abstracts, *XXVIth Congress of the European Dialysis and Transplant Association–European Renal Association*, Göteborg, Sweden, June 11–15, p. 101.

Ab 59 Nolph KD, Twardowski Z, Khanna R. (1989) Tidal peritoneal dialysis (TPD) with racemic or L-lactate solutions. Program and Abstracts, *22nd Annual Meeting of the American Society of Nephrology*, December 3–6, p. 144A.

Ab 59a Nolph KD, Twardowski Z, Khanna R. (1990) Tidal peritoneal dialysis (TPD) with racemic or L-lactate solutions. Reprinted in: Abstracts, American Society of Nephrology, Washington, D.C., December 3–6, 1989. *Kidney Int* **37**: 332.

Ab 60 Dobbie JW, Twardowski ZJ, Algrim C, *et al.* (1990) Clinical evaluation of tidal PD (TPD) as a long term dialysis therapy. Abstracts, 10th Annual Conference on Peritoneal Dialysis, Dallas, TX, February 8–10. *Perit Dial Int* **10**(Suppl 1): 50.

Ab 61 Twardowski ZJ, Prowant BF, Nolph KD, *et al.* (1990) Culture results of peritoneal catheter peri-exit smears (S) and sinus tract washouts (W). Abstracts, *American Society for Artificial Internal Organs, 36th Annual Meeting*, Washington, D.C., April 24–27, p. 80.

Ab 62 Twardowski ZJ, Prowant BF, Khanna R, *et al.* (1990) Long term experience with Swan Neck Missouri 2 (SN-M2) & Swan Neck Missouri 3 (SN-M3) peritoneal dialysis catheters. Abstracts, *American Society for Artificial Internal Organs, 36th Annual Meeting*, Washington, D.C., April 24–27, p. 80.

Ab 63 Twardowski ZJ, Prowant BF, Nolph KD, Khanna R. (1990) Chronic nightly tidal peritoneal dialysis (NTPD). Abstracts, *American Society for Artificial Internal Organs, 36th Annual Meeting*, Washington, D.C., April 24–27, p. 81.

Ab 64 Twardowski ZJ, Dobbie JW, Moore HL, *et al.* (1990) Morphology of peritoneal dialysis (PD) catheter tunnels (CT) — Macroscopy and light microscopy. Abstracts, *American Society for Artificial Internal Organs, 36th Annual Meeting*, Washington, D.C., April 24–27, p. 81.

Ab 65 Twardowski ZJ, Tully RJ, Ersoy FF, Dedhia NM. (1990) Computerized tomographic peritoneography (CTP) in peritoneal dialysis (PD) patients. Abstracts, *American Society for Artificial Internal Organs, 36th Annual Meeting*, Washington, D.C., April 24–27, p. 81.

Ab 66   Twardowski ZJ, Prowant BF, Nolph KD, *et al.* (1990) Key factors in exit site(s) (ES) evaluation. Abstracts, *American Society for Artificial Internal Organs, 36th Annual Meeting*, Washington, D.C., April 24–27, p. 81.

Ab 67   Nolph KD, Twardowski Z, Khanna R. (1990) Tidal peritoneal dialysis (TPD) with racemic or L-lactate solutions. Abstracts, *XIth International Congress of Nephrology*, Tokyo, Japan, July 15–20, p. 25A.

Ab 68   Twardowski ZJ, Prowant BF, Nolph KD, *et al.* (1990) Key factors in exit site(s) (ES) evaluation. Abstracts, *XIth International Congress of Nephrology* Tokyo, Japan, July 15–20, p. 26A.

Ab 69   Twardowski ZJ, Prowant BF, Khanna R, *et al.* (1990) Long term experience with Swan Neck Missouri 2 (SN-M2) and Swan Neck Missouri 3 (SN-M3) peritoneal dialysis catheters. Abstracts, *XIth International Congress of Nephrology*, Tokyo, Japan, July 15–20, p. 257A.

Ab 70   Twardowski ZJ, Dobbie JW, Moore HL, *et al.* (1990) Morphology of peritoneal dialysis (PD) catheter tunnels (CT) — Macroscopy and light microscopy. Abstracts, *XIth International Congress of Nephrology*, Tokyo, Japan, July 15–20, p. 259A.

Ab 71   Twardowski ZJ, Prowant BF, Nolph KD, *et al.* (1990) Culture results of peritoneal catheter peri-exit smears (S) and sinus tract washouts (W). Abstracts, *XIth International Congress of Nephrology*, Tokyo, Japan, July 15–20, p. 259A.

Ab 72   Twardowski ZJ, Prowant BF, Nolph KD, Khanna R. (1990) Chronic nightly tidal peritoneal dialysis (NTPD). Abstracts, *XIth International Congress of Nephrology*, Tokyo, Japan, July 15–20, p. 259A.

Ab 73   Twardowski ZJ, Tully RJ, Ersoy FF, Dedhia NM. (1990) Computerized tomographic peritoneography (CTP) in peritoneal dialysis (PD) patients. Abstracts, *XIth International Congress of Nephrology*, Tokyo, Japan, July 15–20, p. 262A.

Ab 74   Twardowski ZJ. (1990) Reduced complications with Swan Neck peritoneal dialysis catheters. Abstracts, *Vth Congress of the International Society for Peritoneal Dialysis*, Kyoto, Japan, July 21–24, p. 10.

Ab 75   Khanna R, Moore HL, Mactier R, *et al.* (1990) Effect of increased intraperitoneal hydrostatic pressure (PCHP) on Starling's forces during a peritoneal dialysis exchange (PDEX) in rat. Abstracts, *Vth Congress of the International Society for Peritoneal Dialysis*, Kyoto, Japan, July 21–24, p. 22.

Ab 76   Nolph KD, Twardowski ZJ, Khanna R. (1990) Tidal peritoneal dialysis (TPD) with racemic or L-lactate solutions. Abstracts, *Vth Congress of the International Society for Peritoneal Dialysis*, Kyoto, Japan, July 21–24, p. 25.

Ab 77   Twardowski ZJ, Tully RJ, Ersoy FF, Dedhia NM. (1990) Computerized tomography (CT) and CT peritoneography (CTP) in peritoneal dialysis (PD)

Ab 78   patients. Abstracts, *Vth Congress of the International Society for Peritoneal Dialysis*, Kyoto, Japan, July 21–24, p. 26.

Ab 78   Twardowski ZJ, Dobbie JW, Moore HL, *et al.* (1990) Macroscopic and light microscopic morphology of peritoneal dialysis (PD) catheter tunnels (CT). Abstracts, *Vth Congress of the International Society for Peritoneal Dialysis*, Kyoto, Japan, July 21–24, p. 28.

Ab 79   Twardowski ZJ, Prowant BF, Nolph KD, *et al.* (1990) Exit site(s) (ES) healing and classification. Abstracts, *Vth Congress of the International Society for Peritoneal Dialysis*, Kyoto, Japan, July 21–24, p. 36.

Ab 80   Ersoy FF, Moore HL, Khanna R, *et al.* (1990) The effect of respiration on peritoneal cavity lymphatic absorption. Abstracts, *Vth Congress of the International Society for Peritoneal Dialysis*, Kyoto, Japan, July 21–24, p. 44.

Ab 81   Twardowski ZJ, Prowant BF, Nolph KD, Khanna R. (1990) Nightly tidal peritoneal dialysis (NTPD). Abstracts, *Vth Congress of the International Society for Peritoneal Dialysis*, Kyoto, Japan, July 21–24, p. 45.

Ab 82   Twardowski ZJ, Prowant BF, Khanna R, *et al.* (1990) Three-year experience with Swan Neck Missouri 2 (SN-M2) and Swan Neck Missouri 3 (SN-M3) peritoneal dialysis catheters. Abstracts, *Vth Congress of the International Society for Peritoneal Dialysis*, Kyoto, Japan, July 21–24, p. 52.

Ab 83   Twardowski ZJ, Prowant BF, Nolph KD, *et al.* (1990) Culture results in peri-exit smears (S), and sinus tract washouts (W) of peritoneal catheters, and swabs from nares (N). Abstracts, *Vth Congress of the International Society for Peritoneal Dialysis*, Kyoto, Japan, July 21–24, p. 60.

Ab 84   Twardowski ZJ. (1990) Peritoneal access — Methods and complications. Abstracts, *2nd International Congress on Access Surgery*, Maastricht, The Netherlands, November 14–17, p. 19.

Ab 85   Chen TW, Khanna R, Moore HL, *et al.* (1990) Contribution of intraperitoneal (IP) hydrostatic pressure to ultrafiltration (UF) kinetics during peritoneal dialysis (PD). *Clin Res* **38**: 826A.

Ab 86   Chen TW, Khanna R, Moore HL, *et al.* (1990) Contribution of intraperitoneal (IP) hydrostatic pressure to ultrafiltration (UF) kinetics during peritoneal dialysis (PD). Abstracts, 23rd Annual Meeting of the American Society of Nephrology, December 2–5. *J Am Soc Nephrol* **1**: 385.

Ab 87   Chen TW, Khanna R, Nolph KD, Twardowski ZJ. (1990) The kinetics of hydraulic (H) ultrafiltration (UF) during peritoneal dialysis (PD) exchanges (EXS) in rats. Abstracts, 23rd Annual Meeting of the American Society of Nephrology, December 2–5. *J Am Soc Nephrol* **1**: 385.

Ab 88   Chen TW, Khanna R, Moore HL, *et al.* (1991) Contribution of intraperitoneal (IP) hydrostatic pressure to ultrafiltration (UF) kinetics during peritoneal dialysis (PD). Abstracts, 11th Annual CAPD Conference. *Perit Dial Int* **11**(Suppl 1): 50.

Ab 89   Chen TW, Khanna R, Nolph KD, Twardowski ZJ. (1991) The kinetics of hydraulic (H) ultrafiltration (UF) during peritoneal dialysis (PD) exchanges (EXS) in rats. Abstracts, 11th Annual CAPD Conference. *Perit Dial Int* **11**(Suppl 1): 51.

Ab 90   Schmidt LM, Prowant BF, Twardowski ZJ, Craig PS. (1991) Preventing accidental disconnection at the peritoneal catheter-adapter junction. Abstracts, 11th Annual CAPD Conference. *Perit Dial Int* **11**(Suppl 1): 235.

Ab 91   Twardowski ZJ, Prowant BF, Khanna R, *et al.* (1991) Long term experience with Swan Neck Missouri 2 (SN-M2) and Swan Neck Missouri 3 (SN-M3) peritoneal dialysis catheters. Abstracts, 11th Annual CAPD Conference. *Perit Dial Int* **11**(Suppl 1): 276.

Ab 92   Twardowski ZJ, Dobbie JW, Moore HL, *et al.* (1991) Morphology of peritoneal dialysis catheter tunnels. Abstracts, 11th Annual CAPD Conference. *Perit Dial Int* **11**(Suppl 1): 277.

Ab 93   Khanna R, Chen TW, Moore HL, *et al.* (1991) Contribution of intraperitoneal (IP) hydrostatic pressure to ultrafiltration (UF) kinetics during peritoneal dialysis (PD). Abstracts, *American Society for Artificial Internal Organs, 37th Annual Meeting*, Chicago Hilton and Towers, Chicago, Illinois, April 25–27, p. 101.

Ab 94   Khanna R, Chen TW, Moore HL, *et al.* (1991) Reflection coefficients for sodium salts ($\sigma_{Na\,salt}$ & glucose$_{(\sigma_G)}$) during peritoneal dialysis in rats: A simple clinical method. Abstracts, *American Society for Artificial Internal Organs, 37th Annual Meeting*, Chicago Hilton and Towers, Chicago, Illinois, April 25–27, p. 101.

Ab 95   Twardowski ZJ. (1991) The CAPD Option. Program and Book of Abstracts, *Renal Update '91, Singapore Society of Nephrology 3rd Scientific Meeting*, College of Medicine Building, Singapore, September 28–29, p. 15.

Ab 96   Nolph KD, Moore HL, Khanna R, Twardowski ZJ. (1992) Cross-sectional assessment of weekly urea and creatinine clearances in CAPD patients. Abstracts, VIth Congress of the International Society for Peritoneal Dialysis, Thessaloniki, Greece, October 1–4. *Perit Dial Int* **12**(Suppl 2): S15.

Ab 97   Nolph KD, Keshaviah P, Prowant BF, *et al.* (1992). Assessment of lean body mass (LBM) from creatinine kinetics (CK). Abstracts, VIth Congress of the International Society for Peritoneal Dialysis, Thessaloniki, Greece, October 1–4. *Perit Dial Int* **12**(Suppl 2): S15.

Ab 98   Ersoy FF, Twardowski ZJ, Satalowich RJ, Ketchersid T. (1992) A retrospective analysis of peritoneal dialysis catheter (PDC) position and function in 91 patients. Abstracts, VIth Congress of the International Society for Peritoneal Dialysis, Thessaloniki, Greece, October 1–4. *Perit Dial Int* **12**(Suppl 2): S49.

Ab 99   Twardowski ZJ, Nichols WK, Nolph K, Khanna R. (1992) Swan Neck presternal catheter for peritoneal dialysis. Abstracts, VIth Congress of the

International Society for Peritoneal Dialysis, Thessaloniki, Greece, October 1–4. *Perit Dial Int* **12** (Suppl 2): S54.

Ab 100 Nolph KD, Khanna R, Twardowski ZJ, Moore HL. (1992) Predictors of serum albumin concentration (SA) in CAPD. *Clin Res* **40**(3): 700.

Ab 101 Twardowski ZJ, Van Stone JC, Jones ME, Klusmeyer MS. (1992) Blood recirculation (REC) in intravenous catheters (IVC) for hemodialysis (HD). Abstracts, 25th Annual Meeting of the American Society of Nephrology, November 15–18. *J Am Soc Nephrol* **3**(3): 399.

Ab 102 Nolph KD, Khanna R, Twardowski ZJ, Moore HL. (1992) Correlations with KT/V urea in CAPD. Abstracts, 25th Annual Meeting of the American Society of Nephrology, November 15–18. *J Am Soc Nephrol* **3**(3): 415.

Ab 103 Nolph KD, Khanna R, Twardowski ZJ, Moore HL. (1992) Predictors of serum albumin concentration (SA) in CAPD. Abstracts, 25th Annual Meeting of the American Society of Nephrology, November 15–18. *J Am Soc Nephrol* **3**(3): 417.

Ab 104 Vassa N, Twardowski ZJ, Campbell J. (1993) Hyperbaric oxygen (HBO) chamber therapy in calciphylaxis induced skin necrosis in peritoneal dialysis (PD) patient. Abstracts, XIIIth Annual CAPD Conference, San Diego, CA, March 7–9. *Perit Dial Int* **13**(Suppl 1): S5.

Ab 105 Nolph KD, Khanna R, Twardowski ZJ, Moore HL. (1993) Correlations with KT/V Urea in CAPD. Abstracts, XIIIth Annual CAPD Conference, San Diego, CA, March 7–9. *Perit Dial Int* **13**(Suppl 1): S12.

Ab 106 Twardowski ZJ, Nichols WK, Nolph K, Khanna R. (1993) One year experience with Swan Neck presternal catheters for peritoneal dialysis. Abstracts, XIIIth Annual CAPD Conference, San Diego, CA, March 7–9. *Perit Dial Int* **13**(Suppl 1): S60.

Ab 107 Nolph K, Moore H, Prowant B, *et al.* (1993) CAPD with a high flux membrane. Abstracts, *American Society for Artificial Internal Organs, 39th Annual Meeting*, New Orleans Hilton Hotel, New Orleans, LA, April 29–30, May 1, p. 110.

Ab 108 Twardowski ZJ, Prowant BF, Nolph KD, *et al.* (1993) Peritoneal catheter (PC) exit site (ES): Appearance, and factors influencing healing. Abstracts, *XIIth International Congress of Nephrology*, Jerusalem, Israel, June 13–19, p. 311.

Ab 109 Twardowski ZJ, Nichols WK, Nolph KD, Khanna R. (1993) Swan Neck presternal catheter for peritoneal dialysis — Eighteen month experience in adults. Abstracts, *XIIth International Congress of Nephrology*, Jerusalem, Israel, June 13–19, p. 335.

Ab 110 Ersoy FF, Twardowski ZJ, Ketchersid T. (1993) A retrospective analysis of peritoneal dialysis catheter (PDC) position and function in 91 patients. Abstracts, *XIIth International Congress of Nephrology*, Jerusalem, Israel, June 13–19, p. 341.

Ab 111 Trivedi HS, Khanna RK, Prowant BF, et al. (1993) Reproducibility of the peritoneal equilibration test (PET). Abstracts, 26th Annual Meeting of the American Society of Nephrology, Boston, MA, November 14–17. *J Am Soc Nephrol* **4**: 419.

Ab 111a Trivedi HS, Khanna RK, Prowant BF, et al. (1993) Reproducibility of the peritoneal equilibration test (PET). *Clin Res* **41**(3): 655A.

Ab 112 Trivedi HS, Khanna RK, Gamboa S, et al. (1994) How reproducible is the peritoneal equilibration test (PET)? Abstracts, XIVth Annual Conference on Peritoneal Dialysis, Orlando, FL, January 24–26. *Perit Dial Int* **14**(Suppl 1): S3.

Ab 113 Trivedi HS, Twardowski ZJ. (1994) Successful NIPD for 10 years — A case report. Abstracts, XIVth Annual Conference on Peritoneal Dialysis, Orlando, FL, January 24–26. *Perit Dial Int* **14** (Suppl 1): S3.

Ab 114 Suzuki K, Twardowski ZJ, Moore HL, Nolph KD. (1993) Absorption of iron from peritoneal cavity of rats. Abstracts, XIVth Annual Conference on Peritoneal Dialysis, Orlando, FL, January 24–26. *Perit Dial Int* **14**(Suppl 1): S73.

Ab 115 Kathuria P, Moore HL, Twardowski ZJ, Prowant BF. (1994) Evaluation of silver coated peritoneal catheters as a barrier to early exit site infection in rats. Abstracts, 27th Annual Meeting of the American Society of Nephrology, Orange County Convention Center, Orlando, FL, October 26–29. *J Am Soc Nephrol* **5**: 418.

Ab 116 Suzuki K, Khanna R, Moore HL, et al. (1995) Alteration of peritoneal function of rats on 9 weeks of PD. Abstracts, XVth Annual Conference on Peritoneal Dialysis, Baltimore, MD, February 12–14. *Perit Dial Int* **15**(Suppl 1): S14.

Ab 117 Suzuki K, Twardowski ZJ, Moore HL, et al. (1995) Absorption of iron dextran from the peritoneal cavity of rats. Abstracts, XVth Annual Conference on Peritoneal Dialysis, Baltimore, MD, February 12–14. *Perit Dial Int* **15**(Suppl 1): S15.

Ab 118 Wieczorowska K, Khanna R, Moore HL, et al. (1995) Rat model of peritoneal fibrosis: Preliminary observations. Abstracts, XVth Annual Conference on Peritoneal Dialysis, Baltimore, MD, February 12–14. *Perit Dial Int* **15**(Suppl 1): S15.

Ab 119 Kathuria P, Moore HL, Mehrotra R, et al. (1995) Preliminary evaluation of silver coated peritoneal catheters in rats. Abstracts, XVth Annual Conference on Peritoneal Dialysis, Baltimore, MD, February 12–14. *Perit Dial Int* **15**(Suppl 1): S28.

Ab 120 Suzuki K, Khanna R, Moore HL, et al. (1995) Spontaneous peritonitis in rats on peritoneal dialysis. Abstracts, XVth Annual Conference on Peritoneal Dialysis, Baltimore, MD, February 12–14. *Perit Dial Int* **15**(Suppl 1): S33.

Ab 121 Suzuki K, Khanna R, Moore HL, et al. (1995) Factors that affect peritoneal equilibration test (PET) results in rats. Abstracts, 7th Congress of the International Society for Peritoneal Dialysis, Stockholm, Sweden, June 18–21. *Perit Dial Int* **15**(Suppl 1): S23.

Ab 122 Nolph KD, Keshaviah P, Emerson P, et al. (1995) A new nutritional approach to optimizing KT/V in hemodialysis (HD) and continuous ambulatory peritoneal dialysis (CAPD). Abstracts, 7th Congress of the International Society for Peritoneal Dialysis, Stockholm, Sweden, June 18–21. *Perit Dial Int* **15**(4) (Suppl 1): S30.

Ab 123 Twardowski ZJ, Prowant BF, Pickett B, et al. (1995) Swan Neck presternal catheter (SN-PC) for peritoneal dialysis. Abstracts, 7th Congress of the International Society for Peritoneal Dialysis, Stockholm, Sweden, June 18–21. *Perit Dial Int* **15**(4) (Suppl 1): S61.

Ab 124 Bhatla B, Nolph KD, Moore H, et al. (1995) Residual renal function in hemodialysis (HD) and continuous ambulatory peritoneal dialysis (CAPD) patients. *J Am Soc Nephrol* **6**(3): 592.

Ab 125 Khanna R, Twardowski ZJ, Prowant BF, et al. (1991) Reproducibility of the peritoneal equilibration test results in sequential exchanges in a CAPD patient. *Clin Res* **39**(3): 776A.

Ab 126 Lo WK, Brendolan A, Prowant B, et al. (1994) Serial peritoneal equilibration tests (PETs) in chronic peritoneal dialysis (CPD). Abstracts, *American Society for Artificial Internal Organs, 40th Anniversary Meeting,* San Francisco Hilton Hotel, San Francisco, CA, April 14–16, p. 105.

Ab 127 Goel S, Kathuria P, Mehrotra R, et al. (1996) A study on the effect of peritonitis on the peritoneal membrane transport properties in patients on CAPD. Abstracts, XVIth Annual CAPD Conference. *Perit Dial Int* **16** (Suppl 2): S6.

Ab 128 Kathuria P, Goel S, Moore HL, et al. (1996) Protein losses during CAPD. Abstracts, XVIth Annual CAPD Conference. *Perit Dial Int* **16**(Suppl 2): S9.

Ab 129 Suzuki K, Khanna R, Moore HL, et al. (1996) Effects of bicarbonate dialysis solution on peritoneal transport in rats. Abstracts, XVIth Annual CAPD Conference. *Perit Dial Int* **16**(Suppl 2): S13.

Ab 130 Suzuki K, Khanna R, Moore HL, et al. (1996) Effects of manidipine hydrochloride (MH) on peritoneal transport in rats. Abstracts, XVIth Annual CAPD Conference. *Perit Dial Int* **16**(Suppl 2): S13.

Ab 131 Mehrotra R, Khanna R, Yang TK, et al. (1996) A mathematical model to predict 6 hour D/P creatinine using the 4 hour D/P from the peritoneal equilibration test. Abstracts, XVIth Annual CAPD Conference. *Perit Dial Int* **16**(Suppl 2): S27.

Ab 132 Kathuria P, Moore HL, Mehrotra R, et al. (1996) Evaluation of healing and sinus tract histology of silver coated peritoneal catheter in rats. Abstracts, XVIth Annual CAPD Conference. *Perit Dial Int* **16**(Suppl 2): S52.

Ab 133 Trivedi HS, Twardowski ZJ. (1996) Use of double lumen hemodialysis catheters: Loading with locked heparin. Abstracts, XVIth Annual CAPD Conference. *Perit Dial Int* **16**(Suppl 2): S100.

Ab 134 Twardowski ZJ. (1996) Current approach to exit site infection in patients of peritoneal dialysis. Book of Abstracts, *1st Slovene Congress of Nephrology*, Portoroñ, Slovenia, October 23-26, pp. 148-149.

Ab 135 Usha K, Kathuria P, Khanna R, *et al.* (1996) Long term experience with peritoneal dialysis. *J Am Soc Nephrol* **7**(9): 1467.

Ab 136 Twardowski ZJ. (1996) Swan Neck Missouri peritoneal dialysis catheters — Design, insertion and break-in. *Videomed '96, X Certamen Internacional De Videocine Médico*, Badajoz, Spain, November 22, p. 232.

Ab 137 Usha K, Kathuria P, Nolph KD, *et al.* (1997) The relationship of nPNA to weekly Kt/V urea in chronic PD. *Perit Dial Int* **17**(Suppl 1): S24.

Ab 138 Goel S, Ribby KJ, Khanna R, *et al.* (1997) Temporary stoppage of peritoneal dialysis when laparoscopic procedures are performed on patients undergoing CAPD/CCPD: A change in policy. *Perit Dial Int* **17**(Suppl 1): S60.

Ab 139 Park SE, Twardowski ZJ, Moore HL, *et al.* (1997) Chronic injections of iron dextran into the peritoneal cavity of rats. *Perit Dial Int* **17**(Suppl 1): S99.

Ab 140 Twardowski ZJ. (1997) High dose intradialytic urokinase to restore the patency of permanent central vein hemodialysis catheters. Abstracts, XIVth International Congress of Nephrology, Sydney, Australia, May 25-29. *Nephrology* **3**(Suppl 1): S420.

Ab 141 Twardowski ZJ, Prowant BF, Nichols WK. (1997) Swan Neck presternal catheter for peritoneal dialysis — Five year experience in adults. Abstracts, XIVth International Congress of Nephrology, Sydney, Australia, May 25-29. *Nephrology* **3**(Suppl 1): S428.

Ab 142 Twardowski ZJ, Prowant BF, Nichols WK, *et al.* (1997) Six-year experience with Swan Neck presternal peritoneal dialysis catheter. Abstracts, XXXth Annual Meeting, San Antonio, TX, November 2-5. *J Am Soc Nephrol* **8**: 183A.

Ab 143 Pecoits R, Twardowski ZJ, Kim YL, *et al.* (1997) Intraperitoneal iron dextran toxicity: A functional and histological analysis. Abstracts, XXXth Annual Meeting, San Antonio, TX, November 2-5. *J Am Soc Nephrol* **8**: 270A.

Ab 144 Pecoits R, Twardowski ZJ, Khanna R, *et al.* (1997) The effect of antibiotic prophylaxis on the healing of exit-sites of peritoneal dialysis catheters in rats. Abstracts, *American Society for Artificial Internal Organs, 43rd Annual Meeting*, Atlanta, GA, May 1-3, p. 80.

Ab 145 Kim YL, Khanna R, Moore HL, *et al.* (1997) Effects of dialysis solution PH on peritoneal transport of glucose in rats. Abstracts, *American Society for Artificial Internal Organs, 43rd Annual Meeting*, Atlanta, GA, May 1-3, p. 80

Ab 146   Williams AW, Ting G, Blagg C, et al. Daily Hemodialysis Study Group, Mayo Clinic, Rochester, MN. (1999) Early clinical, quality of life, and biochemical changes of daily hemodialysis. Abstracts, 32nd Annual Meeting, Miami Beach, FL, November 1–8. *J Am Soc Nephrol* **10**: 270A.

Ab 147   Ing TS, Williams AW, Ting GO, et al. (1999) Daily Hemodialysis Study Group, Hines, IL. Factors influencing agreement between blood urea nitrogen levels obtained thirty minutes before and thirty minutes after the end of hemodialysis. Abstracts, 32nd Annual Meeting, Miami Beach, FL, November 1–8. *J Am Soc Nephrol* **10**: 330A.

Ab 148   Kjellstrand CM, Williams AW, Ting GO, et al. (1999) Daily Hemodialysis Study Group, Loyola University, Chicago, IL. Dialysis quantification made accurate, simple and inexpensive. Abstracts, 32nd Annual Meeting, Miami Beach, FL, November 1–8. *J Am Soc Nephrol* **10**: 332A.

Ab 149   Kondle V, Twardowski Z, Nolph KD, Khanna R. (2000) Is PD catheter removal a solution for alcaligenes peritonitis (P). Abstracts, 20th Annual PD Conference, San Francisco, CA, February 27–29. *Perit Dial Int* **20**(Suppl 1): S38.

Ab 150   Agrawal A, Katyal A, Khanna R, Twardowski ZJ. (2000) Successful peritoneal dialysis (PD) after cardiac surgery in patients with Swan-Neck presternal catheter. Abstracts, 20th Annual PD Conference, San Francisco, CA, February 27–29. *Perit Dial Int* **20**(Suppl 1): S46.

Ab 151   Lee JH, Reddy D, Moore H, et al. (2000) Advanced glycosylation end-products (AGEs) in diabetic rats on peritoneal dialysis (PD) with different solutions. Abstracts, 20th Annual PD Conference, San Francisco, CA, February 27–29. *Perit Dial Int* **20**(Suppl 1): S57.

Ab 152   Ing TS, Williams AW, Ting GO, et al. (2000) Equilibrated urea reduction ratio (eURR) derived by using blood urea nitrogen levels obtained 30 minutes before the end of dialysis or by using an equation. Abstracts, 20th Annual PD Conference, San Francisco, CA, February 27–29. *Perit Dial Int* **20**(Suppl 1): S104.

Ab 153   Saran R, Venkataraman V, Leavey S, et al. (2000) High-dose urokinase (HDU) restores patency of hemodialysis (HD) catheters: A prospective observational study. Abstracts, 20th Annual PD Conference, San Francisco, CA, February 27–29. *Perit Dial Int* **20**(Suppl 1): S107.

Ab 154   Grushevsky A, Blagg CR, Bower J, et al. (2000) Microbiology of hot water dialyzer reuse and backfiltered dialysate for priming. Abstracts, 33rd Annual Meeting, Toronto, Ontario, Canada, October 10–16. *J Am Soc Nephrol* **11**: 174A.

Ab 155   Reddy DK, Moore HL, Lee JH, et al. (2000) Chronic peritoneal dialysis (PD) in iron deficient rats with solutions containing iron dextran. Abstracts, 33rd Annual Meeting, Toronto, Ontario, Canada, October 10–16. *J Am Soc Nephrol* **11**: 217A.

Ab 156 Brunson P, Pickett B, Hutton J, *et al.* (2000) Reuse of dialyzers by hot water cleaning alone. Abstracts, 33rd Annual Meeting, Toronto, Ontario, Canada, October 10–16. *J Am Soc Nephrol* **11**: 316A.

Ab 157 James J, Twardowski ZJ, Blagg CR, *et al.* (2001) Effect of non-chemical hot water reuse on dialyzer performance. Programs and Abstracts, ASN/ISN World Congress of Nephrology, San Francisco, CA, October 10–17. *J Am Soc Nephrol* **12**: 267A.

Ab 158 Twardowski ZJ, Blagg CR, Bower JD, *et al.* (2001) Bacteriology and endotoxin levels in heat-sanitized dialysis equipment. Programs and Abstracts, ASN/ISN World Congress of Nephrology, San Francisco, CA, October 10–17. *J Am Soc Nephrol* **12**: 278A.

Ab 159 Blagg CR, Bower JD, Twardowski ZJ, Kjellstrand CM. (2001) Well-being during dialysis with biocompatible high flux, high efficiency dialyzers and ultra-pure dialysate. Programs and Abstracts, ASN/ISN World Congress of Nephrology, San Francisco, CA, October 10–17. *J Am Soc Nephrol* **12**: 371A.

Ab 160 Blagg CR, Eschbach J, Bower JD, *et al.* (2002) LDH and haptoglobin changes by polysulphone membranes. Abstracts, 22nd Annual Conference on Dialysis, Tampa, FL, March 4–6. *Perit Dial Int* **22**(Suppl 1): S61.

Ab 161 James J, Twardowski ZJ, Blagg CR, *et al.* (2002) Effect of non-chemical hot water reuse on dialyzer performance. Abstracts, 22nd Annual Conference on Dialysis, Tampa, FL, March 4–6. *Perit Dial Int* **22**(Suppl 1): S61.

Ab 162 Twardowski ZJ, Blagg CR, Bower JD, Kjellstrand CM. (2002) Well-being during dialysis with biocompatible high flux, high efficiency (BIOHFHE) membranes: Influence of ultrapure dialysate. Abstracts, 22nd Annual Conference on Dialysis, Tampa, FL, March 4–6. *Perit Dial Int* **22**(Suppl 1): S62.

Ab 163 Twardowski ZJ, Blagg CR, Bower JD, *et al.* (2002) Bacteriology and endotoxin levels in heat-sanitized hemodialysis equipment. Abstracts, 22nd Annual Conference on Dialysis, Tampa, FL, March 4–6. *Perit Dial Int* **22**(Suppl 1): S62.

Ab 164 Twardowski ZJ, Pawlak K, Colburn D, *et al.* (2002) Blood tubing sets for extended use in hemodialysis. Abstracts, 22nd Annual Conference on Dialysis, Tampa, FL, March 4–6. *Perit Dial Int* **22**(Suppl 1): S62.

Ab 165 Pickett B, Prowant BF, Twardowski ZJ. (2002) Daily hemodialysis as a rescue therapy in a patient with severe cardiovascular disease and multiple medical problems. Abstracts, 22nd Annual Conference on Dialysis, Tampa, FL, March 4–6. *Perit Dial Int* **22**(Suppl 1): S65.

Ab 166 James J, McComb T, Twardowski ZJ, *et al.* (2002) Multiple reuses of dialysis — Filters and bloodlines *in situ* for daily hemodialysis. ERA/EDTA 2002. *Nephrol Dial Transplant* **17**(Suppl 1): 292.

Ab 167 Moore HL, Twardowski ZJ. (2003) Bactericidal properties of acidified (pH 2.0), concentrated (27%) NaCl (ACS), a potentially useful agent for locking hemodialysis catheters. Abstracts, 23rd Annual Conference on Dialysis, Seattle, WA, March 2-4. *Hemodial Int* **7**(1): 74-75.

Ab 168 Twardowski ZJ, Reams G, Prowant B, et al. (2003) Air-bubble method of locking central-vein catheters: A pilot study. Abstracts, 23rd Annual Conference on Dialysis, Seattle, WA, March 2-4. *Hemodial Int* **7**(1): 75.

Ab 169 Kjellstrand C, Twardowski Z, Bower J, Blagg CR. (2003) A comparison of CV-catheters (CV), grafts (GR) and fistulae (FI) in quotidian hemodialysis. Abstracts, 23rd Annual Conference on Dialysis, Seattle, WA, March 2-4. *Hemodial Int* **7**(1): 76-77.

Ab 170 Twardowski ZJ, Prowant BF, Moore HL, et al. (2003) Short peritoneal equilibration test: Impact of preceding dwell time. Abstracts, 23rd Annual Conference on Dialysis, Seattle, WA, March 2-4. *Perit Dial Int* **23**(Suppl 1): S11.

Ab 171 Kjellstrand C, Twardowski ZJ, Bower J, Blagg CR. (2003) Hot water reuse (HWR) of dialysis filters gives smoother dialysis than single use (SU) or chemical reuse (CRU). *J Am Soc Nephrol* **14**: 502A.

Ab 172 Kjellstrand CM, Twardowski ZJ, Bower J, Blagg CR. (2004) What influences cardiovascular instability and discomfort during daily hemodialysis? Abstracts, 24th Annual Dialysis Conference, San Antonio, TX, February 9-11. *Hemodial Int* **8**(1): 96.

Ab 173 Kjellstrand CM, Twardowski ZJ, Bower J, et al. (2004) Hot water reuse (HWR) of dialyzers gives smoother dialysis than single use (SU) or chemical reuse (CR). Abstracts, 24th Annual Dialysis Conference, San Antonio, TX, February 9-11. *Hemodial Int* **8**(1): 98-99.

Ab 174 Kjellstrand C, Blagg CR, Twardowski ZJ, Bower J. (2004) Cardiovascular instability during dialysis — Relative influence of dialysis purity, clearance and ultrafiltration speed: Experience with the Aksys PHD system. Abstract Book, European Renal Association-European Dialysis and Transplant Association, XLI Congress, Lisbon, Portugal, May 15-18, p. 332.

Ab 175 Kjellstrand C, Blagg CR, Twardowski ZJ, Bower J. (2004) Cardiovascular stability during daily hemodialysis — Relative influence of dialysis purity, clearance and ultrafiltration speed: Experience with the Aksys PHD system. Canadian Society of Nephrology, Program, Annual Meeting, May 27-31, Abstract 89, p. 81.

Ab 176 Kjellstrand C, Blagg CR, Twardowski ZJ, Bower J. (2004) Cardiovascular stability (CVI) during daily hemodialysis (DHD) — Relative influence of dialysis purity, clearance and ultrafiltration speed: Experience with the Aksys PHD system. *ASAIO J* **50**: 177.

Ab 177 Kjellstrand C, Blagg CR, Young B, et al. (2005) 106 patient-years experience with the AKSYS PHD system for quotidian home hemodialysis. *Hemodial Int* **9**(1): 80.

Ab 178 Prowant BF, Moore HL, Twardowski ZJ, Khanna R. (2008) High serum glucose distorts peritoneal equilibration test results. Abstracts, 12th Congress of the ISPD (PP. 363). *Perit Dial Int* **28**(Suppl 4): 107.

Ab 179 Prowant BF, Moore HL, Twardowski ZJ, Khanna R. (2008) Discrepancies in peritoneal equilibration test results between the peritoneal membrane classification indicated by the 4-hour dialysate to plasma creatinine ratio and the 4-hour dialysate glucose/glucose at time 0. Abstracts, 12th Congress of the ISPD (PP. 382). *Perit Dial Int* **28**(Suppl 4): 112.

Ab 180 Prowant B, Moore H, Khanna R, Twardowski Z. (2009) Discrepancies in peritoneal equilibration test (PET) results between the peritoneal membrane classification indicated by ratios of dialysate to plasma creatinine (Cr D/P) and the 4-hour dialysate glucose/glucose at time 0 (Gluc D/D0). *Perit Dial Int* **29**(Suppl 1): S3.

Ab 181 Twardowski Z, Prowant B, Moore H, Satalowich R. (2009) Continuous ambulatory peritoneal dialysis (CAPD) technique survival and body size. *Perit Dial Int* **29**(Suppl 1): S8.

Ab 182 Twardowski ZJ. (2010) Possible detrimental role of high dialyzer blood flow on blood access. *J Vasc Access* **11**(Suppl 3): S39.

Ab 183 Twardowski ZJ. (2010) The history of buttonhole technique. *J Vasc Access* **11**(Suppl 3): S39.

Ab 184 Twardowski ZJ. (2010) Intravenous catheter design and problems. *J Vasc Access* **11**(Suppl 3): S39–S40.

Ab 185 Twardowski ZJ. (2010) Buttonhole method of fistula cannulation. *J Vasc Access* **11**(Suppl 3): S39.

Selected Presentations

Pr 1   Twardowski ZJ. (1962) Leczenie ostrej niewydolności nerek. (Treatment of acute renal failure.) *Posiedzenie Krakowskiego Oddziału Polskiego Towarzystwa Lekarskiego* (*Meeting of the Kraków Chapter of the Polish Medical Association*), Kraków, Poland.

Pr 2   Twardowski ZJ. (1964) Ostra niewydolność nerek. (Acute renal failure.) *Posiedzenie Bytomskiego Koła Polskiego Towarzystwa Lekarskiego* (*Meeting of the Bytom Chapter of the Polish Medical Association*), Bytom, Poland.

Pr 3   Twardowski ZJ. (1966) Dwa przypadki przeszczepienia nerki. (Two cases of kidney transplantation.) *Posiedzenie Sekcji Nefrologicznej Wydziału Nauk Medycznych Polskiej Akademii Nauk* (*Meeting of the Polish Academy of Science, Department of Medical Science, Renal Section*), Warsaw, Poland.

Pr 4   Twardowski ZJ. (1967) Przeszczepienie nerki od żywego dawcy. (Kidney transplantation from a living donor.) *Posiedzenie Katowickiego Oddziału Polskiego Towarzystwa Lekarskiego* (*Meeting of the Katowice Chapter of the Polish Medical Association*), Katowice, Poland.

Pr 5   Twardowski ZJ. (1969) Zespół nerczycowy. (Nephrotic syndrome.) *Posiedzenie Katowickiego Oddziału Polskiego Towarzystwa Lekarskiego*, Konferencja Okrągłego Stołu (*Meeting of the Katowice Chapter of the Polish Medical Association, Panel Discussion*), Katowice, Poland.

Pr 6   Twardowski ZJ. (1969) Leczenie przewlekłej niewydolności nerek za pomocą dializ. (Treatment of chronic renal failure with dialysis.) *Posiedzenie Krakowskiego Oddziału Towarzystwa Internistów Polskich* (*Meeting of the Kraków Chapter of the Polish Society of Internal Medicine*), Kraków, Poland.

Pr 7   Twardowski ZJ. (1970) Leczenie przewlekłej niewydolności nerek. (Treatment of chronic renal failure.) *Posiedzenie Katowickiego Oddziału Towarzystwa Internistów Polskich* (*Meeting of the Katowice Chapter of the Polish Society of Internal Medicine*), Katowice, Poland.

Pr 8   Twardowski ZJ. (1970) Przeszczepianie nerek. (Kidney transplantation.) *Posiedzenie Katowickiego Oddziału Polskiego Towarzystwa Urologicznego*, Konferencja Okrągłego Stołu (*Meeting of the Katowice Chapter of the Polish Society of Urology, Panel Discussion*), Katowice, Poland.

Pr 9   Twardowski ZJ. (1971) Ostra niewydolność nerek. (Acute renal failure.) *Posiedzenie Bytomskiego Koła Polskiego Towarzystwa Lekarskiego* (*Meeting of the Bytom Chapter of the Polish Medical Association*), Bytom, Poland.

Pr 10   Twardowski ZJ. (1971) Odmiedniczkowe zapalenie nerek. (Pyelonephritis.) *Posiedzenie Bytomskiego Koła Polskiego Towarzystwa Lekarskiego* (*Meeting of the Bytom Chapter of the Polish Medical Association*), Bytom, Poland.

Pr 11   Twardowski ZJ. (1971) Leczenie ostrej niewydolności nerek. (Treatment of acute renal failure.) *Sympozjum Sekcji Nefrologicznej Towarzystwa Internistów Polskich*, Konferencja Okrągłego Stołu (*Symposium of the Nephrology Section of the Polish Society of Internal Medicine*, Panel Discussion), Gdańsk, Poland.

Pr 12   Twardowski ZJ, Lebek R. (1971) Wielokrotne użycie dializatora zwojowego. (Repeated use of coil dialyzers.) *Sympozjum Sekcji Nefrologicznej Towarzystwa Internistów Polskich* (*Symposium of the Nephrology Section of the Polish Society of Internal Medicine*), Gdańsk, Poland.

Pr 13   Twardowski ZJ. (1972) Immunologiczne aspekty chorób nerek. (Immunological aspects of kidney diseases.) *Posiedzenie Bytomskiego Koła Polskiego Towarzystwa Lekarskiego* (*Meeting of the Bytom Chapter of the Polish Medical Association*), Bytom, Poland.

Pr 14   Twardowski ZJ. (1973) Przewlekła niewydolność nerek. (Chronic renal failure.) *Posiedzenie Bytomskiego Koła Polskiego Towarzystwa Lekarskiego* (*Meeting of the Bytom Chapter of the Polish Medical Association*), Bytom, Poland.

Pr 15   Twardowski Z. (1975) Leczenie hemodializami przewlekłej niewydolności nerek. (Treatment of chronic renal failure with haemodialysis.) *XV Zjazd Polskiego Towarzystwa Urologicznego* (*XVth Congress of the Polish Society of Urology*), Wisla-Jawornik, Poland, May 28.

Pr 16   Twardowski ZJ, Nolph KD, Popovich RP, Hopkins CA. (1977) Comparison of polymer, glucose and hydrostatic pressure induced ultrafiltration in a hollow fiber dialyzer: Effects on convective solute transport. Presented at: *10th Annual Meeting of the American Society of Nephrology*, Washington, D.C., November 22.

Pr 17   Twardowski Z. (1977) Transport konwekcyjny i dyfuzyjny w systemach dializacyjnych. (Convective and diffusive transport in dialysis systems.) *Posiedzenie Sekcji Nefrologicznej Wydziału Nauk Medycznych Polskiej Akademii Nauk* (*Meeting of the Polish Academy of Science*, Department of Medical Science, Renal Section), Warsaw, Poland, November 16.

Pr 18   Twardowski Z. (1977) (Invited Lecturer) Dializoterapia łuszczycy. (Dialysis for psoriasis.) *Posiedzenie Polskiego Towarzystwa Dermatologicznego* (*Meeting of the Polish Society of Dermatology*), Warsaw, Poland, October 14.

Pr 19   Twardowski Z. (1978) Transport konwekcyjny i dyfuzyjny w systemach dializacyjnych. (Convective and diffusive transport in dialysis systems.) *Posiedzenie Poznańskiego Oddziału Towarzystwa Patologów Polskich* (*Meeting of the Polish Society of Pathology, Poznań Section*), Poland, March 18.

Pr 20   Nolph KD, Hopkins C, Rubin J, Twardowski Z, Poporich R. (1978) Polymer induced ultrafiltration in hollow fiber dialyzers (HFK): High osmotic pressure due to impermeant polymer sodium. *24th Annual Meeting of the American Society for Artificial Internal Organs*, The Palmer House, Chicago, IL, April 28.

Pr 21   Twardowski Z. (1978) Ciągła ambulatoryjna dializa otrzewnowa. (Continuous ambulatory peritoneal dialysis.) *Posiedzenie Sekcji Nefrologicznej Wydziału Nauk Medycznych Polskiej Akademii Nauk* (*Meeting of the Polish Academy of Sciences, Department of Medical Science, Renal Section*), Warsaw, Poland, May 22.

Pr 22   Twardowski Z. (1979) Dalsze badania nad dializoterapią łuszczycy. (Further experience in dialysis for psoriasis.) *Posiedzenie Wydziału Terapii Doświadczalnej Polskiej Akademii Nauk* (*Meeting of the Polish Academy of Science, Department of Experimental Therapy*), Warsaw, Poland, January 14.

Pr 23   Janicka L, Twardowski Z, Sokołowska G. (1979) Wpływ płynu dwuwęglanowego i octanowego na przebieg hemodializy w przewlekłej niewydolności nerek. (Influence of bicarbonate and acetate dialysis solutions on patients treated with repeated hemodialysis.) *Posiedzenie Sekcji Nefrologicznej Wydziału Nauk Medycznych Polskiej Akademii Nauk* (*Meeting of the Polish Academy of Science, Department of Medical Science, Renal Section*), Warsaw, Poland, March 12.

Pr 24   Twardowski Z, Książek A. (1979) Farmakokinetyka leków w niewydolności nerek. (Pharmacokinetics of drugs in renal failure.) *Sesja Naukowa: XXXV lat Wydziałów Lekarskiego i Farmaceutycznego w Lublinie oraz XX Lat Współpracy ze Zjednoczeniem Przemysłu Farmaceutycznego "Polfa"* (*Scientific Session: 35 Years of Schools of Medicine and Pharmacology in Lublin and 20 Years of Cooperation Between the Pharmaceutical Industry "Polfa" and the Medical Academy in Lublin*), Akademia Medyczna w Lublinie, Lublin, Poland, November 25.

Pr 25   Twardowski Z, Książek A, Majdan M, et al. (1979) Kinetyka ciągłej ambulatoryjnej dializy otrzewnowej. (Kinetics of continuous ambulatory peritoneal dialysis.) *Posiedzenie Sekcji Nefrologicznej Wydziału Nauk Medycznych Polskiej Akademii Nauk* (*Meeting of the Polish Academy of Science*, Department of Medical Science, Renal Section), Warsaw, Poland, December 12.

Pr 26   Twardowski Z. (1980) Dializoterapia łuszczycy. (Dialysis for psoriasis.) *Posiedzenie Wydziału Terapii Doświadczalnej Polskiej Akademii Nauk* (*Meeting of the Polish Academy of Science*, Department of Experimental Therapy), Warsaw, Poland, January 25.

Pr 27   Twardowski Z, Dmoszyńska A, Janicka L, et al. (1980) Liczba płytek w żyle łokciowej, tętnicy udowej, żyle udowej i przetoce tętniczo-żylnej. (Platelet counts in cubital vein, femoral artery, femoral vein, and arteriovenous fistula.) *Posiedzenie Polskiego Towarzystwa Hematologicznego* (*Annual Meeting of the Polish Society of Hematology*), Nałęczów, Poland, June 7.

Pr 28   Twardowski Z. (1980) (Invited Lecturer) Leczenie ostrej niewydolności nerek. (Treatment of acute renal failure.) *Posiedzenie Sekcji Nefrologicznej Towarzystwa Internistów Polskich* (*Annual Meeting of the Polish Society of Internal Medicine*, Renal Section), Lublin, Poland, September 18.

Pr 29   Twardowski Z. (1981) Ostra niewydolność nerek. (Acute renal failure.) *Posiedzenie Polskiego Towarzystwa Pediatrycznego, Konferencja Okrągłego Stołu* (*Meeting of the Polish Pediatric Society*, Panel Discussion), Warsaw, Poland, March 20.

Pr 30   Twardowski Z, Janicka L, Majdan M, et al. (1981) Efficiency of continuous ambulatory peritoneal dialysis with three 2.5 L exchanges per day. *2nd International Symposium on Peritoneal Dialysis*, Berlin-West, West Germany, June 18.

Pr 31   Twardowski ZJ. (1981) Studies on the new osmotic agents for peritoneal dialysis. Travenol Corporate Headquarters, Deerfield, IL, November 12.

Pr 32   Twardowski ZJ. (1981) Three liter exchanges for continuous ambulatory peritoneal dialysis. Travenol Corporate Headquarters, Deerfield, IL, November 12.

Pr 33   Twardowski ZJ. (1981) Influence of time on dialysate cell count. Travenol Corporate Headquarters, Deerfield, IL, November 12.

Pr 34   Twardowski ZJ, Nolph KD, McGary TJ, Moore HL. (1981) Sustained ultrafiltration with polymer dialysate during long dwell peritoneal dialysis exchanges (Poster Presentation). *14th Annual Meeting of the American Society of Nephrology*, Washington, D.C., November 23.

Pr 35   Twardowski ZJ, Nolph KD, McGary TJ, Moore HL. (1982) Comparison of glucose and polyacrylate as osmotic agents for peritoneal dialysis: *In vitro* and rat studies. The Southern Section, American Federation for Clinical Research, New Orleans, LA, The Hilton Hotel, Durham Room, January 14.

Pr 36   Twardowski ZJ. (1982) CAPD kinetics and clearances. *2nd Annual National Conference Pediatric and Adult Continuous Ambulatory Peritoneal Dialysis*, Centennial Room, Crown Center Hotel, Kansas City, MO, February 15.

Pr 37   Twardowski ZJ, Gutman RA, Moncrief JW, Gallagher N. (1982) Panel discussion: Catheter break-in. *2nd Annual National Conference: Pediatric and Adult Continuous Ambulatory Peritoneal Dialysis*, Centennial Room, Crown Center Hotel, Kansas City, MO, February 15.

Pr 38   Twardowski ZJ, Nolph KD. (1982) Clinical management and complications of the CAPD patient. *2nd Annual National Conference: Pediatric and Adult Continuous Ambulatory Peritoneal Dialysis*, Centennial Room, Crown Center Hotel, Kansas City, MO, February 16.

Pr 39   Nolph KD, Twardowski ZJ. (1982) Current concepts of the physiology of peritoneal dialysis (Invited Lecturers). *1st International Symposium on Peritoneal Dialysis*, sponsored by University of British Columbia, Faculty of Medicine, Vancouver, British Columbia, Canada, May 6.

Pr 40   Twardowski ZJ. (1982) Peritoneal dialysis system. *American Association of Nephrology Nurses and Technicians Seminar*, Hyatt Regency Hotel, New Orleans, LA, June 12.

Pr 41   Twardowski ZJ. (1982) CAPD: An overview. *Home Hemodialysis and CAPD Symposium*, Southern Illinois University School of Medicine, Hilton Hotel, Century Room, Springfield, IL, September 23.

Pr 42   Twardowski ZJ. (1982) Clinical experience with polyacrylonitrile membrane dialyzers in Lublin, Poland. *1st Annual AN69 Membrane Scientific Exchange*, Atlantic City, NJ, October 28–29.

Pr 43   Twardowski ZJ, Alpert MA, Gupta RC, et al. (1982) Circulating immune complexes: A possible toxin responsible for serositis (pericarditis, pleuritis, and peritonitis) in renal failure. *IX Annual Meeting, ESAO*, Brussels, Belgium, September 3.

Pr 44   Twardowski ZJ. (1982) Insulin adsorption into peritoneal dialysis bags. *Travenol CAPD Consultants Meeting*, San Diego, CA, November 9.

Pr 45   Twardowski ZJ. (1983) Catheter break-in. Simultaneous Session I, *3rd National CAPD Conference*, Crown Center, Kansas City, MO, February 14.

Pr 46   Twardowski ZJ. (1983) High volume-low frequency CAPD. Simultaneous Session V, *3rd National CAPD Conference*, Crown Center, Kansas City, MO, February 15.

Pr 47   Twardowski ZJ. (1983) Insulin binding. Simultaneous Session VI, *3rd National CAPD Conference*, Crown Center, Kansas City, MO, February 15.

Pr 48   Twardowski ZJ. (1983) Theory of peritoneal dialysis. *Peritoneal Dialysis Seminar for Health Professionals (IPD, CCPD, CAPD): Theory and Skills*, The University of Colorado Health Sciences Center, Denver, CO, March 17.

Pr 49   Twardowski ZJ. (1983) Review of the kinetics of peritoneal dialysis. MO/KS Council on Renal Nutrition, Columbia, MO, April 1.

Pr 50   Twardowski ZJ. (1983) Efficiency of high volume, low frequency continuous ambulatory peritoneal dialysis (CAPD). *American Society for Artificial Internal Organs*, Sheraton Centre Hotel, Toronto, Canada, April 28.

Pr 51   Twardowski ZJ. (1983) Individualized dialysis for CAPD patient. *American Association of Nephrology Nurses and Technicians National Meeting*, Franklin Plaza Hotel, Philadelphia, PA, June 2.

Pr 52   Twardowski ZJ. (1983) Gelatin as an osmotic agent for peritoneal dialysis. Rat studies. Travenol meeting, Lincolnshire Marriott Resort, Chicago, IL, June 3.

Pr 53   Alpert MA, Van Stone J, Twardowski ZJ, et al. (1983) Comparative effects of hemodialysis and continuous ambulatory peritoneal dialysis on left ventricular volume and performance. *4th Congress of the International Society of Artificial Organs*, Kyoto, Japan, September 17.

Pr 54   Twardowski ZJ. (1984) Catheter break-in: Which method to use? Basic Concepts-New Ideas I. 4th National Conference on CAPD, Crown Center, Kansas City, MO, February 8.

Pr 55   Twardowski ZJ. (1984) Polymers as osmotic agents. *Basic Concepts-New Ideas II. 4th National Conference on CAPD*, Crown Center, Kansas City, MO, February 8.

Pr 56   Twardowski ZJ. (1984) Individualization of exchange volume. *Basic Concepts-New Ideas II. 4th National Conference on CAPD*, Crown Center, Kansas City, MO, February 8.

Pr 57   Twardowski ZJ. (1984) Blood purification in acute renal failure. Grand Rounds, Department of Surgery, University of Missouri, Columbia, MO, April 21.

Pr 58   Twardowski ZJ. (1984) Continuous ambulatory peritoneal dialysis for psoriasis. Travenol Corporate Headquarters, Deerfield, IL, June 6.

Pr 59   Twardowski ZJ. (1984) Gelatin derivatives as osmotic agents for peritoneal dialysis. Travenol Corporate Headquarters, Deerfield, IL, June 6.

Pr 60   Twardowski ZJ, Hain H, Moore HL, *et al.* (1984) Sustained ultrafiltration (UF) with gelatin dialysate during long dwell peritoneal dialysis exchanges in rats. *3rd International Symposium on Peritoneal Dialysis*, Washington, D.C., Capital Hilton Hotel, Presidential Room, June 18.

Pr 61   Twardowski ZJ, Khanna R, Burrows LN, *et al.* (1984) Two years experience with high volume low frequency continuous ambulatory peritoneal dialysis (CAPD). *3rd International Symposium on Peritoneal Dialysis*, Washington, D.C., Capital Hilton Hotel, Presidential Room, June 19.

Pr 62   Twardowski ZJ. (1984) USA CAPD Registry with special emphasis on diabetes mellitus. *4th Benelux Symposium on Continuous Ambulatory Peritoneal Dialysis*, Lecture Room 7, Medical Faculty of the Erasmus University, Rotterdam, The Netherlands, November 24.

Pr 63   Twardowski ZJ. (1984) Oxypolygelatin as an osmotic agent for peritoneal dialysis in rats. Travenol meeting, Round Lake, IL, December 19.

Pr 64   Twardowski ZJ. (1985) Osmotic agents and ultrafiltration in peritoneal dialysis. *5th National Conference on CAPD*, Crown Center, Kansas City, MO, February 6.

Pr 65   Oreopoulos DG, Faller B, Twardowski ZJ. (1985) Peritonitis treatment. *5th National Conference on CAPD*, Crown Center, Kansas City, MO, February 7, 1985.

Pr 66   Twardowski ZJ. (1985) Tunnel bent peritoneal dialysis catheter. Travenol meeting, Deerfield, IL, March 5.

Pr 67   Twardowski ZJ. (1985) Complications and tolerance of long-term intraperitoneal therapy in renal disease. *Gastrointestinal Tumor Study Group Workshop on Intraperitoneal Therapy*, Marriott Inn, Orlando, FL, March 17.

Pr 68   Twardowski ZJ. (1985) Ultrafiltration properties and absorption rates of gelatin derivatives as osmotic agents during long dwell peritoneal dialysis exchanges in rats. Travenol meeting. Deerfield, IL, July 9.

Pr 69   Twardowski ZJ. (1985) Selected aspects of peritoneal dialysis. Surgical Grand Round, Department of Surgery, University of Missouri, Columbia, MO, September 21.

Pr 70   Twardowski ZJ, Nolph KD, Khanna R, *et al.* (1985) Charged polymers as osmotic agents for peritoneal dialysis. *Biomedical Materials Symposium*, organized by Materials Research Society, America Ballroom, Westin Hotel, Boston, MA, December 5.

Pr 71   Twardowski ZJ, Nolph KD, Khanna R, *et al.* (1985) The need for Swan Neck Tunnel peritoneal dialysis catheter. *18th Annual Meeting, American Society of Nephrology*, South Hall, Rivergate Convention Center, New Orleans, LA, December 15.

Pr 72   Twardowski ZJ. (1986) Variation in peritoneal membrane permeability in renal failure patients. General Session I, *6th National Conference on CAPD*, Centennial Room, Crown Center, Kansas City, MO, February 5.

Pr 73   Twardowski ZJ. (1986) Intraabdominal pressure during activity and implications for catheter break-in. Simultaneous Session I, *6th National Conference on CAPD*, Crown Center, Kansas City, MO, February 5.

Pr 74   Franklin JO, Alpert MA, Twardowski ZJ, Khanna R. (1986) Effect of posture and intraperitoneal infusion volume on left ventricular systolic function in patients on continuous ambulatory peritoneal dialysis. Simultaneous Session I, *6th National Conference on CAPD*, Crown Center, Kansas City, MO, February 5.

Pr 75   Twardowski ZJ. (1986) Catheter placement and exit site infections. Special Session on Preventing Infections, *6th National Conference on CAPD*, Centennial Room, Crown Center, Kansas City, MO, February 7.

Pr 76   Twardowski ZJ. (1986) Pregnancy and renal disease. Medical Grand Rounds, Department of Medicine, University of Missouri, Columbia, MO, March 21.

Pr 77   Prowant B, Ryan LP, Twardowski ZJ. (1986) Effect of dialysis solution volume, position and activity on intraabdominal pressure in continuous ambulatory peritoneal dialysis patients. *17th National Symposium of American Nephrology Nurses' Association*, New Orleans, LA, April 11.

Pr 78   Nolph KD, Twardowski ZJ, Khanna R. (1986) Clinical pathology conference: Peritoneal dialysis. *32nd Annual Meeting of American Society for Artificial Internal Organs*, Disneyland Hotel, Anaheim, CA, May 7.

Pr 79   Twardowski ZJ, Khanna R, Nolph KD, *et al.* (1986) Preliminary experience with the Swan Neck peritoneal dialysis catheter. *32nd Annual Meeting of American Society for Artificial Internal Organs*, Disneyland Hotel, Anaheim, CA, May 7.

Pr 80   Lampainen E, Khanna R, Schaefer R, Twardowski ZJ, Nolph KD. (1986) Is air under the diaphragm a significant finding in CAPD patients? *32nd Annual Meeting of American Society for Artificial Internal Organs*, Disneyland Hotel, Anaheim, CA, May 9.

Pr 81   Franklin JO, Alpert MA, Twardowski ZJ, Khanna R. (1986) Effect of intraperitoneal infusion volume and posture on left ventricular systolic function in patients on continuous ambulatory peritoneal dialysis. *32nd Annual*

Pr 82   *Meeting of American Society for Artificial Internal Organs*, Disneyland Hotel, Anaheim, CA, May 9.

Pr 82 Twardowski ZJ, Nolph KD, Khanna R et al. (1986) Daily clearances with continuous ambulatory peritoneal dialysis and nightly peritoneal dialysis. *32nd Annual Meeting of American Society for Artificial Internal Organs*, Disneyland Hotel, Anaheim, CA, May 9.

Pr 83 Twardowski ZJ. (1986) Tidal peritoneal dialysis. Preliminary experience. Travenol meeting, O'Hare Hilton Hotel, Chicago, IL, June 4.

Pr 84 Twardowski ZJ, Nolph KD, Khanna R, et al. (1986) The need for Swan Neck Tunnel peritoneal dialysis catheter. *Annual Network No. 9 Coordinating Council Meeting*, Bear's Den, Wohl Center, Washington University, St. Louis, MO, June 12.

Pr 85 Twardowski ZJ, Khanna R, Nolph KD, et al. (1986) Preliminary experience with the Swan Neck peritoneal dialysis catheter. *Annual Network No. 9 Coordinating Council Meeting*, Bear's Den, Wohl Center, Washington University, St. Louis, MO, June 12.

Pr 86 Twardowski ZJ, Nolph KD, Khanna R, et al. (1986) Daily clearances with continuous ambulatory peritoneal dialysis and nightly peritoneal dialysis. *Annual Network No. 9 Coordinating Council Meeting*, Bear's Den, Wohl Center, Washington University, St. Louis, MO, June 12.

Pr 87 Twardowski ZJ. (1986) Clinical case studies. *Peritoneal Dialysis Seminar — Advances in the Therapy*, The Charles Hotel, Cambridge, MA, September 24.

Pr 88 Twardowski ZJ. (1986) Advances in catheter selection and placement. *Peritoneal Dialysis Seminar — Advances in the Therapy*, Hyatt Regency, Memphis, TN, October 1.

Pr 89 Twardowski ZJ. (1986) Clinical case studies. *Peritoneal Dialysis Seminar — Advances in the Therapy*, Crystal City Marriott Hotel, Arlington, VA, October 8.

Pr 90 Mactier RA, Nolph KD, Khanna R, Twardowski ZJ, Moore H, McGary T. (1986) Lymphatic absorption in peritoneal dialysis in the rat. *Founder Bi-Annual Meeting of the North American Society of Lymphology*, Marriott Hotel, St. Louis, October 17.

Pr 91 Twardowski ZJ. (1986) Clinical case studies. *Peritoneal Dialysis Seminar*, Hilton Hotel, New Orleans, LA, October 29.

Pr 92 Twardowski ZJ. (1987) Tidal peritoneal dialysis. Travenol meeting, Allgaures Hotel, Wheeling, IL, January 22.

Pr 93 Twardowski ZJ. (1987) Is tidal peritoneal dialysis the most effective way to use a cycler. *7th National Conference on CAPD*, The Westin Crown Center Hotel, Kansas City, MO, February 4.

Pr 94 Schreiber M, Vas S, Twardowski ZJ. (1987) Recommendations for preventing and treating exit site infections. Panel presentation and discussion: *7th National Conference on CAPD*, The Westin Crown Center Hotel, Kansas City, MO, February 4.

Pr 95   Twardowski Z. (1987) Update on the Swan Neck catheter. *7th National Conference on CAPD*, The Westin Crown Center Hotel, Kansas City, MO, February 5.

Pr 96   Twardowski Z. (1987) Peritoneal dialysis modifications to avoid CAPD dropouts. *7th National Conference on CAPD*, The Westin Crown Center Hotel, Kansas City, MO, February 6.

Pr 97   Twardowski Z. (1987) Proteinuria. Medical Grand Rounds, Department of Medicine, University of Missouri, Columbia, MO, March 12.

Pr 98   Prowant BF, Schmidt LM, Twardowski ZJ, et al. (1987) A randomized prospective evaluation of three procedures for peritoneal dialysis catheter exit site care. *American Nephrology Nurses' Association's 18th National Symposium*, Marriott Marquis, S. Broadway Ballroom, New York, NY, May 17.

Pr 99   Nolph KD, Dobbie JW, Khanna R, Rippe B, Twardowski Z. (1987) Peritoneal dialysis — Prevention and treatment of catheter problems. Panel discussion, *International Conference on Peritoneum and Peritoneal Access*, Lund University Hospital, Lund, Sweden, June 22.

Pr 100   Twardowski ZJ. (1987) Advances in peritoneal catheter selection, placement, and break-in. *International Conference on Peritoneum and Peritoneal Access*, Lund University Hospital, Lund, Sweden, June 24.

Pr 101   Buchwald H, Jeppsson B, Twardowski ZJ, Updike SJ. (1987) Implantable pumps and catheters for intraperitoneal delivery. Panel discussion, *International Conference on Peritoneum and Peritoneal Access*, Lund University Hospital, Lund, Sweden, June 24.

Pr 102   Mactier RA, Khanna R, Nolph KD, Twardowski Z, Moore H. (1987) Neostigmine increases ultrafiltration and solute clearances in peritoneal dialysis by reducing lymphatic drainage. *IV Congress of the International Society for Peritoneal Dialysis*, Venice, Italy, Palazzo del Cinema, June 30.

Pr 103   Mactier RA, Khanna R, Twardowski Z, Nolph KD. (1987) Lymphatic absorption in CAPD. *IV Congress of the International Society for Peritoneal Dialysis*, Venice, Italy, Palazzo del Cinema, June 30.

Pr 104   Nolph KD, Mactier RA, Khanna R, Twardowski Z, Moore H. (1987) Kinetics of peritoneal ultrafiltration (UF): The role of lymphatics. *IV Congress of the International Society for Peritoneal Dialysis*, Venice, Italy, Palazzo del Cinema, June 30.

Pr 105   Prowant B, Twardowski Z, Schmidt L, et al. (1987) Use of smears for diagnosis of peritoneal catheter exit site (ESO) infection (INF). *IV Congress of the International Society for Peritoneal Dialysis*, Venice, Italy, Palazzo del Cinema, June 30.

Pr 106   Twardowski ZJ, Khanna R, Nichols WK, et al. (1987) Low complication rates with Swan Neck Short Tunnel Missouri (SNSTM) peritoneal catheter. *IV Congress of the International Society for Peritoneal Dialysis*, Venice, Italy, Palazzo del Cinema, July 1.

Pr 107   Twardowski Z, Nolph K, Khanna R, et al. (1987) Eight hr tidal peritoneal dialysis (TPD) matches 24 hr CAPD and surpasses 8 hr nightly intermittent peritoneal dialysis (NIPD) clearances (C). *IV Congress of the International Society for Peritoneal Dialysis*, Venice, Italy, Palazzo del Cinema, July 1.

Pr 108 Cheek TR, Twardowski ZJ, Moore HL, Nolph KD. (1987) High molecular weight (MW) gelatin isocyanate absorption from the peritoneal cavity of rats. *IV Congress of the International Society for Peritoneal Dialysis*, Venice, Italy, Palazzo del Cinema, July 1.

Pr 109 Alpert MA, Franklin JO, Twardowski ZJ, Khanna R. (1987) Impact of increasing intraperitoneal volume on left ventricular function in CAPD patients. *IV Congress of the International Society for Peritoneal Dialysis*, Venice, Italy, Palazzo del Cinema, July 2.

Pr 110 Twardowski ZJ. (1987) (Visiting Professor) Postępy w dializie otrzewnowej. (Advances in peritoneal dialysis.) Centrum Zdrowia Dziecka — Szpital Pomnik (Center of the Child Health — Hospital Monument), Warsaw, Poland, July 15.

Pr 111 Twardowski ZJ. (1987) (Invited Lecturer) Postępy w dializie otrzewnowej. (Advances in peritoneal dialysis.) *Posiedzenie Oddziału Poznańskiego Polskiego Towarzystwa Nefrologicznego (Conference of the Poznań Chapter of the Polish Society of Nephrology)*, Klinika Nefrologii Akademii Medycznej, Poznań, Poland, July 21.

Pr 112 Twardowski ZJ. (1987) Tidal dialysis. *Seminar of Renal Education Program: Current Research in Nephrology*, Ramada Inn Executive Center, Columbia, MO, November 19.

Pr 113 Mactier RA, Khanna R, Moore H, Twardowski Z, Nolph K. (1987) Phosphatidylcholine enhances the efficiency of peritoneal dialysis by reducing lymphatic absorption. *20th Annual Meeting of the American Society of Nephrology*, Washington Ballroom, Sheraton-Washington, Washington, D.C., December 16.

Pr 114 Twardowski ZJ. (1988) Absorption of gelatin isocyanate and inulin from the peritoneal cavity of rats. Workshop on lymphatic absorption from the peritoneal cavity, *8th National Conference on CAPD*, The Westin Crown Center Hotel, Kansas City, MO, February 9.

Pr 115 Twardowski ZJ. (1988) Update on equilibrium kinetics. *8th National Conference on CAPD*, The Westin Crown Center Hotel, Kansas City, MO, February 10.

Pr 116 Twardowski ZJ. (1988) Update on tidal peritoneal dialysis. *8th National Conference on CAPD*, The Westin Crown Center Hotel, Kansas City, MO, February 11.

Pr 117 Gallagher N, Schmidt L, Schreiber M, Twardowski ZJ. (1988) Panel on exit site care. *8th National Conference on CAPD*, The Westin Crown Center Hotel, Kansas City, MO, February 11.

Pr 118 Twardowski ZJ. (1988) Raging controversies related to peritoneal catheter design, placement and management. *8th National Conference on CAPD*, The Westin Crown Center Hotel, Kansas City, MO, February 12.

Pr 119   Twardowski ZJ. (1988) New approaches to cycler dialysis and adequacy. Tutorial: Peritoneal dialysis update. Presiding: Nolph KD. *34th Annual Meeting American Society for Artificial Internal Organs*, Reno, NV, May 3.

Pr 120   Twardowski ZJ. (1988) Peritoneal catheter development: Currently used catheters — advantages/disadvantages/complications — and catheter tunnel morphology in humans. Panel: Percutaneous access. Presiding: Kantrowitz A. *34th Annual Meeting American Society for Artificial Internal Organs*, Reno, NV, May 3.

Pr 121   Twardowski ZJ. (1988) Effectiveness of the peritoneal access — Implantation and post-op care. *Peritoneal Dialysis Seminar: Peritoneal Dialysis Services — Organization and Management*, New Jersey Renal Network Council, Hyatt Regency, New Brunswick, May 10.

Pr 122   Twardowski ZJ. (1988) The catheter — Therapeutic decisions regarding usage and catheter design. *Peritoneal Dialysis Seminar: Peritoneal Dialysis Services — Organization and Management*, Hyatt Regency, New Brunswick, May 11.

Pr 123   Twardowski ZJ. (1988) Proteinuria. Medical Grand Round, Department of Medicine, University of Missouri, Columbia, MO, June 9.

Pr 124   Twardowski ZJ. (1988) Stan obecny i perspektywy użyteczności dializy otrzewnowej. (Current status and practical perspectives of peritoneal dialysis.) *IVth Conference of the Polish Society of Nephrology*, City Council Auditorium, Poznań, Poland, June 25.

Pr 125   Twardowski ZJ. (1988) Dializa otrzewnowa. (Peritoneal dialysis.) Nephrology Grand Round, Klinika Nefrologii Instytutu Chorób Wewnętrznych Akademii Medycznej w Lublinie (Department of Nephrology, Institute of Internal Medicine, Medical Academy in Lublin), Poland, June 29.

Pr 126   Twardowski ZJ. (1988) Achieving adequate dialysis using CAPD. *Perspectives on Peritoneal Dialysis*, seminar organized by Baxter Healthcare, Inc., The Ritz-Carlton, Naples, FL, August 18.

Pr 127   Multiple Authors. (1988) Cross sectional malnutrition study. Poster, *5th International Congress on Nutrition and Metabolism in Renal Disease*, Strasbourg, France, September 3.

Pr 128   Twardowski ZJ. (1988) New advances in automated peritoneal dialysis. *Peritoneal Dialysis Seminar*, organized by Baxter Limited, Hotel Plaza, Sendai, Japan, October 15.

Pr 129   Twardowski ZJ. (1988) Swan Neck peritoneal dialysis catheter. *Peritoneal Dialysis Seminar*, organized by Baxter Limited, Hotel Plaza, Sendai, Japan, October 15.

Pr 130   Twardowski ZJ. (1988) Peritoneal access — History and current advances. Grand Round, invited by Prof. Kazuo Ota, Director of Kidney Center, Tokyo Women's Medical College, Tokyo, Japan, October 18.

Pr 131   Twardowski ZJ. (1988) Tidal peritoneal dialysis. *Peritoneal Dialysis Seminar*, organized by Baxter Limited for Saitama Medical School, Palace Hotel Omiya, Sonic City Building, Omiya, Japan, October 18.

Pr 132 Twardowski ZJ. (1988) Swan Neck peritoneal dialysis catheter. *Peritoneal Dialysis Seminar*, organized by Baxter Limited for Saitama Medical School, Palace Hotel Omiya, Sonic City Building, Omiya, Japan, October 18.

Pr 133 Twardowski ZJ. (1988) Peritoneal access — History and current advances. Grand Round, invited by Dr. Yoshihei Hirasawa, Vice President of Shinrakuen Hospital, Niigata, Japan, October 19.

Pr 134 Twardowski ZJ. (1988) Peritoneal access — History and current advances. Grand Round, invited by Prof. Akira Shinoda, Director, Division of Nephrology, Kanazawa Medical University, Kanazawa, Ishikawa, Japan, October 20.

Pr 135 Twardowski ZJ. (1988) Tidal peritoneal dialysis. *Peritoneal Dialysis Seminar*, organized by Baxter Limited and Hayashidera Medinol, Kanazawa Miyako Hotel, Kanazawa, Ishikawa, Japan, October 20.

Pr 136 Twardowski ZJ. (1988) Swan Neck peritoneal dialysis catheter. *Peritoneal Dialysis Seminar*, organized by Baxter Limited and Hayashidera Medinol, Kanazawa Miyako Hotel, Kanazawa, Ishikawa, Japan, October 20.

Pr 137 Twardowski ZJ. (1988) New advances in automated peritoneal dialysis. *Peritoneal Dialysis Seminar*, organized by Baxter Limited and Hayashidera Medinol, Meitetsu Toyama Hotel, Toyama, Japan, October 21.

Pr 138 Twardowski ZJ. (1988) Peritoneal dialysis. Grand Round, invited by Prof. Hiroshi Kida, The First Department of Internal Medicine, School of Medicine, Kanazawa University, Kanazawa, Ishikawa, Japan, October 24.

Pr 139 Twardowski ZJ. (1988) Peritoneal access — History and current advances. Grand Round, invited by Dr. Dairoku Shirai, Director, Division of Nephrology, Osaka Koseinenkin Hospital, Osaka, Japan, October 25.

Pr 140 Twardowski ZJ. (1988) New advances in automated peritoneal dialysis. *Peritoneal Dialysis Seminar*, organized by Baxter Limited, ANA Hotel, Hiroshima, Japan, October 26.

Pr 141 Twardowski ZJ. (1988) Swan Neck peritoneal dialysis catheter. *Peritoneal Dialysis Seminar*, organized by Baxter Limited, ANA Hotel Hiroshima, Hiroshima, Japan, October 26.

Pr 142 Twardowski ZJ. (1988) Patient tailored peritoneal dialysis for adequate treatment. *The 6th Benelux CAPD Symposium*, RAI Congrescentrum, Amsterdam, The Netherlands, December 2.

Pr 143 Twardowski ZJ, Khanna R, Nichols WK, Nolph KD. (1988) Swan Neck peritoneal dialysis catheters — Design, insertion, break-in, and chronic care, Second Edition, Video presentation. *The 6th Benelux CAPD Symposium*, RAI Congrescentrum, Amsterdam, The Netherlands, December 2.

Pr 144 Oreopoulos DG (and multiple authors including Twardowski ZJ). (1988) Nutritional status of CAPD patients: An International Study. *21st Annual Meeting of the American Society of Nephrology*, Convention Center, San Antonio, TX, December 13.

Pr 145 Artis AK, Alpert MA, Van Stone J, Twardowski ZJ, Khanna R. (1988) Effect of beta blockade on LV systolic function in patients undergoing hemodialysis. *21st Annual Meeting of the American Society of Nephrology*, Convention Center, San Antonio, TX, December 13.

Pr 146 Twardowski ZJ. (1989) Morphology of the catheter exit site and tunnel. *Baxter Healthcare Corporation Peritoneal Dialysis Consultants Meeting*, The Ritz-Carlton Naples, Naples, FL, January 5.

Pr 147 Twardowski ZJ. (1989) Update on Tidal PD Study. *Baxter Healthcare Corporation Peritoneal Dialysis Consultants Meeting*, The Ritz-Carlton Naples, Naples, FL, January 6.

Pr 148 Twardowski ZJ. (1989) Clinical experience with tidal peritoneal dialysis. Baxter Healthcare Corporation Headquarters, Round Lake, IL, January 25.

Pr 149 Oreopoulos GD, Everett ED, Gokal R, Khanna R, Twardowski ZJ. (1989) Quiz the experts. *9th Annual Conference on Peritoneal Dialysis*, The Loews Anatole Hotel, Senators Lecture Hall, Dallas, TX, February 23.

Pr 150 Twardowski ZJ. (1989) Morphology of the catheter exit site and tunnel. *9th Annual Conference on Peritoneal Dialysis*, The Loews Anatole Hotel, Chantilly Ballroom East, Dallas, TX, February 24.

Pr 151 Twardowski ZJ. (1989) Patient tailored peritoneal dialysis for adequate treatment. *Peritoneal Dialysis Seminar*, organized by Baxter Healthcare, Inc., The Breckenridge Frontenac Hotel, St. Louis, MO, March 13.

Pr 152 Twardowski ZJ. (1989) Morphology of the peritoneal catheter tunnel. Research meeting, Department of Medicine, School of Medicine, University of Missouri, Columbia, MO, March 16.

Pr 153 Twardowski ZJ. (1989) Results and complications with Swan Neck peritoneal dialysis catheters. Danville Urologic Clinic, Danville, Virginia, April 5.

Pr 154 Twardowski ZJ. (1989) Adequacy of dialysis and new cycler techniques. Danville Urologic Clinic, Danville, Virginia, April 5.

Pr 155 Twardowski ZJ. (1989) Patient tailored peritoneal dialysis for adequate treatment. *3rd Annual Symposium on Renal Disease*, Pecora Auditorium, Community Medical Center, Toms River, NJ, April 12.

Pr 156 Twardowski ZJ. (1989) Achieving adequate dialysis using CAPD. *PD Perspectives*, seminar organized by Baxter Healthcare, Inc., The Hyatt Regency Scottsdale, Scottsdale, AZ, April 27.

Pr 157 Twardowski ZJ. (1989) Mesna — Dimesna — Mesna. Friday Morning Matinee, Department of Medicine, University of Missouri, VA Auditorium, Columbia, MO, May 12.

Pr 158 Twardowski ZJ. (1989) Achieving adequate dialysis using CAPD. *PD Perspectives*, seminar organized by Baxter Healthcare, Inc., Rancho Bernardo Inn, San Diego, CA, June 8.

Pr 159 Twardowski ZJ. (1989) Patient tailored peritoneal dialysis for adequate treatment. *Cruise Symposium "Fresh Perspectives in Automated Peritoneal Dialysis"*, organized by Baxter Sweden in connection with the XXVIth Congress of the European Dialysis and Transplant Association, European Renal Association, Göteborg Archipelago, Önnered Conference Center, Sweden, June 12.

Pr 160 Twardowski ZJ. (1989) Tidal peritoneal dialysis. *XVIIIth Annual Conference of the European Dialysis Technician and Nurses Association–European Renal Care Association*, Hall N, Liseberg, Göteborg, Sweden, June 13.

Pr 161 Twardowski ZJ. (1989) Morphology of the peritoneal catheter tunnel. *Workshop on Peritoneal Access in CAPD Patients*, organized by Percuseal Medical AB, Park Avenue Hotel, Kungsportsavenyn 36–38, Göteborg, Sweden, June 15.

Pr 162 Twardowski ZJ. (1989) Exit site healing and infection evaluation in CAPD — Preliminary results. *Workshop on Peritoneal Access in CAPD Patients*, organized by Percuseal Medical AB, Park Avenue Hotel, Kungsportsavenyn 36–38, Göteborg, Sweden, June 15.

Pr 163 Twardowski ZJ. (1989) Results with the Swan Neck peritoneal dialysis catheters. Grand Round, Rigshospitalet, Copenhagen, Denmark, June 20.

Pr 164 Twardowski ZJ. (1989) Results with the Swan Neck peritoneal dialysis catheters. Grand Round, Aarhus Kommunehospital, Denmark, June 21.

Pr 165 Twardowski ZJ. (1989) Exit site healing and infection evaluation. Grand Round, Nottingham City Hospital, Nottingham, England, June 22.

Pr 166 Twardowski ZJ. (1989) Peritoneal catheter implantation and conditioning. Grand Round, Cantonal University Hospital of Geneva, Switzerland, June 23.

Pr 167 Twardowski ZJ. (1989) Peritoneal catheter implantation and conditioning. Grand Round, Cantonal University Hospital of Lausanne, Switzerland, June 23.

Pr 168 Twardowski ZJ. (1989) Current issues in peritoneal dialysis. *Concepts in Peritoneal Dialysis*, seminar sponsored by Hazel Taylor Chapter of American Nephrology Nurses' Association and Baxter Healthcare Corporation, Wynfrey Hotel, 1000 Riverchase Galleria, Birmingham, Alabama, August 15.

Pr 169 Twardowski ZJ. (1989) Optimizing dialysis using CAPD. *PD Perspectives*, seminar organized by Baxter Healthcare, Inc., Ballroom G, Marriott Harbor Beach, Fort Lauderdale, FL, August 24.

Pr 170 Twardowski ZJ. (1989) Tidal peritoneal dialysis. *XIII Annual Chronic Renal Disease Symposium*, Searle Continuing Education Center, Duke University Medical Center, Durham, North Carolina, October 2.

Pr 171 Twardowski ZJ. (1989) Optimizing dialysis using CAPD. *PD Perspectives*, seminar organized by Baxter Healthcare, Inc., The Westin Hotel, Hilton Head Island, South Carolina, November 4.

Pr 172 Twardowski ZJ. (1989) Preventing and managing complications — Catheters. *PD Perspectives*, seminar organized by Baxter Healthcare, Inc., The Westin Hotel, Hilton Head Island, South Carolina, November 4.

Pr 173 Twardowski ZJ. (1989) Catheter implantation and exit site care. *Peritoneal Dialysis 1989: A State-of-the-Art Practicum*, sponsored by School of Medicine,

University of Missouri, Division of Nephrology and Office of Continuing Education, Hudson River Inn and Conference Center, 321 North Highland Avenue, Ossining, New York, November 10.

Pr 174 Twardowski ZJ, Nolph KD. (1989) Achieving optimal dialysis on CAPD, CCPD, Nightly PD, and TPD. *Peritoneal Dialysis 1989: A State-of-the-Art Practicum*, sponsored by School of Medicine, University of Missouri, Division of Nephrology and Office of Continuing Education, Hudson River Inn and Conference Center, 321 North Highland Avenue, Ossining, New York, November 10.

Pr 175 Twardowski ZJ. (1989) Tailoring peritoneal dialysis for special patients: Physically impaired. *Peritoneal Dialysis 1989: A State-of-the-Art Practicum*, sponsored by School of Medicine, University of Missouri, Division of Nephrology and Office of Continuing Education, Hudson River Inn and Conference Center, 321 North Highland Avenue, Ossining, New York, November 11.

Pr 176 Twardowski ZJ. (1989) Patient tailored peritoneal dialysis for adequate therapy. Grand Round, The Bowman Gray School of Medicine, Wake Forrest University, 300 South Hawthorne Road, Winston-Salem, North Carolina, November 15.

Pr 177 Twardowski ZJ, Khanna R, Nichols WK, Nolph KD. (1989) Swan Neck peritoneal dialysis catheters — Design, insertion, break-in, and chronic care. Video, Second Edition, Academic Support Center, The Curators of the University of Missouri, 1988, presented at VIDEOMED-89, V Semana Internacional de Videocine Médico, Hospital Provincial, Badajoz, 13–18 November.

Pr 178 Nolph KD, Twardowski ZJ, Khanna R. (1989) Tidal peritoneal dialysis with racemic or L-lactate solutions. *22nd Annual Meeting of the American Society of Nephrology*, Exhibit Hall A, Sheraton Washington, Washington, D.C., December 3.

Pr 179 Twardowski ZJ. (1990) Pathophysiology of exit site and tunnel infections — New insights. *10th Annual Conference on Peritoneal Dialysis*, The Loews Anatole Hotel, Dallas, TX, February 8.

Pr 180 Twardowski ZJ. (1990) The PET — A simpler approach for determining recipes for any peritoneal dialysis therapy. *10th Annual Conference on Peritoneal Dialysis*, The Loews Anatole Hotel, Dallas, TX, February 9.

Pr 181 Dobbie JW, Twardowski ZJ, Algrim C, *et al.* (1990) Clinical evaluation of tidal PD (TPD) as a long term dialysis therapy. *10th Annual Conference on Peritoneal Dialysis*, The Loews Anatole Hotel, Dallas, TX, February 9.

Pr 182 Moore HL, Ellersieck MR, Prowant BF, *et al.* (1990) Stability of clinical analytes in peritoneal dialysate. *10th Annual Conference on Peritoneal Dialysis*, The Loews Anatole Hotel, Dallas, TX, February 9.

Pr 183 Twardowski ZJ. (1990) The current status of tidal peritoneal dialysis. *10th Annual Conference on Peritoneal Dialysis*, The Loews Anatole Hotel, Dallas, TX, February 10.

Pr 184 Twardowski ZJ. (1990) Adequacy of peritoneal dialysis — PET and other quantitative indicators. *8th Annual Meeting of the California Dialysis Council*, The Spa Hotel, Palm Springs, CA, April 3.

Pr 185 Twardowski ZJ, Prowant BF, Khanna R, et al. (1990) Long term experience with Swan Neck Missouri 2 (SN-M2) and Swan Neck Missouri 3 (SN-M3) peritoneal dialysis catheters. *36th Annual Meeting American Society for Artificial Internal Organs*, International Ballroom West, Slide Forum #12, Washington Hilton & Towers, Washington, D.C., April 26.

Pr 186 Twardowski ZJ, Prowant BF, Nolph KD, et al. (1990) Culture results of peritoneal catheter peri-exit smears (S) and sinus tract washouts (W). *36th Annual Meeting American Society for Artificial Internal Organs*, International Ballroom West, Slide Forum #12, Washington Hilton & Towers, Washington, D.C., April 26.

Pr 187 Twardowski ZJ, Tully RJ, Ersoy FF, Dedhia NM. (1990) Computerized tomographic peritoneography (CTP) in peritoneal dialysis (PD) patients. *36th Annual Meeting American Society for Artificial Internal Organs*, Exhibit Hall, Poster Session #7, Washington Hilton & Towers, Washington, D.C., April 26.

Pr 188 Twardowski ZJ, Prowant BF, Nolph KD, Khanna R. (1990) Chronic nightly tidal peritoneal dialysis (NTPD). *36th Annual Meeting American Society for Artificial Internal Organs*, Exhibit Hall, Poster Session #7, Washington Hilton & Towers, Washington, D.C., April 26.

Pr 189 Twardowski ZJ. (1990) Tidal Peritoneal Dialysis — What? why? who? how? and when? Minnesota Kidney Club, Minneapolis, MN, May 3.

Pr 190 Twardowski ZJ. (1990) Patient tailored peritoneal dialysis for adequate treatment. Grand Round, Hennepin County Medical Center, Minneapolis, MN, May 4.

Pr 191 Twardowski ZJ. (1990) Pathophysiology of exit site and tunnel infections — New insights. Colorado Society of Nephrology, Hyatt Regency Hotel, Denver, CO, May 9.

Pr 192 Twardowski ZJ. (1990) Patient tailored peritoneal dialysis for adequate treatment. Grand Round, Division of Nephrology, Department of Medicine, University of Colorado, Denver, CO, May 10.

Pr 193 Twardowski ZJ. (1990) Prevention, diagnosis and treatment of exit site and tunnel infections. Grand Round, Division of Nephrology, Department of Medicine, Fitzsimmons Army Medical Center, Aurora, CO, May 10.

Pr 194 Twardowski ZJ. (1990) Automated peritoneal dialysis, tidal peritoneal dialysis. *1990 Nephrology Conference of Tri-State Renal Network*, Inc., Hilton on the Circle, Indianapolis, IN, May 17.

Pr 195 Twardowski ZJ. (1990) How do we optimize peritoneal dialysis prescription? *1st Western Canada Conference on Peritoneal Dialysis*, Walter C. Mackenzie Health Sciences Centre, University of Alberta, Edmonton, Alberta, Canada, May 24.

Pr 196 Twardowski ZJ, Schmidt LM. (1990) PET Workshop. *1st Western Canada Conference on Peritoneal Dialysis*, Walter C. Mackenzie Health Sciences Centre, University of Alberta, Edmonton, Alberta, Canada, May 24.

Pr 197 Twardowski ZJ. (1990) A new approach to diagnosis and treatment of exit site infection. *1st Western Canada Conference on Peritoneal Dialysis*, Walter C. Mackenzie Health Sciences Centre, University of Alberta, Edmonton, Alberta, Canada, May 24.

Pr 198 Twardowski ZJ, Schmidt LM. (1990) Workshop on exit site infection. *1st Western Canada Conference on Peritoneal Dialysis*, Walter C. Mackenzie Health Sciences Centre, University of Alberta, Edmonton, Alberta, Canada, May 24.

Pr 199 Twardowski ZJ. (1990) Peritoneal equilibration test and adequacy of peritoneal dialysis. Kidney Club Meeting, Marriott Mountain Shadow Hotel, Phoenix, AZ, June 13.

Pr 200 Twardowski ZJ. (1990) Percutaneous access in CAPD: Exit site histopathology. *Sneak Previews — 2nd Annual Science and Technology Conference*, organized by Renal Division of Baxter Healthcare Corporation, Willow Conference Room, Holiday Inn, Crystal Lake, IL, June 20.

Pr 201 Twardowski ZJ. (1990) Percutaneous access in CAPD: Swan Neck Catheter — U.S. Experience. *Sneak Previews — 2nd Annual Science and Technology Conference*, organized by Renal Division of Baxter Healthcare Corporation, Willow Conference Room, Holiday Inn, Crystal Lake, IL, June 20.

Pr 202 Twardowski ZJ, Prowant BF, Khanna R, *et al.* (1990) Long term experience with Swan Neck Missouri 2 (SN-M2) and Swan Neck Missouri 3 (SN-M3) peritoneal dialysis catheters. *XIth International Congress of Nephrology*, Takanawa Prince Hotel, Hiten Room, Tokyo, Japan, July 20.

Pr 203 Twardowski ZJ, Dobbie JW, Moore HL, *et al.* (1990) Morphology of peritoneal dialysis (PD) catheter tunnel (CT) — Macroscopy and light microscopy. *XIth International Congress of Nephrology*, Takanawa Prince Hotel, Hiten Room, Tokyo, Japan, July 20.

Pr 204 Twardowski ZJ, Prowant BF, Nolph KD, *et al.* (1990) Culture results of peritoneal catheter peri-exit smears (S) and sinus tract washouts (W). *XIth International Congress of Nephrology*, Takanawa Prince Hotel, Hiten Room, Tokyo, Japan, July 20.

Pr 205 Twardowski ZJ, Prowant BF, Nolph KD, Khanna R. (1990) Chronic nightly tidal peritoneal dialysis (NTPD). *XIth International Congress of Nephrology*, Takanawa Prince Hotel, Hiten Room, Tokyo, Japan, July 20.

Pr 206 Twardowski ZJ, Tully RJ, Ersoy FF, Dedhia NM. (1990) Computerized tomographic peritoneography (CTP) in peritoneal dialysis (PD) patients. *XIth International Congress of Nephrology*, Takanawa Prince Hotel, Hiten Room, Tokyo, Japan, July 20.

Pr 207 Twardowski ZJ, Prowant BF, Nolph KD, *et al.* (1990) Key factors in exit site(s) (ES) evaluation. *XIth International Congress of Nephrology*, Takanawa Prince Hotel, Asuka Room, Tokyo, Japan, July 20.

Pr 208 Khanna R, Nolph KD, Twardowski ZJ. (1990) Manipulation of ultrafiltration in peritoneal dialysis. *XIth International Congress of Nephrology*, Takanawa Prince Hotel, Asuka Room, Tokyo, Japan, July 20.

Pr 209 Khanna R, Moore HL, Mactier R, *et al.* (1990) Effect of increased intraperitoneal hydrostatic pressure (PCHP) on Starling's forces during a peritoneal dialysis exchange (PDEX) in rat. *Vth Congress of the International Society for Peritoneal Dialysis*, Kyoto Grand Hotel, Room A-2, Kyoto, Japan, July 22.

Pr 210 Nolph KD, Twardowski ZJ, Khanna R. (1990) Tidal peritoneal dialysis with racemic or L-lactate solutions. *Vth Congress of the International Society for Peritoneal Dialysis*, Kyoto Grand Hotel, Room A-2, Kyoto, Japan, July 22.

Pr 211 Twardowski ZJ, Tully RJ, Ersoy FF, Dedhia NM. (1990) Computerized tomography (CT) and CT peritoneography (CTP) in peritoneal dialysis (PD) patients. *Vth Congress of the International Society for Peritoneal Dialysis*, Kyoto Grand Hotel, Room A-2, Kyoto, Japan, July 22.

Pr 212 Ersoy FF, Moore HL, Khanna R, Nolph KD, Twardowski ZJ. (1990) The effect of respiration on peritoneal cavity lymphatic absorption. *Vth Congress of the International Society for Peritoneal Dialysis*, Kyoto Grand Hotel, Room C, Kyoto, Japan, July 22.

Pr 213 Twardowski ZJ, Prowant BF, Nolph KD, Khanna R. (1990) Nightly tidal peritoneal dialysis (NTPD). *Vth Congress of the International Society for Peritoneal Dialysis*, Kyoto Grand Hotel, Room C, Kyoto, Japan, July 22.

Pr 214 Twardowski ZJ, Prowant BF, Khanna R, *et al.* (1990) Three-year experience with Swan Neck Missouri 2 (SN-M2) and Swan Neck Missouri 3 (SN-M3) peritoneal dialysis catheters. *Vth Congress of the International Society for Peritoneal Dialysis*, Kyoto Grand Hotel, Room E, Kyoto, Japan, July 22.

Pr 215 Twardowski ZJ, Dobbie JW, Moore HL, *et al.* (1990) Macroscopic and light microscopic morphology of peritoneal dialysis (PD) catheter tunnel (CT). *Vth Congress of the International Society for Peritoneal Dialysis*, Kyoto Grand Hotel, Room A-2, Kyoto, Japan, July 23.

Pr 216 Twardowski ZJ, Prowant BF, Nolph KD, *et al.* (1990) Culture results in peri-exit smears (S), and sinus tract washouts (W) of peritoneal catheters, and swabs from nares (N). *Vth Congress of the International Society for Peritoneal Dialysis*, Kyoto Grand Hotel, Room C, Kyoto, Japan, July 23.

Pr 217 Twardowski ZJ, Prowant BF, Nolph KD, *et al.* (1990) Exit site(s) (ES) healing and classification. *Vth Congress of the International Society for Peritoneal Dialysis*, Kyoto Grand Hotel, Room A-2, Kyoto, Japan, July 24.

Pr 218 Twardowski ZJ. (1990) Reduced complications with Swan Neck peritoneal dialysis catheters. *Vth Congress of the International Society for Peritoneal Dialysis*, Kyoto Grand Hotel, Room A-1, Kyoto, Japan, July 24.

Pr 219 Twardowski ZJ. (1990) PET — A simpler approach for determining recipes for any peritoneal dialysis therapy. *Peritoneal Dialysis Seminar*, organized by Hayashidera Medinol and Toyama Medical and Pharmaceutical University, Meitetsu Toyama Hotel, Toyama, Japan, July 25.

Pr 220 Twardowski ZJ. (1990) PET — A simpler approach for determining recipes for any peritoneal dialysis therapy. Grand Round, invited by Prof. Akira Shinoda, Director, Division of Nephrology, Kanazawa Medical University, Kanazawa Miyako Hotel, Kanazawa, Ishikawa, Japan, July 26.

Pr 221 Twardowski ZJ. (1990) Pathophysiology of exit site and tunnel infections — New insights. *Peritoneal Dialysis Seminar*, organized by Baxter Japan, Hakata Zen-Nikku Hotel, Fukuoka, Japan, July 28.

Pr 222 Twardowski ZJ. (1990) Overview of Missouri CAPD Program. *Advanced Topics in Peritoneal Dialysis, Taiwan PD Symposium*, Regent Hotel, Taipei, Taiwan, July 31.

Pr 223 Twardowski ZJ. (1990) Exit site care. *Advanced Topics in Peritoneal Dialysis, Taiwan PD Symposium*, Regent Hotel, Taipei, Taiwan, July 31.

Pr 224 Twardowski ZJ. (1990) Patient tailoring and adequacy of dialysis. *Advanced Topics in Peritoneal Dialysis, Taiwan PD Symposium*, Regent Hotel, Taipei, Taiwan, July 31.

Pr 225 Twardowski ZJ. (1990) Morphology of the peritoneal dialysis catheter tunnel. *The 11th International Congress of Nephrology, Satellite Symposium of Nephrology in Taipei*, Clinical Research Center, Veterans General Hospital, Taipei, Taiwan, August 1.

Pr 226 Twardowski ZJ. (1990) Prescription dialysis. *Perspectives on Peritoneal Dialysis*, seminar organized by Baxter Healthcare, Inc., The Ritz-Carlton, Naples, FL, August 9.

Pr 227 Twardowski ZJ. (1990) Diagnosis and treatment of infectious complications. *CAPD no Brasil — 10 Anos, 1980–1990, Simposio Comemorativo* (*Ten years of CAPD in Brazil, 1980–1990, Commemorative Symposium*), Auditorio Bourbon, Bourbon & Tower Hotel, Curitiba, Parana, Brazil, August 24.

Pr 228 Twardowski ZJ. (1990) Management of exit site infections: Practical aspects. *CAPD no Brasil — 10 Anos, 1980–1990, Simposio Comemorativo* (*Ten years of CAPD in Brazil, 1980–1990, Commemorative Symposium*), Auditorio Bourbon, Bourbon & Tower Hotel, Curitiba, Parana, Brazil, August 24.

Pr 229 Twardowski ZJ, Nissenson AR. (1990) Quiz the experts. *CAPD no Brasil — 10 Anos, 1980–1990, Simposio Comemorativo* (*Ten years of CAPD in Brazil, 1980–1990, Commemorative Symposium*), Auditorio Bourbon, Bourbon & Tower Hotel, Curitiba, Parana, Brazil, August 24.

Pr 230 Nissenson AR, Twardowski ZJ. (1990) Quiz the experts. *CAPD no Brasil — 10 Anos, 1980–1990, Simposio Comemorativo* (*Ten years of CAPD in Brazil, 1980–1990, Commemorative Symposium*), Auditorio Bourbon, Bourbon & Tower Hotel, Curitiba, Parana, Brazil, August 24.

Pr 231 Twardowski ZJ. (1990) Adequacy of peritoneal dialysis. *CAPD no Brasil — 10 Anos, 1980-1990, Simposio Comemorativo (Ten years of CAPD in Brazil, 1980-1990, Commemorative Symposium)*, Auditorio Bourbon, Bourbon & Tower Hotel, Curitiba, Parana, Brazil, August 25.

Pr 232 Twardowski ZJ. (1990) Practical aspects of adequacy of peritoneal dialysis: Individualization of treatment. *CAPD no Brasil — 10 Anos, 1980-1990, Simposio Comemorativo (Ten years of CAPD in Brazil, 1980-1990, Commemorative Symposium)*, Auditorio Bourbon, Bourbon & Tower Hotel, Curitiba, Parana, Brazil, August 25.

Pr 233 Twardowski ZJ, Nissenson AR. (1990) Quiz the experts. *CAPD no Brasil — 10 Anos, 1980-1990, Simposio Comemorativo (Ten years of CAPD in Brazil, 1980-1990, Commemorative Symposium)*, Auditorio Bourbon, Bourbon & Tower Hotel, Curitiba, Parana, Brazil, August 25.

Pr 234 Twardowski ZJ. (1990) Preventing and managing complications — Catheters. *PD Perspectives*, seminar organized by Baxter Healthcare, Inc., The Registry, Scottsdale, AZ, October 4.

Pr 235 Nolph KD, Schreiber MJ, Twardowski ZJ, *et al.* (1990) Panel discussion, Clinical management. *PD Perspectives*, seminar organized by Baxter Healthcare, Inc., The Registry, Scottsdale, AZ, October 4.

Pr 236 Twardowski ZJ. (1990) Clinical aspects of dialysis adequacy. *2nd CAPD Expert Meeting*, Sun Hotel Phoenix, Miyazaki, Japan, October 20.

Pr 237 Twardowski ZJ. (1990) Swan Neck Catheter — Missouri experience. *2nd CAPD Expert Meeting*, Sun Hotel Phoenix, Miyazaki, Japan, October 20.

Pr 238 Chen TW, Khanna R, Moore HL, Nolph KD, Twardowski ZJ. (1990) Contribution of intraperitoneal (IP) hydrostatic pressure to ultrafiltration (UF) kinetics during peritoneal dialysis (PD). *Central Society for Clinical Research*, Gild Coast and French Rooms, Drake Hotel, Chicago, IL, October 31.

Pr 239 Twardowski ZJ. (1990) Postępy w dializie otrzewnowej (State of the art in peritoneal dialysis). *Posiedzenie Oddziału Krakowskiego Polskiego Towarzystwa Nefrologicznego (Kraków Chapter of the Polish Society of Nephrology Meeting)*, Klinika Nefrologii Akademii Medycznej im. M. Kopernika, Kraków, Poland, November 9.

Pr 240 Twardowski ZJ (presented by Nolph KD). (1990) Tunnel morphology, exit site healing, and clinical results with Missouri Swan Neck catheters. *2nd International Interdisciplinary Symposium*, Hotel Hilton International, Vienna, Austria, November 14.

Pr 241 Twardowski ZJ. (1990) Peritoneal access methods and complications. *2nd International Congress on Access Surgery*, MECC Congress Centre, Maastricht, The Netherlands, November 16.

Pr 242 Twardowski ZJ. (1990) Prevention and treatment of exit/tunnel infection in peritoneal dialysis patients. *40th Anniversary Annual Meeting, The National Kidney Foundation, Inc.-Council of Nephrology Nurses and Technicians,*

Baltimore/Annapolis Room, Sheraton Washington, Washington, D.C., December 1.

Pr 243 Chen TW, Khanna R, Nolph KD, Twardowski ZJ. (1990) The kinetics of hydraulic (H) ultrafiltration (UF) during peritoneal dialysis (PD) exchanges (EXS) in rats. *American Society of Nephrology 23rd Annual Meeting*, Hampton Room, Omni Shoreham, Washington, D.C., December 3.

Pr 244 Twardowski ZJ. (1991) Swan Neck Missouri Catheter. Wednesday Morning Matinee, Department of Medicine, University of Missouri, VA Auditorium, Columbia, MO, January 9.

Pr 245 Twardowski ZJ. (1991) Preventing and managing complications — Catheters. *PD Perspectives*, seminar organized by Baxter Healthcare, Inc., The Ritz Carlton, Palm Springs, CA, January 17.

Pr 246 Nolph KD, Schreiber MJ, Twardowski ZJ, et al. (1991) Panel discussion, Clinical management. *PD Perspectives*, seminar organized by Baxter Healthcare, Inc., The Ritz Carlton, Palm Springs, CA, January 17.

Pr 247 Schreiber MJ, Twardowski ZJ, Soderblom R, Nortman DF. (1991) Panel discussion, Clinical management. *PD Perspectives*, seminar organized by Baxter Healthcare, Inc., The Ritz Carlton, Palm Springs, CA, January 18.

Pr 248 Twardowski ZJ. (1991) Classification of exit site appearance, medical aspects of therapy. *11th Annual Conference on Peritoneal Dialysis*, Presidential Room, Opryland Hotel, Nashville, TN, February 6.

Pr 249 Twardowski ZJ, Dobbie JW, Moore HL, et al. (1991) Morphology of peritoneal dialysis catheter tunnels. *11th Annual Conference on Peritoneal Dialysis*, Opryland Hotel, Nashville, TN, February 6.

Pr 250 Twardowski ZJ. (1991) Long-term experience with Swan Neck Missouri 2 and Swan Neck Missouri 3 peritoneal dialysis catheters. *11th Annual Conference on Peritoneal Dialysis*, Centennial A Room, Opryland Hotel, Nashville, TN, February 7.

Pr 251 Twardowski ZJ. (1991) Controversy: Which is better for predicting peritoneal dialysis adequacy — Weekly creatinine clearance or KT/V urea? Weekly creatinine clearance (opposing view: Keshaviah P), *11th Annual Conference on Peritoneal Dialysis*, Adams Room, Opryland Hotel, Nashville, TN, February 8.

Pr 252 Twardowski ZJ. (1991) Controversy: Nasal carriage of *Staphylococcus aureus* is associated with an increased incidence of exit site infection with the same organism. Disagree (opposing view: Luzar MA), *11th Annual Conference on Peritoneal Dialysis*, Adams Room, Opryland Hotel, Nashville, TN, February 8.

Pr 253 Chen TW, Khanna R, Nolph KD, Twardowski ZJ. (1991) The kinetics of hydraulic (H) ultrafiltration (UF) during peritoneal dialysis (PD) exchanges (EXS) in rats. Oral Presentation, *11th Annual Conference on Peritoneal Dialysis*, Nashville, TN, February 6–8.

Pr 254   Chen TW, Khanna R, Moore HL, Nolph KD, Twardowski ZJ. (1991) Contribution of intraperitoneal (IP) hydrostatic pressure to ultrafiltration (UF) kinetics during peritoneal dialysis (PD). Poster Presentation, *11th Annual Conference on Peritoneal Dialysis*, Nashville, TN, February 6-8.

Pr 255   Twardowski ZJ. (1991) Peritoneal dialysis. *3rd Annual National Kidney Foundation — Update 1991*, Salon ABC, The Astrodome Marriott, Houston, TX, March 1.

Pr 256   Twardowski ZJ (substituting for Nolph KD). (1991) Keynote address, State of the art in peritoneal dialysis. *PD Perspectives*, seminar organized by Baxter Healthcare, Inc., Rancho Bernardo Inn, San Diego, CA, March 14.

Pr 257   Twardowski ZJ. (1991) Preventing and managing complications — Catheters. *PD Perspectives*, seminar organized by Baxter Healthcare, Inc., Rancho Bernardo Inn, San Diego, CA, March 14.

Pr 258   Schreiber MJ, Burkart J, Hamburger R, Moncrief JW, Twardowski ZJ. (1991) Panel discussion, Clinical management. *PD Perspectives*, seminar organized by Baxter Healthcare, Inc., Rancho Bernardo Inn, San Diego, CA, March 14.

Pr 259   Twardowski ZJ. (1991) Principal Discussant in Peritoneal Dialysis Case Forum, Hematuria and blood tinged peritoneal dialysate in 55 year old man with end stage renal disease secondary to polycystic renal disease. Presenter: Schreiber MJ. *PD Perspectives*, seminar organized by Baxter Healthcare, Inc., Rancho Bernardo Inn, Catalina West Room, San Diego, CA, March 14.

Pr 260   Twardowski ZJ. (1991) Overview of peritoneal dialysis. Grand Round, Department of Medicine, Fitzsimmons Army Medical Center, Aurora, CO, March 21.

Pr 261   Twardowski ZJ. (1991) Exit site studies. Baxter Corporate Headquarters, Deerfield, IL, April 1.

Pr 262   Twardowski ZJ. (1991) Swan Neck catheter studies. Baxter Corporate Headquarters, Deerfield, IL, April 1.

Pr 263   Twardowski ZJ. (1991) Ultrafiltration in CAPD. Course on Dialysis, *37th Annual Meeting of American Society for Artificial Internal Organs*, Conrad International Ballroom North, Chicago Hilton and Towers, Chicago, IL, April 25.

Pr 264   Twardowski ZJ. (1991) Management of exit site infection. Peritoneal Access and Devices, *37th Annual Meeting of American Society for Artificial Internal Organs*, Williford Room A, Chicago Hilton and Towers, Chicago, IL, April 26.

Pr 265   Twardowski ZJ. (1991) Peritoneal dialysis of the future. *37th Annual Meeting of American Society for Artificial Internal Organs*, Private Dining Room 2, Chicago Hilton and Towers, Chicago, IL, April 27.

Pr 266   Khanna R, Chen TW, Moore HL, Nolph KD, Twardowski ZJ. (1991) Contribution of intraperitoneal (IP) hydrostatic pressure to ultrafiltration (UF) kinetics during peritoneal dialysis (PD). *37th Annual Meeting American Society for Artificial Internal Organs*, Chicago Hilton and Towers, April 25-27.

Pr 267 Khanna R, Chen TW, Moore HL, Nolph KD, Twardowski ZJ. (1991) Reflection coefficients for sodium salts & glucose during peritoneal dialysis in rats: A simple clinical method. *37th Annual Meeting of American Society for Artificial Internal Organs*, Chicago Hilton and Towers, April 25–27.

Pr 268 Twardowski ZJ. (1991) Peritoneal dialysis — Adequacy and new directions. *End Stage Renal Disease: Issues and Answers, Miami Chapter ANNA Meeting*, Baptist Hospital Auditorium, Miami, FL, May 4.

Pr 269 Twardowski ZJ. (1991) Prescription dialysis. *PD Perspectives*, seminar organized by Baxter Healthcare, Inc., Sheraton Tucson El Conquistador, Tucson, AZ, May 16.

Pr 270 Nolph KD, Burkart J, Helfrich B, Prichard S, Twardowski ZJ. (1991) Panel discussion, Clinical management. *PD Perspectives*, seminar organized by Baxter Healthcare, Inc., Sheraton Tucson El Conquistador, Tucson, AZ, May 16.

Pr 271 Twardowski ZJ. (1991) Preventing and managing complications — Catheters. *PD Perspectives*, seminar organized by Baxter Healthcare, Inc., Haleakala Ballroom, The Westin Maui, Lahaina, Maui, Hawaii, June 19.

Pr 272 Nolph KD, Hamburger RJ, Suki W, Twardowski ZJ. (1991) Panel discussion, Clinical management. *PD Perspectives*, seminar organized by Baxter Healthcare, Inc., Haleakala Ballroom, The Westin Maui, Lahaina, Maui, Hawaii, June 19.

Pr 273 Twardowski ZJ. (1991) Prescription dialysis. *PD Perspectives*, seminar organized by Baxter Healthcare, Inc., Haleakala Ballroom, The Westin Maui, Lahaina, Maui, Hawaii, June 19.

Pr 274 Gokal R, Twardowski ZJ. (1991) Indications for CAPD, APD & HD. *CAPD Doctor Seminar*, Ramada Renaissance Hotel, Seoul, Korea, September 24.

Pr 275 Twardowski ZJ. (1991) Workshop: Catheters/Exit Sites, *CAPD Doctor Seminar*, Ramada Renaissance Hotel, Seoul, Korea, September 24.

Pr 276 Twardowski ZJ. (1991) Workshop: Adequacy of Peritoneal Dialysis, *CAPD Doctor Seminar*, Ramada Renaissance Hotel, Seoul, Korea, September 24.

Pr 277 Twardowski ZJ. (1991) Recent advancement in CAPD. *CAPD Doctor Seminar*, Ramada Renaissance Hotel, Seoul, Korea, September 24.

Pr 278 Twardowski ZJ. (1991) Recent advancement in CAPD. *Seminar "Advancement in CAPD"*, Room Salon 5, JW Marriott Hotel, Hong Kong, September 25.

Pr 279 Twardowski ZJ, Gokal R. (1991) Indications for CAPD, APD & HD. *The Hong Kong Society of Nephrology Peritoneal Dialysis Symposium, 1991*, Grand Ballroom, Shangri-La Hotel, Kowloon, Hong Kong, September 26.

Pr 280 Twardowski ZJ. (1991) Catheters/exit sites. *The Hong Kong Society of Nephrology Peritoneal Dialysis Symposium, 1991*, Grand Ballroom, Shangri-La Hotel, Kowloon, Hong Kong, September 26.

Pr 281 Twardowski ZJ. (1991) Adequacy of peritoneal dialysis. *The Hong Kong Society of Nephrology Peritoneal Dialysis Symposium, 1991*, Grand Ballroom, Shangri-La Hotel, Kowloon, Hong Kong, September 26.

Pr 282 Twardowski ZJ. (1991) Plenary Lecture, The CAPD option. *Renal Update '91, Singapore Society of Nephrology 3rd Scientific Meeting*, Auditorium, College of Medicine Building, Singapore, September 28.

Pr 283 Twardowski ZJ. (1991) Assessment of adequacy of peritoneal dialysis. CAPD Workshop, *Renal Update '91, Singapore Society of Nephrology 3rd Scientific Meeting*, Auditorium, College of Medicine Building, Singapore, September 28.

Pr 284 Twardowski ZJ. (1991) Catheter-related complications and exit site infection. CAPD Workshop, *Renal Update '91, Singapore Society of Nephrology 3rd Scientific Meeting*, Auditorium, College of Medicine Building, Singapore, September 28.

Pr 285 Twardowski ZJ. (1991) Peritoneal dialysis tailoring. CAPD Workshop, *Renal Update '91, Singapore Society of Nephrology 3rd Scientific Meeting*, Auditorium, College of Medicine Building, Singapore, September 28.

Pr 286 Twardowski ZJ. (1991) Pathology and the management of the exit site. *Toward Optimal Peritoneal Access*, conference organized by MEDED, Turnbury Isle Yacht and Country Club, Aventura, FL, October 11.

Pr 287 Twardowski ZJ. (1991) Worldwide status of PD and emerging trends. State of the Art Lecture, *2nd Congress of the Latin American Society of Peritoneal Dialysis*, Salon Isabel la Catolica, Hotel Colon, Quito, Ecuador, October 18.

Pr 288 Twardowski ZJ. (1991) Infectious complications of peritoneal dialysis. *2nd Congress of the Latin American Society of Peritoneal Dialysis*, Salon Isabel la Catolica, Hotel Colon, Quito, Ecuador, October 19.

Pr 289 Twardowski ZJ. (1991) Catheter and exit site management. *2nd Congress of the Latin American Society of Peritoneal Dialysis*, Salon Isabel la Catolica, Hotel Colon, Quito, Ecuador, October 19.

Pr 290 Twardowski ZJ. (1991) Adequacy of peritoneal dialysis and prescription dialysis. *2nd Congress of the Latin American Society of Peritoneal Dialysis*, Salon Isabel la Catolica, Hotel Colon, Quito, Ecuador, October 20.

Pr 291 Twardowski ZJ. (1991) State-of-the-art in dialysis with emphasis on peritoneal dialysis. *3rd Baxter Peritoneal Dialysis Symposium*, Park Hotel, Vitznau, Switzerland, October 24.

Pr 292 Twardowski ZJ. (1991) Tailored dialysis and adequacy. *3rd Baxter Peritoneal Dialysis Symposium*, Park Hotel, Vitznau, Switzerland, October 25.

Pr 293 Twardowski ZJ. (1991) Prescription dialysis. *PD Perspectives*, seminar organized by Baxter Healthcare, Inc., Ritz Carlton Hotel, Naples, FL, November 7.

Pr 294 Nolph KD, Burkhart J, Helfrich B, Hamburger RJ, Twardowski ZJ. (1991) Panel discussion, Clinical management. *PD Perspectives*, seminar organized by Baxter Healthcare, Inc., Ritz Carlton Hotel, Naples, FL, November 7.

Pr 295 Twardowski ZJ. (1991) Catheter implantation and exit site care. *Peritoneal Dialysis Workshop*, Hotel Europa & Regina on the Grand Canal, Venice, Italy, November 11.

Pr 296 Twardowski ZJ. (1991) Optimizing peritoneal dialysis. *Peritoneal Dialysis Workshop*, Hotel Europa & Regina on the Grand Canal, Venice, Italy, November 11.

Pr 297 Twardowski ZJ. (1991) Optimization of peritoneal dialysis. *Seminar for the Central PD*, sponsored by Amgen, Inc., The Plaza Club at the First Bank, San Antonio, TX, December 5.

Pr 298 Twardowski ZJ. (1991) Overview of peritoneal dialysis. Nephrology Grand Round, Pedi Conference Room, Beach Pavilion, Brooke Army Medical Center, San Antonio, TX, December 6.

Pr 299 Twardowski ZJ. (1992) New information on exit site healing. General Session I, *12th Annual Conference on Peritoneal Dialysis*, Ballroom ABC, Washington State Convention and Trade Center, Seattle, WA, February 19.

Pr 300 Twardowski ZJ. (1992) Clinical assessment of PD adequacy is the gold standard. Special Session on Peritoneal Dialysis Prescription for Adequate Dialysis, *12th Annual Conference on Peritoneal Dialysis*, Ballroom BC, Washington State Convention and Trade Center, Seattle, WA, February 19.

Pr 301 Keshaviah P, Twardowski ZJ, Gotch F, *et al.* (1992) Quiz the Experts: Issues Related to Adequacy, *12th Annual Conference on Peritoneal Dialysis*, Room 606–609, Washington State Convention and Trade Center, Seattle, WA, February 19.

Pr 302 Twardowski ZJ. (1992) In search for the ideal catheter. Clinical Topics, *12th Annual Conference on Peritoneal Dialysis*, Room 606–609, Washington State Convention and Trade Center, Seattle, WA, February 20.

Pr 303 Twardowski ZJ. (1992) Peritoneal dialysis today. *4th Annual Kidney Foundation Symposium — Update 1992*, High Chaparral, Astrodome Marriott, Houston, TX, February 28.

Pr 304 Twardowski ZJ. (1992) Adequacy of peritoneal dialysis. *4th Annual Kidney Foundation Symposium — Update 1992*, Salon ABC, Astrodome Marriott, Houston, TX, February 28.

Pr 305 Twardowski ZJ. (1992) Morphology of peritoneal dialysis catheter tunnel — Macroscopy and light microscopy. University of Missouri Colloquium, MA217 Health Sciences Center, University of Missouri, March 11.

Pr 306 Twardowski ZJ. (1992) Peritoneal dialysis: Adequacy and prescription. *Practical Aspects of Chronic Peritoneal Dialysis Therapy*, conference organized by the National Kidney Foundation of the National Capital Area, Inc., Loews L'Enfant Plaza Hotel, Washington, D.C., March 13.

Pr 307 Twardowski ZJ. (1992) Designer peritoneal dialysis: Prescribing peritoneal dialysis for the needs of the individual patient. *Symposium: New Developments in Peritoneal Dialysis*, The First National Kidney Foundation (NKF) Spring Clinical Meetings, Chicago Ballroom, The Chicago Downtown Marriott, Chicago, IL, April 10.

Pr 308 Twardowski ZJ. (1992) Exit site care. Panel 8: Peritoneal access devices, *38th Annual Meeting of the American Society for Artificial Internal Organs*, Sumner B Room, Opryland Hotel, Nashville, TN, May 7.

Pr 309 Twardowski ZJ. (1992) Swan Neck Missouri catheter. Panel 8: Peritoneal access devices, *38th Annual Meeting of the American Society for Artificial Internal Organs*, Sumner B Room, Opryland Hotel, Nashville, TN, May 7.

Pr 310 Twardowski ZJ. (1992) Future of peritoneal dialysis: Advances in catheters and connectors. State-of-the-art lecture, *VIII Congreso Argentino de Nefrologia* (*8th Argentine Congress of Nephrology*), Salon A, Hotel de la Federacion de Luz y Fuerza "13 de Julio," Mar del Plata, Argentina, June 6.

Pr 311 Twardowski ZJ. (1992) Peritoneal catheter exit site care. *Symposium: Complications of the Exit Site in Peritoneal Dialysis, VIII Congreso Argentino de Nefrologia* (*8th Argentine Congress of Nephrology*) (chairman: Locatelli A, other panelists: Piantanida JJ, Barone R), Salon A, Hotel de la Federacion de Luz y Fuerza "13 de Julio," Mar del Plata, Argentina, June 6.

Pr 312 Twardowski ZJ. (1992) Peritoneal dialysis catheter and care. *Issues in Peritoneal Dialysis — Annual Symposium: National Kidney Foundation of Virginia*, Salon E, Richmond Marriott, Richmond, Virginia, June 25.

Pr 313 Twardowski ZJ. (1992) Designer peritoneal dialysis — Prescription peritoneal dialysis for needs of individual patients. *Issues in Peritoneal Dialysis — Annual Symposium: National Kidney Foundation of Virginia*, Salon E, Richmond Marriott, Richmond, Virginia, June 25.

Pr 314 Twardowski ZJ. (1992) Catheter insertion. *Peritoneal Dialysis Workshop*, organized by Baxter S.A. de C.V., Hotel Sierra, Manzanillo, Colima, Mexico, August 7.

Pr 315 Twardowski ZJ. (1992) Peritonitis management. *Peritoneal Dialysis Workshop*, organized by Baxter S.A. de C.V., Hotel Sierra, Manzanillo, Colima, Mexico, August 7.

Pr 316 Twardowski ZJ. (1992) Adequacy of peritoneal dialysis. *Peritoneal Dialysis Workshop*, organized by Baxter S.A. de C.V., Hotel Sierra, Manzanillo, Colima, Mexico, August 8.

Pr 317 Twardowski ZJ. (1992) Peritoneal catheter care and infections. *Aspects of Peritoneal Dialysis — Peritoneal Update, Hazel Taylor Chapter of the American Nephrology Nurses' Association*, Salon D, The Wynfrey Hotel, Birmingham, Alabama, August 20.

Pr 318 Twardowski ZJ. (1992) Calcium/phosphorus balance in the peritoneal dialysis patient. *Aspects of Peritoneal Dialysis — Peritoneal Update, Hazel Taylor Chapter of the American Nephrology Nurses' Association*, Salon D, The Wynfrey Hotel, Birmingham, Alabama, August 20.

Pr 319 Twardowski ZJ. (1992) Complications of peritoneal catheters and exit site care. *25th Anniversary Symposium of the Colombian Society of Nephrology*, Salon Sugamuxi A, Paipa Hotel Centro de Convenciones, Paipa, Colombia, September 4.

Pr 320   Twardowski ZJ. (1992) Peritoneal equilibration test. *25th Anniversary Symposium of the Colombian Society of Nephrology*, Salon Sugamuxi A, Paipa Hotel Centro de Convenciones, Paipa, Colombia, September 4.

Pr 321   Twardowski ZJ. (1992) Disconnect system for peritoneal dialysis. *25th Anniversary Symposium of the Colombian Society of Nephrology*, Salon Sugamuxi A, Paipa Hotel Centro de Convenciones, Paipa, Colombia, September 4.

Pr 322   Twardowski ZJ. (1992) PET, Kt/V, and creatinine clearance. *III Congress of the Panamerican Dialysis and Transplantation Society, I Venezuelan Congress of Transplantation*, Gran Salon, Seccion A, Hotel Caracas Hilton, Caracas, Venezuela, September 6.

Pr 323   Twardowski ZJ. (1992) Diverse peritoneal dialysis modalities. *III Congress of the Panamerican Dialysis and Transplantation Society, I Venezuelan Congress of Transplantation*, Gran Salon, Seccion A, Hotel Caracas Hilton, Caracas, Venezuela, September 6.

Pr 324   Twardowski ZJ. (1992) The management of the Tenckhoff catheter exit site pathology. *III Congress of the Panamerican Dialysis and Transplantation Society, I Venezuelan Congress of Transplantation*, Gran Salon, Seccion A, Hotel Caracas Hilton, Caracas, Venezuela, September 6.

Pr 325   Twardowski ZJ. (1992) State-of-the-Art Lecture: Alternate peritoneal dialysis solutions. *Peritoneal Dialysis Symposium*, Medizinische Klinik und Poliklinik, Universität Ulm, Ulm, Germany, September 23.

Pr 326   Twardowski ZJ. (1992) Reasons for the loss of ultrafiltration. *Peritoneal Dialysis Symposium*, Medizinische Klinik und Poliklinik, Universität Ulm, Ulm, Germany, September 23.

Pr 327   Twardowski ZJ. (1992) Success of the CAPD method in patients with no urine output. *Peritoneal Dialysis Symposium*, Medizinische Klinik und Poliklinik, Universität Ulm, Ulm, Germany, September 23.

Pr 328   Twardowski ZJ. (1992) Identification of patients with insufficient clearances. *Peritoneal Dialysis Symposium*, Medizinische Klinik und Poliklinik, Universität Ulm, Ulm, Germany, September 23.

Pr 329   Twardowski ZJ. (1992) Exit site infections: Causes and treatment. *Peritoneal Dialysis Symposium*, Medizinische Klinik und Poliklinik, Universität Ulm, Ulm, Germany, September 23.

Pr 330   Twardowski ZJ. (1992) The advantages of the Swan Neck catheter. *Peritoneal Dialysis Symposium*, Medizinische Klinik und Poliklinik, Universität Ulm, Ulm, Germany, September 23.

Pr 331   Twardowski ZJ. (1992) Experience with the Swan Neck presternal catheter. *Peritoneal Dialysis Symposium*, Medizinische Klinik und Poliklinik, Universität Ulm, Ulm, Germany, September 23.

Pr 332   Ersoy FF, Twardowski ZJ, Satalowich RJ, Ketchersid T. (1992) A retrospective analysis of peritoneal catheter (PDC) position and function in 91 patients.

Poster presentation, *VIth Congress of the International Society for Peritoneal Dialysis*, Philip II Room, Helexpo Congress Center, Thessaloniki, Greece, October 2.

Pr 333 Twardowski ZJ, Nichols WK, Nolph K, Khanna R. (1992) Swan Neck presternal catheter for peritoneal dialysis. Poster presentation, *VIth Congress of the International Society for Peritoneal Dialysis*, Philip II Room, Helexpo Congress Center, Thessaloniki, Greece, October 2.

Pr 334 Nolph KD, Moore HL, Khanna R, Twardowski ZJ. (1992) Cross sectional assessment of weekly urea and creatinine clearances in CAPD patients. Slide forum, *VIth Congress of the International Society for Peritoneal Dialysis*, Macedonia Room, Helexpo Congress Center, Thessaloniki, Greece, October 3.

Pr 335 Nolph KD, Keshaviah P, Prowant BF, Emerson P, Twardowski ZJ, Khanna R. (1992) Assessment of lean body mass (LBM) from creatinine kinetics. Slide forum, *VIth Congress of the International Society for Peritoneal Dialysis*, Macedonia Room, Helexpo Congress Center, Thessaloniki, Greece, October 3.

Pr 336 Twardowski ZJ. (1992) Exit site. Lecture, *VIth Congress of the International Society for Peritoneal Dialysis*, Philip II Room, Helexpo Congress Center, Thessaloniki, Greece, October 3.

Pr 337 Herwaldt LA, Twardowski ZJ. (1992) (Controversies) Nasal carriage of *Staphylococcus aureus* is associated with an increased incidence of exit site infection with the same organism (Yes: Herwaldt LA, No: Twardowski ZJ). *VIth Congress of the International Society for Peritoneal Dialysis*, Alexander the Great Room, Helexpo Congress Center, Thessaloniki, Greece, October 3.

Pr 338 Twardowski ZJ. (1992) Exit site care. Lecture, *VIth Congress of the International Society for Peritoneal Dialysis*, Verginia Room, Helexpo Congress Center, Thessaloniki, Greece, October 4.

Pr 339 Nolph KD, Khanna R, Twardowski ZJ, Moore HL. (1992) Predictors of serum albumin concentration (SA) in CAPD. *65th Annual Meeting of the Central Society for Clinical Research*, Chicago, IL, November 4.

Pr 340 Twardowski ZJ, Van Stone JC, Jones ME, et al. (1992) Blood recirculation (REC) in intravenous catheters (IVC) for hemodialysis (HD). *25th Annual Meeting of the American Society of Nephrology*, Festival Hall, Baltimore Convention Center, Baltimore, MD, November 15.

Pr 341 Nolph KD, Khanna R, Twardowski ZJ, Moore HL. (1992) Correlations with KT/V urea in CAPD. *25th Annual Meeting of the American Society of Nephrology*, Rooms 319, 321, 323, Baltimore Convention Center, Baltimore, MD, November 15.

Pr 342 Nolph KD, Khanna R, Twardowski ZJ, Moore HL. (1992) Predictors of serum albumin concentration (SA) in CAPD. *25th Annual Meeting of the American Society of Nephrology*, Festival Hall, Baltimore Convention Center, Baltimore, MD, November 15.

Pr 343   Twardowski ZJ. (1993) Diagnosing reduced ultrafiltration secondary to abdominal wall leaks. *XIIIth Annual Conference on Peritoneal Dialysis*, Exhibit Hall A, Convention Center, San Diego, CA, March 7.

Pr 344   Bargman J, Boeschoten E, Nichols WK, Twardowski ZJ, Winchester J, Burkart J. (1993) Quiz the Experts: Issues related to peritoneal fluid leaks. *XIIIth Annual Conference on Peritoneal Dialysis*, Meeting Room 15 A–B, Convention Center, San Diego, CA, March 7.

Pr 345   Vassa N, Twardowski ZJ, Campbell J. (1993) Hyperbaric oxygen (HBO) chamber therapy in calciphylaxis induced skin necrosis in peritoneal dialysis (PD) patient. *XIIIth Annual CAPD Conference*, Exhibition Hall B2, Convention Center, San Diego, CA, March 7.

Pr 346   Nolph KD, Khanna R, Twardowski ZJ, Moore HL. (1993) Correlations with KT/V Urea in CAPD. *XIIIth Annual CAPD Conference*, Manchester Ballroom D, Hyatt Regency Hotel, San Diego, CA, March 7.

Pr 347   Twardowski ZJ, Nichols WK, Nolph K, Khanna R. (1993) One year experience with Swan Neck presternal catheters for peritoneal dialysis. *XIIIth Annual CAPD Conference*, Exhibition Hall B2, Convention Center, San Diego, CA, March 7.

Pr 348   Twardowski ZJ, Nichols WK, Dobbie JW, Krediet RT. (1993) Peritoneal Dialysis Case Forum: A 39 year old white male with loss of ultrafiltration. *XIIIth Annual Conference on Peritoneal Dialysis*, Manchester Ballroom A, Hyatt Regency Hotel, San Diego, CA, March 8.

Pr 349   Twardowski ZJ. (1993) Issues and answers on peritoneal dialysis. *The National Kidney Foundation of Southeast Texas Fifth Annual Symposium — Update 1993*, Salon ABC, Astrodome Marriott, Houston, TX, March 18–20.

Pr 350   Twardowski ZJ. (1993) Adequacy of peritoneal dialysis. *7th Annual Symposium on Renal Disease of the Society of Nephrology of New Jersey*, Quality Inn, Toms River, NJ, March 31.

Pr 351   Twardowski ZJ. (1993) Patient tailored peritoneal dialysis. Visiting Professor's lecture at the University of Utah. Aspen Room, University Park Hotel, Salt Lake City, Utah, April 22.

Pr 352   Nolph KD, Moore H, Prowant B, Twardowski ZJ, Khanna R, Pornferrada L. (1993) CAPD with a high-flux membrane. *39th Annual Meeting of the American Society for Artificial Internal Organs*, New Orleans, LA, April 30, 1993.

Pr 353   Twardowski ZJ. (1993) Peritoneal dialysis catheter exit site care and infections. Invited lecturer, *Program on Dialysis Dilemmas*, organized by Mass Bay Chapter of the American Nephrology Nurses' Association, Hampton Room, Holiday Inn Crowne Plaza, Natick, Massachusetts, May 2.

Pr 354   Twardowski ZJ. (1993) Techniques and regimens of peritoneal dialysis. Curso Dialisis Peritoneal, *II Congreso Uruguayo de Nefrologia* (Course on Peritoneal Dialysis, *2nd Congress of the Uruguayan Society of Nephrology*), Salon A (Azul), Intendencia Municipal de Montevideo, Montevideo, Uruguay, May 12.

Pr 355   Twardowski ZJ. (1993) Adequacy of peritoneal dialysis. Curso Dialisis Peritoneal, *II Congreso Uruguayo de Nefrologia* (Course on Peritoneal Dialysis, 2nd Congress of the Uruguayan Society of Nephrology), Salon A (Azul), Intendencia Municipal de Montevideo, Montevideo, Uruguay, May 12.

Pr 356   Twardowski ZJ. (1993) State of the art in peritoneal dialysis. *PD Perspectives*, seminar organized by Baxter Healthcare, Inc., Ballroom Acapulco A, The Pointe Hilton Resort at Tapatio Cliffs, Phoenix, AZ, June 10.

Pr 357   Twardowski ZJ. (1993) Preventing and managing complications — Catheters. *PD Perspectives*, seminar organized by Baxter Healthcare, Inc., Ballroom Acapulco A, The Pointe Hilton Resort at Tapatio Cliffs, Phoenix, AZ, June 10.

Pr 358   Twardowski ZJ, Prowant BF, Nolph KD, *et al.* (1993) Peritoneal catheter (PC) exit site (ES): Appearance, and factors influencing healing. *XIIth International Congress of Nephrology*, Hall F, "Binyanei Ha'ooma" The Jerusalem Convention Center/Jerusalem Hilton Complex, Jerusalem, Israel, June 14.

Pr 359   Twardowski ZJ, Nichols WK, Nolph KD, Khanna R. (1993) Swan Neck presternal catheter for peritoneal dialysis — Eighteen month experience in adults. *XIIth International Congress of Nephrology*, Poster Hall, "Binyanei Ha'ooma" The Jerusalem Convention Center/Jerusalem Hilton Complex, Jerusalem, Israel, June 14.

Pr 360   Ersoy FF, Twardowski ZJ, Satalowich RJ, Ketchersid T. (1993) A retrospective analysis of peritoneal catheter (PDC) position and function in 91 patients. *XIIth International Congress of Nephrology*, Poster Hall, "Binyanei Ha'ooma" The Jerusalem Convention Center/Jerusalem Hilton Complex, Jerusalem, Israel, June 14.

Pr 361   Guerrero PA, Luger A, Lal S, Twardowski ZJ, Nolph KD. (1993) Membranous nephropathy. Internal Medicine Grand Rounds, Acuff Auditorium, MA 217 Health Sciences Center, University of Missouri, Columbia, MO, July 21, 1993.

Pr 362   Twardowski ZJ. (1993) State of the art in peritoneal dialysis. *Reunión de Nefrológos del Bajío* (Conference of Nephrologists of Bajío), Rooms Turquesa & Diamante, Fiesta Americana Hotel, Leon, Ganajuato, Mexico, August 26.

Pr 363   Twardowski ZJ. (1993) Diverse peritoneal dialysis techniques and regimens. *Reunión de Nefrológos del Bajío* (Conference of Nephrologists of Bajío), Rooms Turquesa & Diamante, Fiesta Americana Hotel, Leon, Ganajuato, Mexico, August 26.

Pr 364   Twardowski ZJ. (1993) Preventing and managing peritoneal catheter exit/tunnel infections. *Reunión de Nefrológos del Bajío* (Conference of Nephrologists of Bajío), Rooms Turquesa & Diamante, Fiesta Americana Hotel, Leon, Ganajuato, Mexico, August 26.

Pr 365   Twardowski ZJ. (1993) Effects of inadequate dialysis. *Reunión de Nefrológos del Bajío* (Conference of Nephrologists of Bajío), Rooms Turquesa & Diamante, Fiesta Americana Hotel, Leon, Ganajuato, Mexico, August 26.

Pr 366   Twardowski ZJ. (1993) Daily home hemodialysis — Personal perspective, Aksys LTD, Investors' Meeting, Hyatt Deerfield, Deerfield, IL, September 24.

Pr 367 Twardowski ZJ. (1993) Keynote address, State of the art in peritoneal dialysis. *PD Perspectives*, organized by Baxter Japan, Hana Room, The Westin Maui, Kaanapali Beach, Maui, Hawaii, October 23.

Pr 368 Twardowski ZJ. (1993) Prescription dialysis. *PD Perspectives*, organized by Baxter Japan, Hana Room, The Westin Maui, Kaanapali Beach, Maui, Hawaii, October 25.

Pr 369 Twardowski ZJ. (1993) Peritoneal access. *Consensus Conference on Morbidity and Mortality of Dialysis*, Masur Auditorium, Clinical Center, National Institutes of Health, Bethesda, MD, November 1.

Pr 370 Twardowski ZJ. (1993) Conditions for revival of home hemodialysis: Medical, and general technical requirements. Aksys LTD, Scientific Advisory Board Meeting, Chesapeake Room, Bethesda Marriott, Bethesda, MD, November 2.

Pr 371 Trivedi HS, Khanna R, Prowant B, *et al.* (1993) Reproducibility of the peritoneal equilibration test. Central Society for Clinical Research, Chicago, IL, November 3.

Pr 372 Twardowski ZJ. (1993) Clinical trials with vein shape catheters. Engineering Conference Room E2, Quinton Instruments Co., 2121 Terry Avenue, Seattle, WA, December 7.

Pr 373 Twardowski ZJ. (1994) Workshop B: The diagnosis and treatment of exit site infections. *XIVth Annual Conference on Peritoneal Dialysis*, Northern Hemisphere E-2 Room, Dolphin Hotel, Orlando, FL, January 24.

Pr 374 Twardowski ZJ. (1994) Swan Neck catheters, abdominal and presternal: The concept and the results. General Session II, Special Session on Peritoneal Access, *XIVth Annual Conference on Peritoneal Dialysis*, Northern Hemisphere B–D Room, Dolphin Hotel, Orlando, FL, January 25.

Pr 375 Suzuki K, Twardowski ZJ, Moore HL, Nolph KD. (1994) Absorption of iron from peritoneal cavity of rats. *XIVth Annual Conference on Peritoneal Dialysis*, Exhibit Hall Perimeter, Dolphin Hotel, Orlando, FL, January 24.

Pr 376 Trivedi HS, Khanna RK, Gamboa S, Prowant BE, Nolph KD, Twardowski ZJ. (1994) How reproducible is the peritoneal equilibration test (PET)? *XIVth Annual Conference on Peritoneal Dialysis*, Exhibit Hall Perimeter, Dolphin Hotel, Orlando, FL, January 24.

Pr 377 Trivedi HS, Twardowski ZJ. (1994) Successful NIPD for 10 years — A case report. *XIVth Annual Conference on Peritoneal Dialysis*, Northern Hemisphere A-1 Room, Dolphin Hotel, Orlando, FL, January 26.

Pr 378 Twardowski ZJ. (1994) Classification of PD catheter exit sites. *3rd Annual Spring Clinical Nephrology Meetings, Nurse and Technician Program*, Ohio Room, Sheraton Chicago Hotel & Towers, April 9.

Pr 379 Twardowski ZJ. (1994) Exit site care in PD patients. *5th International Course on Peritoneal Dialysis*, Convention Hall, Banco Ambrosiano Veneto, Vicenza, Italy, May 25.

Pr 380 Twardowski ZJ. (1994) Searching for the optimal peritoneal access devices. *34th Annual Scientific Symposium on Kidney Disease, National Kidney Foundation of Southern California*, Hotel La Jolla Marriott, La Jolla, CA, September 17.

Pr 381 Twardowski ZJ. (1994) Nephrotic syndrome. Medicine Grand Rounds, Myers Auditorium, Indiana University School of Medicine, 1120 South Drive, Indianapolis, IN, October 19.

Pr 382 Twardowski ZJ. (1994) Percutaneous access for hemodialysis. Renal Grand Rounds, University Hospital Conference Room (UH 3175), Indiana University School of Medicine, 1120 South Drive, Indianapolis, IN, October 20.

Pr 383 Twardowski ZJ. (1994) New advances in access for peritoneal dialysis and hemodialysis. *Advances in Nephrology*, workshop organized by the Silesian School of Medicine to celebrate the 65th birthday of Prof. Dr. med. Dr. h.c. mult. Franciszek Kokot, Hotel Orle Gniazdo, ul. Wrzosowa 28A, Szczyrk, Poland, Nevember 19.

Pr 384 Twardowski ZJ. (1994) Postępy w dostępie dla dializy otrzewnowej i hemodializy (New advances in access for peritoneal dialysis and hemodialysis). *Posiedzenie Oddziału Krakowskiego Polskiego Towarzystwa Nefrologicznego* (*A meeting of the Kraków Chapter of the Polish Society of Nephrology*), Krakowski Szpital Specjalistyczny im. Ludwika Rydygiera, Os. Złotej Jesieni 1, Kraków, Poland, Nevember 21.

Pr 385 Trivedi H, Twardowski ZJ, Nolph KD, Arfeen S. (1994) Autosomal dominant polycystic kidney disease. Internal Medicine Grand Rounds, Acuff Auditorium, MA 217 Health Sciences Center, University of Missouri, Columbia, MO, December 22.

Pr 386 Twardowski ZJ. (1995) Physiology of the peritoneal membrane related to peritoneal dialysis. New York Medical College New York City Nephrology Programs Monthly Education Day, Sixth Floor Auditorium, Metropolitan Hospital Center, New York, NY, January 19.

Pr 387 Kathuria P, Moore HL, Mehrotra R, Twardowski ZJ, Prowant BF. (1995) Preliminary evaluation of silver coated peritoneal catheters in rats. *XVth Annual Conference on Peritoneal Dialysis*, Baltimore, Maryland, February 12.

Pr 388 Suzuki K, Khanna R, Moore HL, Nolph KD, Twardowski ZJ. (1995) Alteration of peritoneal function of rats on 9 weeks of PD. *XVth Annual Conference on Peritoneal Dialysis*, Baltimore, Maryland, February 12.

Pr 389 Suzuki K, Twardowski ZJ, Moore HL, et al. (1995) Absorption of iron dextran from the peritoneal cavity of rats. *XVth Annual Conference on Peritoneal Dialysis*, Baltimore, Maryland, February 12.

Pr 390 Suzuki K, Khanna R, Moore HL, Nolph KD, Twardowski ZJ. (1995) Spontaneous peritonitis in rats on peritoneal dialysis. *XVth Annual Conference on Peritoneal Dialysis*, Baltimore, Maryland, February 12.

Pr 391 Twardowski ZJ. (1995) Exit site infections, importance of and classification. *XVth Annual Conference on Peritoneal Dialysis*, Hall A, Baltimore Convention Center, Baltimore, Maryland, February 12.

Pr 392 Tranaeus A, Tank E, Done G, Twardowski ZJ. (1995) Case studies in pediatric peritoneal access. *XVth Annual Conference on Peritoneal Dialysis*, Room 310, Baltimore Convention Center, Baltimore, Maryland, February 12.

Pr 393 Twardowski ZJ. (1995) Prescribing ultrafiltration strategies from PET results. *XVth Annual Conference on Peritoneal Dialysis*, Hall A, Baltimore Convention Center, Baltimore, Maryland, February 13.

Pr 394 Twardowski ZJ. (1995) DHHD — A hybrid of HD and CAPD. *1st International Symposium on Daily Home Hemodialysis, XVth Annual Conference on Peritoneal Dialysis*, Hall A, Baltimore Convention Center, Baltimore, Maryland, February 13.

Pr 395 Twardowski ZJ. (1995) Swan Neck internal jugular (SNIJ): A new intravenous catheter for hemodialysis. *1st International Symposium on Daily Home Hemodialysis, XVth Annual Conference on Peritoneal Dialysis*, Hall A, Baltimore Convention Center, Baltimore, Maryland, February 13.

Pr 396 Wieczorowska K, Khanna R, Moore HL, Nolph KD, Twardowski ZJ. (1995) Rat model of peritoneal fibrosis. *XVth Annual Conference on Peritoneal Dialysis*, Baltimore, Maryland, February 13.

Pr 397 Twardowski ZJ. (1995) Four problems in peritoneal dialysis — Nutrition, hyperlipidemia, peritonitis, and adequacy. *National Kidney Foundation of Southeast Texas — Update 1995*, La Salle Room, Doubletree Allen Center, Houston, TX, February 24.

Pr 398 Twardowski ZJ. (1995) How to do daily hemodialysis. *Vanguard in Dialysis, 41st Annual Conference of the American Society for Artificial Internal Organs*, Boulevard Room, The Chicago Hilton, Chicago, IL, May 5.

Pr 399 Twardowski ZJ. (1995) Peritoneal access for dialysis. *Regional Nephrology Conference*, Robert Wood Johnson University Hospital, New Brunswick, NJ, May 16.

Pr 400 Twardowski ZJ. (1995) The prescription of peritoneal dialysis. Nephrological Society of New Jersey, Overlook Hospital, Summit, May 16.

Pr 401 Twardowski ZJ. (1995) Current status of renal replacement therapy for ESRD. Grand Round, Robert Wood Johnson University Hospital, New Brunswick, NJ, May 17.

Pr 402 Suzuki K, Khanna R, Moore HL, Nolph KD, Twardowski ZJ. (1995) Factors that affect peritoneal equilibration test (PET) results in rats. Poster session 2, *7th Congress of the International Society for Peritoneal Dialysis*, Exhibition Hall, Stockholm International Fairs (Älvsjö Mässan), Stockholm, Sweden, June 20.

Pr 403 Twardowski ZJ, Prowant BF, Pickett B, *et al.* (1995) Swan Neck presternal catheter (SNPC) for peritoneal dialysis. Poster session 2, *7th Congress of the*

Pr 404   *International Society for Peritoneal Dialysis*, Exhibition Hall, Stockholm International Fairs (Älvsjö Mässan), Stockholm, Sweden, June 20.

Pr 404   Nolph K D, Keshaviah P, Emerson P, Vanstone JC, Twardowski ZJ, Khanna R, Moore HL, Colins A, Edward A. (1995) A new nutritional approach to optimizing KT/V in hemodialysis (HD) and continuous ambulatory peritoneal dialysis (CAPD). *7th Congress of the International Society for Peritoneal Dialysis*, Hall K1, Stockholm International Fairs (Älvsjö Mässan), Stockholm, Sweden, June 21.

Pr 405   Twardowski ZJ. (1995) Selection of a PD regimen. CAPD Club Meeting, Wysowa Zdrój, Poland, June 24.

Pr 406   Twardowski ZJ. (1995) Daily home hemodialysis: An important future therapy for ESRD. *7th Annual Network #12 Network Coordinating Council Meeting*, Crowne Plaza Hotel, Kansas City, MO, September 29.

Pr 407   Twardowski ZJ. (1996) Nephrotic syndrome. Medicine Grand Rounds, Acuff Auditorium, MA 217 Health Sciences Center, University of Missouri, Columbia, MO, January 17.

Pr 408   Twardowski ZJ. (1996) The Kt/V concept is faulty-Kt should not be proportional to V. Special Session: Adequacy and Survival in CAPD and Hemodialysis, *XVIth Annual Conference on Peritoneal Dialysis and 2nd International Symposium on Daily Home Hemodialysis*, Washington State Convention and Trade Center, Rooms 606–609, Seattle, WA, February 21.

Pr 409   Prowant BF, Twardowski ZJ. (1996) Special Session on Exit-Sites: The Prevention and Management of Complications, *XVIth Annual Conference on Peritoneal Dialysis and 2nd International Symposium on Daily Home Hemodialysis*, Washington State Convention and Trade Center, Ballroom 6C, Seattle, WA, February 21.

Pr 410   Twardowski ZJ. (1996) Introduction. *2nd International Symposium on Daily Home Hemodialysis, XVIth Annual Conference on Peritoneal Dialysis*, Washington State Convention and Trade Center, Ballroom 6B, Seattle, WA, February 22.

Pr 411   Twardowski ZJ. (1996) An update on intravenous access for daily home hemodialysis. *2nd International Symposium on Daily Home Hemodialysis, XVIth Annual Conference on Peritoneal Dialysis*, Washington State Convention and Trade Center, Ballroom 6B, Seattle, WA, February 22.

Pr 412   Twardowski ZJ. (1996) Quality assurance in peritoneal dialysis. *Qualitätssicherung in der Nierenersatztherapie: Ein amerikanisch-deutscher Dialog*, Stadthaus zu Ulm, Münsterplatz, Ulm, Germany, April 26.

Pr 413   Twardowski ZJ. (1996) Same site puncturing of vascular access. *Vanguard in Dialysis, 42nd Annual Conference of the American Society for Artificial Internal Organs*, International Ballroom East, The Washington Hilton, Washington, D.C., May 3.

Pr 414   Twardowski ZJ. (1996) Daily home hemodialysis. Research Conference, Department of Medicine, School of Medicine, University of Missouri, Columbia, MA 406B Health Sciences Center, Columbia, MO, August 6.

Pr 415 Twardowski ZJ. (1996) Daily home hemodialysis. *Kansas-Western Missouri and Missouri Joint CRN Meeting*, University of Missouri, Columbia, Alumni Center, Columns 208 A–B, Columbia, MO, September 6.

Pr 416 Twardowski ZJ. (1996) Peritoneal dialysis access exit sites. *8th Annual Network Coordinating Council Meeting*, Empire Ballroom A, Hyatt Regency Crown Center, Kansas City, MO, September 13.

Pr 417 Twardowski ZJ. (1996) Current approach to exit site infections in patients on peritoneal dialysis. *1st Slovene Congress of Nephrology*, Grand Hotel Emona, Bernardin, Obala 2, Portorož, Slovenia, October 26.

Pr 418 Twardowski ZJ. (1996) Patient tailored prescription of peritoneal dialysis. *1st International Postgraduate Course of Nephrology*, Grand Hotel Emona, Bernardin, Obala 2, Portorož, Slovenia. October 26.

Pr 419 Twardowski ZJ. (1996) Catheter exit site observation and care. *II Jornadas Nefrológicas sobre Avances en Diálisis Peritoneal*, Hospital Universitario La Paz, Palacio de Congresos, Madrid, Spain, November 21.

Pr 420 Twardowski ZJ. (1996) Prescription based on peritoneal solute kinetics. *II Jornadas Nefrológicas sobre Avances en Diálisis Peritoneal*, Hospital Universitario La Paz, Palacio de Congresos, Madrid, Spain, November 21.

Pr 421 Twardowski ZJ. (1996) Swan Neck Missouri peritoneal dialysis catheters — Design, insertion and break-in. *Videomed '96, X Certamen Internacional de Videocine Médico*, Sala A, Hospital "San Sebastián", Badajoz, Spain, November 22.

Pr 422 Twardowski ZJ. (1996) Influence of different APD schedules on solutes and water removal. *Dialysis Schedule in Hemodialysis and Peritoneal Dialysis*, Aula Magna — Universitá degli Studi, Perugia, Italy, November 25.

Pr 423 Twardowski ZJ. (1997) Kinetics of APD. Special Session on Automated Peritoneal Dialysis (APD), *XVIIth Annual Conference on Peritoneal Dialysis*, Colorado Convention Center, Rooms A205–209, Denver, Colorado, February 16.

Pr 424 Prowant BF, Twardowski ZJ. (1997) Exit-site care — Case studies. Workshop B, *XVIIth Annual Conference on Peritoneal Dialysis*, Colorado Convention Center, Rooms C207–209, Denver, Colorado, February 16.

Pr 425 Twardowski ZJ, Harper G. (1997) Buttonhole method of needle insertion into arteriovenous fistulas. *Blood Access, 3rd International Symposium on Daily Home Hemodialysis, XVIIth Annual Conference on Peritoneal Dialysis*, Colorado Convention Center, Ballrooms 3–4, Denver, Colorado, February 17.

Pr 426 Twardowski ZJ. (1997) Exit-site care recommendations. Special Session on New Clinical Guidelines, *3rd International Symposium on Daily Home Hemodialysis, XVIIth Annual Conference on Peritoneal Dialysis*, Colorado Convention Center, Ballrooms 1–2, Denver, Colorado, February 17.

Pr 427 Twardowski ZJ. (1997) When to initiate dialysis and how to achieve adequate treatment. *National Kidney Foundation of Southeast Texas — Update 1997*, Granger B Room, Doubletree Allen Center, Houston, TX, February 28.

Pr 428 Twardowski ZJ. (1997) Rationale for and feasibility of daily home hemodialysis. Aksys Ltd. Meeting, Aksys Headquarters, Two Marriott Drive, Lincolnshire, IL, March 14.

Pr 429 Twardowski ZJ. (1997) Rationale for and feasibility of daily home hemodialysis. *Symposium on Daily Home Hemodialysis*, Raum Hohenzollern, Hotel Holiday Inn Crown Plaza, Köln, Germany, April 12.

Pr 430 Twardowski ZJ. (1997) Daily home hemodialysis: A rationale and feasibility. Medical Grand Rounds, Acuff Auditorium, MA 217 Health Sciences Center, University of Missouri, Columbia, MO, May 8.

Pr 431 Twardowski ZJ. (1997) High dose intradialytic urokinase to restore the patency of permanent central vein hemodialysis catheters. *XIVth International Congress of Nephrology*, Sydney Convention & Exhibition Centre, Sydney, Australia, May 28.

Pr 432 Twardowski ZJ, Prowant BF, Nichols WK. (1997) Swan Neck presternal catheter for peritoneal dialysis — Five year experience in adults. *XIVth International Congress of Nephrology*, Sydney Convention & Exhibition Centre, Sydney, Australia, May 28.

Pr 433 Twardowski ZJ. (1997) Vascular access in renal failure. *Nephrology Summer School*, Kraków's Academy of Agriculture, Kraków, Poland, August 30.

Pr 434 Twardowski ZJ. (1997) The Belding H. Scribner Award Presentation Address to Dr. K. D. Nolph. Plenary session, *30th Annual Meeting & Scientific Exposition, The American Society of Nephrology*, Plaza A/B, San Antonio Convention Center, San Antonio, TX, November 2.

Pr 435 Pecoits-Filho RFS, Twardowski ZJ, Kim Y-L, et al. (1997) Intraperitoneal iron dextran toxicity: A functional and histological analysis. *30th Annual Meeting & Scientific Exposition, The American Society of Nephrology*, Plaza A/B, San Antonio Convention Center, San Antonio, TX, November 2.

Pr 436 Twardowski ZJ, Prowant BF, Nichols WK, et al. (1997) Six-year experience with Swan Neck presternal peritoneal dialysis catheter. *30th Annual Meeting & Scientific Exposition, The American Society of Nephrology*, North Exhibit Hall, San Antonio Convention Center, San Antonio, TX, November 3.

Pr 437 Twardowski ZJ. (1998) Three squatting men. Medical Grand Rounds, Acuff Auditorium, MA 217 Health Sciences Center, University of Missouri, Columbia, MO, February 12.

Pr 438 Twardowski ZJ. (1998) Special award presentation address for Prof. Vittorio Bonomini. Special Session on Clinical Results, *4th International Symposium on Home Hemodialysis, 18th Annual Conference on Peritoneal Dialysis*, Presidential Ballroom, Opryland Hotel, Nashville, TN, February 23.

Pr 439 Twardowski ZJ, Prowant BF. (1998) Exit-site healing — Case studies. Workshop C, *18th Annual Conference on Peritoneal Dialysis*, Bayou A/B Room, Opryland Hotel, Nashville, TN, February 23.

Pr 440 Twardowski ZJ. (1998) Prevention and treatment of hemodialysis catheter thrombosis. Simultaneous Hemodialysis Sessions, *Blood Access, 4th International Symposium on Home Hemodialysis, 18th Annual Conference on Peritoneal Dialysis*, Presidential B Room, Opryland Hotel, Nashville, TN, February 24.

Pr 441 Twardowski ZJ. (1998) Peritoneal dialysis techniques, regimens, fundamentals of PD — Board Review. *18th Annual Conference on Peritoneal Dialysis*, Johnson A/B Room, Opryland Hotel, Nashville, TN, February 24.

Pr 442 Twardowski ZJ. (1999) Special award presentation address for Prof. Paul E. Teschan. Special Session on Acute Renal Failure, *5th International Symposium on Home Hemodialysis, 19th Annual Conference on Peritoneal Dialysis*, Room 207 ABC, Charlotte Convention Center, Charlotte, North Carolina, February 28.

Pr 443 Twardowski ZJ. (1999) Blood flow, circuit pressures, and hemolysis during hemodialysis. Blood Access Session, *Blood Access, Fifth International Symposium on Home Hemodialysis, 19th Annual Conference on Peritoneal Dialysis*, Room 207 ABC, Charlotte Convention Center, Charlotte, North Carolina, March 1.

Pr 444 Twardowski ZJ. (1999) Frequency vs. time of dialysis — Lessons from the past. Simultaneous Hemodialysis Sessions, *Measure of Optimal Dialysis: Theoretical Indications and Implications for Prescriptions, 5th International Symposium on Home Hemodialysis, 19th Annual Conference on Peritoneal Dialysis*, Room 207 ABC, Charlotte Convention Center, Charlotte, North Carolina, March 2.

Pr 445 Twardowski ZJ. (1999) Intravenous catheters for hemodialysis. Vascular Access Training Agenda, Kendall Healthcare Headquarters, Mansfield, MA, June 10.

Pr 446 Twardowski ZJ. (1999) Peritoneal dialysis access care. Vascular Access Training Agenda, Kendall Healthcare Headquarters, Mansfield, MA, June 11.

Pr 447 Ing TS, Williams AW, Ting GO, Blagg CR, Twardowski ZJ, Woredekal YW, Delano BG, Gandhi VC, Kjellstrand CM. Daily Hemodialysis Study Group, Hines, IL. (1999) Factors influencing agreement between blood urea nitrogen levels obtained thirty minutes before and thirty minutes after the end of hemodialysis. *32nd Annual Meeting & 1999 Renal Week, The American Society of Nephrology*, Halls B & C, Miami Beach Convention Center, Miami Beach, FL, November 5.

Pr 448 Williams AW, Ting G, Blagg C, Twardowski Z, Woredekal Y, Delano B, Gandhi V, Ing T, Kjellstrand C. Daily Hemodialysis Study Group,

Rochester, MN. (1999) Early clinical, quality of life and biochemical changes of daily hemodialysis. *32nd Annual Meeting & 1999 Renal Week, The American Society of Nephrology*, Halls B & C, Miami Beach Convention Center, Miami Beach, FL, November 7.

Pr 449 Kjellstrand CM, Williams AW, Ting GO, Blagg CR, Twardowski ZJ, Woredekal YW, Delano BG, Ing TS, Gandhi VC. Daily Hemodialysis Study Group, Chicago, iL. (1999) Daily quantification made accurate, simple and inexpensive. *32nd Annual Meeting & 1999 Renal Week, The American Society of Nephrology*, Room D234, Miami Beach Convention Center, Miami Beach, FL, November 5.

Pr 450 Twardowski ZJ. (2000) Quotidian hemodialysis: Hemeral and nocturnal. *1st International Congress of Nephrology Via Internet*, www.uninet.edu/cin2000, February 15–March 15.

Pr 451 Twardowski ZJ. (2000) Lifetime achievement award for Carl Kjellstrand, M.D., Ph.D. General Session, *20th Annual Conference on Peritoneal Dialysis*, Esplanade Ballroom, Moscone Convention Center, San Francisco, CA, February 27.

Pr 452 Twardowski ZJ. (2000) Presentation of award for best hemodialysis abstract, General Session, *20th Annual Conference on Peritoneal Dialysis*, Esplanade Ballroom, Moscone Convention Center, San Francisco, CA, February 27.

Pr 453 Twardowski ZJ. (2000) Welcome. *6th International Symposium on Home Hemodialysis, 20th Annual Conference on Peritoneal Dialysis*, Esplanade Ballroom, Moscone Convention Center, San Francisco, CA, February 27.

Pr 454 Twardowski ZJ: Anticoagulation with Warfarin. *6th International Symposium on Home Hemodialysis, 20th Annual Conference on Peritoneal Dialysis*, Room 135, Moscone Convention Center, San Francisco, CA, February 27, 2000.

Pr 455 Twardowski ZJ. (2000) History of peritoneal catheter development, Special Session: Peritoneal Catheters, *20th Annual Conference on Peritoneal Dialysis*, Room 134, Moscone Convention Center, San Francisco, CA, February 28.

Pr 456 Twardowski ZJ. (2000) Overview of available catheters for chronic dialysis. Chronic Intravenous Catheters for Hemodialysis, *6th International Symposium on Home Hemodialysis, 20th Annual Conference on Peritoneal Dialysis*, Room 131, Moscone Convention Center, San Francisco, CA, February 29.

Pr 457 Reddy DK, Moore HL, Lee JH, Saran R, Nolph KD, Khanna R, Twardowski ZJ. (2000) Chronic peritoneal dialysis (PD) in iron deficient rats with solutions containing iron dextran. *33rd Annual Meeting and 2000 Renal Week, The American Society of Nephrology*, Halls D & E, Metro Toronto Convention Centre, Toronto, Ontario, Canada, October 14.

Pr 458 Grushevsky A, Blagg CR, Bower J, Twardowski Z, Brunson P, Pickett B, Hutton J, Meyers, Priester-Coary A, Lascio M, Driscoll M, Kjellstrand C. (2000) Microbiology of hot water dialyzer reuse and backfiltered dialysate for priming. *33rd Annual Meeting and 2000 Renal Week, The American Society of Nephrology*, Room 701A, Metro Toronto Convention Centre, Toronto, Ontario, Canada, October 14.

Pr 459 Brunson P, Pickett B, Hutton J, Meyers J, Priester-Coary A, Lascio M, Driscoll M, Blagg CR, Bower J, Twardowski Z, Kjellstrand C. (2000) Reuse of dialyzers by hot water cleaning alone. *33rd Annual Meeting and 2000 Renal Week, The American Society of Nephrology*, Halls D & E, Metro Toronto Convention Centre, Toronto, Ontario, Canada, October 15.

Pr 460 Twardowski ZJ. (2001) Lifetime achievement award for Bernard Charra, M.D. General Session, *21st Annual Dialysis Conference*, Auditorium, Morial Convention Center, New Orleans, LA, February 19.

Pr 461 Twardowski ZJ. (2001) Welcome. *New Development in Hemodialysis, 7th International Symposium on Hemodialysis, 21st Annual Dialysis Conference*, Room 293–294, Morial Convention Center, New Orleans, LA, February 19.

Pr 462 Twardowski ZJ. (2001) Daily home dialysis. *Renal Care in the 21st Century*, Saint Joseph Health Center, Community Center for Health & Education, Kansas City, MO, May 15.

Pr 463 Twardowski ZJ. (2001) Codzienna hemodializa jest optymalną hemodializą. (Daily hemodialysis is an optimal hemodialysis.) *VII Zjazd Polskiego Towarzystwa Nefrologicznego*, Nowohuckie Centrum Kultury, Kraków, Poland, September 6.

Pr 464 Twardowski ZJ. (2002) Lifetime achievement award for Belding H. Scribner, M.D. General Session, *22nd Annual Dialysis Conference*, Auditorium, Tampa Convention Center, Tampa, FL, March 4.

Pr 465 Twardowski ZJ. (2002) Should we tailor hemodialysis catheters to the patient's anthropometrics? *8th International Symposium on Hemodialysis, 22nd Annual Dialysis Conference*, Room 15–16, Tampa Convention Center, Tampa, FL, March 4.

Pr 466 Twardowski ZJ. (2002) Holistic approach to dialysis adequacy. *8th International Symposium on Hemodialysis, 22nd Annual Dialysis Conference*, Room 15–16, Tampa Convention Center, Tampa, FL, March 4.

Pr 467 Twardowski ZJ. (2002) Daily home hemodialysis. *Renal Care in the 21st Century*, Ballroom DEF, St. Louis Marriott West, St. Louis, MO, May 9.

Pr 468 James J, McComb T, Twardowski ZJ, et al. (2002) Multiple reuses of dialysis-filters and bloodlines *in situ* for daily hemodialysis, Aksys Ltd., Lincolnshire, IL, Northwest Kidney Centers and University of Washington, Seattle, WA, University of Missouri, Columbia, MO, University of Mississippi, Jackson, MS. Poster presentation, ERA/EDTA, Copenhagen, Denmark, July.

Pr 469 Twardowski ZJ. (2002) Moja przygoda z dializoterapią. (My adventure with dialysis therapy.) *V Krakowskie Dni Dializoterapii*, Sala A. Nowohuckie Centrum Kultury, Kraków, Poland, September 7.

Pr 470 Twardowski ZJ. (2003) Blood access in SDHD. *International Short Daily Hemodialysis (SDHD) Symposium*, Sheraton Seattle Hotel & Towers, Seattle, Washington, March 1.

Pr 471 Twardowski ZJ. (2003) Fallacies of high-speed hemodialysis. Keynote address, General Session, *23rd Annual Dialysis Conference*, Room 6 ABC, Washington State Convention & Trade Center, Seattle, WA, March 2.

Pr 472 Twardowski ZJ. (2003) Lifetime achievement award for Albert Leslie Babb, Ph.D., PE. General Session, *23rd Annual Dialysis Conference*, Room 6 ABC, Washington State Convention & Trade Center, Seattle, WA, March 2.

Pr 473 Twardowski ZJ, Prowant BF, Moore HL, *et al.* (2003) Short peritoneal equilibration test: Impact of preceding dwell time. Poster 9, *23rd Annual Dialysis Conference*, Room 4C, Washington State Convention & Trade Center, Seattle, WA, March 2.

Pr 474 Kjellstrand C, Twardowski Z, Bower J, Blagg CR. (2003) A comparison of CV-catheters, grafts and fistulae in quotidian hemodialysis. Poster 99, *23rd Annual Dialysis Conference*, Room 4C, Washington State Convention & Trade Center, Seattle, WA, March 2.

Pr 475 Moore HL, Twardowski ZJ. (2003) Bactericidal properties of acidified (pH 2.0), concentrated (27%) NaCl (ACS), a potentially useful agent for locking hemodialysis catheters. Poster 100, *23rd Annual Dialysis Conference*, Room 4C, Washington State Convention & Trade Center, Seattle, WA, March 2.

Pr 476 Twardowski ZJ, Reams G, Prowant B, *et al.* (2003) Air-bubble method of locking central-vein catheters: A Pilot Study. Poster 101, *23rd Annual Dialysis Conference*, Room 4C, Washington State Convention & Trade Center, Seattle, WA, March 2.

Pr 477 Twardowski ZJ. (2003) Fallacies of high-speed hemodialysis. Clinical, ethical, and regulatory issues in the care of ESRD patient. ANNA North Central, Inc (318) Central Missouri Chapter, Days Inn 1900 I-70 Drive SW, Columbia, MO, March 11.

Pr 478 Kjellstrand C, Twardowski ZJ, Bower J, Blagg CR. (2003) Hot water reuse of dialysis filters gives smoother dialysis than single use or chemical reuse. Poster presentation, *American Society of Nephrology Renal Week*, San Diego Convention Center, San Diego, CA, November 15.

Pr 479 Twardowski ZJ. (2004) Using a batch system to produce ultrapure renal replacement fluids. *International "Ultrafiltration and Beyond" Symposium, International Society for Hemodialysis*, Sheraton Gunter Hotel, San Antonio, TX, February 7.

Pr 480 Twardowski ZJ. (2004) Lifetime achievement award for Claudio Ronco. General Session, *24th Annual Dialysis Conference*, Ballroom A, Henry B. Gonzales Convention Center, San Antonio, TX, February 9.

Pr 481 Twardowski ZJ. (2004) To reuse or not to reuse: Historical background. *24th Annual Dialysis Conference*, Room 006C, Henry B. Gonzales Convention Center, San Antonio, TX, February 10.

Pr 482 Kjellstrand CM, Twardowski ZJ, Bower J, Blagg CR. (2004) What influences cardiovascular instability (CVI) and discomfort (DIS) during daily hemodialysis (DHD)? Slide Forum V, *24th Annual Dialysis Conference*, Room 001B, Henry B. Gonzalez Convention Center, San Antonio, TX, February 10.

Pr 483 Kjellstrand CM, Twardowski ZJ, Bower J, Blagg CR. (2004) Hot water reuse (HWR) of dialysis filters gives smoother dialysis than single use (SU) or chemical reuse (CRU). Slide Forum VI, *24th Annual Dialysis Conference*, Room 101B, Henry B. Gonzalez Convention Center, San Antonio, TX, February 10.

Pr 484 Twardowski ZJ. (2004) Global clinical assessment or medical doctor time per patient. *24th Annual Dialysis Conference*, Room 006A, Henry B. Gonzales Convention Center, San Antonio, TX, February 11.

Pr 485 Kjellstrand C, Blagg CR, Twardowski ZJ, Bower J. (2004) Cardiovascular instability during dialysis: Relative influence of dialysis purity, clearance and ultrafiltration speed — Experience with the Aksys PHD system. Poster session II: Intradialytic complications, *XLI Congress European Renal Association–European Dialysis and Transplant Association*, Lisbon Congress Centre, Praça das Indústrias, 1300–307 Lisbon, Portugal, May 17.

Pr 486 Kjellstrand C, Blagg CR, Twardowski ZJ, Bower J. (2004) Cardiovascular stability during daily hemodialysis: Relative influence of dialysis purity, clearance and ultrafiltration speed — Experience with the Aksys PHD system. Poster presentation, *Canadian Society of Nephrology — Program Annual Meeting/ Société Canadienne de Néphrologie — Programme L'assemblée Annuelle*, May 27–31, Concert Hall, The Fairmont Royal York Hotel Toronto, Ontario, May 31.

Pr 487 Kjellstrand CM, Blagg CR, Twardowski ZJ, Bower J. (2004) Cardiovascular stability during daily hemodialysis: Relative influence of dialysis purity, clearance and ultrafiltration speed — Experience with the Aksys PHD System. Slide presentation in Renal A, *50th Anniversary Conference of the American Society for Artificial Internal Organs*, Jefferson East – Concourse Level, Washington Hilton, Washington, D.C., June 17.

Pr 488 Twardowski ZJ. (2004) Wady szybkiej hemodializy. (Fallacies of speedy dialysis.) *VI Krakowskie Dni Dializoterapii*, Sala A, Nowohuckie Centrum Kultury, Kraków, September 4.

Pr 489 Twardowski ZJ. (2004) Fallacies of short, thrice-weekly hemodialysis. *Dialysis in the 21st Century, The National Kidney Foundation of Illinois and Swedish Medical Center*, Standard Club, 320 Plymouth Ct. Chicago, IL, September 19.

Pr 490 Twardowski ZJ. (2005) Welcome. *Fundamentals of Extracorporeal Therapies, Annual Dialysis Conference*, Tampa Convention Center, Ballroom C. Tampa, FL, February 27.

Pr 491   Twardowski ZJ. (2005) If I were to go on dialysis, what therapy I would choose and why? Quotidian Hemeral, *11th International Symposium on Hemodialysis, 25th Annual Dialysis Conference*, Tampa Convention Center, Room 18-19, Tampa, FL, February 28.

Pr 492   Twardowski ZJ. (2005) Maximizing fistula creation and preservation — Introduction and Historical Background. *11th International Symposium on Hemodialysis, 25th Annual Dialysis Conference*, Tampa Convention Center, Room 22-23, Tampa, FL, March 1.

Pr 493   Twardowski ZJ. (2005) Fistula creation and use: Historical perspective. Monday Noon Conference, Division of Nephrology, Department of Medicine, University of Missouri, Columbia, MO, Dialysis Clinic Inc., 3300 LeMone Industrial Blvd., Columbia, MO, March 7.

Pr 494   Twardowski ZJ. (2005) Fistula creation and use: Historical perspective. *Annual Nephrology Update*, sponsored by ANNA North Central, Inc. 318, Ramada Inn Conference Center, 1100 Vandiver Drive, Columbia, MO, March 15.

Pr 495   Twardowski ZJ. (2005) The importance of ultrapure hemodialysis solution and renal replacement fluids. Monday Noon Lecture, Division of Nephrology, University of Missouri, Columbia, MO, Board Room, Dialysis Clinic Inc., Columbia, MO, May 11.

Pr 496   Twardowski ZJ. (2006) The perfect dialysis access. *12th International Symposium on Hemodialysis, 26th Annual Dialysis Conference*, Room 2005, Moscone West Convention Center, San Francisco CA, February 27.

Pr 497   Twardowski ZJ. (2006) The perfect dialysis access. Monday Noon Lecture, Division of Nephrology, University of Missouri, Columbia, MO, Board Room, Dialysis Clinic Inc., Columbia, MO, May 1.

Pr 498   Twardowski ZJ. (2006) Pathophysiology of peritoneal transport. *15th International Vicenza Course on Peritoneal Dialysis*, Convention Center Ente Fiera, Vicenza, Italy, May 30.

Pr 499   Twardowski ZJ. (2006) The MIA syndrome in PD: Prevention and treatment (substituted for Nolph KD). *15th International Vicenza Course on Peritoneal Dialysis*, Convention Center Ente Fiera, Vicenza, Italy, May 31.

Pr 500   Twardowski ZJ. (2006) Peritoneal access: The past, present, and the future. *15th International Vicenza Course on Peritoneal Dialysis*, Convention Center Ente Fiera, Vicenza, Italy, June 1.

Pr 501   Twardowski ZJ. (2006) Buttonhole method of needle insertion into AV fistula. *Progress in Nephrology Symposium*, organized jointly by Chair and Department of Nephrology, Jagiellonian University Foundation for the Development of Dialytic Treatment in Kraków, International Society for Hemodialysis, and Polish Society of Nephrology, Auditorium Maximum, Jagiellonian University, 33 Krupnicza Str., Kraków, Poland, September 7.

Pr 502   Twardowski ZJ. (2006) Sodium is a uremic toxin: Explanation of the "lag phenomenon" in blood pressure treatment. Division of Nephrology,

Department of Medicine, University of Missouri, Columbia, MO, Dialysis Clinic Inc., 3300 LeMone Industrial Blvd., Columbia, MO, December 18.

Pr 503 Twardowski ZJ. (2007) Treatment time and ultrafiltration rate are more important in dialysis prescription than small molecule clearance. Debate with Dr. Frank Gotch. *Advances in CKD 2007*, Grand Ballroom, Hilton Downtown, Austin, TX, January 26.

Pr 504 Twardowski ZJ. (2007) An ideal intravenous catheter for HD. *Annual Dialysis Conference*, Room 506–507, Colorado Convention Center, Denver, Colorado, February 18.

Pr 505 Twardowski ZJ. (2007) Sodium is a uremic toxin: The "lag phenomenon" finally explained. *Annual Dialysis Conference*, Room 503–504, Colorado Convention Center, Denver, Colorado, February 19.

Pr 506 Twardowski ZJ. (2007) Understanding of the "lag phenomenon" is essential for blood pressure control in dialysis patients. *Medical Accreditation Meeting*, Klassis Hotel Silviri, Istanbul, Turkey, May 13.

Pr 507 Twardowski ZJ. (2007) How to achieve optimal versus adequate hemodialysis. *Medical Accreditation Meeting*, Klassis Hotel Silviri, Istanbul, Turkey, May 13.

Pr 508 Twardowski ZJ. (2008) Effects of blood flow on blood access survival. *28th Annual Dialysis Conference*, Room Suwannee 15, Rosen Shingle Creek Resort, Orlando, FL, March 2.

Pr 509 Twardowski ZJ. (2009) Urea transport in dialysis is unlike any uremic toxin. *29th Annual Dialysis Conference, 15th International Symposium on Hemodialysis, 20th Annual Symposium on Pediatric Dialysis*, Room 310, George R. Brown Convention Center, Houston, TX, March 7.

Pr 510 Twardowski ZJ. (2009) PD catheters: Evolution toward optimal design. *29th Annual Dialysis Conference, 15th International Symposium on Hemodialysis, 20th Annual Symposium on Pediatric Dialysis*, Room 351 D/E, George R. Brown Convention Center, Houston, TX, March 8.

Pr 511 Twardowski ZJ. (2009) Clinical observations and randomized controlled trials (RCTs) in dialysis research: How can they supplement each other? Genesis of this Session, *29th Annual Dialysis Conference, 15th International Symposium on Hemodialysis, 20th Annual Symposium on Pediatric Dialysis*, Room 340, George R. Brown Convention Center, Houston, TX, March 8.

Pr 512 Twardowski ZJ. (2009) Commentary on the role of the PET. *29th Annual Dialysis Conference, 15th International Symposium on Hemodialysis, 20th Annual Symposium on Pediatric Dialysis*, Room 340, George R. Brown Convention Center, Houston, TX, March 8.

Pr 513 Twardowski ZJ. (2009) Przyszłość hemodializ. (Future of hemodialysis.) *XVIII Konferencja Naukowo-Szkoleniowa Polskiego Towarzystwa Nefrologicznego*, Filharmonia Narodowa, Warszawa (*Warsaw National Philharmonic, 18th Scientific-Teaching Conference of the Polish Society of Nephrology*, National Philharmonic, Warsaw), June 4.

Pr 514 Twardowski ZJ. (2009) Why Kt/V_{urea} cannot be a measure of dialysis adequacy? Visiting Professor, Department of Nephrology, Ege University, Izmir, Turkey, August 20.

Pr 515 Twardowski ZJ. (2010) RCT is redundant if observational studies consistently show that daily HD is superior. *30th Annual Dialysis Conference, 16th International Symposium on Hemodialysis, 21st Annual Symposium on Pediatric Dialysis*, Room 609, Washington State Convention & Trade Center, Seattle, WA, March 8.

Pr 516 Twardowski Z. (2010) Global dialysis in the Sixties: Down memory lane, Part 2: Memories from other locations and the impact of development in Seattle. *30th Annual Dialysis Conference, 16th International Symposium on Hemodialysis, 21st Annual Symposium on Pediatric Dialysis*, Room 6A, Washington State Convention & Trade Center, Seattle, WA, March 9.

Pr 517 Twardowski Z. (2010) Statistics in dialysis research. Monday Noon Conference, Division of Nephrology, Department of Medicine. University of Missouri, Columbia, MO. Dialysis Clinic Inc., 3300 LeMone Industrial Blvd., Columbia, MO. March 29.

Pr 518 Twardowski Z. (2010) Traumatic interocular test (TIT). Internal Medicine Grand Rounds, Acuff Auditorium, MA 217 Health Sciences Center, University of Missouri, Columbia, MO, April 8.

Pr 519 Twardowski Z. (2010) The history of buttonhole technique. *Angioaccess for Hemodialysis*, Plenary Session 3, AV Access Auditorium, Centre International, Vinci, Tours, France, June 15.

Pr 520 Twardowski Z. (2010) Buttonhole method of fistula cannulation. *Angioaccess for Hemodialysis*, Workshop 3rd, Session W20, AV Access Auditorium, Centre International, Vinci, Tours, France, June 15.

Pr 521 Twardowski Z. (2010) Intravenous catheter design and problems. *Angioaccess for Hemodialysis*, Workshop 3rd, Session W20, AV Access Auditorium, Centre International, Vinci, Tours, France, June 15.

Pr 522 Twardowski Z. (2010) Possible detrimental role of high dialyzer blood flow on blood access. *Angioaccess for Hemodialysis*, Workshop 3rd, Session W20, AV Access Auditorium, Centre International, Vinci, Tours, France, June 15.

Pr 523 Twardowski ZJ. (2010) Technika wkłuwania w stałe miejsca (buttonhole): Historia i stan obecny. [Constant site (buttonhole) method of needle insertions. History and current status.] *IX Krakowskie Dni Dializoterapii*, Sala 4, Nowohuckie Centrum Kultury, Kraków, Poland.

Pr 524 Twardowski Z. (2011) Treatment time–blood pressure interaction on HD: The transcontinental experience — Summary. *31st Annual Dialysis Conference, 17th International Symposium on Hemodialysis, 22nd Annual Symposium on Pediatric Dialysis*, Phoenix Convention Center, Phoenix, AZ, Room 230, February 20.

Pr 525   Twardowski Z. (2011) Best practices for PD catheter exit-site care: The role of exit site classification. *31st Annual Dialysis Conference, 17th International Symposium on Hemodialysis, 22nd Annual Symposium on Pediatric Dialysis*, Phoenix Convention Center, Phoenix, AZ, Room 224A–B, February 20.

Pr 526   Twardowski Z. (2011) A wide angle view of HD access and blood flow across continents: What can we learn? Summary. *31st Annual Dialysis Conference, 17th International Symposium on Hemodialysis, 22nd Annual Symposium on Pediatric Dialysis*, Phoenix Convention Center, Phoenix, AZ, Room 231A, February 21.

Pr 527   Twardowski Z. (2011) Is it time to give up on Kt/V urea on PD and HD? *31st Annual Dialysis Conference, 17th International Symposium on Hemodialysis, 22nd Annual Symposium on Pediatric Dialysis*, Phoenix Convention Center, Phoenix, AZ, Room 232C, February 21.

Pr 528   Twardowski Z. Prescribed Dialyzer Blood Flow Influences Access Location and Performance. 32nd Annual Dialysis Conference, 18th International Symposium on Hemodialysis. The Henry B. Gonzales Convention Center, San Antonio, TX, February 26, 2012.

Pr 529   Twardowski Z. History of Buttonhole Technique. 32nd Annual Dialysis Conference, 18th International Symposium on Hemodialysis. The Henry B. Gonzales Convention Center, San Antonio, TX, February 26, 2012.

Pr 530   Twardowski Z. (2012) My reminiscence from the 1st hemodialysis in Kraków. Conference on the 50th Anniversary of the First Hemodialysis in Kraków and an educational course on dialysis therapy and kidney transplantation, Hotel Qubus, Krakow, May 11, 2012.

Pr 531   Gellert R, Klinger M, Tattersal J, Twardowski Z, Wańkowicz. (2012) Meet the experts: New Options in Dialysis Therapy. Conference on the 50th Anniversary of the First Hemodialysis in Kraków and an educational course on dialysis therapy and kidney transplantation, Hotel Qubus, Kraków, May 12, 2012.

Videos

Vi 1 Twardowski ZJ, Khanna R, Nichols WK, Nolph KD. (1987) Swan Neck peritoneal dialysis catheters. Educational Resources Group, The Curators of the University of Missouri. Registered in the United States Copyright Office, The Library of Congress, Registration Number: PAu 1 053 272, April 3.

Vi 2 Twardowski ZJ, Khanna R, Nichols WK, Nolph KD. (1988) Swan Neck peritoneal dialysis catheters — Design, insertion, break-in, and chronic care, 2nd ed. Academic Support Center, The Curators of the University of Missouri.

Vi 2a Twardowski ZJ, Khanna R, Nichols WK, Nolph KD. (1988) Swan Neck peritoneal dialysis catheters — Design, insertion, break-in, and chronic care, 2nd ed. Academic Support Center, The Curators of the University of Missouri (Japanese version).

Vi 3 Oreopoulos DG, Helfrich GB, Khanna R, Lum GM, Mathews R, Paulsen K, Twardowski ZJ, Vas SI. (1988) Peritoneal dialysis catheter implantation. Developed by Baxter's Catheter and Exit Site Advisory Committee, Baxter Healthcare Corporation.

Vi 4 Twardowski ZJ, Khanna R, Nolph KD, Nichols WK. (1993) Peritoneal dialysis catheter: Principles of design, implantation, and early care. Academic Support Center, The Curators of the University of Missouri.

Vi 5 Twardowski ZJ, Nichols WK, Khanna R, Nolph KD. (1993) Swan Neck Missouri peritoneal dialysis catheters: Design, insertion, and break-in. Academic Support Center, The Curators of the University of Missouri.

Vi 6 Twardowski ZJ, Nichols WK, Khanna R, Nolph KD. (1993) Swan Neck presternal peritoneal dialysis catheter: Design, insertion, and break-in. Academic Support Center, The Curators of the University of Missouri.

Vi 7 Twardowski ZJ, Harper G. (1997) Buttonhole method of needle insertion into arteriovenous fistulas. Academic Support Center, The University of Missouri.

Index

In the Index '*n*' refers notes and '*f*' refers figure

Ackerman, Jadwiga   25
Acta Medica Polona   42, 47, 52–53, 86
Accurate Surgical Instruments *See also* Zellerman, Elisabeth (Lisa)   187–191*n*5
Acute hepatic failure   55
Acute renal failure   34, 39, 46*n*1, 54–55, 57–59, 63, 64–65, 77, 81, 120, 124, 155, 170, 195, 235
Adam Karol Twardowski, *See also* Adam   133, 402, 405*f*, 406*f*, 407*f*, 408*f*, 410*f*, 411, 412*f*, 413*f*, 415*f*, 416*f*, 417*f*, 480, 503, 504*f*, 574*f*, 580
Adamkiewicz K.   73, 95, 95*n*60
The Administrative Patent Judge (APJ)   208
A. H. Robins Company   196
Akdeniz University Medical   144
Aksys Ltd   220
Aleksander Marian (Alek) Twardowski   133, 574*f*
Aleksandrowicz, Julian   26
Alpha Omega Alpha Honor Medical Society   135
Alport's syndrome   77

Alwall, Nils   34, 34*n*15
Alwall's dialyzer   35*f*, 38*n*21, 46
American Heritage Dictionary   98
American military hospital   8
American Society of Artificial Internal Organs (ASAIO)   91, 102, 103, 221*n*20
Anderson, Philip C.   102, 102*n*5
Annals of Internal Medicine   101, 139
Anna (Ania) Twardowska, *See also* Anna Burke   133, 402, 406*f*, 407*f*, 411, 413*f*, 416*f*, 417*f*, 574*f*, 575*f*, 576*f*
Annual conference on peritoneal dialysis   193
Annual dialysis conference   270–279, 385
Annual Meeting of the American Society of Nephrology   146, 218, 304, 306, 321
Annual Meeting of the Polish Society of Hematology   118
Annual Meeting of the Renal Section   120
Appearance of constant and different sites in patients   244*f*

Austin Biomedical Corporation   189

Bączyk, Kazimierz   47
Başçi, Ali   361, 362f
Baillod, Rosemary   71
Ball thrombus, removed with catheter   200f
Baltic Sea   31
Bannock, Selkirk   72
Baptize   3
Barbara (Basia), Halina's sister   26, 510
Batory, Chorzów   11
Battle of Britain   89, 89n56
Battle of Klewan   2
The Battle of the Milvian Bridge   282
Battle of Poitiers   371n29
Battle of Vienna   282
Bauer, John F.   98, 100
Baxter Healthcare Corporation   218
Baxter Travenol   217
Bednarek-Skublewska, Anna   119
Bellco Company   102
Bengmark, Stig   280
Berkefeld Company   46
Berlin's Kaiser Freidrich Museum   18
BioHole needle   246
Biolink Corporation   245
Black Sea   359
Blagg, Christopher R.   223
Bloat   9n6
Blood Purification   354
Blood urea nitrogen (BUN)   38
Bocheńska-Nowacka, Elżbieta   118
Bogusz, Józef   25
Bolesław Kłosowski   56

Bonomini, Vittorio   88
Boursane, Marquis   18
Bourquelot, Pierre   371, 373, 374f
Bowman capsule proliferation   31
Brooks, Steve   98
Brown, Paul   103
Buckingham Palace   71
Burke, Sean   570f, 575f
Burroughs Wellcome & Company   69, 70n31
Burton, Robert   225f
Buttonhole needle   245–246
   technique of   245

Cadaveric kidney transplant   176
Capillary artificial kidney   40, 41, 47, 50, 51, 53, 116, 186
Carbon monoxide   78
Catheters   186–216
   flat tip, *See* Flat tip catheter
   with inflow bore directed toward outflow tubing   199, 200f
   intravenous   195
      clot resistant multiple lumen catheter   203–206
   multiple lumen catheter for hemodialysis   195–203
   palindrome   205f
      prototype of   210f
      worldwide usage   206f
   patient tailored   211–216
   retrograde tunneling (catheter implantation)   201
   straight catheter complications   186f
   swan neck   186–191
      abdominal catheter Worldwide usage   191f
      design   186f

swan neck presternal
catheter   191–195
   Schematic drawing after
     implantation   192f
   worldwide usage   194f
   wire models   198f
Catheters, swan neck   186–195
Cellophane tubing   36
Center for Postgraduate Medical
   Education, Warsaw   88
Champollion, Jean-François
   417n20
Château d'Azay-le-Rideau   376f
Chorzów   11, 13, 14–15, 15n13
Chronic glomerulonephritis   61
Chronic peritoneal dialysis   64,
   66, 93, 101, 115, 146
Chronic renal failure   51
     See also Hollow-fiber artificial
      kidney (HFAK)
Church of the Annunciation   324
Church of Beatitudes   324
Church of Saint Nicholas   26
Church of Saint Roch, Paris   380f
Cikowice   3
Cimino–Brescia fistulas   71
Circulating immune complexes
   (CIC)   152
Clark Colton   53
Classical indication for
   dialysis   54
Clinical Nephrology   122
Clot catcher   59
Column of Napoleon   379f
Comparison of regular and tidal
   peritoneal dialysis   167f
Composition of dialysis solution
   (in mEq/L)   122
Computed tomography (CT)
   scan   174
     to detect a leak site   175f

Congress Center Ente Fiera   341f
Congress of the International
   Society of Nephrology,
   Amsterdam   118
Constant Site (Buttonhole)
   method of needle insertion
   171–173
Continuous ambulatory peritoneal
   dialysis (CAPD)   103, 115,
   158–161
Continuous cyclic peritoneal
   dialysis (CCPD)   156, 281
Continuous intra-abdominal
   pressure, experimental
   set-up   159
Continuous Medical Education
   (CME)   270
Cooper, Susan   128
Cordis Dow Artificial Kidney
   capillary dialyzer (CDAK 4)   89
Covidien   190n5, 194, 202, 207,
   209–211, 213
Crista terminalis   212
The Crown Center Hotel   270
Crystal Lake, Illinois   307
Cum eximia laude (with special
   praise)   22, 28
Cybulski, Napoleon Nikodem
   23n4
Czartoryski Museum   17

Dairy Queen   109, 109n12
Dalton Research Center   147
Damienice, Bochnia County   2
Danforth, John C.   132
Davanzo, W. J.   202n14
Dave Ramsey   132
Daytime ambulatory peritoneal
   dialysis (DAPD)   179
DEKA   237
Denaturat   78

Dialysis & Transplantation 128, 172, 242, 247
Dialysis Clinic Inc. (DCI) 138
Dialysis Outcome and Practice Patterns Study (DOPPS) 373
Dialysis on serum albumin (frequency and duration) 85*f*
Dialyzer module 228*f*
Diuresis 83, 83*n*47
Docent position in Lublin (appointment order) 113, 113*f*
Domine Quo Vadis Church 284
Dow Chemical Company 50, 51, 53
Dow Corning Corporation 51
Duke of Milan 17
Dutkiewicz, Jerzy 59

Edinburgh Military Tattoo 72
Educational Commission for Foreign Medical Graduates (ECFMG) examination 91, 135
Eiffel Tower, Paris 378*f*
Endogenous creatinine clearance 83
Epithelial-granulation tissue junction types 251*f*
Equilibration curves 104*f*
Ersoy, Fevzi 144, 360*n*24, 362, 363*f*
Ether anesthesia 3
Eugenia (Gena) Nowosielska 27, 134–136
European Renal Association-European Dialysis and Transplant Association (ERA-EDTA) 389
European Society for Artificial Organs 153
European Vascular Access Course, Maastricht 373
Exit site healing
  early infected exit 268*f*
  fast healing exit 266*f*
  interrupted healing 267*f*
  slow healing exit 267*f*
Exit site study (after peritoneal catheter implantation)
  care and treatment recommendations 262–265
  exit site healing 265–268
  healed exits, 253–262, *See also* Exit site and visible sinus characteristics
Exit site and visible sinus characteristics 255–256
  acutely infected exit 256, 256*f*, 257*f*
  chronic catheter exit site infection 256–257, 257*f*
  equivocally infected catheter exit site 257–258, 258*f*, 259*f*
  external cuff infection without exit infection 260–261, 261*f*, 262*f*
  good catheter exit 258–259, 259*f*, 260*f*
  perfect catheter exit 259–260, 260*f*, 261*f*
  traumatized exit 261–262
External cuff under light microscopy 252*f*
Exuberant granulation tissue (proud flesh) 263
  cauterization of 264*f*
ExxTended Catheter 194

Fałda–Deczkowski shunt 37, 54
Fałda, Zbigniew 34, 34n17, 37n20, 54, 332
Fabryka Samochodów Osobowych (FSO) 30
Factory for Passenger Automobiles 30
Faculty Council of the Medical Academy 86
Federal Licensing Examination (FLEX) 129, 130
Feinstein, Alvan R. 233
FIFA World Cup 313
Fistula creation 79f
Fitzsimons Army Medical Center, Colorado 307
Flat tip catheter 203f
  with extended septum 205f
    recirculation with 204f
Florian Satalowich (Roberta's husband) 365, 365f
Fluid spaces 386
Food and Drug Administration (FDA) 193
Forum des Halles, Paris 381f
Frank, Hans 18
Franz H.E. 320, 321, 329, 332
Frequent Hemodialysis Network (FHN) 231n31
From Russia with Love 358

Gallerani, Cecilia 17
The Gardens of the Château de Villandry 376f
Gauntner, Wallace C. 98
Genbaku Domu (Atomic Bomb Dome) 302f
Generic computer 138–139
  harvard Graphics 139
  method of transferring files 139
  Microsoft office 139
  progress in computing power 139
  texan monitor 138
Geruzja 15
Gibbs–Donnan effect 94
Gibiński, Kornel 55, 55n16, 86
Giędosz, Bronisław 25
Giza, Stanisław 27
GlaxoSmithKline 70n31
  See also Glaxo Wellcome; SmithKline Beecham
Glaxo Wellcome 70n31
Glucose-free dialysate 77
Gottner, Stanisław 115
Gram-positive organisms 262, 265
Gross-Rosen concentration camp 55n16
Gutka, Anna 92, 113

Habilitated Doctor certificate 88f
Hammersmith Hospital 68–69
Ham test (acidified serum lysis) 65
Hana highway 315
Hanicki, Zygmunt 33, 93
Harasiewicz, Adam 22
Harasiewicz, Barbara 22
Harper, George 242–243, 245
Harry S. Truman Memorial Veterans Hospital 131
Hawiger, Jacek 22, 26, 33, 90n57, 100
Hawthorne effect 231
Hayashidera, Hiroshi 286, 288n3, 296, 302f, 308
Heart structure (Netter, F. H) 211f

Hel peninsula   31
Hemodialyses   59
Hemodialysis International   76, 223*n*25, 278, 401, 418, 425, 449
Hemodialysis sessions (Ultra-flo 145 dialyzers)   94
Hemp (*Cannabis sativa*)   50
Hepatitis B virus   55
Highland Cradle Song   72
High Noon   60
Hillbilly   99, 99*n*2
Hirosaka Church, Kanazawa   297*f*
Hirszel, Przemysław (Przemek)   33, 34, 36–40, 46, 47, 54, 57, 65, 90–91, 154
Hoeltzenbein J.   74*n*37
Hollow-fiber artificial kidney (HFAK)   51
    See also capillary artificial kidney
Holy Trinity Column   353*f*
Home army (Armia Krajowa)   6
Home hemodialysis machine   216–239
Home Hemodialysis Today   277
Home of Sherlock Holmes   71
Honorary Member Diploma of Colombian Society of Nephrology   320*f*
Hoover Dam   337
Hopkins, Carole A.   98
Hospital for Miners   53
Hoszowska, Danuta   316
The Hôtel Lambert   18
House of Brokers Realty   132
House of Pancakes   109, 109*n*12
House of Venus in the Shell, Italy   348f
Hyde Park   71

Ice skating   9
Ikinaritei Restaurant   292–293
Infected intercuff segment   253*f*
Institute of the Organic Technology I (Warsaw University)   37*n*20
Intercuff under light microscopy   252*f*
Intermittent peritoneal dialysis (IPD)   104
International Journal for Artificial Organs   216
International Symposium on Peritoneal Dialysis   124
Intra-abdominal pressures (IAP)   160
Investigational device exemption (IDE)   193, 224
Ishikawa (*Ishi*: rock; *kawa*: river), with Dr. Sakai   292
"I Survived the Road to Hana" (T-shirt)   316

Jabłońska, Stefania   117
Jagiellonian Dynasty   2*n*1
Jagiellonian University   2
Jakliński, Andrzej   120
Janicka, Lucyna   113
Jan z Twardowa   2*n*1
Jinrikisha, Kanazawa Castle   309*f*
Joanna (Halina's Sister)   26, 136
Jolanta Ostrowska Jaźwiecka (Jola)   133, 285, 447, 449*f*
Joseph, Donald W.   217
Journal of the American Society of Artificial Internal Organs   221*n*20
Journal of Vascular Access   202, 216
Judogi (traditional judo uniform)   89

Jugular catheter   197f
  reverse tunneling   201f

Kagaya Ryokan (Japanese inn)   298f
Karol Nowosielski ("Lolek")   27, 68
Karski, Jerzy   116
Katowice   5, 13, 54–55, 57–58, 86, 334
Kaulbersz, Jerzy   23, 23n5, 25
Kendall Healthcare Company   204
Kelly, Lara C.   207–209
Kenley, Rodney S. (Rod)   218–222, 220f, 226, 227f, 236–239, 242
Kenrokuen, Japan (oldest fountain)   296f
Khanna, Ramesh   137, 137f, 138, 143, 156, 183, 187, 190, 192, 270, 277, 307, 308f, 312, 336, 364, 575, Epilogue 3
Kidney machine
    insufficient   59–61
    Rhodial   75, 113
    Travenol RSP   113
    Unimat (with Vita 2 HF dialyzers)   113–114
Kidney transplant   58, 61, 65, 71, 93, 103, 164, 171, 174, 176, 222, 248, 290, 389
Kiil dialyzers   71
Kirchmayer, Stanisław   41, 33
Kliniki Akademii Medycznej (Departments of the Medical Academy)   24
Koebner, Heinrich   177, 177n8
Koebner phenomenon   178f
Kobiela, Stanisław   577f

Kokot, Franciszek   55, 55n17, 86, 334f, Epilogue 3
Kolff, Willem J.   52n10, 69
Konturek, Stanisław Jan   23n5
Kosecki, Henryk   76
Kostrzewski, Józef Karol   26
Kotlińska (Twardowska), Małgorzata (Gosia)   133, 576f, 580
Kowalczykowa, Janina   25, 25n7
Kraków   2, 22–43, 98, 134–136, 139, 173, 238, 284–285, 311–312, 314, 328, 334, 336, 338–340, 352, 354, 367, 368, 370–371, 385, 388, 400–402, 418–420, 449–509
Kraków Academy for Mining and Metallurgy   22
Kręciołek (spinner)   85
Krönung, Gerhard   242n3, 332
Krzyżanowski Arek   135
Krzyżanowski, Włodzimierz   135, 395
Książek, Andrzej   113
Kubara, Helena 81, *See also* Sister Helena   172
Kubiczek, Mieczysław   24, 33
Kumamoto Castle   312f
Kuopio University Hospital, Kuopio   143
Kyungpook National University Hospital, Daegu   149

Lady with an Ermine (*Weasel*)   17
Lake Łabap   30
Lake Dobskie   30
Lake Kisajno   30
The Last Supper   324, 327
Least expensive dialysis methods   86

Lebek, Roman   79f
Lee–White method   38
Legend of Sisyphus (King of Corinth)   12n10
Lejman, Kazimierz   26, 26n8
Le Macchine di Leonardo da Vinci (exhibition)   342
   automated roasting spit   343f
   Glider, arched bridge   344f
Lem, S.   341n14
Leonardo da Vinci: The Tragic Pursuit of Perfection   16–17, 17f
L'Ermellino   18
Lesław Andrzej Twardowski
   See also Lesław   3, 5n4, 26, 396, 399f, 586
Letter of congratulations from President Clinton   274f
Liceum Muzyczne (Musical Lyceum)   13
Life or Death Committee   62
The life and work of Napoleon Cybulski   23n4
Litomerice   8
Livonian War   14
Lobeck, Charles C.   130
Łotkowski, Kazimierz   171
Lublin Pharmaceutical Industry   121n5
Lundin, A. Peter   222n22, 242

Maastricht University, Netherlands   389f
Madame Tussauds museum   71
Magda van Loon   247, 389f
Magnetic resonance imaging (MRI)   213
The Magnificent Seven   60
Maher, John F.   91, 91n58
Mahon, Henry I.   51
Maid of the Mist   337
Majdan, Maria   119
Malignant hypertension   61
Maneki Neko   303f
Marciana, Biblioteca   282
Marczewski Krzysztof   119
Marquette School of Medicine   51
Massachusetts Institute of Technology   53
Massalski, Jerzy Michał   41n24
Massry, Shaul   334n13, 334f
Mass transfer coefficient (MTC)   104–105, 104n9
Matsushima (*matsu*: pine; *shima*: island)   288
Matsuzaki, Kimihiko   285, 286, 288, 288f, 292, 296, 297, 302f
Matteson, Charles R.   188
Matthews, Dawn   220, 220f, 227f
McCurdy, Barbara Clarke   207–209
Mean forced vital capacity (supine position)   158f
Mean forced vital capacity (three position)   158f
MEDED (Medical Education)   317
Medical Academy, Kraków   16
Medical Academy, Lublin   120
Medical Sciences Knowledge Profile (MSKP) exam   130, 133, 135
Medisystems Research Corporation   245
Mediterranean Sea   362
Meduna's mixture   35
Mees, Evert Doorhout   367, 367f
Mesh welded   75f
Michejda, Kornel   25

Miodoński, Jan   26
Misra, Madhukar   146, 147, 231, 278, 575
Missouri Medical Review   50, 223
Model of the Saturn V rocket   365*f*
Molotov–Ribbentrop Pact   3*n*3
Mona Lisa   379
Montelupi prison   6
Monument Hospital Children's Health Center   281
Moore, Harold F.   103, 137*f*
Moorhead, John   71
Motokoji Church, Japan   287*f*
Mount Cook (Aoraki)   333
Mount Fuji (Fujiyama; *yama*: mountain)   304
Muller, Thomas E.   217
Musical talent   13–14
Mustela erminea   18
Mustela nivalis   17

Nalidixic acid   70*n*31
NASA's Lyndon Johnson Space Center   365
National Kidney Foundation Kidney Disease Outcomes Quality Initiative guidelines   181
NegGram   69–70, 70*n*31
Nephrology Committee of the Polish Academy of Science   65
Nerve conduction velocity   85*f*
New England Journal of Medicine   147, 216, 231, 393
Newnam, William   89
Nichols, W. Kirt   103
Niepołomice forest (Puszcza Niepołomicka)   5
Nightly Intermittent Peritoneal Dialysis (NIPD)   165, 173–177

Niigata University   291
Nijubashi (*ni*: two; *ju*: arch; *bashi*: bridge), double-arch bridge   288–289
Ninja Derra   293
Nissenson, Allen R.   223
Nolph, Georgia   272*f*, 315, 326, 341*f*
Nolph, Karl   91*n*59, 98–99, 101, 108–109, 118, 124, 128–131, 137*f*, 138, 144–145, 147–148, 153, 187, 189–190, 192–193, 222, 270, 272–273, 272*f*, 275, 279, 314–315, 322, 326, 340, 341*f*, 363, 394, 575, Epilogue 3
Northwestern University, Chicago   135
Northwest Kidney Center, Seattle   235
Nose, Yukihiko   52, 52*n*10
Notre Dame, Paris   382*f*
Nowosielski, Adolf   68
Nowosielski, Włodzimierz   39
NxStage system   236

Ok, Ercan   361, 362*f*, 366
Olbrycht, Jan Stanisław   26
Oldsmobile Delta   88, 134, 135
Orłowski, Tadeusz   34*n*17, 49, 65
Orawski, Lech   56
Order of the Ermine   18
Osaka Castle, Japan   300*f*

Palais Garnier   381*f*
Paliwoda, Tadeusz   73
Parochial institution   11*n*8
Paroxysmal nocturnal hemoglobinuria   64

Patients inspired or contributed
to progress 170–183
    Balicka, Alicja 170–171
    Blattner, Hugh 179
    Brodhacker, Joe 177–179
    columbia district award of
      excellence for outstanding
      vocational achievement
      176f
    Rosen, Mitzi 173–177
    Shirley, Lucille 179–183, 182f
    Zieleniec, Maria 171–173
Pence, Thomas 306
Penson, Jakub 49
Periodontitis 186
Peritoneal cavity 67
Peritoneal dialysis 93, 136
    catheters 186–191,
      See also Catheters
    diagram of the experimental
      set-up 154
    research 137, 137f
    saving blood in patients
      on 93
Peritoneal Dialysis International
    253, 270
Peritoneal equilibration curves
    162f
Peritoneal equilibration test (PET)
    67, 161
    results 163f
Personal hemodialysis system
    (PHD) 181
    aksys machine
      first version 224f
      second version 227f
    diagram of fluid paths
      in 229f
    general view of the "Phase 2,"
      228f

machine overview 226,
    229–230
"Pharmacokinetics of drugs
    in renal failure," 121
Piazza San Marco 282
Pierratos, A. 254n6
Pizzeria 109, 109n12
Poland 2
Policy of prophylactic dialysis
    54
Polish Academy of Science 65
Polish Archives of Internal
    Medicine 121
Polish Medical Journal 86
The Polish postal service 130
Polish United Worker's Party 67
Polish war cemetery, Italy 346f
Politowski, Mieczysław 93
Polyester fibers surrounded by
    multinucleated giant cells
    252f
Polyvinyl chloride 64
Potato diet
    treatment of chronic renal
      failure 8n5
Premature ventricular complexe
    (PVC) 318
Presentations on dialysis related
    topics 279–390
Prince Adam Kazimierz
    Czartoryski 18
Princes Street Gardens 72
Probability of Fistula Survival 80f
Prowant, Barbara F. ("Barb")
    107n11, 137f, 270–271, 277,
    Epilogue 3
Przemysław Wiktor Twardowski,
    (Przemek) 26, 574f
    Alpha Omega Alpha Honor
      Medical Society 135

passed the MSKP   135,
    See also Medical Sciences Knowledge Profile (MSKP) exam
passion for swimming   90
Przybyłkiewicz, Zdzisław   25
Psoriatic lesions   178*f*
Psychiatry hospital (Kobierzyn)   31

A Question of Honor. The Kosciuszko Squadron: Forgotten Heroes of World War II   89*n*56
Quinton Instruments Company   196, 196*n*11
Quinton–Scribner arteriovenous shunts   54
Quinton, W E.   196, 198*f*
"Quiz the Expert,"   318, 322
Quo Vadis?   284

Raba River   9, 10
Radomysł Marian Twardowski (Radek)   26, 30, 133, 574*f*
    Honor Graduate Award   133
    passed the MSKP   133,
        See also Medical Sciences Knowledge Profile (MSKP) exam
Ramie (*Boehmeria nivea*)   50
Randomized controlled trial (RCT)   230–234, 364–365, 367, 369
Recirculating single pass (RSP)   76
"Red Diploma,"   22, 22*n*1, 28, 29*f*
Renal arteriography   58
"Renal Care in the 21st Century,"   338
Retrograde pyelography   58
Retrograde tunneling   201
Reverse osmosis system   51

Rio Bravo   60
Ritz, Eberhard   334*f*
Riverdance   409*f*
Rogalski, Tadeusz   25
Rothamsted Agricultural Experimental Station   232
Royal Canadian Mounted Police   72
Royal Free Hospital   68–69
Royal Infirmary Hospital   70
Rudka, Roman   172
Rue Foyatier, Paris   383*f*
Ruins of Smyrna, Turkey   369*f*
Ryan, Daniel D.   188

Sacré-Coeur Basilica, Paris   384*f*
St. Lazarus Hospital   24
St. Peter's Catholic Church   287
Satalowich, Roberta   274*f*, 365
Schechter, H.   177*n*9
Schematic of the dialyzing unit   43, 42*f*
The School of Athens   282
Scientific Committee of the symposium   124
Scribner, Belding H.   242
Scything   9*n*7
Sea of Marmara   359
Selection of patients for chronic dialysis   62
Sendai medical school   286
Separable peritoneal dialysis catheter   193
Shatsk District Hospital   581–583, 581*f*
Shepherding cattle   9
Shimkus, E. M.   102*n*6
Siemdaj, Antoni   3, 4*n*1

Sieniawska, Maria   194
Sieving coefficient   105–106, 105n10
Sigismundus Augustus   2n1
    See also Zygmunt August
Silastic-Teflon bypass cannulas   58n21
Silesian Medical Academy   54
Sil-Med Corporation   188
Silverman, I   56n20
Singapore   317
Skarżyński, Bolesław   25
Skeggs–Leonards dialyzer   42
    sheet dialyzer   71n34
    See also Warsaw Artificial Kidney
Skierniewice   2
Skowron, Stanisław   25, 25n6
Sleeping Beauty   374
SmithKline Beecham   70n31
Smoking (smokers)   392, 393n2
SNIJ 3, *See* Swan Neck Internal Jugular Catheter Model, 3 (SNIJ 3)
Société Francaise des Abords Vasculaires (SFAV)   371
Sorkin, Michael   98
Soviet–Polish Non-Aggression Pact   3n3
Soviet Union   4
Spartan Senate   15n12
Square-meter hour hypothesis   87
Sroczyński, J.   86
Stanisławice, Bochnia County   3, 5–6, 10
Starzl, T. E.   56n19
Starzycka, Maria   30n11, 41
Statue of the faun, Pompeii   348f
Statue of Octavian Augustus, Italy   351f

Stephen Báthory (Prince of Transylvania and King of Poland)   14n11
    honor award statuette   19f
Stewart, Richard D.   52f
Stobhill General Hospital, Glasgow   143
Struzik, Tadeusz   33
Study on complications in relation to catheter implantation   188
Study on the influence of hypophysectomy on gastric ulcer development   23
Study on osmotic ultrafiltration   118
Stukas (German military aircraft)   5
Sułowicz, Władysław   352, 389
Summa cum laude (with highest praise)   22, 28
Summa technologiae (Sum of Technology)   341
Supniewski, Janusz   25
Susan Molumphy   273
Swan Neck Internal Jugular Catheter Model 3 (SNIJ 3)   199, 276, 292f
Swan Neck Pigtail Double Lumen Intravenous Catheter   196
Sweden Freezer Company   54
Szack   3
Szkodny, Adam   86
Szopienice   4

Tacrolimus   176
Tarnawski, Andrzej S.   98
Tempka, Tadeusz   26, 27, 33
Tenckhoff, H.   177n9
Tenon   250
Teschan, Paul   54, 54n15

Testimonium ortus et baptismi (Certificate of birth and baptism) 4*f*
   3:10 to *Yuma* 60
Tidal peritoneal dialysis (TPD) 166
Tiger Motor Hotel 98, 109, 128, 131
Tlałka, Wiesław 576, 577*f*
Tochowicz, Leon 26
Toilet paper and flight 112
Tokyo Women's Medical College 290
Topkapi Palace 357
Torchbearer Award Dinner Program 271*f*, 272*f*
   present from Ram Gokal 273*f*
Tordoir, Jan H.M. 314, 387
Toronto Western Hospital 188
The Total Money Makeover 132
Toyama Pharmaceutical University 294
Transfer of urea 386
Transmembrane pressure (TMP) 105
Transplantation Committee of the Ministry of Health 65
Trans World Airlines (TWA) 285
Trans World Express (TWE) 284–285
Traumatic Interocular Test (T.I.T.) 233, 370
Traumatized exit
   cauterization of proud flesh 264*f*
   external appearance 263*f*
   sinus appearance 263*f*
"Treatment of chronic renal failure with hemodialysis," 94

The Tri-State Renal Network 307
Tuskegee Syphilis Experiment 370
Twardowska, Halina 2, 26, 27*f*, 65, 289*f*, 297*f*, 378*f*, 339*f*, 380*f*, 383*f*
Twardowski, Józef 2, 7*f*
Twardowski, Zbylut J. 27*f*, 52*f*, 79*f*, 137*f*, 198*f*, 220*f*, 288*f*, 289*f*, 294*f*, 296*f*, 297*f*, 308*f*, 341*f*, 375*f*
   British Museum 417*f*
   career development 66–67
   certificate of honorary membership (Polish Society of Nephrology) 366
   certificate of recognition from the mayor of Matto 311*f*
   childhood 2–10
   congratulatory card from Halinka 226*f*
   cooperation with fellows 142–147
   cooperation with laboratory visitors 147–149
   cooperation with nurses and technicians 149
   debated with Dr. Frank Gotch 236
   Doktor Medycyny certificate 48*f*
   conferring the title 48*f*
   fellowship in america 98–110
   genbaku domu (Atomic Bomb Dome) 302*f*
   graduation 14–15, 16*f*, 22
   Hiroshima lecture 303*f*
   in Ikinaritei Restaurant with Geisha girls 293*f*
   Kagaya Ryokan (Japanese inn) 298*f*

king of peritoneal dialysis 273, 274f
lecture in Kanazawa 309f, 310f
letter of congratulations from President Clinton 274f
major research 242–268
marriage 26, 27f
medical school and career 22–43
Osaka Castle, Japan 300f
permanent residence in the United States 131
Polish citizenship 140
presenting the history of the buttonhole technique 372, 372f
professional life (Bytom) 46–95
Red Diploma 29f
return to Poland (The Lublin years) 112–125
with Rod and Dawn 220f, 227f
schooling 10
specialist in Nephrology 88
sports 22–23
study on complications in relation to catheter implantation 188
Susan Molumphy presents the Torchbearer Award 275f
token of appreciation, Rosen, Mitzi 176, 176f
Tokyo women school lecture 290f
U.S. citizenship 131, 140
vacations and travel 392–586, See also Vacations and travel unrelated to business

visit to Dr. Sakai, Shinji home 291f
Two methods of needle insertion (comparison) 244f

Ukraine 2n2, 3, 454n37, 507, 577, 580–586
Ulleval Hospital 71n34
Ulm, University of 320, 321, 329, 332
Ulster Medical Journal 101
Ultrafiltration (UF) 105, 106f
Umberto Buoncristiani 223
UNESCO World Heritage city 330
University of California 98n1
University of Colorado 152
  school of medicine and surgical service 56
University of Connecticut 91
University of Hokkaido 52n10
University of Louisiana 133
University of Michigan 51, 146
University of Missouri 90, 102, 104, 107, 120, 128, 131, 133, 152, 187–189, 194, 204, 206–207, 209, 213, 254, 270, 305–306
  clinical research center 107
  dalton research center 131
Uremia, signs and symptoms 82
Uremic Pericarditis 170
Urologia Polska 95
U.S. Independence Day 134

Vacations and travel unrelated to business
  Adam and Gosia to Kraków and Ukraine 580
  Ania's wedding in Minneapolis 575–576

712   Around the World with Nephrology

Ballestas Islands   520*f*
Bieszczady   576–580
Blarney Castle   406*f*
Branson   393–394
Canada and Alaska tour and cruise   394–396
Capela dos Ossos   462*f*
Cardiff Castle   405*f*
Celsus Library, Ephesus   565*f*
chalky deposit   560*f*
Christ on a Donkey   411*f*
Church of St. Lawrence   459*f*
Clay pithoi   513*f*
cliff of Paracas Peninsula   520*f*
Clinton Square, Syracuse   499*f*
clock that stopped at the beginning of Bolshevik Revolution   433*f*
copy of the Bull-Leaping Fresco   511*f*
Crete, Peru tour   509–545
cuneiform writing   550*f*
Den Lille Havfrue (The Little Mermaid)   447*f*
England tour   480–506
enormous Malbork Castle   420*f*
the espy house   482*f*
Father Edvin Cole's Kraków visit and our Portugal tour   449–480
father John Long in Kraków   418–420
fifteen graduates from the class of 1952   423*f*
Great Britain and Ireland   402–417

Great Samson Sea Canal, Peterhof   434*f*
Gustave Eiffel's Maria Pia railway bridge, Porto   469*f*
Hadrian's Wall   414*f*
Herodotus, 560*n*60, 571*n*61
huldra   442*n*34
  at Kjosfossen 442*f*
island of Helgeandsholmen   428*f*
Illia   526, 527*f*
"Jesus I trust in you" (painting) 521*f*
Jurata, Slovakia and New York   420–425
Keystone   392–393
Killarney National Park, Kerry   407*f*
Korean War Memorial, Albany   498*f*
Kraków, Zamość, Puławy   507–509
Kuźnica   392
Larco Museum   524*f*
Les Lettres portugaises   461*f*
The Liberty Bell (symbol of American Independence)   486*f*
lighthouse at Cabo   458*f*
London, Turkey   545–575
Lviv's Latin Cathedral   585*f*
Machu Picchu's Temple of the Sun   533*f*
Metropolitan Museum of Art   425*f*
models of churches, Myczkowce   579*f*
monument to Frédéric Chopin   505*f*

Index   713

monument to Nikola
    Tesla   502f
monument to Peter the
    Great   435f
Mother Mary's House,
    Meryemana Evi   568f
mushroom shaped fairy
    chimneys   554f
        Neptune's fountain   419f
Niagara Falls   501f
obligatory photo in the Trojan
    horse   571f
old faithful geyser in
    Yellowstone blows its
    top   398f
Pavlovsk Palace   434f
peace monument on Swedish-
    Norwegian border   437f
plague column   422f
Prince Czartoryski's Palace,
    Puławy   509f
retirement and apartment,
    Kraków   400–402
sandboarders   518f
Scandinavia, St. Petersburg
    and Estonia   425–449
Shatsk District Hospital
    581f
sleeping beauty   424f
St. Kinga's Chapel   452f
St. Lawrence on a grate,
    Almancil   459f
St. Margaret's Chapel   412f
statue of Christ overlooking
    Cusco   540f
statue of D. Dinis   470f
statue of Dom Nuno Álvares
    Pereira   474f
statue of King Afonso
    Henriques   466f

statue of Pope John Paul II
    484f
statue of the Virgin
    Mary   567f
Syv Søstrene (Seven Sisters),
    The   440f
theater at Aspendos   558f
throne room with gypsum
    throne   512f
Tree of Life sculpture, Vigeland
    Park in Oslo   445f
trip with my brother, Lesław,
    through the American
    Midwest   396–400
trolls   439n33
    typically Scandinavian
    warning sign   440f
Urubamba Valley, Andes
    525f
Vasa and Riks bridge   428f
Vasa ship comprising Vasa
    emblem   429f
village of Chinchero   537f
wedding anniversary   547f
Vanderbilt University, Nashville
    90
Van Stone, John C.   98, 100,
    129, 195, 197n13, 204n15, 272f,
    332, 392
Vas-Cath Inc   190, 209
Venous system of chest and neck
    (selected points)   214
    formula to measure selected
    points   215
Ventricular needle   100n3
Veterans Administration
    Hospital   51, 56, 98, 128, 179
Vim–Silverman biopsy needle   56
Voivodeship   2n2, 31n12, 55,
    63–64, 115, 583–584

Volume changes at long hemodialysis   388*f*
Volume changes at short hemodialysis   387*f*

Waitomo Glowworm Caves   333
Warsaw Academy of Medicine   34
Warsaw Artificial Kidney   42
Warszawa
  See also Factory for Passenger Automobiles
Wawszczak (Twardowska), Katarzyna (Kasia)   135, 546, 574*f*
West Edmonton Mall   307
Western General Hospital   70
  Nuffield Transplant Unit   71
Weston–Roberts catheter   63
"White Surgery" (The First Department of Surgery)   28
Wierzynek Restaurant   284
Wojtczak, Andrzej   47, 91
Wood Veterans Administration Hospital   51

World Trade Center   277
World War II   3*n*3, 5, 69, 72, 89*n*56, 72, 136, 301, 324, 333, 415
Wrocław University   49

Yale University School of Medicine   204
Yalta Conference   3
Yamabiko (*yama*: mountain; *biko*: echo)   286
Yamanoo Restaurant, Kanazawa   297*f*
Yashica Dental Eye camera   255*f*
Young, Thomas   417*n*19

Zakuro Restaurant   289
Zborowska, Matylda   3, 4*n*1
Zbylut (*zby*- "to get rid of"; *lut*- "anger, cruelty, and bad temper")   5*n*4
Zeiss prism loupe   254*f*
Zellerman, Elisabeth (Lisa)   187–191*n*5, 193, 196, 323*f*
Zygmunt August   2*n*1

Index   715